Tuberculosis Treatment: The Search for New Drugs

Tuberculosis Treatment: The Search for New Drugs

Edited by Megan Durham

hayle medical

New York

Hayle Medical,
750 Third Avenue, 9th Floor,
New York, NY 10017, USA

Visit us on the World Wide Web at:
www.haylemedical.com

ISBN: 978-1-64647-525-4

Cataloging-in-Publication Data

Tuberculosis treatment : the search for new drugs / edited by Megan Durham.
p. cm.
Includes bibliographical references and index.
ISBN 978-1-64647-525-4
1. Tuberculosis. 2. Tuberculosis--Research. 3. Chest--Diseases.
4. Lungs--Diseases. 5. Mycobacterial diseases. I. Durham, Megan.
RC311.4 .R43 2023
616.995--dc23

Table of Contents

Preface

Tuberculosis (TB) refers to a type of infectious disease generally caused by Mycobacterium tuberculosis. Lungs are the primary target of this disease, but it can also affect the other parts of the body. It can be treated with a combination of antibacterial medications. However, the evolution of drug-resistant tuberculosis necessitates the development of effective, novel and safe drug regimens. Drug discovery and development is a difficult, expensive and time-consuming process. One of the popular frameworks used in drug discovery is model-informed drug discovery and development (MID3). It aims to provide an informative prediction of drug efficacy and exposure in people for choosing innovative anti-tuberculosis drug combinations. This book is compiled in such a manner, that it will provide in-depth knowledge about drug discovery for treating tuberculosis. Those with an interest in this area of pharmaceutical science would find it helpful.

Significant researches are present in this book. Intensive efforts have been employed by authors to make this book an outstanding discourse. This book contains the enlightening chapters which have been written on the basis of significant researches done by the experts.

Finally, I would also like to thank all the members involved in this book for being a team and meeting all the deadlines for the submission of their respective works. I would also like to thank my friends and family for being supportive in my efforts.

Editor

1

In Silico Strategies in Tuberculosis Drug Discovery

Stephani Joy Y. Macalino [1,2], Junie B. Billones [2,*], Voltaire G. Organo [2] and Maria Constancia O. Carrillo [2]

1 Chemistry Department, De La Salle University, 2401 Taft Avenue, Manila 0992, Philippines; stephanimacalino@gmail.com

2 OVPAA-EIDR Program, "Computer-Aided Discovery of Compounds for the Treatment of Tuberculosis in the Philippines", Department of Physical Sciences and Mathematics, College of Arts and Sciences, University of the Philippines Manila, Manila 1000, Philippines; vgorgano@up.edu.ph (V.G.O.); mtobrerocarrillo@up.edu.ph (M.C.O.C.)

* Correspondence: jbbillones@up.edu.ph.

Academic Editor: Rainer Riedl

Abstract: Tuberculosis (TB) remains a serious threat to global public health, responsible for an estimated 1.5 million mortalities in 2018. While there are available therapeutics for this infection, slow-acting drugs, poor patient compliance, drug toxicity, and drug resistance require the discovery of novel TB drugs. Discovering new and more potent antibiotics that target novel TB protein targets is an attractive strategy towards controlling the global TB epidemic. *In silico* strategies can be applied at multiple stages of the drug discovery paradigm to expedite the identification of novel anti-TB therapeutics. In this paper, we discuss the current TB treatment, emergence of drug resistance, and the effective application of computational tools to the different stages of TB drug discovery when combined with traditional biochemical methods. We will also highlight the strengths and points of improvement in *in silico* TB drug discovery research, as well as possible future perspectives in this field.

Keywords: tuberculosis; druggability; docking; pharmacophore; MD simulation; QSAR; DFT

---

1. Introduction

In 1882, *Mycobacterium tuberculosis* (*Mtb*) was identified by Robert Koch as the causative agent of tuberculosis (TB), an infectious disease that continuous to be a relevant threat to global public health, especially in low- to middle-income countries. The pathogenesis of TB has several risk factors, including HIV infection, malnutrition, air pollution, type 2 diabetes, alcoholism, and smoking [1–5].

TB is encountered either as latent TB infection (LTBI), which is non-communicable and asymptomatic [6], or active TB, which is communicable and has symptoms such as fever, weight loss, productive cough, and hemoptysis [7]. Active infection is also classified depending on the strain: (1) drug-sensitive, (2) multidrug-resistant TB (MDR-TB), which is resistant to isoniazid and rifampicin, and (3) extensively drug-resistant TB (XDR-TB), which shows resistance to isoniazid, rifampicin, any fluoroquinolone, and aminoglycoside. Around 1.7 billion people are projected to suffer from LTBI and are at risk of progressing into active TB infection [8]. The World Health Organization (WHO) stated that active TB disease can be found in approximately 10 million people and has caused approximately 1.5 million deaths in 2018. An estimated half million individuals have rifampicin-resistant TB (RR-TB), of which 78% had MDR-TB. Furthermore, approximately 6.2% are suggested to have XDR-TB from these MDR cases [8].

2. Current Tuberculosis Management

One of the major challenges in managing TB is the estimated three million 'missing' individuals who have developed active infections but remained undetected or undiagnosed. TB can be deadly if not treated. With the help of conventional regimen, an estimated 58 million infected individuals were saved from 2000 to 2018. Global treatment outcome in 2017 shows a success rate of 85% for new TB cases and 56% for those with drug-resistant TB [8].

2.1. Latent Tuberculosis Infection

Treatment for LTBI are only provided for select groups that have a high risk of transitioning to active TB infection, including HIV-positive patients, people who were exposed to those with active TB, patients undergoing dialysis for end-stage renal disease, taking anti-tumor necrosis factor (TNF) medications, preparing for transplant surgery, or those with silicosis. Depending on whether it is beneficial or not, especially for children below 5 years of age, exposure to patients with active MDR-TB would require personalized treatment regimens and close observation. WHO recommended several different treatment regimens for LTBI, including 3 months of rifapentine and isoniazid, 3–4 months of isoniazid and rifampicin, 3–4 months of rifampicin, and 6–9 months of isoniazid [9,10]. While all these have established efficacy, poor patient compliance continues to be an issue especially with long treatment periods [9–11].

2.2. Active Drug-Sensitive Tuberculosis

In the last several decades, the treatment strategy for active drug-sensitive TB has not changed from the standard regimen of first-line drugs rifampicin, isoniazid, pyrazinamide and ethambutol (Figure 1) for the first 2 months continued by isoniazid and rifampicin for the next 4 months [12,13]. While this treatment procedure is highly efficacious and successful, its long duration primarily leads to poor patient compliance. This has long been an issue in TB management, necessitating monitoring protocols like the directly observed therapy (DOT), wherein a health professional directly supervises each dose intake [14]. Another issue brought about by the prolonged treatment is drug toxicity resulting in numerous adverse effects such as skin rash, gastrointestinal intolerance, neuropathy, arthralgia, increase in liver enzymes, hepatitis, immune thrombocytopaenia, agranulocytosis, haemolysis, renal failure, optic neuritis, and ototoxicity [15,16].

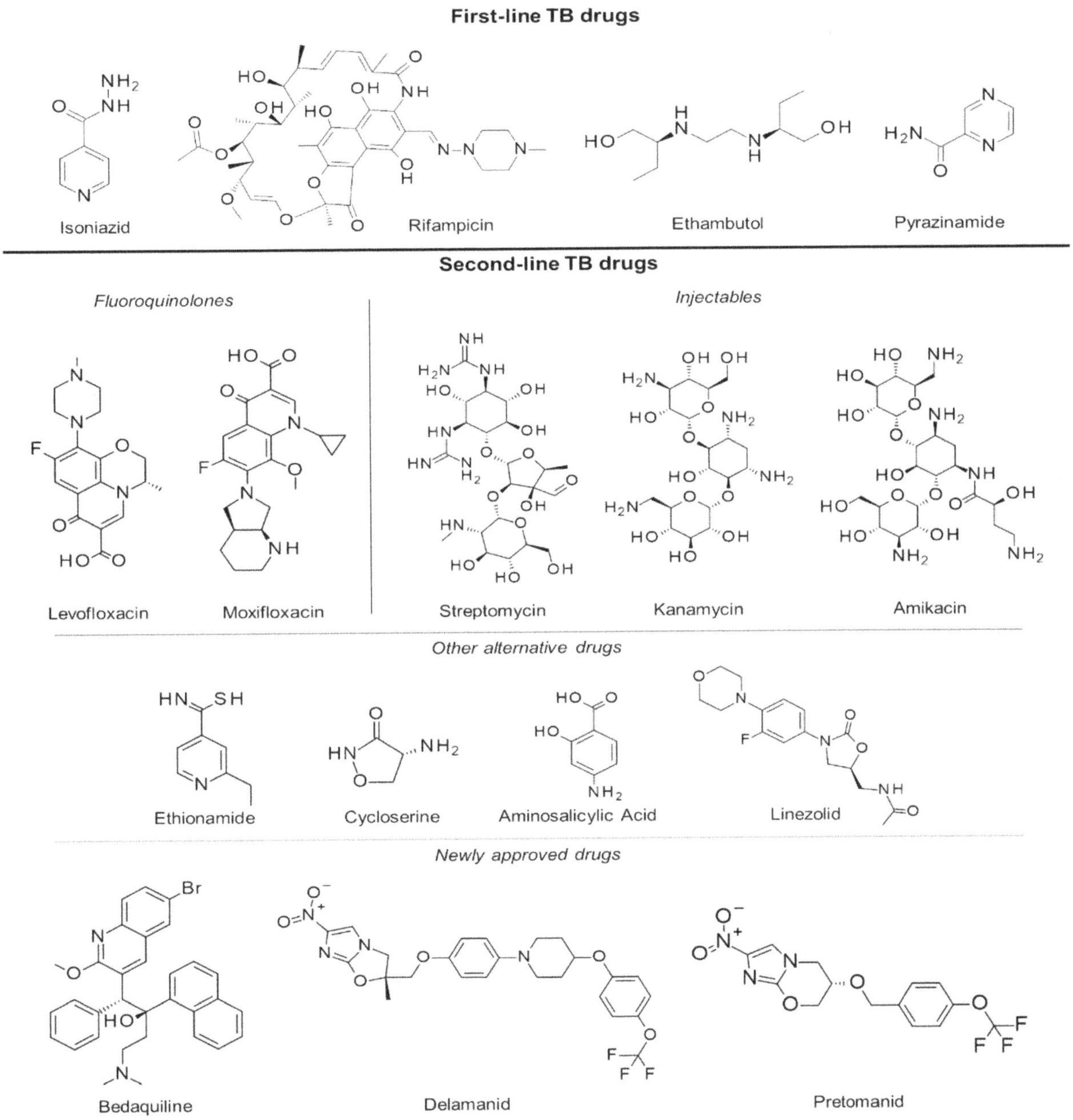

Figure 1. First- and second-line drugs approved for tuberculosis treatment.

2.3. *Multiple and Extensively Drug-Resistant Tuberculosis*

Failure to complete the full TB regimen leads to disease relapse and drug resistance, which is more challenging to treat. A specific regimen can be designed depending on the resistance profile of the TB strain in a patient [17,18]. These treatments are often of longer duration (18 months or more) and utilize the more expensive second-line drugs (Figure 1) which have uncertain efficacy and high toxicity, resulting in poorer compliance and undesirable outcomes. To mitigate these issues, an updated seven-drug regimen guideline for the treatment of drug-resistant TB lasting 9 to 12 months was released by the WHO last 2016 [19].

With the increasing threat of treatment-resistant TB infection, a number of drugs have been fast-tracked to aid with the efforts in controlling TB worldwide. At the end of 2012, the US Food and Drug Administration (FDA) conferred accelerated approval to the drug bedaquiline for the treatment of resistant TB [20]. Bedaquiline's anti-mycobacterial activity is due to its inhibition of the mycobacterial ATP synthase, a key enzyme in ATP synthesis, resulting in bacterial death. However, its use was shown to have an increased risk of death, thereby causing concerns about its approval. During clinical trials, roughly 11.4% of patients who took bedaquiline died as compared with 2.5% of those who took placebo treatments [21]. In 2014, the use of delamanid, a nitro-dihydro-imidazooxazole derivative, in the treatment of MDR-TB in adults was given conditional approval by the European Medicines Agency (EMA) [22]. Delamanid inhibits mycolic acid biosynthesis to block the formation of mycobacterial cell wall leading to improved drug permeation and more effective treatment [23]. Just recently, pretomanid in combination with bedaquiline and linezolid has also been approved by the FDA for treatment-resistant TB [24]. Pretomanid is a prodrug activated by nitroreductase, which reduces pretomanid's imidazole ring to generate active metabolites. Specifically, a des-nitro metabolite leads to elevated levels of nitric oxide, which displays antimycobacterial activities due to its work as a poison for bacterial respiration under anaerobic conditions [25]. In aerobic conditions, it works like delaminid by targeting cell wall mycolic acid biosynthesis [26], and while there were several potential targets for this drug, its exact protein target is not yet known [27].

An increasing number of XDR-TB cases, such as in India, China, South Africa, Russia, and in eastern Europe, have proved difficult to treat even with the more intensive drug-resistant TB treatment regimen [18]. Novel therapeutics such as bedaquiline, delamanid, and pretomanid might help in curing these patients, though a suitable treatment regimen still has to be carefully designed. However, there is an additional difficulty in acquiring these drugs, especially in developing countries, resulting in a pool of patients that may remain untreated. Essentially, TB can be cured completely with the use of currently available and newly approved anti-tubercular drugs. However, difficulties in diagnosing and reporting infection, long treatment durations leading to drug toxicity and poor patient compliance, emergence of drug resistant strains, and limited acquisition of required treatment urgently necessitates the discovery and development of newer and effective drugs for TB.

3. Rise of Computer-Aided Drug Design in TB Drug Discovery

The drug discovery paradigm covers a wide range of fields, including biochemistry, chemical and structural biology, chem- and bioinformatics, computational chemistry, physical chemistry, organic synthesis, and others. The whole process entails large investments of time, money, and effort in order to produce promising candidates for the pipeline. Over the years, the drug discovery process for new antitubercular therapeutics have changed due to the increase in biological and chemical data, number of identified and validated targets, and advances in high-throughput screening technologies and software development. Moreover, the progress in data storage capacities, supercomputing powers, and parallel processing in the last several years allowed computer-aided drug design (CADD) to become an integral part of TB pharmaceutical research. This continuing expansion in computing power can soon potentially allow the exploration of the vast chemical space, thought to comprise of approximately 10^{60} organic molecules below 500 Da, in order to identify therapeutically interesting scaffolds [28]. Moreover, the boom in protein structural data, including over 150,000 macromolecular structures found in the Protein Data Bank (PDB, www.rcsb.org) [29], proved beneficial in elucidating important molecular and computational concepts for drug design studies. As with any other disease, TB has been the subject of continuous and numerous drug discovery studies, including thousands of published CADD investigations. Despite this, a paper by Ekins et al. noted gaps in the application of these methods in TB research [30], resulting in the slow output of candidates into the TB drug pipeline despite the apparent need and urgency for this disease. This suggests that more rigorous efforts are needed in TB drug discovery to maximize the advantages provided by computational tools.

Computational or *in silico* methods are knowledge-driven, rationally exploring available data to investigate protein function and design new molecular entities (NMEs) that can effectively regulate its behavior. Computational drug discovery approaches are generally divided into structure—(SBDD) and ligand-based drug design (LBDD), depending on the availability of structural data (Figure 2). However, it has been a common practice to integrate these methods in a complementary manner in order to increase the success rate of current drug discovery projects (Figure 2). SBDD requires the target's three-dimensional (3D) structure to be able to examine and use the binding pocket for screening and design of suitable ligands, which can then be experimentally validated and optimized. In the absence of protein structural data, LBDD utilizes knowledge gained from a collection of diverse ligands with known activity to create predictive models for hit discovery and lead optimization [31]. Different types of SB and LB strategies, or a combination thereof, can be applied at different stages of TB drug discovery and development in order to alleviate the challenges involved with experimental methods. With the availability of TB genome and proteome, as well as abundant structural data, data mining and docking strategies can be employed for target identification. Virtual screening (VS) can then be applied to pick out the best potential candidates from a database containing millions of molecules for a chosen TB target. After validation of candidates, structure-activity or -property relationship (SAR/SPR) studies can be implemented to understand mechanism of action and ADMET (absorption, distribution, metabolism, excretion, and toxicity) properties in order to design compounds with better activity and pharmacokinetics. Data (both positive and negative results) taken from these investigations can be kept and used for further iteration and method optimization in the design of novel TB compounds. Both commercial and free software and webservers have been developed covering different SBDD and LBDD techniques, some of which are listed in Table 1.

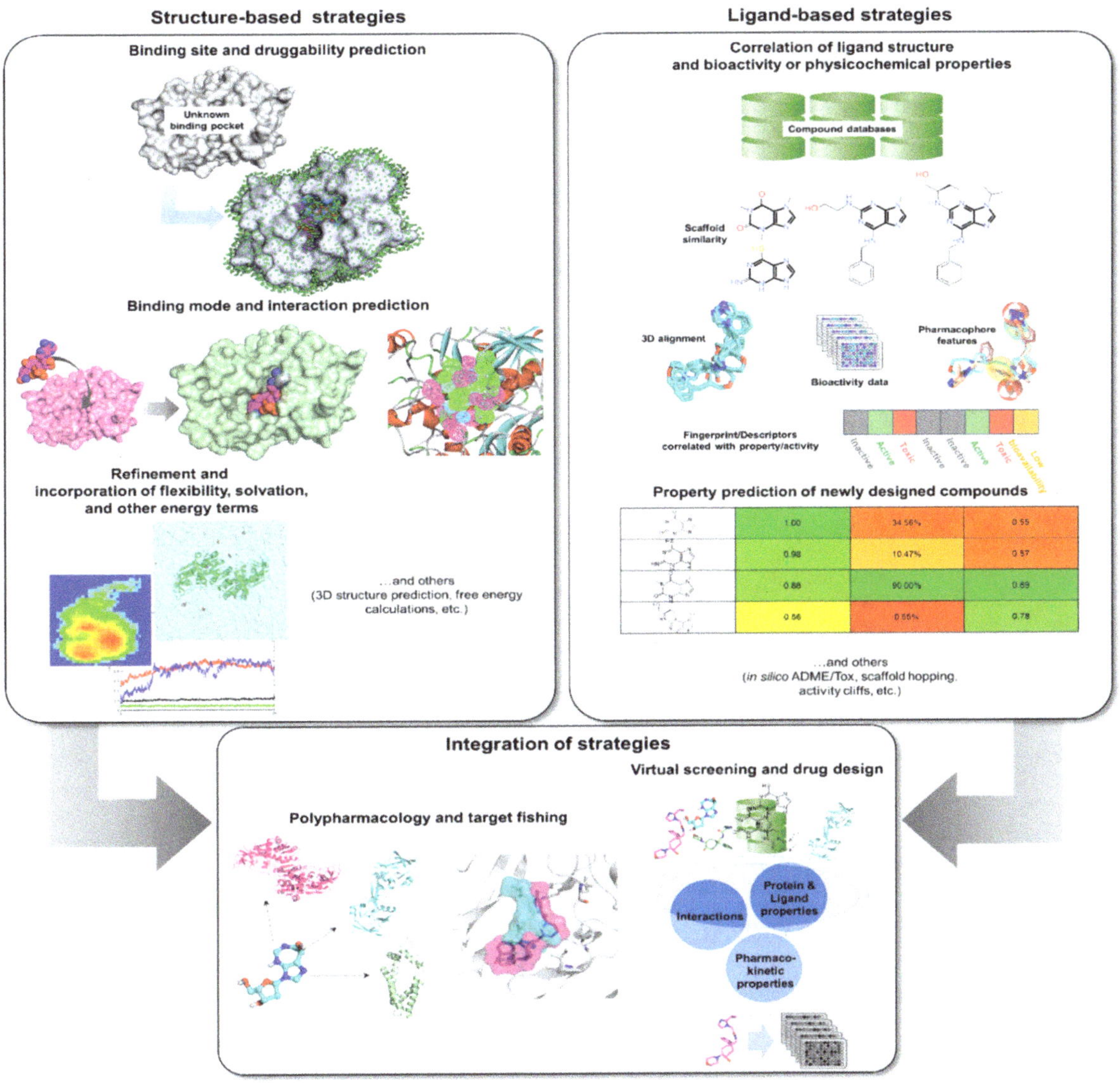

Figure 2. *In silico* tools that can be applied to TB drug design and development.

Table 1. Free and commercially available programs, webservers, and source codes for SBDD and LBDD.

Function	Software/ Webserver Name	Availability	Website
Comparative modeling	SWISS-MODEL [32]	Free webserver	https://swissmodel.expasy.org/
Structural geometry confirmation	MODELLER [33]	Free standalone program for academic license or commercially available through BIOVIA	https://salilab.org/modeller/ https://www.3dsbiovia.com/
	Robetta [34]	Free webserver	http://new.robetta.org/
	Prime [35]	Commercially available through Schrödinger	https://www.schrodinger.com/prime
	I-TASSER [36–41]	Free webserver or standalone program for academic license	https://zhanglab.ccmb.med.umich.edu/I-TASSER/
	HHPred [42–44]	Free webserver	https://toolkit.tuebingen.mpg.de/tools/hhpred
Structural geometry confirmation	PROCHECK [45]	Free webserver and source code	https://www.ebi.ac.uk/thornton-srv/software/ PROCHECK/
Druggability and binding site prediction Druggability and binding site prediction	ProSA [46]	Free webserver	https://prosa.services.came.sbg.ac.at/prosa.php
	VERIFY3D [47]	Free webserver	https://servicesn.mbi.ucla.edu/Verify3D/
	ERRAT [48]	Free webserver	https://servicesn.mbi.ucla.edu/ERRAT/
	PockDrug [49]	Free webserver	http://pockdrug.rpbs.univ-paris-diderot.fr/cgi-bin/index.py?page=home
	DoGSiteScorer [50]	Free webserver	https://proteins.plus/
	fpocket [51,52]	Free/open source platform	https://github.com/Discngine/fpocket
	CASTp [53–55]	Free webserver	http://sts.bioe.uic.edu/castp/calculation.html
	PocketQuery [56]	Free webserver	http://pocketquery.csb.pitt.edu/
	PASS [57]	Free/open source platform	http://www.ccl.net/cca/software/UNIX/pass/ overview.html
	SiteMap [58]	Commercially available through Schrödinger	https://www.schrodinger.com/sitemap
Docking, pharmacophore, and virtual screening Docking, pharmacophore, and virtual screening	ConCavity [59]	Free webserver	https://compbio.cs.princeton.edu/concavity/
	PrankWeb [60]	Free webserver	http://prankweb.cz/
	ProFunc [61]	Free webserver	http: //www.ebi.ac.uk/thornton-srv/databases/ProFunc/
	AutoDock [62] and AutoDock Vina [63]	Free standalone program	http://autodock.scripps.edu/
	DOCK [64]	Free/open source platform	http://dock.compbio.ucsf.edu/
	GOLD [65]	Commercially available through CCDC	https://www.ccdc.cam.ac.uk/solutions/csd-discovery/components/gold/
	Glide [66]	Commercially available through Schrödinger	https://www.schrodinger.com/glide/
	Induced Fit [67]	Commercially available through Schrödinger	https://www.schrodinger.com/induced-fit
	FlexX [68]	Commercially available through BioSolveIT	https://www.biosolveit.de/flexx/index.html
	RosettaLigand [69]	Free/open source platform for academic license	https://www.rosettacommons.org/software
	CDOCKER [70]	Commercially available through BIOVIA	https://www.3dsbiovia.com/
	SwissDock [71,72]	Free webserver	http://www.swissdock.ch/docking
	Pharmer [73]	Free/open source platform	http://smoothdock.ccbb.pitt.edu/pharmer/
	CATALYST [74]	Commercially available through BIOVIA	https://www.3dsbiovia.com/products/ collaborative-science/biovia-discovery-studio/ pharmacophore-and-ligand-based-design.html
	PharmGist [75]	Free webserver	http://bioinfo3d.cs.tau.ac.il/pharma/php.php
	LigandScout [76]	Commercially available through Inte:Ligand	http://www.inteligand.com/ligandscout/
	SwissSimilarity [77]	Free webserver	http://www.swisssimilarity.ch/

Table 1. *Cont.*

Function	Software/ Webserver Name	Availability	Website
	LEA3D [78]	Free webserver	https://chemoinfo.ipmc.cnrs.fr/LEA3D/index.html
	PyRx [79]	Free (no support) or commercially available	https://pyrx.sourceforge.io/
	Phase [80]	Commercially available through Schrödinger	https://www.schrodinger.com/phase
Molecular Dynamics	AMBER [81,82]	Commercially available	https://ambermd.org/
	CHARMM [83]	Free or commercially available through CHARMM or BIOVIA	http://charmm.chemistry.harvard.edu/ https: //www.3dsbiovia.com/products/collaborative-science/biovia-discovery-studio/simulations.html
	CHARMMing [84]	Free webserver	https://www.charmming.org/charmming
	GROMACS [85,86]	Free/open source platform	http://www.gromacs.org/
	NAMD [87]	Free/open source platform	https://www.ks.uiuc.edu/Research/namd/
	Desmond [88]	Commercially available through Schrödinger	https://www.schrodinger.com/desmond
	SwissParam [89]	Free webserver	http://www.swissparam.ch/
	CHARMM-GUI [90]	Free webserver	http://www.charmm-gui.org/
	ParamChem CGenFF [91–93]	Free webserver	https://cgenff.umaryland.edu/
	VMD [94]	Free/open source platform	https://www.ks.uiuc.edu/Research/vmd/
Molecular Descriptors, Fingerprints, and Quantitative Structure-Activity Relationship	Dragon [95]	Commercially available through Talete	http://www.talete.mi.it/products/dragon_description.htm
	E-Dragon [96]	Free webserver	http://146.107.217.178/lab/edragon/start.html
	Canvas [97]	Commercially available through Schrödinger	https://www.schrodinger.com/canvas
	RDKit [98]	Free/open source platform	https://www.rdkit.org/docs/source/rdkit.ML.Descriptors.MoleculeDescriptors.html
	PyDescriptor [99]	Free/open source platform	https://ochem.eu/home/show.do
	Mordred [100]	Free/open source platform	https://github.com/mordred-descriptor/mordred
	Open3DQSAR [101]	Free/open source platform	http://open3dqsar.sourceforge.net/?Home
	ChemSAR [102]	Free webserver	http://chemsar.scbdd.com/
	SeeSAR [103]	Commercially available through BioSolveIT	https://www.biosolveit.de/SeeSAR/
Pharmacokinetic properties	QikProp [104]	Commercially available through Schrödinger	https://www.schrodinger.com/qikprop
	ADMET Predictor [105]	Commercially available through SimulationsPlus, Inc.	https: //www.simulations-plus.com/software/overview/
	ACD Percepta [106]	Commercially available through ACD/Labs	https: //www.acdlabs.com/products/percepta/index.php
	FAF-Drugs4 [107]	Free webserver	http://fafdrugs4.mti.univ-paris-diderot.fr/
	PatchSearch [108]	Free webserver	http://mobyle.rpbs.univ-paris-diderot.fr/cgi-bin/portal.py#forms::PatchSearch
	TOPKAT [109] and ADMET [110]	Commercially available through BIOVIA	https://www.3dsbiovia.com/products/collaborative-science/biovia-discovery-studio/qsar-admet-and-predictive-toxicology.html
	PASS Online [111]	Free webserver or commercially available standalone program	http://pharmaexpert.ru/Passonline/index.php
	SwissADME [112]	Free webserver	http://www.swissadme.ch/
	MetaSite [113]	Commercially available through Molecular Discovery	https://www.moldiscovery.com/software/metasite/
	ToxPredict [114]	Free webserver	https://apps.ideaconsult.net/ToxPredict#
	VirtualToxLab [115–118]	Free standalone software	http://www.biograf.ch/index.php?id=home
	admetSAR [119–121]	Free webserver	http://lmmd.ecust.edu.cn/admetsar1/home/
	MetaTox [122,123]	Free webserver	http://way2drug.com/mg2/

More available tools and detailed descriptions for the programs and servers can be found at https://www.click2drug.org/.

3.1. Databases

The era of big data has greatly affected the current drug discovery paradigm through innovations in data storage, management, and mining. Moreover, drastic cost reductions in sequencing technologies allowed the study of multi-omics (e.g., genomics, transcriptomics, proteomics, and metabolomics) for several species including *M. tuberculosis* [124–129]. In order to take advantage of the benefits provided by SB and LB techniques, these biological and/or chemical data must be acquired for analysis via numerous publicly accessible databases on the internet [130–132]. Given that TB is an old disease, vast amounts of data points have already been gathered and are waiting to be used in the fight against this infection.

One of the most extensive and widely-used protein information resource is UniProt (https://www.uniprot.org/) [133], which consists of annotations from several other databases for protein function, omics, and structural data. More specific to TB, the TB Database (http://tbdb.bu.edu/tbdb_sysbio/MultiHome.html) [134,135] contains information on mycobacterium genomes, genes, gene expression correlation, gene epitopes, and experimental and computational models of TB molecular pathways. Alternatively, genomic and proteomic data for various pathogenic mycobacteria can also be found in the Mycobrowser (https://mycobrowser.epfl.ch/) [136], which is linked to UniProt for mycobacterium protein information. On the other hand, patient clinical data is provided by the TB Portals (https://tbportals.niaid.nih.gov/) [137], which is an open-access platform containing socioeconomic, geographic, clinical, laboratory, radiological, and genomic data from patients infected with drug-resistant TB, from the National Institute of Allergy and Infectious Diseases (NIAID) in collaboration with data scientists and clinicians and scientists from countries suffering from heavy TB burden.

Advances in structural and computational biology techniques led to the surge in structural data, resulting in thousands of three-dimensional protein structures generated from X-ray crystallography, nuclear magnetic resonance (NMR), cryo-electron microscopy (EM), homology modeling, and molecular dynamics (MD) simulations. Data from these experiments are customarily deposited to structure databases such as PDB [29], PDBsum [138], etc. Associated with this, the size of the virtual chemical space [28] and improvements in combinatorial chemistry [139] also permitted the availability of chemical libraries (Table 2).

Table 2. Publicly available compound libraries.

Database	Size (Approximate)	Website
GDB-17 [140]	166 billion	http://gdb.unibe.ch/
Enamine REAL [141]	700 million	https://enamine.net/
PubChem [131]	97 million	https://pubchem.ncbi.nlm.nih.gov/
ChemSpider [142]	77 million	http://www.chemspider.com/
ZINC [143]	230 million	http://zinc.docking.org/
ChEMBL [144]	1.9 million	https://www.ebi.ac.uk/chembl/
NCI [145]	460,000	https://cactus.nci.nih.gov/download/roadmap/

Protein subcellular localization databases are also available for study, such as eSLDB (eukaryotic Subcellular Localization database) for general eukaryotes [146], LOCATE for human and other mammals [147], and PSORTdb for bacteria and archaea [148]. Lead optimization and drug repurposing researches can also benefit from protein binding databases like ReLiBase, which consists of interaction information for receptor-ligand complexes from PDB [149], BindingDB, which describes interactions and affinity information between protein target and drug-like molecules [150,151], and Database of Interacting Proteins (DIP) [152], Biological General Repository for Interaction Datasets (BioGRID) [153] and Search Tool for the Retrieval of Interacting Genes/Proteins (STRING) [154], which contains data on protein-protein interactions.

3.2. *Structure-Based Tools*

3.2.1. Comparative Modeling, Binding Site Prediction, and Druggability

Employment of SBDD tools (Figure 2 and Table 1) require not only the availability of 3D structural data but also information on its druggability and potential binding sites. In the absence of structural data obtained from experiments, such as X-ray crystallography and NMR, a computational model can also be generated either through homology modeling or protein threading techniques (Table 1), which are well-established methods in protein comparative modeling. Homology modeling entails the use of a structural template with suitably similar sequence as the target protein [155]. The most critical stage of any homology modeling procedure is the initial sequence alignment. While there are numerous bioinformatics tools available for this, such as NCBI Blast [156–158], COBALT [159], Clustal Omega [160], KAlign [161], etc., manual inspection and modification of the alignment is crucial, especially if a researcher's knowledge about specific protein folds and domains need to be further incorporated. Then, the secondary structures (i.e., alpha helices, beta strands, loops, etc.) are copied from the template based on the final sequence alignment in order to approximate the target structure. The final model is then refined through minimization or MD and its stereochemical quality is checked using tools like those listed in Table 1 until the structure has improved and is suitable for further computational studies.

Druggability is the capacity of a protein target to be modulated by a ligand. It is important to characterize this property as it helps avoid intractable proteins and allows the identification and prioritization of significant targets. Some predictive approaches that include this property are listed in Table 1. A druggability database, the Druggable Cavity Directory (DCD), is also publicly available to allow researchers to submit protein pocket and druggability information, which is later verified and made available to other researchers [162]. After ascertaining that a given target is indeed tractable, binding pocket information should be acquired either from protein structures complexed with natural substrates or known inhibitors, or from mutational data distinguishing key interaction residues. Ideally, a binding pocket is a concave area in the receptor that is characterized by chemical features with which a ligand can desirably interact to attain the required receptor behavior (e.g., inhibition or activation) [163]. However, if binding information is unknown, several *in silico* methods and webservers (Table 1) are available to identify potential receptor binding sites from a given structure and have been described in detail elsewhere [31]. Otherwise, a number of studies have also used 'blind' docking [164], wherein the whole protein is set as the binding site, allowing ligands to freely bind anywhere in the structure in the hopes of finding a suitable pocket.

It is also prudent to remember that other potential binding sites may be present on the target surface, i.e., allosteric sites. Conventional drug discovery efforts often target the primary (orthosteric) binding site to block substrate binding. But, as in the case of uncompetitive and noncompetitive inhibitors, ligands can also allosterically modulate activity within the protein structure. Such is the case in the study done by Shi and colleagues, where they identified a second druggable binding site in *Mtb* UDP-galactopyranose mutase (UGM) [165]. NMR and kinetics studies classified MS-208, a known *Mtb*UGM inhibitor, as a noncompetitive/mixed inhibitor and therefore binds in another site in the enzyme to allosterically affect substrate binding. Blind docking in AutoDock Vina [63] was performed to identify possible allosteric sites for MS-208. Two regions, A- and S-site, were initially identified and docked complexes featuring binding to either sites were further subjected to simulation studies using Amber [81]. The A-site-bound structure exhibited the most stable complex formation with excellent interaction energy, as well as the most number of contacts, suggesting that this is the second druggable binding site in *Mtb*UGM [165].

3.2.2. Pharmacophore Modeling and Molecular Docking

Virtual screening is one of the most popular *in silico* drug discovery approaches as it allows researchers to quickly extract data from unexplored chemical space in a cost-effective manner. It has become customary to complement high-throughput screening with VS for the prioritization and identification of novel ligands with the most potential as starting points for drug discovery efforts [166]. Two of the most common VS methods are pharmacophore modeling [167] and docking [168].

Pharmacophore models can be generated from a receptor alone or a receptor-ligand complex. Previously, due to lack of protein structural data, ligand-based pharmacophore has been more customarily used (see Section 3.3.2). A pharmacophore is a group of geometrically-mapped chemical features, such as *H*-bond donors and acceptors, hydrophobicity, and ionizable groups, required for optimal interactions to elicit a response between a receptor target and its partner molecule [169,170]. In line with 3D-mapping in a pharmacophore, exclusion volumes can also be included in the model to incorporate binding site shape [171]. After generating a 3D model, large chemical databases can be efficiently searched for candidates that match pharmacophore elements. However, the pharmacophore database screen only provides a fit score that cannot be translated as affinity. The fit score weighs the alignment quality between the ligand substructures and center of model features. Weights and penalties can also be employed for features deemed significant to activity [171]. These models can also be used for scaffold hopping, allowing for the discovery of novel chemotypes based on fit of interaction and geometric characteristics [171,172].

Another well-established *in silico* method is docking, which can be used to facilitate the investigation of how ligands can fit and complement receptor binding pocket features in order to modulate its activity [168]. Numerous docking methods (Table 1) have been developed and comparative studies and detailed reviews about these have been published elsewhere [173–177]. In the early days of computational drug discovery, docking was developed to be able to predict the bioactive conformation within a set of docking results. However, protein-ligand interactions need to be evaluated using a scoring function to find the best pose using estimated affinity, distinguish actives from inactives, and prioritize candidates for further testing and optimization. This was soon discovered to be the most challenging part of docking due to approximations applied to other crucial factors, such as protein flexibility, solvent involvement, and system entropy [168]. Despite advances in scoring functions through increased understanding of protein-ligand interactions, it is difficult to handle all these aspects while still maintaining method efficiency. Moreover, scoring functions often depend on the protein families and ligand sets from which it was generated and validated [31,178]. And while there is currently no ideal scoring function that can be utilized across all druggable targets, implementation of method validation before starting any VS project establishes whether a chosen docking method and scoring function can be applicable or not [171].

Both pharmacophore modeling and docking have been applied in combination with other *in silico* tools for the identification of novel antimycobacterial agents. Pharmacophore screening followed by docking can be employed as complementary screening tools, resulting in faster processing and more optimized results. A recent study published by our group exemplifies both pharmacophore-based and docking VS by targeting *Mtb* 7,8-diaminopelargonic acid aminotransferase (BioA), an important enzyme in its lipid biosynthesis pathway with no corresponding human ortholog [179]. A receptor-based pharmacophore was generated in Discovery Studio [180] using the BioA structure, characterizing 25 functionalities (nine hydrophobic, nine H-bond donors, and seven *H*-bond acceptors), and was employed to screen 4.5 million compounds from the Enamine REAL database. Compounds with good pharmacophore fit, as well as the co-crystallized inhibitor, were subsequently docked to the BioA protein via CDOCKER [70] and ligands with better binding energy values than the known inhibitor were chosen for the TOPKAT protocol [109] to filter out potentially toxic compounds. This step-by-step screening led to the identification of 45 virtual hits, 17 of which were available for purchasing and validation. Whole-cell assay was performed to eliminate compounds that cannot penetrate the distinctive thick, waxy lipid layer of the mycobacterium, identifying compound **7** ((*Z*)-*N*-(2-isopropoxyphenyl)-2-oxo-2-((3-(trifluoromethyl)-cyclohexyl)amino)acetimidic acid) as a potential BioA inhibitor with a minimum inhibitory concentration of ~25 μM [179].

Throughout the years, various improvements have been harnessed to enhance ranking performance, such as rescoring or consensus scoring. Given the different strengths and limitations of each scoring function, rescoring with the help of a separate scoring function not used in a docking study provides users with a different perspective for selection of final hits. For instance, a faster scoring function can be employed for pose prediction while another one is used for affinity prediction and ranking [171]. Currently, consensus scoring is more commonly used for docking studies and has already been examined by several groups in the last couple of decades as an improved protocol for finding potential hits [181–185]. This strategy aims to characterize the intricacy of target molecular recognition based on various energy functions which can be covered by several scoring schemes, resulting in decrease in false positives [184].

However, there is also a risk of rejecting true positives, which have favorable scores in only 1 function used. Thus, it is also imperative to validate a consensus scoring workflow against specific targets [171]. An exemplary case features salicylate synthase MbtI, a critical enzyme in the biosynthesis of siderophore mycobactins, which is used by *Mtb* to chelate iron required for growth and survival in the host. Absence of siderophores prevents bacterial growth in the persistent state after engulfment by macrophages [186]. Previously identified MbtI inhibitors include those based on the MbtI reaction intermediate isochorismate [187], benzimidazole-2-thione [188], and chromane scaffolds [189]. Chiarelli et al. [190] discovered furan-based MbtI inhibitors through structure-based pharmacophore and consensus docking.

The pharmacophore model was generated from important binding features in the MbtI-inhibitor complex, including interaction with the conserved Y385, lipophilic interactions, and ionizable interaction with the Mg^{2+} ion. Screening of 1.5 M compounds from Enamine [141] led to over 2,000 pharmacophore hits which were subjected to consensus docking. Docking methods including AutoDock [62], AutoDock Vina [63], DOCK [64], FRED [191], GOLD [65] (comprising four scoring functions), and PLANT [192] were first evaluated using several MbtI-inhibitor complexes to identify which methods are most reliable. GOLD and PLANT were employed for the consensus procedure of the pharmacophore hits, and those with similar binding modes and consistent scores across all scoring functions were further examined if the docked conformation still matched the 3D arrangement of the pharmacophore model. From these, five virtual hits progressed to bioassays, wherein two compounds showed potent MbtI inhibitory activity. MD simulation was additionally applied to study enzyme-ligand interactions and provide information for further optimization. The furan scaffold from the more potent hit was used as a starting point for lead optimization, resulting in a candidate with promising activity against MbtI and suitable antimycobacterial activity [190].

Inclusion of limited protein flexibility, such as in the binding pocket, while still maintaining efficiency has been considered in methods like induced fit docking (IFD) and ensemble docking. IFD incorporates the principle that ligand binding induces changes in residue side chain conformations within the specified pocket, thereby inciting tighter binding with the receptor [193,194]. However, backbone movement should also be considered as it increases the accuracy of side chain positioning and orientations [31]. An example of this is shown in Figure 3, in which *Mtb* InhA exhibits backbone and side chain conformational differences between its apo (PDB ID: 4DRE) [195], fatty acyl substrate-bound (PDB ID: 1BVR) [196] and isoniazid (INH)-bound (PDB ID: 4TRO) structures [197]. These movements can change the binding pocket shape and volume, potentially affecting VS results. The utilization of several experimentally—(X-ray crystallography, NMR, or cryo-electron microscopy) or computationally-derived (MD trajectory) protein structures to integrate both backbone and side chain movements has also been employed in ensemble docking [198]. Structural ensembles provide better reproducibility of experimental conditions as rigid protein structures, such as those obtained from X-ray crystallography experiments, only provide a snapshot of a dynamic ensemble of conformations.

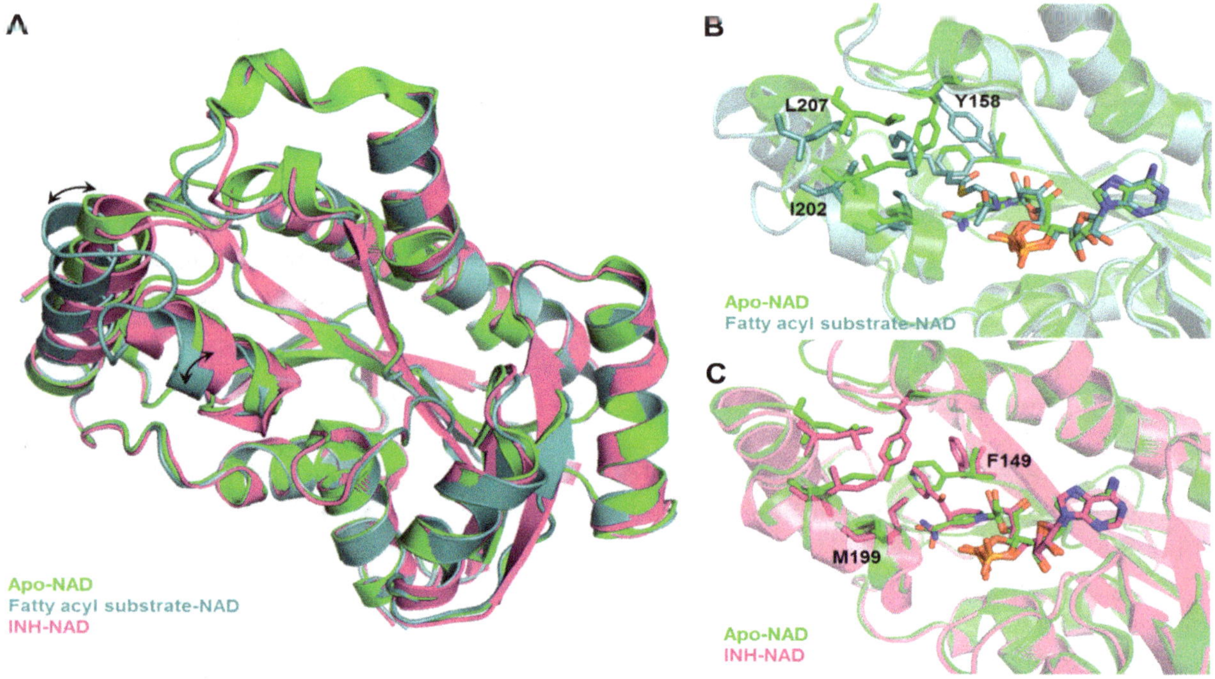

Figure 3. Backbone and sidechain flexibility shown by Mtb InhA, apo vs. fatty acyl-bound vs. INH-bound. (**A**) Structural overlay of apo, fatty acyl-bound, INH-bound Mtb InhA shows backbone movement upon substrate (fatty acyl) binding. Binding site comparison of (**B**) fatty acyl-bound and (**C**) INH-bound vs. apo Mtb InhA structure shows distinct changes in residue side chain positions and conformations. Black arrows indicate movement of alpha helices, side chains that showed large conformational change upon fatty acyl or INH binding are labelled in black.

Various docking approaches were applied by Brindha et al. [199] for drug repurposing against *Mtb* murE, which is an attractive target due to its significance in the peptidoglycan biosynthesis of tuberculosis bacteria and lack of eukaryotic homolog. VS of compounds from DrugBank [200] was first implemented through the parallel use of Glide Standard Precision (SP) [66] and AutoDock Vina [63]. To improve prioritization of compounds through the incorporation of binding site flexibility, common hits from both methods were further subjected to IFD [67]. Final rankings were done using Glide eXtra Precision (XP) scoring and AutoDock Vina binding energy prediction, resulting in 17 common top hits identified as repurposed antitubercular drug candidates [199]. In another example, ensemble docking using three enzyme structures was performed to better elucidate ligand binding interactions, especially due to the binding site flexibility of the *Mtb* Type II dehydroquinase (MtDHQase), an essential virulence factor in TB [201]. Conformation of key residues were determined by analyzing superimposed MtDHQase structures and rotamer distribution of each residue from the penultimate rotamer library [202]. The benzene sulfonamide containing compound with the best activity, a Schaeffer's acid amide, was docked using GOLD [65] and scored using ChemPLP [203]. Varying the side chain flexibility during the docking procedure led to the identification of residues that are required to transition the binding site into an open conformation, which is the preferred conformation of the inhibitor to display its activity. Along with the interaction and flexibility data, Schaeffer's acid amide can be optimized into a potent antitubercular therapeutic compound [201].

3.2.3. Molecular Dynamics

The availability of 3D structural information has greatly helped in structure-based drug design by presenting atomic-level insights into molecular interactions. Nonetheless, these provide only partial interpretations of biomolecular structures, as well as related aspects of molecular recognition and binding. In physiological conditions, proteins frequently undergo conformational changes upon binding with a partner, such as a small molecule, peptide, or another protein, to perform a specific function. At times, these transformations only involve side chain conformations and small to medium movements in the backbone. However, there are cases in which significant deviations are seen in the overall protein fold and/or subunit arrangement [204–207].

Molecular dynamics simulation, a method that was first developed in the 70s [208], can be employed to analyze these protein dynamics and study the binding energy landscape. The availability of MD platforms (Table 1) allowed for the routine assimilation of simulation studies for systems containing ~50,000–100,000 atoms. The investigation of even larger systems is made possible using graphics processing units (GPUs), which are high-performance processors that can support heavy computational load, and high-performance computing (HPC) technologies featuring messaging passing interface (MPI), a system which employs multiple cores in parallel to distribute computational load and reduce the time required for simulation [206,209]. Popular MD packages have been adapted for these tools, and while MD simulation projects commonly use a combination of both, the speedy development of more advanced GPUs increasingly allows for the use of personal workstations [206].

To start an MD simulation, a 3D protein structure of the required system (e.g., apo protein, protein-ligand or protein-protein complex) must be obtained experimentally or through homology modeling, and represented based on the duration and details of study [206,210]. Another critical aspect of system preparation in MD is the solvent model, which can be explicit or implicit. Explicit solvent is more frequently used due to its simplicity and its proficiency in recovering native solvent effects to protein structure [211]. However, large system size resulting from this model makes conformational sampling challenging. To speed up conformational sampling, an implicit solvent model can be generated by adding approximations to the system, but this may affect the free energy landscapes [212]. Once a solvent model has been chosen, the next step is to select an appropriate force field, which is used to define the forces acting on every atom in the system and to calculate the potential energy within the molecular structure. While there are numerous force fields that have been and are still being developed and improved, some of the most popular force fields applied in simulation systems are currently CHARMM [213], Amber [214], GROMOS [215], and OPLS-AA [216,217]. Different force fields use different parameterization to characterize atomistic molecular simulations, distinguishing their applicability in atomistic molecular simulations of diverse target structures and systems, but are often equivalent [206]. To ensure efficiency while keeping the calculations accurate, simple molecular representations in force fields include springs depicting bond length and angles, periodic functions depicting rotations and Lennard-Jones potentials, and Coulomb's law characterizing van der Waals and electrostatic interactions within the system [206]. Newton's law of motion is then employed for the computation of accelerations and velocities during atom movement. Minimization and equilibration are typically performed ahead of a production run to adjust the system to the applied force field, relax steric clashes, and to stabilize system temperature and pressure. Once the prepared system is correctly minimized and equilibrated, the production run can be performed for a suitable amount of time (ps, ns, μs, etc.) depending on research needs (Figure 4). A timestep of 1 or 2 fs is frequently used for atomistic MD simulations [206].

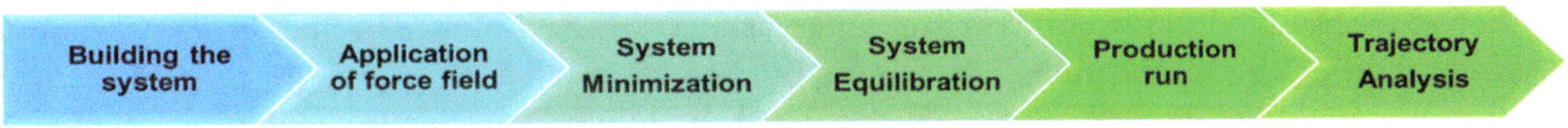
Building the system
Application of force field
System Minimization
System Equilibration
Production run
Trajectory Analysis

Figure 4. Typical molecular dynamics simulation workflow.

After obtaining simulation trajectories, this information can be used for additional analyses, including but not limited to: (1) verifying stability through root-mean-square deviation (RMSD), root-mean-square fluctuation (RMSF), or radius of gyration (RoG) [218,219], which can identify critical components for protein flexibility, (2) investigating protein structural or energy networks through network analysis [220], which can pinpoint residues that are pivotal in allosteric or long-range communications within the protein, (3) studying protein energy landscape by mapping trajectories [221], providing information about protein folding and function, as well as most stable populations within a given trajectory. Findings from each analysis provide crucial information that would otherwise be imperceptible with other techniques, thereby increasing our understanding of a given system.

With current computational capabilities, simulation times are nearly of biological relevance, allowing researchers to observe biological events, such as allosteric regulation, transient protein changes and binding, and enzyme catalysis. A number of MD studies have already been done for the structural and functional elucidation of validated TB targets and design new antitubercular agents [222–224]. One such study investigated the differences of inhibitor binding against wild-type and mutant structures of InhA, a very well-known TB target [223]. Mutations for this protein led to lower affinity for its co-factor, NADH, resulting in isoniazid resistance. MD simulations of the wild-type and mutant structures of InhA bound to NADH were performed using Amber [81] to understand the underlying aspects affected by structural mutations. Schroeder and colleagues found that mutations in the glycine-rich loop (I21V and I16T) disturbed the NADH binding conformation, specifically that of its pyrophosphate moiety, and decreased its direct and indirect *H*-bond contacts within the binding pocket. Isoniazid requires the formation of a covalent adduct with NADH within the InhA binding site. Changes in binding interactions and conformation of NADH can negatively affect this, hence, contributing to isoniazid resistance [223]. A very recent MD study for TB drug discovery using Amber [81] has been published by Cruz et al. [224], wherein the binding mechanisms of Tam1 and its analogs against polyketide synthase 13 (Pks13), an enzyme that carries out the final step in mycolic acid biosynthesis [225], were investigated to obtain insights that can aid in the design of new antitubercular agents [224]. Fluctuation analysis revealed distinct flexibility in the protein lid domain of *Mtb* Pks13, which was decreased upon ligand binding, suggesting that residues from this domain are critical for ligand interaction. Binding free energy calculations from trajectory data agreed with experimental data, identifying Tam16 as the most potent of the Tam analogs due to conformational stability offered by *H*-bond interactions at both ends of the ligand structure that was not observed for other compounds. Energy decomposition analysis further specifically identified residues that greatly contributed to inhibitor binding, which can then be targeted for optimization of Tam16 and the design of other analogs [224].

3.3. *Ligand-Based Tools*

3.3.1. Similarity-Based and Quantitative Structure-Activity/Property Relationship Methods

Even before the upsurge of available target structural data, rational inhibitor design has been employed with the help of substrate or product structures, and thus termed as ligand-based drug discovery and design (Figure 2). The simplest and most inexpensive LBDD approach is the similarity-based method, wherein compound candidates were designed and optimized through the principle of chemical similarity, i.e., similar (untested) ligand structures are posited to have similar activities as known inhibitors or modulators [226,227]. A typical workflow requires one or more reference structures with existing bioactivity information against a specific target. This is then used as a template to select new potential candidates from a chemical database to prioritize for assay testing.

Different molecular descriptors and parameterizations can be employed to characterize compounds and efficiently determine similarities. Descriptors can be generated as one-, two- or three-dimensional (1D, 2D, or 3D), wherein 1D descriptors comprise of global ligand properties (e.g., molecular weight, logP, number of *H*-bonds, etc.), 2D descriptors include topological and connectivity properties (e.g., aromaticity, degree of branching, etc.), and 3D descriptors involve geometrical properties (e.g., shape, volume, surface area, etc.) [228,229]. Additionally, fingerprints can also be used to depict template and database compounds by rendering structural features, such as those based on substructure (i.e., scaffold or functional groups), topology or path (i.e., fragmentation following a linear path of bonds), circular or radial (i.e., surrounding features of an atom up to a certain radius), and pharmacophoric (i.e., distance-based features, incorporating molecular shape, and interactions required for biological activity) elements [230]. Well-known platforms that generate molecular descriptors and fingerprints are listed in Table 1.

To compare structural similarity after obtaining simplified molecular features, similarity coefficient and weighing scheme are required to measure and highlight the importance of certain aspects of a compound's structure in relation with its activity. Given that there are multiple tools available for both components, careful selection of analysis tools is crucial to have successful VS campaign. Tanimoto coefficient, which uses the ratio of shared features in both fingerprints to the total number of features between each fingerprint sets, is used as a standard for similarity evaluation of any two vectors. This coefficient returns values between 1 and 0 to depict chemical similarity [231]. Other known similarity measures include Manhattan distance, Euclidean distance, Dice index, Cosine coefficient, and others [232]. In terms of weighing schemes, some features may be 'silenced' or set as optional depending on its importance for a specific activity. There is not one method that can be considered the best for the full range of known targets and chemicals, as each method have their own data set applicability [233,234]. In this case, data fusion can be employed to obtain a consensus of outputs from different methods [235,236]. Both 2D and 3D similarity methods have been successful in identifying hits for various targets and have been established to have comparable or even better enrichment than docking [237]. While similarity-based approaches are known for their efficiency, there is a risk of obtaining low diversity hits as most similarity methods are highly dependent on the input structures used to calculate descriptors [238]. Moreover, there is a potential occurrence of 'activity cliffs,' in which small modifications in a ligand structure lead to significant difference in activity [239–241].

The similarity concept is also applied in studies involving quantitative structure-activity/property relationship (QSAR/QSPR), a method which is used to investigate the correlation between structural and physicochemical properties of ligands with known biological activities. QSAR modeling depends on the premise that ligand 2D and 3D properties can provide information to establish a statistical model of the desired biological activity, which can then be employed for activity prediction of ligand candidates [242,243]. The statistical model is generated based on an appropriate data set, consisting of compound structures with known bioactivity against a specific target, which must be checked and pre-processed. This data set should contain an adequate number of samples (i.e., a minimum of 20 experimentally-validated compounds) and, if from separate studies, identified using same assay protocols such that equivalent activities are obtained. Included in the data set preparation, especially for higher dimensions of QSAR modeling, is the conformational selection and alignment which allows the identification of scaffolds and functional groups that are critical to activity and therefore has more weight in the statistical model [242]. In this case, it is important to remember that the lowest energy conformation is not always equivalent to the bioactive conformation [244,245] and that ligands chosen for the training set should interact with the same binding site [242]. Typical alignment methods include the analysis of molecular fields, structural shapes, or pharmacophores. Pharmacophore generation for ligand alignment is more favorable as it aligns compounds based on feature similarity rather than chemical substructure [246]. As with similarity-based methods, QSAR makes use of molecular descriptors with dimensionality depending on the information available. Descriptors applied to the model should be carefully chosen to avoid autocorrelation and over-fitting. Before proceeding with and *in silico* prediction study, the model must be validated with internal and/or external data sets to establish its predictivity and applicability against a desired target [31,247].

Different QSAR methods have been developed and incorporated in various open-source platforms and commercial software (Table 1). The earliest QSAR-based algorithms include Comparative Molecular Field Analyses (CoMFA) [248] and Comparative Molecular Similarity Indices Analysis (CoMSIA) [249], both of which are still widely used today for various drug discovery endeavors [250–253]. 3D-QSAR CoMFA was used by Singh and Supuran [252] for the discovery of novel *Mtb* carbonic anhydrase inhibitors. A number of sulfonamides that target *Mtb* carbonic anhydrase 2 to regulate bacterial growth were used as the data set for QSAR modeling. The best developed model had excellent predictivity and good fit with an r^2 value of 0.93 and cross-validated coefficient q^2 value of 0.88. From the CoMFA results, it was also determined that several steric and electrostatic features play critical roles in the inhibition of *Mtb* carbonic anhydrase 2. Using this information, nine compounds were designed and later observed to have better predicted inhibitory activities compared to the test set used. However, experimental validation is still required to determine the feasibility of these findings [252].

3.3.2. Ligand-Based Pharmacophore Modeling

Pharmacophore modelling have already demonstrated its value in ligand-based drug discovery studies. Ligand substructures required for optimal bioactivity can be aligned and characterized as a spatial arrangement of features in 3D space, which can be directly used for screening or applied to 3D-QSAR modeling [169,170,246]. Several software and webservers (Table 1) are available for the generation of ligand-based pharmacophores.

As with any other ligand-based methods, a data set of diverse ligands with known bioactivity against a specific target is required for pharmacophore generation. The training ligands used for ligand-based pharmacophore modeling must bind to the same pocket and have similar binding interactions, much like in QSAR studies. After obtaining a pharmacophore, its validity is assessed using a separate test set. It is then employed for virtual search of candidate compounds from libraries of untested molecules, wherein compounds are taken as potential hits if it 'fits' well with the pharmacophore (Figure 5). The main advantage of pharmacophore modeling is the use of molecular features rather than structural groups in depicting critical functionalities for activity, which allows for the identification of novel ligands with diverse structures (i.e., scaffold hopping) [172]. Moreover, pharmacophores can also be used for target profiling and polypharmacological studies to avoid adverse effects resulting from off-target binding [254]. This is especially useful when designing antitubercular and other antibiotic or antiviral agents as to avoid harmful interactions with human proteins.

Due to the numerous parallels between pharmacophore and 3D-QSAR modeling, these methods have been used in combination for a number of ligand-based drug discovery efforts. A study by Tawari et al. used PHASE [80] to target the *Mtb* aryl acid adenylating enzymes known as MbtA, which are involved in siderophore biosynthesis in tuberculosis [255]. A set of nucleoside bisubstrate analogs with known whole cell assay activity and bioactivity against siderophore biosynthesis in *Mtb* were used for pharmacophore and QSAR model development. *H*-bond donor, *H*-bond acceptor, and aromatic features were found to be critical for the inhibition of MbtA. The pharmacophore was also used to align molecules for the 3D-QSAR model, which exhibited suitable predictability and applicability with a Q^2 value of 0.71, RMSE of 0.65, and Pearson-R of 0.85 when assessed against a test set. The SAR studies additionally revealed the disadvantageous effects of bulky groups at the adenyl moiety *C*-6 position. Information taken from these models can be used for the rational design of new MbtA bisubstrate inhibitors as antitubercular agents [255].

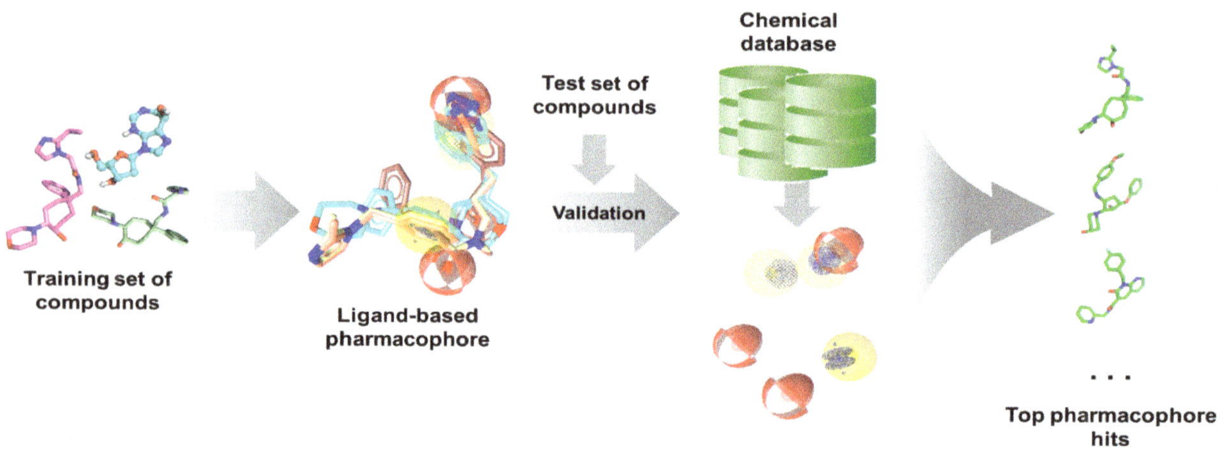

Figure 5. Typical ligand-based pharmacophore generation and screening workflow.

3.3.3. Density Functional Theory

Density functional theory (DFT) is quantum mechanical method established in the 1960s [256,257], which can be used in material science, computational chemistry, and computational physics to study the electronic properties of a many-particle (e.g., atom, molecule, condensed phase) system. DFT is based on two Hohenberg-Kohn (HK) theorems. First, the ground state properties of the many-particle system can be determined using only three spatially determined electron densities. Second, the HK theorem describes an energy functional, which can be minimized by the correct ground state electron density [258]. The use of DFT circumvents the computational expense of conventional methods like Hartree-Fock (HF) Theory since DFT relies on the premise that energies, intricate motions, and pair correlations can be derived directly from the electron probability density alone, instead of using wavefunctions. Theoretically, quantum mechanical wavefunctions consist of all the information required from a target system, and while the Schrödinger equation can be solved for a simple system, such as that of a hydrogen atom, it needs extensive computational efforts and it is impossible to solve this for a many-body system. In this case, DFT is used as an equivalent and efficient alternative to the Schrödinger equation [259], making DFT a popular tool in several computational fields [260].

In tuberculosis research, DFT has found uses in studies involving catalytic mechanisms [261,262], structure-activity relationship analysis [263], and inhibitor potency [264]. Chi and colleagues applied DFT to support their initial observations regarding a change in inhibitor binding mode in the MbtI enzyme after the addition of a substituted enolpyruvyl group to the parent compound structure previously designed from isochorismate [264]. X-ray crystal structures of MbtI complexed with its inhibitors depicted two different binding modes (Mode 1 and 2), suggesting binding site flexibility to accommodate ligand binding. The global minimum conformation of (*E*)-3-(1-carboxyprop-1-enyloxy)-2-hydroxybenzoic acid (AMT), *Z*-methyl-AMT, and *E*-methyl-AMT inhibitors in solution were calculated using Gaussian09 [265] with the B3LYP hybrid functional [266,267]. Global minimum conformation of free *Z*- and *E*-methyl-AMT were found to be similar to its bound conformation (Mode 2), indicating prearranged conformations to facilitate its binding to MbtI. Calculation of conformational entropy values for the three compounds revealed that *Z*-methyl-AMT is the least disordered, which may be due to the methyl conformational lock in its structure. Although a pure *Z*-isomer has not yet been obtained to experimentally differentiate it from the *E*-isomer, this finding rationalizes potent binding of methyl-AMT to MbtI and offers more information for the future design of novel and potent MbtI inhibitors [264].

Despite the success and popularity of DFT, it still has deficiencies due to approximations used in the development of functionals. Systems predominantly comprised of dispersion (van der Waals) forces, such as gaseous systems, or those wherein dispersion has a considerable contribution, such as biomolecular systems, are challenging to characterize using DFT [268]. However, several studies have already investigated the inclusion of van der Waals to improve this method [269–271]. Other major limitations of DFT application in computational chemistry include the characterization of charge transfer excitations, transition states, and global potential energy surfaces [272].

3.4. Integrated Tools

With the variety of available tools and structural data for drug discovery nowadays, it is more common to find studies that employ a combination of structure- and ligand-based approaches rather than exclusive application of each (Figure 2). Additionally, integration of these strategies often produces better results owing to more effective exploration of chemical and biological space. Moreover, the strengths of one method can overcome the limitations of the other, resulting in a highly complementary drug discovery process [171,238,273]. Integrated *in silico* workflows include sequential and parallel or data fusion methods [274–276], though hybrid methods have also already been developed [277,278]. Sequential methods involve the successive use of computational methods with the aim of increasing the selectivity of the VS workflow by continually reducing the number of potential hits before experimental evaluation [31]. However, it has been established that structure- and ligand-based methods have similar enrichment and frequently yield hits with different scaffolds [276], indicating that these methods are better applied in parallel rather than sequentially [279]. Parallel application, through simultaneous employment of various computational tools, often produce a more diverse hit profile [31,280]. Nonetheless, since results from these methods are often fused to produce a final ranking, a large number of virtual hits is obtained from this approach [31].

In silico methods have already been applied to tuberculosis studies in several different ways and combinations depending on the goal of the study implemented, such as for drug discovery [179,281], understanding protein structure and function [282,283], and others [284]. One example showing the integration of computational methods is a study implemented by Li et al. involving 3D-QSAR, binding pocket prediction, docking, and MD simulation studies for FtsZ, which is a validated *Mtb* target and plays a significant role in cell division [285]. Trisubstituted benzimidazoles were found to target this protein and used for 3D-QSAR CoMFA [248] analysis in order to elucidate important structural factors related to their inhibitory activities. Homology modeling using the SWISS-MODEL server [32] was required to obtain the GDP-bound structure of *Mtb* FtsZ using *S. aureus* FtsZ as template. Afterwards, binding site prediction using ProFunc [61] was performed to identify potential binding pockets (other than the GDP binding site) for the candidate compounds. Selected trisubstituted benzimidazole analogs were docked into the *Mtb* FtsZ model using AutoDock, after which the lowest binding energy docked complex was refined using MD simulation. Using the MD-refined *Mtb* FtsZ structure, all trisubstituted benzimidazoles were docked using Surflex-Dock [286]. In the lowest energy state of the compounds, the benzimidazole scaffold and cyclohexyl group were located in a highly hydrophobic pocket within FtsZ, while the carbamate groups were oriented towards the hydrophilic area. These interactions are posited to be crucial for ligand binding stabilization and inhibition of *Mtb* FtsZ. The results of this study display how the concerted application of different *in silico* methods can lead to better understanding of protein structure, ligand design, and inhibitory activities [285].

4. Edges and Pitfalls of *In Silico* Methods

There are roughly 2500 protein structures for tuberculosis in the PDB and perhaps thousands of ligand candidates published. All these pieces of information are available with a few keyboard strokes and a click of the mouse. Along with existing technologies, it is now possible to analyze TB enzymes and lead candidates at the atomic level in order to understand their function and how to regulate them. While computational methods have been widely used in drug discovery nowadays due to their successful applications [287–289], it is still important to remember that these tools are like any other experimental approaches—prone to limitations dependent on the system and other various parameters being studied [290–292].

VS has been known to successfully screen millions of compounds to identify potential inhibitors for a given target [287,289]. This lends efficiency to cost, time, and efforts used in drug discovery projects as only the most promising compounds are brought forward for more rigorous experimental testing and drug development. However, optimization and validation of these methods are far from perfect and are highly dependent on the protein system and compound classes used, leading to possible bias in the computational model. Thus, it is challenging to determine which method has the advantage over another; many benchmark studies have been published regarding this matter [293,294]. Other major limitations include difficulties in incorporating protein flexibility and solvent effects due to the computational burden attached to these factors [31]. Fortunately, available technologies seem to be catching up as enhance sampling methods, HPC, and MD platforms are now routinely applied in drug discovery projects and are known to calculate up to milliseconds of simulations for various protein targets [295–297]. In terms of ligand-based drug design, its main advantage is its simplicity and efficiency. Indeed, LBDD has a long history and numerous candidates have already been discovered even with the lack of protein structural information [298–300]. Nonetheless, several factors should be considered when applying ligand-based tools. Firstly, ligand alignments are based on the lowest conformation energy, which is often different from the bioactive conformation [244,245], as well as on the assumption that ligands bind in the same site and display the same conformation. Secondly, compounds should be evaluated by the same group (preferred) or tested using the same assay with the same parameters to be considered comparable [242]. Thirdly, the basic premise of 'similar structures display similar activities' are contradicted by the existence of activity cliffs [239–241], and so care should be taken when selecting potential candidates from a pool of virtual hits. Finally, it is also a challenge to incorporate the effects of solvation and protein flexibility due to the nature of the analysis.

As mentioned in the previous section, integration of several *in silico* methods have become common practice when designing and optimizing lead candidates to overcome the shortcomings of each individual tools. Despite requiring more computational resources, assimilation of computational methods result in better accuracy and enrichment of hits. In addition, the combination of a researcher's innate knowledge with the computational efficiency of these tools is perhaps the best integration of all, as a human's touch continues to be irreplaceable in the interpretation of all the data produced by *in silico* methods.

5. Conclusions and Future Perspectives

TB remains to be a relevant public health threat worldwide, necessitating accelerated discovery and design of novel antimycobacterial agents. Computer-aided drug design has become one of anchors of drug discovery research and continues to be a formidable tool in the hunt for promising drug leads, especially for tuberculosis. Continuous advancements in computing power and available software can enhance current computational tools and their application to different stages in the drug discovery pipeline. Nonetheless, these methods are not invincible as each tool have their own restrictions, and approximations are often used during the analysis. To overcome these, it is best to assimilate several *in silico* tools to complement the strength and limitations of each method used. The application of CADD in TB research has led to the identification of several antimycobacterial compounds that have already reached clinical evaluations, promoting its value in the drug discovery paradigm. Nonetheless, more work has to be done in order to expedite the discovery of anti-TB therapeutics.

Machine learning (ML) methods are making a comeback in drug discovery studies due to the upsurge in available data and enhanced computational powers. This has resulted in a wave drug discovery studies involving artificial intelligence (AI), wherein ML and deep learning (DL) techniques are applied to efficiently and 'intelligently' solve problems. This new shift in the drug discovery landscape is observed in personalized medicine and a number of relevant illnesses like cancer. While there are already several FDA-approved uses of AI in healthcare and diagnostics [301], it has yet to produce a successful drug candidate but it might not be far off. Currently, AI studies involving TB frequently covers diagnostics and treatment outcomes. This is perhaps one of the gaps that needs to be filled to be able to fast-track the discovery of novel and efficacious anti-TB drugs and finally alleviate the heavy burden of this infection around the globe.

Author Contributions: S.J.Y.M. and J.B.B. conceptualized and prepared the manuscript draft; J.B.B., V.G.O., and M.C.O.C. provided critical comments; all authors reviewed, edited, and approved the manuscript. All authors have read and agreed to the published version of the manuscript.

References

1. Pai, M.; Behr, M.A.; Dowdy, D.; Dheda, K.; Divangahi, M.; Boehme, C.C.; Ginsberg, A.; Swaminathan, S.; Spigelman, M.; Getahun, H.; et al. Tuberculosis. *Nat. Rev. Dis. Primers* **2016**, *2*, 16076. [CrossRef] [PubMed]
2. Havlir, D.V.; Getahun, H.; Sanne, I.; Nunn, P. Opportunities and challenges for HIV care in overlapping HIV and TB epidemics. *JAMA* **2008**, *300*, 423–430. [PubMed]

3. Leung, C.C.; Yew, W.W.; Chan, C.K.; Chang, K.C.; Law, W.S.; Lee, S.N.; Tai, L.B.; Leung, E.C.; Au, R.K.; Huang, S.S.; et al. Smoking adversely affects treatment response, outcome and relapse in tuberculosis. *Eur. Respir. J.* **2015**, *45*, 738–745. [CrossRef] [PubMed]
4. Imtiaz, S.; Shield, K.D.; Roerecke, M.; Samokhvalov, A.V.; Lonnroth, K.; Rehm, J. Alcohol consumption as a risk factor for tuberculosis: Meta-analyses and burden of disease. *Eur. Respir. J.* **2017**, *50*, 1700216. [CrossRef] [PubMed]
5. Restrepo, B.I. Diabetes and Tuberculosis. In *Understanding the Host Immune Response against Mycobacterium tuberculosis Infection*; Springer International Publishing: Cham, Switzerland, 2018; pp. 1–21.
6. Getahun, H.; Matteelli, A.; Chaisson, R.E.; Raviglione, M. Latent *Mycobacterium tuberculosis* infection. *N. Engl. J. Med.* **2015**, *372*, 2127–2135. [CrossRef]
7. Miller, L.G.; Asch, S.M.; Yu, E.I.; Knowles, L.; Gelberg, L.; Davidson, P. A population-based survey of tuberculosis symptoms: How atypical are atypical presentations? *Clin. Infect. Dis.* **2000**, *30*, 293–299. [CrossRef]
8. World Health Organization (WHO). *Global Tuberculosis Report 2019*; World Health Organization (WHO): Geneva, Switzerland, 2019.
9. World Health Organization (WHO). *Guidelines on the Management of Latent Tuberculosis Infection*; World Health Organization (WHO): Geneva, Switzerland, 2015.
10. World Health Organization (WHO). *Latent Tuberculosis infection: Updated and Consolidated Guidelines for Programmatic Management*; World Health Organization (WHO): Geneva, Switzerland, 2018.
11. Getahun, H.; Matteelli, A.; Abubakar, I.; Aziz, M.A.; Baddeley, A.; Barreira, D.; Den Boon, S.; Borroto Gutierrez, S.M.; Bruchfeld, J.; Burhan, E.; et al. Management of latent *Mycobacterium tuberculosis* infection: WHO guidelines for low tuberculosis burden countries. *Eur. Respir. J.* **2015**, *46*, 1563–1576. [CrossRef]
12. World Health Organization (WHO). *Treatment of Tuberculosis: Guidelines*; World Health Organization (WHO): Geneva, Switzerland, 2010.
13. Nahid, P.; Dorman, S.E.; Alipanah, N.; Barry, P.M.; Brozek, J.L.; Cattamanchi, A.; Chaisson, L.H.; Chaisson, R.E.; Daley, C.L.; Grzemska, M.; et al. Official American Thoracic Society/Centers for Disease Control and Prevention/Infectious Diseases Society of America Clinical Practice Guidelines: Treatment of Drug-Susceptible Tuberculosis. *Clin. Infect. Dis.* **2016**, *63*, e147–e195. [CrossRef]
14. Volmink, J.; Garner, P. Directly observed therapy for treating tuberculosis. *Cochrane Database Syst. Rev.* **2007**, CD003343. [CrossRef]
15. Horsburgh, C.R., Jr.; Barry, C.E., 3rd; Lange, C. Treatment of Tuberculosis. *N. Engl. J. Med.* **2015**, *373*, 2149–2160. [CrossRef]
16. Saukkonen, J.J.; Cohn, D.L.; Jasmer, R.M.; Schenker, S.; Jereb, J.A.; Nolan, C.M.; Peloquin, C.A.; Gordin, F.M.; Nunes, D.; Strader, D.B.; et al. An official ATS statement: Hepatotoxicity of antituberculosis therapy. *Am. J. Respir. Crit. Care Med.* **2006**, *174*, 935–952. [CrossRef]
17. Dheda, K.; Barry, C.E., 3rd; Maartens, G. Tuberculosis. *Lancet* **2016**, *387*, 1211–1226. [CrossRef]
18. Dheda, K.; Gumbo, T.; Gandhi, N.R.; Murray, M.; Theron, G.; Udwadia, Z.; Migliori, G.B.; Warren, R. Global control of tuberculosis: From extensively drug-resistant to untreatable tuberculosis. *Lancet. Respir. Med.* **2014**, *2*, 321–338. [CrossRef]
19. World Health Organization (WHO). *WHO Treatment Guidelines for Drug-Resistant Tuberculosis 2016 Update*; World Health Organization (WHO): Geneva, Switzerland, 2016.
20. Walker, J.; Tadena, N. J&J Tuberculosis Drug Gets Fast-Track Clearance. *Wall St. J.* **2013**. Available online: https://www.wsj.com/articles/SB10001424127887323320404578213421059138236 (accessed on 27 November 2019).
21. Mahajan, R. Bedaquiline: First FDA-approved tuberculosis drug in 40 years. *Int. J. Appl. Basic Med. Res.* **2013**, *3*, 1–2. [CrossRef]
22. European Medicines Agency (EMA). *Deltyba Delamanid Summary of the European Public Assessment Report (EPAR) for Deltyba*; EMA: Amsterdam, The Netherlands, 2014; pp. 1–3. Available online: https://www.ema.europa.eu/en/medicines/human/EPAR/deltyba (accessed on 15 November 2019).
23. Ryan, N.J.; Lo, J.H. Delamanid: First global approval. *Drugs* **2014**, *74*, 1041–1045. [CrossRef]
24. US FDA. *FDA Approves New Drug for Treatment-Resistant Forms of Tuberculosis That Affects the Lungs*; US FDA: Silver Spring, MD, USA, 2019.

25. Baptista, R.; Fazakerley, D.M.; Beckmann, M.; Baillie, L.; Mur, L.A.J. Untargeted metabolomics reveals a new mode of action of pretomanid (PA-824). *Sci. Rep.* **2018**, *8*, 5084. [CrossRef]
26. Thompson, A.M.; Bonnet, M.; Lee, H.H.; Franzblau, S.G.; Wan, B.; Wong, G.S.; Cooper, C.B.; Denny, W.A. Antitubercular Nitroimidazoles Revisited: Synthesis and Activity of the Authentic 3-Nitro Isomer of Pretomanid. *ACS Med. Chem. Lett.* **2017**, *8*, 1275–1280. [CrossRef]
27. Manjunatha, U.; Boshoff, H.I.; Barry, C.E. The mechanism of action of PA-824: Novel insights from transcriptional profiling. *Commun. Integr. Biol.* **2009**, *2*, 215–218. [CrossRef]
28. Reymond, J.-L.; van Deursen, R.; Blum, L.C.; Ruddigkeit, L. Chemical space as a source for new drugs. *MedChemComm* **2010**, *1*, 30–38. [CrossRef]
29. Berman, H.M.; Westbrook, J.; Feng, Z.; Gilliland, G.; Bhat, T.N.; Weissig, H.; Shindyalov, I.N.; Bourne, P.E. The Protein Data Bank. *Nucleic Acids Res.* **2000**, *28*, 235–242. [CrossRef]
30. Ekins, S.; Freundlich, J.S.; Choi, I.; Sarker, M.; Talcott, C. Computational databases, pathway and cheminformatics tools for tuberculosis drug discovery. *Trends Microbiol.* **2011**, *19*, 65–74. [CrossRef]
31. Macalino, S.J.; Gosu, V.; Hong, S.; Choi, S. Role of computer-aided drug design in modern drug discovery. *Arch. Pharm. Res.* **2015**, *38*, 1686–1701. [CrossRef]
32. Schwede, T.; Kopp, J.; Guex, N.; Peitsch, M.C. SWISS-MODEL: An automated protein homology-modeling server. *Nucleic Acids Res.* **2003**, *31*, 3381–3385. [CrossRef]
33. Webb, B.; Sali, A. Comparative Protein Structure Modeling Using MODELLER. *Curr. Protoc. Protein Sci.* **2016**, *86*, 1–37. [CrossRef]
34. Kim, D.E.; Chivian, D.; Baker, D. Protein structure prediction and analysis using the Robetta server. *Nucleic Acids Res.* **2004**, *32*, W526–W531. [CrossRef]
35. Schrödinger. Prime. Available online: https://www.schrodinger.com/prime (accessed on 26 October 2019).
36. Zheng, W.; Zhang, C.; Bell, E.W.; Zhang, Y. I-TASSER gateway: A protein structure and function prediction server powered by XSEDE. *Future Gener. Comput. Syst.* **2019**, *99*, 73–85. [CrossRef]
37. Zhang, Y. I-TASSER server for protein 3D structure prediction. *BMC Bioinf.* **2008**, *9*, 40. [CrossRef]
38. Yang, J.; Zhang, Y. I-TASSER server: New development for protein structure and function predictions. *Nucleic Acids Res.* **2015**, *43*, W174–W181. [CrossRef]
39. Yang, J.; Yan, R.; Roy, A.; Xu, D.; Poisson, J.; Zhang, Y. The I-TASSER Suite: Protein structure and function prediction. *Nat. Methods* **2015**, *12*, 7–8. [CrossRef]
40. Roy, A.; Kucukural, A.; Zhang, Y. I-TASSER: A unified platform for automated protein structure and function prediction. *Nat. Protoc.* **2010**, *5*, 725–738. [CrossRef] [PubMed]
41. Zhang, Y. I-TASSER: Fully automated protein structure prediction in CASP8. *Proteins* **2009**, *77*, 100–113. [CrossRef] [PubMed]
42. Zimmermann, L.; Stephens, A.; Nam, S.Z.; Rau, D.; Kubler, J.; Lozajic, M.; Gabler, F.; Soding, J.; Lupas, A.N.; Alva, V. A Completely Reimplemented MPI Bioinformatics Toolkit with a New HHpred Server at its Core. *J. Mol. Biol.* **2018**, *430*, 2237–2243. [CrossRef] [PubMed]
43. Hildebrand, A.; Remmert, M.; Biegert, A.; Soding, J. Fast and accurate automatic structure prediction with HHpred. *Proteins* **2009**, *77*, 128–132. [CrossRef] [PubMed]
44. Soding, J.; Biegert, A.; Lupas, A.N. The HHpred interactive server for protein homology detection and structure prediction. *Nucleic Acids Res.* **2005**, *33*, W244–W248. [CrossRef] [PubMed]
45. Laskowski, R.A.; MacArthur, M.W.; Moss, D.S.; Thornton, J.M. PROCHECK: A program to check the stereochemical quality of protein structures. *J. Appl. Cryst.* **1993**, *26*, 283–291. [CrossRef]
46. Wiederstein, M.; Sippl, M.J. ProSA-web: Interactive web service for the recognition of errors in three-dimensional structures of proteins. *Nucleic Acids Res.* **2007**, *35*, W407–W410. [CrossRef]
47. Eisenberg, D.; Luthy, R.; Bowie, J.U. VERIFY3D: Assessment of protein models with three-dimensional profiles. *Methods Enzymol.* **1997**, *277*, 396–404.
48. Colovos, C.; Yeates, T.O. Verification of protein structures: Patterns of nonbonded atomic interactions. *Protein Sci.* **1993**, *2*, 1511–1519. [CrossRef]
49. Hussein, H.A.; Borrel, A.; Geneix, C.; Petitjean, M.; Regad, L.; Camproux, A.C. PockDrug-Server: A new web server for predicting pocket druggability on holo and apo proteins. *Nucleic Acids Res.* **2015**, *43*, W436–W442. [CrossRef]
50. Volkamer, A.; Kuhn, D.; Rippmann, F.; Rarey, M. DoGSiteScorer: A web server for automatic binding site prediction, analysis and druggability assessment. *Bioinformatics* **2012**, *28*, 2074–2075. [CrossRef] [PubMed]

51. Schmidtke, P.; Le Guilloux, V.; Maupetit, J.; Tuffery, P. fpocket: Online tools for protein ensemble pocket detection and tracking. *Nucleic Acids Res.* **2010**, *38*, W582–W589. [CrossRef] [PubMed]
52. Le Guilloux, V.; Schmidtke, P.; Tuffery, P. Fpocket: An open source platform for ligand pocket detection. *BMC Bioinf.* **2009**, *10*, 168. [CrossRef] [PubMed]
53. Tian, W.; Chen, C.; Lei, X.; Zhao, J.; Liang, J. CASTp 3.0: Computed atlas of surface topography of proteins. *Nucleic Acids Res.* **2018**, *46*, W363–W367. [CrossRef] [PubMed]
54. Binkowski, T.A.; Naghibzadeh, S.; Liang, J. CASTp: Computed Atlas of Surface Topography of proteins. *Nucleic Acids Res.* **2003**, *31*, 3352–3355. [CrossRef]
55. Dundas, J.; Ouyang, Z.; Tseng, J.; Binkowski, A.; Turpaz, Y.; Liang, J. CASTp: Computed atlas of surface topography of proteins with structural and topographical mapping of functionally annotated residues. *Nucleic Acids Res.* **2006**, *34*, W116–W118. [CrossRef]
56. Koes, D.R.; Camacho, C.J. PocketQuery: Protein-protein interaction inhibitor starting points from protein-protein interaction structure. *Nucleic Acids Res.* **2012**, *40*, W387–W392. [CrossRef]
57. Brady, G.P., Jr.; Stouten, P.F. Fast prediction and visualization of protein binding pockets with PASS. *J. Comput. Aided Mol. Des.* **2000**, *14*, 383–401. [CrossRef]
58. Halgren, T.A. Identifying and characterizing binding sites and assessing druggability. *J. Chem. Inf. Model.* **2009**, *49*, 377–389. [CrossRef]
59. Capra, J.A.; Laskowski, R.A.; Thornton, J.M.; Singh, M.; Funkhouser, T.A. Predicting protein ligand binding sites by combining evolutionary sequence conservation and 3D structure. *PLoS Comput. Biol.* **2009**, *5*, e1000585. [CrossRef]
60. Jendele, L.; Krivak, R.; Skoda, P.; Novotny, M.; Hoksza, D. PrankWeb: A web server for ligand binding site prediction and visualization. *Nucleic Acids Res.* **2019**, *47*, W345–W349. [CrossRef] [PubMed]
61. Laskowski, R.A.; Watson, J.D.; Thornton, J.M. ProFunc: A server for predicting protein function from 3D structure. *Nucleic Acids Res.* **2005**, *33*, W89–W93. [CrossRef]
62. Morris, G.M.; Huey, R.; Lindstrom, W.; Sanner, M.F.; Belew, R.K.; Goodsell, D.S.; Olson, A.J. AutoDock4 and AutoDockTools4: Automated docking with selective receptor flexibility. *J. Comput. Chem.* **2009**, *30*, 2785–2791. [CrossRef] [PubMed]
63. Trott, O.; Olson, A.J. AutoDock Vina: Improving the speed and accuracy of docking with a new scoring function, efficient optimization, and multithreading. *J. Comput. Chem.* **2010**, *31*, 455–461. [CrossRef] [PubMed]
64. Allen, W.J.; Balius, T.E.; Mukherjee, S.; Brozell, S.R.; Moustakas, D.T.; Lang, P.T.; Case, D.A.; Kuntz, I.D.; Rizzo, R.C. DOCK 6: Impact of new features and current docking performance. *J. Comput. Chem.* **2015**, *36*, 1132–1156. [CrossRef]
65. Verdonk, M.L.; Cole, J.C.; Hartshorn, M.J.; Murray, C.W.; Taylor, R.D. Improved protein–ligand docking using GOLD. *Proteins* **2003**, *52*, 609–623. [CrossRef]
66. Schrödinger. Glide. Available online: https://www.schrodinger.com/glide (accessed on 26 October 2019).
67. Schrödinger. Induced Fit. Available online: https://www.schrodinger.com/induced-fit (accessed on 26 October 2019).
68. Rarey, M.; Kramer, B.; Lengauer, T.; Klebe, G. A fast flexible docking method using an incremental construction algorithm. *J. Mol. Biol.* **1996**, *261*, 470–489. [CrossRef]
69. Davis, I.W.; Baker, D. RosettaLigand docking with full ligand and receptor flexibility. *J. Mol. Biol.* **2009**, *385*, 381–392. [CrossRef]
70. Wu, G.; Robertson, D.H.; Brooks, C.L., 3rd; Vieth, M. Detailed analysis of grid-based molecular docking: A case study of CDOCKER-A CHARMm-based MD docking algorithm. *J. Comput. Chem.* **2003**, *24*, 1549–1562. [CrossRef]
71. Bitencourt-Ferreira, G.; de Azevedo, W.F., Jr. Docking with SwissDock. *Methods Mol. Biol.* **2019**, *2053*, 189–202.
72. Grosdidier, A.; Zoete, V.; Michielin, O. SwissDock, a protein-small molecule docking web service based on EADock DSS. *Nucleic Acids Res.* **2011**, *39*, W270–W277. [CrossRef] [PubMed]
73. Koes, D.R.; Camacho, C.J. Pharmer: Efficient and exact pharmacophore search. *J. Chem. Inf. Model.* **2011**, *51*, 1307–1314. [CrossRef] [PubMed]
74. Dassault Systèmes BIOVIA. *Catalyst*. Available online: https://www.3dsbiovia.com/products/collaborative-science/biovia-discovery-studio/pharmacophore-and-ligand-based-design.html (accessed on 26 October 2019).

75. Schneidman-Duhovny, D.; Dror, O.; Inbar, Y.; Nussinov, R.; Wolfson, H.J. PharmaGist: A webserver for ligand-based pharmacophore detection. *Nucleic Acids Res.* **2008**, *36*, W223–W228. [CrossRef] [PubMed]
76. Inte:Ligand. LigandScout. Available online: http://www.inteligand.com/ligandscout/ (accessed on 26 October 2019).
77. Zoete, V.; Daina, A.; Bovigny, C.; Michielin, O. SwissSimilarity: A Web Tool for Low to Ultra High Throughput Ligand-Based Virtual Screening. *J. Chem. Inf. Model.* **2016**, *56*, 1399–1404. [CrossRef]
78. Douguet, D. e-LEA3D: A computational-aided drug design web server. *Nucleic Acids Res.* **2010**, *38*, W615–W621. [CrossRef]
79. Dallakyan, S.; Olson, A.J. Small-molecule library screening by docking with PyRx. *Methods Mol. Biol.* **2015**, *1263*, 243–250.
80. Schrödinger. PHASE. Available online: https://www.schrodinger.com/phase (accessed on 26 October 2019).
81. Case, D.A.; Cheatham, T.E., 3rd; Darden, T.; Gohlke, H.; Luo, R.; Merz, K.M., Jr.; Onufriev, A.; Simmerling, C.; Wang, B.; Woods, R.J. The Amber biomolecular simulation programs. *J. Comput. Chem.* **2005**, *26*, 1668–1688. [CrossRef]
82. Salomon-Ferrer, R.; Case, D.A.; Walker, R.C. An overview of the Amber biomolecular simulation package. *Wiley Interdiscip. Rev. Comput. Mol. Sci.* **2013**, *3*, 198–210. [CrossRef]
83. Brooks, B.R.; Brooks, C.L., 3rd; Mackerell, A.D., Jr.; Nilsson, L.; Petrella, R.J.; Roux, B.; Won, Y.; Archontis, G.; Bartels, C.; Boresch, S.; et al. CHARMM: The biomolecular simulation program. *J. Comput. Chem.* **2009**, *30*, 1545–1614. [CrossRef]
84. Miller, B.T.; Singh, R.P.; Klauda, J.B.; Hodoscek, M.; Brooks, B.R.; Woodcock, H.L., 3rd. CHARMMing: A new, flexible web portal for CHARMM. *J. Chem. Inf. Model.* **2008**, *48*, 1920–1929. [CrossRef]
85. Van Der Spoel, D.; Lindahl, E.; Hess, B.; Groenhof, G.; Mark, A.E.; Berendsen, H.J. GROMACS: Fast, flexible, and free. *J. Comput. Chem.* **2005**, *26*, 1701–1718. [CrossRef] [PubMed]
86. Abraham, M.J.; Murtola, T.; Schulz, R.; Páll, S.; Smith, J.C.; Hess, B.; Lindahl, E. GROMACS: High performance molecular simulations through multi-level parallelism from laptops to supercomputers. *SoftwareX* **2015**, *1–2*, 19–25. [CrossRef]
87. Phillips, J.C.; Braun, R.; Wang, W.; Gumbart, J.; Tajkhorshid, E.; Villa, E.; Chipot, C.; Skeel, R.D.; Kale, L.; Schulten, K. Scalable molecular dynamics with NAMD. *J. Comput. Chem.* **2005**, *26*, 1781–1802. [CrossRef] [PubMed]
88. Schrödinger. Desmond. Available online: https://www.schrodinger.com/desmond (accessed on 26 October 2019).
89. Zoete, V.; Cuendet, M.A.; Grosdidier, A.; Michielin, O. SwissParam: A fast force field generation tool for small organic molecules. *J. Comput. Chem.* **2011**, *32*, 2359–2368. [CrossRef] [PubMed]
90. Jo, S.; Kim, T.; Iyer, V.G.; Im, W. CHARMM-GUI: A web-based graphical user interface for CHARMM. *J. Comput. Chem.* **2008**, *29*, 1859–1865. [CrossRef] [PubMed]
91. Vanommeslaeghe, K.; Hatcher, E.; Acharya, C.; Kundu, S.; Zhong, S.; Shim, J.; Darian, E.; Guvench, O.; Lopes, P.; Vorobyov, I.; et al. CHARMM general force field: A force field for drug-like molecules compatible with the CHARMM all-atom additive biological force fields. *J. Comput. Chem.* **2010**, *31*, 671–690. [CrossRef] [PubMed]
92. Vanommeslaeghe, K.; MacKerell, A.D., Jr. Automation of the CHARMM General Force Field (CGenFF) I: Bond perception and atom typing. *J. Chem. Inf. Model.* **2012**, *52*, 3144–3154. [CrossRef] [PubMed]
93. Vanommeslaeghe, K.; Raman, E.P.; MacKerell, A.D., Jr. Automation of the CHARMM General Force Field (CGenFF) II: Assignment of bonded parameters and partial atomic charges. *J. Chem. Inf. Model.* **2012**, *52*, 3155–3168. [CrossRef]
94. Humphrey, W.; Dalke, A.; Schulten, K. VMD: Visual molecular dynamics. *J. Mol. Graph.* **1996**, *14*, 27–38. [CrossRef]
95. Helguera, A.M.; Combes, R.D.; Gonzalez, M.P.; Cordeiro, M.N. Applications of 2D descriptors in drug design: A DRAGON tale. *Curr. Top. Med. Chem.* **2008**, *8*, 1628–1655. [CrossRef]
96. Tetko, I.V.; Gasteiger, J.; Todeschini, R.; Mauri, A.; Livingstone, D.; Ertl, P.; Palyulin, V.A.; Radchenko, E.V.; Zefirov, N.S.; Makarenko, A.S.; et al. Virtual computational chemistry laboratory—Design and description. *J. Comput. Aided Mol. Des.* **2005**, *19*, 453–463. [CrossRef] [PubMed]
97. Schrödinger. Canvas. Available online: https://www.schrodinger.com/canvas (accessed on 26 October 2019).
98. Landrum, G. RDKit: Open-Source Cheminformatics. Available online: http://www.rdkit.org (accessed on 26 October 2019).

99. Masand, V.H.; Rastija, V. PyDescriptor: A new PyMOL plugin for calculating thousands of easily understandable molecular descriptors. *Chemom. Intell. Lab. Syst.* **2017**, *169*, 12–18. [CrossRef]
100. Moriwaki, H.; Tian, Y.S.; Kawashita, N.; Takagi, T. Mordred: A molecular descriptor calculator. *J. Cheminform.* **2018**, *10*, 4. [CrossRef] [PubMed]
101. Tosco, P.; Balle, T. Open3DQSAR: A new open-source software aimed at high-throughput chemometric analysis of molecular interaction fields. *J. Mol. Model.* **2011**, *17*, 201–208. [CrossRef]
102. Dong, J.; Yao, Z.J.; Zhu, M.F.; Wang, N.N.; Lu, B.; Chen, A.F.; Lu, A.P.; Miao, H.; Zeng, W.B.; Cao, D.S. ChemSAR: An online pipelining platform for molecular SAR modeling. *J. Cheminform.* **2017**, *9*, 27. [CrossRef]
103. BioSolveIT. SeeSAR version 9.2. Available online: https://www.biosolveit.de/SeeSAR/ (accessed on 26 October 2019).
104. Schrödinger. QikProp. Available online: https://www.schrodinger.com/qikprop (accessed on 26 October 2019).
105. SimulationsPlus. ADMET Predictor. Available online: https://www.simulations-plus.com/software/admetpredictor/ (accessed on 26 October 2019).
106. ACD/Labs. Percepta Platform. Available online: https://www.acdlabs.com/products/percepta/ (accessed on 26 October 2019).
107. Miteva, M.A.; Violas, S.; Montes, M.; Gomez, D.; Tuffery, P.; Villoutreix, B.O. FAF-Drugs: Free ADME/tox filtering of compound collections. *Nucleic Acids Res.* **2006**, *34*, W738–W744. [CrossRef]
108. Rasolohery, I.; Moroy, G.; Guyon, F. PatchSearch: A Fast Computational Method for Off-Target Detection. *J. Chem. Inf. Model.* **2017**, *57*, 769–777. [CrossRef]
109. Dassault Systèmes BIOVIA. DS TOPKAT. Available online: https://www.3dsbiovia.com/products/collaborative-science/biovia-discovery-studio/qsar-admet-and-predictive-toxicology.html (accessed on 26 October 2019).
110. Dassault Systèmes BIOVIA. DS ADMET. Available online: https://www.3dsbiovia.com/products/collaborative-science/biovia-pipeline-pilot/component-collections/adme-tox.html (accessed on 26 October 2019).
111. Poroikov, V.; Filimonov, D.; Lagunin, A.; Gloriozova, T.; Zakharov, A. PASS: Identification of probable targets and mechanisms of toxicity. *SAR QSAR Environ. Res.* **2007**, *18*, 101–110. [CrossRef]
112. Daina, A.; Michielin, O.; Zoete, V. SwissADME: A free web tool to evaluate pharmacokinetics, drug-likeness and medicinal chemistry friendliness of small molecules. *Sci. Rep.* **2017**, *7*, 42717. [CrossRef]
113. Cruciani, G.; Carosati, E.; De Boeck, B.; Ethirajulu, K.; Mackie, C.; Howe, T.; Vianello, R. MetaSite: Understanding metabolism in human cytochromes from the perspective of the chemist. *J. Med. Chem.* **2005**, *48*, 6970–6979. [CrossRef]
114. Tcheremenskaia, O.; Benigni, R.; Nikolova, I.; Jeliazkova, N.; Escher, S.E.; Batke, M.; Baier, T.; Poroikov, V.; Lagunin, A.; Rautenberg, M.; et al. OpenTox predictive toxicology framework: Toxicological ontology and semantic media wiki-based OpenToxipedia. *J. Biomed. Semant.* **2012**, *3*, S7. [CrossRef] [PubMed]
115. Smiesko, M.; Vedani, A. VirtualToxLab: Exploring the Toxic Potential of Rejuvenating Substances Found in Traditional Medicines. *Methods Mol. Biol.* **2016**, *1425*, 121–137.
116. Vedani, A.; Dobler, M.; Smiesko, M. VirtualToxLab—A platform for estimating the toxic potential of drugs, chemicals and natural products. *Toxicol. Appl. Pharmacol.* **2012**, *261*, 142–153. [CrossRef] [PubMed]
117. Vedani, A.; Smiesko, M.; Spreafico, M.; Peristera, O.; Dobler, M. VirtualToxLab—In silico prediction of the toxic (endocrine-disrupting) potential of drugs, chemicals and natural products. Two years and 2000 compounds of experience: A progress report. *ALTEX* **2009**, *26*, 167–176. [CrossRef] [PubMed]
118. Vedani, A.; Dobler, M.; Spreafico, M.; Peristera, O.; Smiesko, M. VirtualToxLab—In silico prediction of the toxic potential of drugs and environmental chemicals: Evaluation status and internet access protocol. *ALTEX* **2007**, *24*, 153–161. [CrossRef]
119. Cheng, F.; Li, W.; Zhou, Y.; Shen, J.; Wu, Z.; Liu, G.; Lee, P.W.; Tang, Y. Correction to "admetSAR: A Comprehensive Source and Free Tool for Assessment of Chemical ADMET Properties". *J. Chem. Inf. Model.* **2019**. [CrossRef]
120. Yang, H.; Lou, C.; Sun, L.; Li, J.; Cai, Y.; Wang, Z.; Li, W.; Liu, G.; Tang, Y. admetSAR 2.0: Web-service for prediction and optimization of chemical ADMET properties. *Bioinformatics* **2019**, *35*, 1067–1069. [CrossRef]
121. Cheng, F.; Li, W.; Zhou, Y.; Shen, J.; Wu, Z.; Liu, G.; Lee, P.W.; Tang, Y. admetSAR: A comprehensive source and free tool for assessment of chemical ADMET properties. *J. Chem. Inf. Model.* **2012**, *52*, 3099–3105. [CrossRef]

122. Rudik, A.; Bezhentsev, V.; Dmitriev, A.; Lagunin, A.; Filimonov, D.; Poroikov, V. Metatox-Web application for generation of metabolic pathways and toxicity estimation. *J. Bioinform. Comput. Biol.* **2019**, *17*, 1940001. [CrossRef] [PubMed]
123. Rudik, A.V.; Bezhentsev, V.M.; Dmitriev, A.V.; Druzhilovskiy, D.S.; Lagunin, A.A.; Filimonov, D.A.; Poroikov, V.V. MetaTox: Web Application for Predicting Structure and Toxicity of Xenobiotics' Metabolites. *J. Chem. Inf. Model.* **2017**, *57*, 638–642. [CrossRef]
124. Cole, S.T.; Brosch, R.; Parkhill, J.; Garnier, T.; Churcher, C.; Harris, D.; Gordon, S.V.; Eiglmeier, K.; Gas, S.; Barry, C.E., 3rd; et al. Deciphering the biology of *Mycobacterium tuberculosis* from the complete genome sequence. *Nature* **1998**, *393*, 537–544. [CrossRef] [PubMed]
125. Rosenkrands, I.; King, A.; Weldingh, K.; Moniatte, M.; Moertz, E.; Andersen, P. Towards the proteome of *Mycobacterium tuberculosis*. *Electrophoresis* **2000**, *21*, 3740–3756. [CrossRef]
126. Jungblut, P.R.; Schaible, U.E.; Mollenkopf, H.J.; Zimny-Arndt, U.; Raupach, B.; Mattow, J.; Halada, P.; Lamer, S.; Hagens, K.; Kaufmann, S.H. Comparative proteome analysis of *Mycobacterium tuberculosis* and Mycobacterium bovis BCG strains: Towards functional genomics of microbial pathogens. *Mol. Microbiol.* **1999**, *33*, 1103–1117. [CrossRef] [PubMed]
127. Kruh, N.A.; Troudt, J.; Izzo, A.; Prenni, J.; Dobos, K.M. Portrait of a pathogen: The *Mycobacterium tuberculosis* proteome in vivo. *PLoS ONE* **2010**, *5*, e13938. [CrossRef]
128. Keren, I.; Minami, S.; Rubin, E.; Lewis, K. Characterization and transcriptome analysis of *Mycobacterium tuberculosis* persisters. *MBio* **2011**, *2*, e00100–e00111. [CrossRef]
129. Rachman, H.; Strong, M.; Ulrichs, T.; Grode, L.; Schuchhardt, J.; Mollenkopf, H.; Kosmiadi, G.A.; Eisenberg, D.; Kaufmann, S.H. Unique transcriptome signature of *Mycobacterium tuberculosis* in pulmonary tuberculosis. *Infect. Immun.* **2006**, *74*, 1233–1242. [CrossRef]
130. Xu, D. Protein databases on the internet. *Curr. Protoc. Protein Sci.* **2012**. [CrossRef]
131. Kim, S.; Thiessen, P.A.; Bolton, E.E.; Chen, J.; Fu, G.; Gindulyte, A.; Han, L.; He, J.; He, S.; Shoemaker, B.A.; et al. PubChem Substance and Compound databases. *Nucleic Acids Res.* **2016**, *44*, D1202–D1213. [CrossRef]
132. Williams, A.J. Public chemical compound databases. *Curr. Opin. Drug Discov. Dev.* **2008**, *11*, 393–404.
133. UniProt, C. Ongoing and future developments at the Universal Protein Resource. *Nucleic Acids Res.* **2011**, *39*, D214–D219.
134. Reddy, T.B.; Riley, R.; Wymore, F.; Montgomery, P.; DeCaprio, D.; Engels, R.; Gellesch, M.; Hubble, J.; Jen, D.; Jin, H.; et al. TB database: An integrated platform for tuberculosis research. *Nucleic Acids Res.* **2009**, *37*, D499–D508. [CrossRef] [PubMed]
135. Galagan, J.E.; Sisk, P.; Stolte, C.; Weiner, B.; Koehrsen, M.; Wymore, F.; Reddy, T.B.; Zucker, J.D.; Engels, R.; Gellesch, M.; et al. TB database 2010: Overview and update. *Tuberculosis* **2010**, *90*, 225–235. [CrossRef] [PubMed]
136. Kapopoulou, A.; Lew, J.M.; Cole, S.T. The MycoBrowser portal: A comprehensive and manually annotated resource for mycobacterial genomes. *Tuberculosis* **2011**, *91*, 8–13. [CrossRef]
137. Rosenthal, A.; Gabrielian, A.; Engle, E.; Hurt, D.E.; Alexandru, S.; Crudu, V.; Sergueev, E.; Kirichenko, V.; Lapitskii, V.; Snezhko, E.; et al. The TB Portals: An Open-Access, Web-Based Platform for Global Drug-Resistant-Tuberculosis Data Sharing and Analysis. *J. Clin. Microbiol.* **2017**, *55*, 3267–3282. [CrossRef] [PubMed]
138. Laskowski, R.A.; Jablonska, J.; Pravda, L.; Varekova, R.S.; Thornton, J.M. PDBsum: Structural summaries of PDB entries. *Protein Sci.* **2018**, *27*, 129–134. [CrossRef] [PubMed]
139. Liu, R.; Li, X.; Lam, K.S. Combinatorial chemistry in drug discovery. *Curr. Opin. Chem. Biol.* **2017**, *38*, 117–126. [CrossRef]
140. Ruddigkeit, L.; van Deursen, R.; Blum, L.C.; Reymond, J.L. Enumeration of 166 billion organic small molecules in the chemical universe database GDB-17. *J. Chem. Inf. Model.* **2012**, *52*, 2864–2875. [CrossRef]
141. Shivanyuk, A.; Ryabukhin, S.; Bogolyubsky, A.V.; Mykytenko, D.M.; Chuprina, A.; Heilman, W.; Kostyuk, A.N.; Tolmachev, A. Enamine real database: Making chemical diversity real. *Chem. Today* **2007**, *25*, 58–59.
142. Williams, A.J. ChemSpider: Integrating Structure-Based Resources Distributed across the Internet. In *Enhancing Learning with Online Resources, Social Networking, and Digital Libraries*; American Chemical Society: Washington, DC, USA, 2010; Volume 1060, pp. 23–39.

143. Sterling, T.; Irwin, J.J. ZINC 15—Ligand Discovery for Everyone. *J. Chem. Inf. Model.* **2015**, *55*, 2324–2337. [CrossRef]
144. Gaulton, A.; Hersey, A.; Nowotka, M.; Bento, A.P.; Chambers, J.; Mendez, D.; Mutowo, P.; Atkinson, F.; Bellis, L.J.; Cibrian-Uhalte, E.; et al. The ChEMBL database in 2017. *Nucleic Acids Res.* **2017**, *45*, D945–D954. [CrossRef]
145. Voigt, J.H.; Bienfait, B.; Wang, S.; Nicklaus, M.C. Comparison of the NCI open database with seven large chemical structural databases. *J. Chem. Inf. Comput Sci.* **2001**, *41*, 702–712. [CrossRef]
146. Pierleoni, A.; Martelli, P.L.; Fariselli, P.; Casadio, R. eSLDB: Eukaryotic subcellular localization database. *Nucleic Acids Res.* **2007**, *35*, D208–D212. [CrossRef]
147. Sprenger, J.; Lynn Fink, J.; Karunaratne, S.; Hanson, K.; Hamilton, N.A.; Teasdale, R.D. LOCATE: A mammalian protein subcellular localization database. *Nucleic Acids Res.* **2008**, *36*, D230–D233. [CrossRef]
148. Peabody, M.A.; Laird, M.R.; Vlasschaert, C.; Lo, R.; Brinkman, F.S. PSORTdb: Expanding the bacteria and archaea protein subcellular localization database to better reflect diversity in cell envelope structures. *Nucleic Acids Res.* **2016**, *44*, D663–D668. [CrossRef]
149. Hendlich, M.; Bergner, A.; Gunther, J.; Klebe, G. Relibase: Design and development of a database for comprehensive analysis of protein-ligand interactions. *J. Mol. Biol.* **2003**, *326*, 607–620. [CrossRef]
150. Chen, X.; Lin, Y.; Liu, M.; Gilson, M.K. The Binding Database: Data management and interface design. *Bioinformatics* **2002**, *18*, 130–139. [CrossRef]
151. Liu, T.; Lin, Y.; Wen, X.; Jorissen, R.N.; Gilson, M.K. BindingDB: A web-accessible database of experimentally determined protein-ligand binding affinities. *Nucleic Acids Res.* **2007**, *35*, D198–D201. [CrossRef]
152. Salwinski, L.; Miller, C.S.; Smith, A.J.; Pettit, F.K.; Bowie, J.U.; Eisenberg, D. The Database of Interacting Proteins: 2004 update. *Nucleic Acids Res.* **2004**, *32*, D449–D451. [CrossRef]
153. Oughtred, R.; Stark, C.; Breitkreutz, B.J.; Rust, J.; Boucher, L.; Chang, C.; Kolas, N.; O'Donnell, L.; Leung, G.; McAdam, R.; et al. The BioGRID interaction database: 2019 update. *Nucleic Acids Res.* **2019**, *47*, D529–D541. [CrossRef]
154. Jensen, L.J.; Kuhn, M.; Stark, M.; Chaffron, S.; Creevey, C.; Muller, J.; Doerks, T.; Julien, P.; Roth, A.; Simonovic, M.; et al. STRING 8—A global view on proteins and their functional interactions in 630 organisms. *Nucleic Acids Res.* **2009**, *37*, D412–D416. [CrossRef]
155. Franca, T.C. Homology modeling: An important tool for the drug discovery. *J. Biomol. Struct. Dyn.* **2015**, *33*, 1780–1793. [CrossRef]
156. McGinnis, S.; Madden, T.L. BLAST: At the core of a powerful and diverse set of sequence analysis tools. *Nucleic Acids Res.* **2004**, *32*, W20–W25. [CrossRef]
157. Ye, J.; McGinnis, S.; Madden, T.L. BLAST: Improvements for better sequence analysis. *Nucleic Acids Res.* **2006**, *34*, W6–W9. [CrossRef]
158. Madden, T. The BLAST Sequence Analysis Tool. In *The NCBI Handbook [Internet]*, 2nd ed.; National Center for Biotechnology Information (US): Bethesda, MD, USA, 2013.
159. Papadopoulos, J.S.; Agarwala, R. COBALT: Constraint-based alignment tool for multiple protein sequences. *Bioinformatics* **2007**, *23*, 1073–1079. [CrossRef]
160. Sievers, F.; Higgins, D.G. Clustal Omega, Accurate Alignment of Very Large Numbers of Sequences. In *Multiple Sequence Alignment Methods*; Russell, D.J., Ed.; Humana Press: Totowa, NJ, USA, 2014; pp. 105–116.
161. Lassmann, T.; Sonnhammer, E.L. Kalign—An accurate and fast multiple sequence alignment algorithm. *BMC Bioinf.* **2005**, *6*, 298. [CrossRef]
162. Schmidtke, P.; Barril, X. Understanding and predicting druggability. A high-throughput method for detection of drug binding sites. *J. Med. Chem.* **2010**, *53*, 5858–5867. [CrossRef]
163. Kalyaanamoorthy, S.; Chen, Y.P. Structure-based drug design to augment hit discovery. *Drug Discov. Today* **2011**, *16*, 831–839. [CrossRef]
164. Hetenyi, C.; van der Spoel, D. Blind docking of drug-sized compounds to proteins with up to a thousand residues. *FEBS Lett.* **2006**, *580*, 1447–1450. [CrossRef]
165. Shi, Y.; Colombo, C.; Kuttiyatveetil, J.R.; Zalatar, N.; van Straaten, K.E.; Mohan, S.; Sanders, D.A.; Pinto, B.M. A Second, Druggable Binding Site in UDP-Galactopyranose Mutase from *Mycobacterium tuberculosis*? *Chembiochem* **2016**, *17*, 2264–2273. [CrossRef]
166. Stahura, F.L.; Bajorath, J. Virtual screening methods that complement HTS. *Comb. Chem. High Throughput Screen.* **2004**, *7*, 259–269. [CrossRef]

167. Steindl, T.M.; Schuster, D.; Wolber, G.; Laggner, C.; Langer, T. High-throughput structure-based pharmacophore modelling as a basis for successful parallel virtual screening. *J. Comput. Aided Mol. Des.* **2006**, *20*, 703–715. [CrossRef]
168. Halperin, I.; Ma, B.; Wolfson, H.; Nussinov, R. Principles of docking: An overview of search algorithms and a guide to scoring functions. *Proteins* **2002**, *47*, 409–443. [CrossRef] [PubMed]
169. Leach, A.R.; Gillet, V.J.; Lewis, R.A.; Taylor, R. Three-dimensional pharmacophore methods in drug discovery. *J. Med. Chem.* **2010**, *53*, 539–558. [CrossRef] [PubMed]
170. Wermuth, C.G.; Ganellin, C.R.; Lindberg, P.; Mitscher, L.A. Glossary of terms used in medicinal chemistry (IUPAC Recommendations 1998). *Pure Appl. Chem.* **1998**, *70*, 1129. [CrossRef]
171. Hein, M.; Zilian, D.; Sotriffer, C.A. Docking compared to 3D-pharmacophores: The scoring function challenge. *Drug Discov. Today Technol.* **2010**, *7*, e229–e236. [CrossRef]
172. Hessler, G.; Baringhaus, K. The scaffold hopping potential of pharmacophores. *Drug Discov. Today Technol.* **2010**, *7*, e263–e269. [CrossRef]
173. Pagadala, N.S.; Syed, K.; Tuszynski, J. Software for molecular docking: A review. *Biophys. Rev.* **2017**, *9*, 91–102. [CrossRef]
174. Cross, J.B.; Thompson, D.C.; Rai, B.K.; Baber, J.C.; Fan, K.Y.; Hu, Y.; Humblet, C. Comparison of several molecular docking programs: Pose prediction and virtual screening accuracy. *J. Chem. Inf. Model.* **2009**, *49*, 1455–1474. [CrossRef]
175. Cummings, M.D.; DesJarlais, R.L.; Gibbs, A.C.; Mohan, V.; Jaeger, E.P. Comparison of automated docking programs as virtual screening tools. *J. Med. Chem.* **2005**, *48*, 962–976. [CrossRef]
176. Annamala, M.K.; Inampudi, K.K.; Guruprasad, L. Docking of phosphonate and trehalose analog inhibitors into *M. tuberculosis* mycolyltransferase Ag85C: Comparison of the two scoring fitness functions GoldScore and ChemScore, in the GOLD software. *Bioinformation* **2007**, *1*, 339–350. [CrossRef]
177. Perola, E.; Walters, W.P.; Charifson, P.S. A detailed comparison of current docking and scoring methods on systems of pharmaceutical relevance. *Proteins* **2004**, *56*, 235–249. [CrossRef]
178. Xu, W.; Lucke, A.J.; Fairlie, D.P. Comparing sixteen scoring functions for predicting biological activities of ligands for protein targets. *J. Mol. Graph. Model.* **2015**, *57*, 76–88. [CrossRef]
179. Billones, J.B.; Carrillo, M.C.; Organo, V.G.; Sy, J.B.; Clavio, N.A.; Macalino, S.J.; Emnacen, I.A.; Lee, A.P.; Ko, P.K.; Concepcion, G.P. In silico discovery and in vitro activity of inhibitors against *Mycobacterium tuberculosis* 7,8-diaminopelargonic acid synthase (Mtb BioA). *Drug Des. Devel. Ther.* **2017**, *11*, 563–574. [CrossRef]
180. Dassault Systèmes BIOVIA. Discovery Studio. Available online: https://www.3dsbiovia.com/products/collaborative-science/biovia-discovery-studio/ (accessed on 26 October 2019).
181. Huang, S.Y.; Grinter, S.Z.; Zou, X. Scoring functions and their evaluation methods for protein-ligand docking: Recent advances and future directions. *Phys. Chem. Chem. Phys.* **2010**, *12*, 12899–12908. [CrossRef]
182. Ericksen, S.S.; Wu, H.; Zhang, H.; Michael, L.A.; Newton, M.A.; Hoffmann, F.M.; Wildman, S.A. Machine Learning Consensus Scoring Improves Performance Across Targets in Structure-Based Virtual Screening. *J. Chem. Inf. Model.* **2017**, *57*, 1579–1590. [CrossRef]
183. Li, D.D.; Meng, X.F.; Wang, Q.; Yu, P.; Zhao, L.G.; Zhang, Z.P.; Wang, Z.Z.; Xiao, W. Consensus scoring model for the molecular docking study of mTOR kinase inhibitor. *J. Mol. Graph. Model.* **2018**, *79*, 81–87. [CrossRef]
184. Charifson, P.S.; Corkery, J.J.; Murcko, M.A.; Walters, W.P. Consensus scoring: A method for obtaining improved hit rates from docking databases of three-dimensional structures into proteins. *J. Med. Chem.* **1999**, *42*, 5100–5109. [CrossRef]
185. Clark, R.D.; Strizhev, A.; Leonard, J.M.; Blake, J.F.; Matthew, J.B. Consensus scoring for ligand/protein interactions. *J. Mol. Graph. Model.* **2002**, *20*, 281–295. [CrossRef]
186. Harrison, A.J.; Yu, M.; Gardenborg, T.; Middleditch, M.; Ramsay, R.J.; Baker, E.N.; Lott, J.S. The structure of MbtI from *Mycobacterium tuberculosis*, the first enzyme in the biosynthesis of the siderophore mycobactin, reveals it to be a salicylate synthase. *J. Bacteriol.* **2006**, *188*, 6081–6091. [CrossRef]
187. Manos-Turvey, A.; Bulloch, E.M.; Rutledge, P.J.; Baker, E.N.; Lott, J.S.; Payne, R.J. Inhibition studies of *Mycobacterium tuberculosis* salicylate synthase (MbtI). *ChemMedChem* **2010**, *5*, 1067–1079. [CrossRef]
188. Vasan, M.; Neres, J.; Williams, J.; Wilson, D.J.; Teitelbaum, A.M.; Remmel, R.P.; Aldrich, C.C. Inhibitors of the salicylate synthase (MbtI) from *Mycobacterium tuberculosis* discovered by high-throughput screening. *ChemMedChem* **2010**, *5*, 2079–2087. [CrossRef]

189. Pini, E.; Poli, G.; Tuccinardi, T.; Chiarelli, L.R.; Mori, M.; Gelain, A.; Costantino, L.; Villa, S.; Meneghetti, F.; Barlocco, D. New Chromane-Based Derivatives as Inhibitors of *Mycobacterium tuberculosis* Salicylate Synthase (MbtI): Preliminary Biological Evaluation and Molecular Modeling Studies. *Molecules* **2018**, *23*, 1506. [CrossRef]
190. Chiarelli, L.R.; Mori, M.; Barlocco, D.; Beretta, G.; Gelain, A.; Pini, E.; Porcino, M.; Mori, G.; Stelitano, G.; Costantino, L.; et al. Discovery and development of novel salicylate synthase (MbtI) furanic inhibitors as antitubercular agents. *Eur. J. Med. Chem.* **2018**, *155*, 754–763. [CrossRef]
191. McGann, M. FRED pose prediction and virtual screening accuracy. *J. Chem. Inf. Model.* **2011**, *51*, 578–596. [CrossRef]
192. Korb, O.; Stützle, T.; Exner, T.E. PLANTS: Application of Ant Colony Optimization to Structure-Based Drug Design. In *ANTS 2006: Ant Colony Optimization and Swarm Intelligence*; Dorigo, M., Gambardella, L.M., Birattari, M., Martinoli, A., Poli, R., Stützle, T., Eds.; Springer: Heidelberg/Berlin, Germany, 2016; pp. 247–258.
193. Koshland, D.E. Application of a Theory of Enzyme Specificity to Protein Synthesis. *Proc. Natl. Acad. Sci. USA* **1958**, *44*, 98–104. [CrossRef]
194. Sotriffer, C.A. Accounting for induced-fit effects in docking: What is possible and what is not? *Curr. Top. Med. Chem.* **2011**, *11*, 179–191. [CrossRef]
195. Hartkoorn, R.C.; Sala, C.; Neres, J.; Pojer, F.; Magnet, S.; Mukherjee, R.; Uplekar, S.; Boy-Rottger, S.; Altmann, K.H.; Cole, S.T. Towards a new tuberculosis drug: Pyridomycin-nature's isoniazid. *EMBO Mol. Med.* **2012**, *4*, 1032–1042. [CrossRef]
196. Rozwarski, D.A.; Vilcheze, C.; Sugantino, M.; Bittman, R.; Sacchettini, J.C. Crystal structure of the *Mycobacterium tuberculosis* enoyl-ACP reductase, InhA, in complex with NAD+ and a C16 fatty acyl substrate. *J. Biol. Chem.* **1999**, *274*, 15582–15589. [CrossRef]
197. Rozwarski, D.A.; Grant, G.A.; Barton, D.H.; Jacobs, W.R., Jr.; Sacchettini, J.C. Modification of the NADH of the isoniazid target (InhA) from *Mycobacterium tuberculosis*. *Science* **1998**, *279*, 98–102. [CrossRef]
198. Amaro, R.E.; Li, W.W. Emerging methods for ensemble-based virtual screening. *Curr. Top. Med. Chem.* **2010**, *10*, 3–13. [CrossRef]
199. Brindha, S.; Sundaramurthi, J.C.; Velmurugan, D.; Vincent, S.; Gnanadoss, J.J. Docking-based virtual screening of known drugs against murE of *Mycobacterium tuberculosis* towards repurposing for TB. *Bioinformation* **2016**, *12*, 359–367. [CrossRef]
200. Wishart, D.S.; Knox, C.; Guo, A.C.; Cheng, D.; Shrivastava, S.; Tzur, D.; Gautam, B.; Hassanali, M. DrugBank: A knowledgebase for drugs, drug actions and drug targets. *Nucleic Acids Res.* **2008**, *36*, D901–D906. [CrossRef]
201. Schmidt, M.F.; Korb, O.; Howard, N.I.; Dias, M.V.B.; Blundell, T.L.; Abell, C. Discovery of Schaeffer's Acid Analogues as Lead Structures of *Mycobacterium tuberculosis* Type II Dehydroquinase Using a Rational Drug Design Approach. *ChemMedChem* **2013**, *8*, 54–58. [CrossRef]
202. Lovell, S.C.; Word, J.M.; Richardson, J.S.; Richardson, D.C. The penultimate rotamer library. *Proteins* **2000**, *40*, 389–408. [CrossRef]
203. Korb, O.; Stutzle, T.; Exner, T.E. Empirical scoring functions for advanced protein-ligand docking with PLANTS. *J. Chem. Inf. Model.* **2009**, *49*, 84–96. [CrossRef]
204. Bhabha, G.; Biel, J.T.; Fraser, J.S. Keep on moving: Discovering and perturbing the conformational dynamics of enzymes. *Acc. Chem. Res.* **2015**, *48*, 423–430. [CrossRef]
205. Goh, C.S.; Milburn, D.; Gerstein, M. Conformational changes associated with protein-protein interactions. *Curr. Opin. Struct. Biol.* **2004**, *14*, 104–109. [CrossRef]
206. Hospital, A.; Goni, J.R.; Orozco, M.; Gelpi, J.L. Molecular dynamics simulations: Advances and applications. *Adv. Appl. Bioinform. Chem.* **2015**, *8*, 37–47.
207. Lee, Y.; Jeong, L.S.; Choi, S.; Hyeon, C. Link between allosteric signal transduction and functional dynamics in a multisubunit enzyme: S-adenosylhomocysteine hydrolase. *J. Am. Chem. Soc.* **2011**, *133*, 19807–19815. [CrossRef]
208. McCammon, J.A.; Gelin, B.R.; Karplus, M. Dynamics of folded proteins. *Nature* **1977**, *267*, 585–590. [CrossRef]
209. Larsson, P.; Hess, B.; Lindahl, E. Algorithm improvements for molecular dynamics simulations. *WIREs Comput. Mol. Sci.* **2011**, *1*, 93–108. [CrossRef]
210. Orozco, M.; Orellana, L.; Hospital, A.; Naganathan, A.N.; Emperador, A.; Carrillo, O.; Gelpi, J.L. Coarse-grained representation of protein flexibility. Foundations, successes, and shortcomings. *Adv. Protein Chem. Struct. Biol.* **2011**, *85*, 183–215.

211. Linge, J.P.; Williams, M.A.; Spronk, C.A.; Bonvin, A.M.; Nilges, M. Refinement of protein structures in explicit solvent. *Proteins* **2003**, *50*, 496–506. [CrossRef]
212. Anandakrishnan, R.; Drozdetski, A.; Walker, R.C.; Onufriev, A.V. Speed of conformational change: Comparing explicit and implicit solvent molecular dynamics simulations. *Biophys. J.* **2015**, *108*, 1153–1164. [CrossRef]
213. MacKerell, A.D.; Bashford, D.; Bellott, M.; Dunbrack, R.L.; Evanseck, J.D.; Field, M.J.; Fischer, S.; Gao, J.; Guo, H.; Ha, S.; et al. All-atom empirical potential for molecular modeling and dynamics studies of proteins. *J. Phys. Chem. B* **1998**, *102*, 3586–3616. [CrossRef]
214. Cornell, W.D.; Cieplak, P.; Bayly, C.I.; Gould, I.R.; Merz, K.M.; Ferguson, D.M.; Spellmeyer, D.C.; Fox, T.; Caldwell, J.W.; Kollman, P.A. A Second Generation Force Field for the Simulation of Proteins, Nucleic Acids, and Organic Molecules. *J. Am. Chem. Soc.* **1995**, *117*, 5179–5197. [CrossRef]
215. Oostenbrink, C.; Villa, A.; Mark, A.E.; van Gunsteren, W.F. A biomolecular force field based on the free enthalpy of hydration and solvation: The GROMOS force-field parameter sets 53A5 and 53A6. *J. Comput. Chem.* **2004**, *25*, 1656–1676. [CrossRef]
216. Jorgensen, W.L.; Maxwell, D.S.; Tirado-Rives, J. Development and Testing of the OPLS All-Atom Force Field on Conformational Energetics and Properties of Organic Liquids. *J. Am. Chem. Soc.* **1996**, *118*, 11225–11236. [CrossRef]
217. Kaminski, G.A.; Friesner, R.A.; Tirado-Rives, J.; Jorgensen, W.L. Evaluation and Reparametrization of the OPLS-AA Force Field for Proteins via Comparison with Accurate Quantum Chemical Calculations on Peptides†. *J. Phys. Chem. B* **2001**, *105*, 6474–6487. [CrossRef]
218. Daggett, V.; Levitt, M. Protein Unfolding Pathways Explored Through Molecular Dynamics Simulations. *J. Mol. Biol.* **1993**, *232*, 600–619. [CrossRef]
219. Alonso, H.; Bliznyuk, A.A.; Gready, J.E. Combining docking and molecular dynamic simulations in drug design. *Med. Res. Rev.* **2006**, *26*, 531–568. [CrossRef]
220. Papaleo, E. Integrating atomistic molecular dynamics simulations, experiments, and network analysis to study protein dynamics: Strength in unity. *Front. Mol. Biosci.* **2015**, *2*, 28. [CrossRef]
221. Prada-Gracia, D.; Gomez-Gardenes, J.; Echenique, P.; Falo, F. Exploring the free energy landscape: From dynamics to networks and back. *PLoS Comput. Biol.* **2009**, *5*, e1000415. [CrossRef]
222. Wahab, H.A.; Choong, Y.S.; Ibrahim, P.; Sadikun, A.; Scior, T. Elucidating isoniazid resistance using molecular modeling. *J. Chem. Inf. Model.* **2009**, *49*, 97–107. [CrossRef]
223. Schroeder, E.K.; Basso, L.A.; Santos, D.S.; de Souza, O.N. Molecular dynamics simulation studies of the wild-type, I21V, and I16T mutants of isoniazid-resistant *Mycobacterium tuberculosis* enoyl reductase (InhA) in complex with NADH: Toward the understanding of NADH-InhA different affinities. *Biophys. J.* **2005**, *89*, 876–884. [CrossRef]
224. Cruz, J.N.; Costa, J.F.S.; Khayat, A.S.; Kuca, K.; Barros, C.A.L.; Neto, A. Molecular dynamics simulation and binding free energy studies of novel leads belonging to the benzofuran class inhibitors of *Mycobacterium tuberculosis* Polyketide Synthase 13. *J. Biomol. Struct. Dyn.* **2019**, *37*, 1616–1627. [CrossRef]
225. Aggarwal, A.; Parai, M.K.; Shetty, N.; Wallis, D.; Woolhiser, L.; Hastings, C.; Dutta, N.K.; Galaviz, S.; Dhakal, R.C.; Shrestha, R.; et al. Development of a Novel Lead that Targets, *M. tuberculosis* Polyketide Synthase 13. *Cell* **2017**, *170*, 249–259. [CrossRef]
226. Nikolova, N.; Jaworska, J. Approaches to Measure Chemical Similarity—A Review. *QSAR Comb. Sci.* **2003**, *22*, 1006–1026. [CrossRef]
227. Johnson, M.A.; Maggiora, G.M. American Chemical Society. In *Concepts and Applications of Molecular Similarity*; Wiley: New York, NY, USA, 1990.
228. Bacilieri, M.; Moro, S. Ligand-based drug design methodologies in drug discovery process: An overview. *Curr. Drug Discov. Technol.* **2006**, *3*, 155–165. [CrossRef]
229. Sukumar, N.; Das, S. Current trends in virtual high throughput screening using ligand-based and structure-based methods. *Comb. Chem. High Throughput Screen.* **2011**, *14*, 872–888. [CrossRef]
230. Cereto-Massague, A.; Ojeda, M.J.; Valls, C.; Mulero, M.; Garcia-Vallve, S.; Pujadas, G. Molecular fingerprint similarity search in virtual screening. *Methods* **2015**, *71*, 58–63. [CrossRef]
231. Bajusz, D.; Racz, A.; Heberger, K. Why is Tanimoto index an appropriate choice for fingerprint-based similarity calculations? *J. Cheminform.* **2015**, *7*, 20. [CrossRef]
232. Faulon, J.-L.; Bender, A. *Handbook of Chemoinformatics Algorithms*; Chapman & Hall/CRC: Boca Raton, FL, USA, 2010; 440p.

233. Haranczyk, M.; Holliday, J. Comparison of similarity coefficients for clustering and compound selection. *J. Chem. Inf. Model.* **2008**, *48*, 498–508. [CrossRef]
234. Al Khalifa, A.; Haranczyk, M.; Holliday, J. Comparison of nonbinary similarity coefficients for similarity searching, clustering and compound selection. *J. Chem. Inf. Model.* **2009**, *49*, 1193–1201. [CrossRef]
235. Ginn, C.M.R.; Willett, P.; Bradshaw, J. Combination of molecular similarity measures using data fusion. *Perspect. Drug Discov. Des.* **2000**, *20*, 1–16. [CrossRef]
236. Medina-Franco, J.L.; Maggiora, G.M.; Giulianotti, M.A.; Pinilla, C.; Houghten, R.A. A similarity-based data-fusion approach to the visual characterization and comparison of compound databases. *Chem. Biol. Drug Des.* **2007**, *70*, 393–412. [CrossRef]
237. Hu, G.; Kuang, G.; Xiao, W.; Li, W.; Liu, G.; Tang, Y. Performance evaluation of 2D fingerprint and 3D shape similarity methods in virtual screening. *J. Chem. Inf. Model.* **2012**, *52*, 1103–1113. [CrossRef]
238. Drwal, M.N.; Griffith, R. Combination of ligand- and structure-based methods in virtual screening. *Drug Discov. Today Technol.* **2013**, *10*, e395–e401. [CrossRef]
239. Hu, Y.; Bajorath, J. Extending the activity cliff concept: Structural categorization of activity cliffs and systematic identification of different types of cliffs in the ChEMBL database. *J. Chem. Inf. Model.* **2012**, *52*, 1806–1811. [CrossRef]
240. Hu, Y.; Stumpfe, D.; Bajorath, J. Advancing the activity cliff concept. *F1000Res* **2013**, *2*, 199. [CrossRef]
241. Stumpfe, D.; de la Vega de Leon, A.; Dimova, D.; Bajorath, J. Advancing the activity cliff concept, part II. *F1000Res* **2014**, *3*, 75. [CrossRef]
242. Verma, J.; Khedkar, V.M.; Coutinho, E.C. 3D-QSAR in drug design—A review. *Curr. Top. Med. Chem.* **2010**, *10*, 95–115. [CrossRef]
243. Exploring QSAR. *Environ. Sci. Technol.* **1995**, *29*, 444A. [CrossRef]
244. Bostrom, J.; Norrby, P.O.; Liljefors, T. Conformational energy penalties of protein-bound ligands. *J. Comput. Aided Mol. Des.* **1998**, *12*, 383–396. [CrossRef]
245. Perola, E.; Charifson, P.S. Conformational analysis of drug-like molecules bound to proteins: An extensive study of ligand reorganization upon binding. *J. Med. Chem.* **2004**, *47*, 2499–2510. [CrossRef]
246. Melo-Filho, C.C.; Braga, R.C.; Andrade, C.H. 3D-QSAR approaches in drug design: Perspectives to generate reliable CoMFA models. *Curr. Comput. Aided Drug Des.* **2014**, *10*, 148–159. [CrossRef]
247. Cherkasov, A.; Muratov, E.N.; Fourches, D.; Varnek, A.; Baskin, II; Cronin, M.; Dearden, J.; Gramatica, P.; Martin, Y.C.; Todeschini, R.; et al. QSAR modeling: Where have you been? Where are you going to? *J. Med. Chem.* **2014**, *57*, 4977–5010. [CrossRef]
248. Cramer, R.D.; Patterson, D.E.; Bunce, J.D. Comparative molecular field analysis (CoMFA). 1. Effect of shape on binding of steroids to carrier proteins. *J. Am. Chem. Soc.* **1988**, *110*, 5959–5967. [CrossRef]
249. Klebe, G.; Abraham, U.; Mietzner, T. Molecular similarity indices in a comparative analysis (CoMSIA) of drug molecules to correlate and predict their biological activity. *J. Med. Chem.* **1994**, *37*, 4130–4146. [CrossRef]
250. Bajpai, A.; Agarwal, N.; Gupta, S.P. A comparative 2D QSAR study on a series of hydroxamic acid-based histone deacetylase inhibitors vis-a-vis comparative molecular field analysis (CoMFA) and comparative molecular similarity indices analysis (CoMSIA). *Indian J. Biochem. Biophys.* **2014**, *51*, 244–252.
251. Chhatbar, D.M.; Chaube, U.J.; Vyas, V.K.; Bhatt, H.G. CoMFA, CoMSIA, Topomer CoMFA, HQSAR, molecular docking and molecular dynamics simulations study of triazine morpholino derivatives as mTOR inhibitors for the treatment of breast cancer. *Comput. Biol. Chem.* **2019**, *80*, 351–363. [CrossRef]
252. Singh, S.; Supuran, C.T. 3D-QSAR CoMFA studies on sulfonamide inhibitors of the Rv3588c beta-carbonic anhydrase from *Mycobacterium tuberculosis* and design of not yet synthesized new molecules. *J. Enzym. Inhib. Med. Chem.* **2014**, *29*, 449–455. [CrossRef]
253. Punkvang, A.; Hannongbua, S.; Saparpakorn, P.; Pungpo, P. Insight into the structural requirements of aminopyrimidine derivatives for good potency against both purified enzyme and whole cells of *M. tuberculosis*: Combination of HQSAR, CoMSIA, and MD simulation studies. *J. Biomol. Struct. Dyn.* **2016**, *34*, 1079–1091. [CrossRef] [PubMed]
254. Schuster, D. 3D pharmacophores as tools for activity profiling. *Drug Discov. Today Technol.* **2010**, *7*, e205–e211. [CrossRef] [PubMed]
255. Tawari, N.R.; Degani, M.S. Predictive models for nucleoside bisubstrate analogs as inhibitors of siderophore biosynthesis in *Mycobacterium tuberculosis*: Pharmacophore mapping and chemometric QSAR study. *Mol. Divers.* **2011**, *15*, 435–444. [CrossRef]

256. Hohenberg, P.; Kohn, W. Inhomogeneous Electron Gas. *Phys. Rev.* **1964**, *136*, B864–B871. [CrossRef]
257. Kohn, W.; Sham, L.J. Self-Consistent Equations Including Exchange and Correlation Effects. *Phys. Rev.* **1965**, *140*, A1133–A1138. [CrossRef]
258. Sharma, S. *Molecular Dynamics Simulation of Nanocomposites Using BIOVIA Materials Studio, Lammps and Gromacs*, 1st ed.; Elsevier: Waltham, MA, USA, 2019.
259. Fiolhais, C.; Nogueira, F.; Marques, M.A.L. *A Primer in Density Functional Theory*; Springer: Berlin, Germany; New York, NY, USA, 2003.
260. Becke, A.D. Perspective: Fifty years of density-functional theory in chemical physics. *J. Chem. Phys.* **2014**, *140*, 18A301. [CrossRef]
261. Rabi, S.; Patel, A.H.G.; Burger, S.K.; Verstraelen, T.; Ayers, P.W. Exploring the substrate selectivity of human sEH and *M. tuberculosis* EHB using QM/MM. *Struct. Chem.* **2017**, *28*, 1501–1511. [CrossRef]
262. Ramalho, T.C.; Caetano, M.S.; Josa, D.; Luz, G.P.; Freitas, E.A.; da Cunha, E.F. Molecular modeling of *Mycobacterium tuberculosis* dUTpase: Docking and catalytic mechanism studies. *J. Biomol. Struct. Dyn.* **2011**, *28*, 907–917. [CrossRef]
263. Oliveira, C.G.; da, S.M.P.I.; Souza, P.C.; Pavan, F.R.; Leite, C.Q.; Viana, R.B.; Batista, A.A.; Nascimento, O.R.; Deflon, V.M. Manganese(II) complexes with thiosemicarbazones as potential anti-*Mycobacterium tuberculosis* agents. *J. Inorg. Biochem.* **2014**, *132*, 21–29. [CrossRef]
264. Chi, G.; Manos-Turvey, A.; O'Connor, P.D.; Johnston, J.M.; Evans, G.L.; Baker, E.N.; Payne, R.J.; Lott, J.S.; Bulloch, E.M. Implications of binding mode and active site flexibility for inhibitor potency against the salicylate synthase from *Mycobacterium tuberculosis*. *Biochemistry* **2012**, *51*, 4868–4879. [CrossRef]
265. Frisch, M.J.; Trucks, G.W.; Schlegel, H.B.; Scuseria, G.E.; Robb, M.A.; Cheeseman, J.R.; Scalmani, G.; Barone, V.; Mennucci, B.; Petersson, G.A.; et al. *Gaussian 09, Revision E.01*; Gaussian, Inc.: Wallingford, CT, USA, 2009.
266. Stephens, P.J.; Devlin, F.J.; Chabalowski, C.F.; Frisch, M.J. Ab Initio Calculation of Vibrational Absorption and Circular Dichroism Spectra Using Density Functional Force Fields. *J. Phys. Chem.* **1994**, *98*, 11623–11627. [CrossRef]
267. Becke, A.D. Density-functional thermochemistry. III. The role of exact exchange. *J. Chem. Phys.* **1993**, *98*, 5648–5652. [CrossRef]
268. Indarto, A. *Theoretical Modelling and Mechanistic Study of the Formation and Atmospheric Transformations of Polycyclic Aromatic Compounds and Carbonaceous Particles*; Universal Publishers: Irvine, CA, USA, 2010.
269. Hamada, I. van der Waals density functional made accurate. *Phys. Rev. B* **2014**, *89*, 121103. [CrossRef]
270. Berland, K.; Cooper, V.R.; Lee, K.; Schroder, E.; Thonhauser, T.; Hyldgaard, P.; Lundqvist, B.I. van der Waals forces in density functional theory: A review of the vdW-DF method. *Rep. Prog. Phys.* **2015**, *78*, 066501. [CrossRef]
271. Grimme, S. Accurate description of van der Waals complexes by density functional theory including empirical corrections. *J. Comput. Chem.* **2004**, *25*, 1463–1473. [CrossRef]
272. Cohen, A.J.; Mori-Sanchez, P.; Yang, W. Insights into current limitations of density functional theory. *Science* **2008**, *321*, 792–794. [CrossRef]
273. Wilson, G.L.; Lill, M.A. Integrating structure-based and ligand-based approaches for computational drug design. *Future Med. Chem.* **2011**, *3*, 735–750. [CrossRef]
274. Polgar, T.; Keseru, G.M. Integration of virtual and high throughput screening in lead discovery settings. *Comb. Chem. High Throughput Screen.* **2011**, *14*, 889–897. [CrossRef]
275. Tanrikulu, Y.; Kruger, B.; Proschak, E. The holistic integration of virtual screening in drug discovery. *Drug Discov. Today* **2013**, *18*, 358–364. [CrossRef]
276. Tan, L.; Geppert, H.; Sisay, M.T.; Gutschow, M.; Bajorath, J. Integrating structure- and ligand-based virtual screening: Comparison of individual, parallel, and fused molecular docking and similarity search calculations on multiple targets. *ChemMedChem* **2008**, *3*, 1566–1571. [CrossRef]
277. Huang, S.Y.; Li, M.; Wang, J.; Pan, Y. HybridDock: A Hybrid Protein-Ligand Docking Protocol Integrating Protein- and Ligand-Based Approaches. *J. Chem. Inf. Model.* **2016**, *56*, 1078–1087. [CrossRef]
278. Lam, P.C.; Abagyan, R.; Totrov, M. Ligand-biased ensemble receptor docking (LigBEnD): A hybrid ligand/receptor structure-based approach. *J. Comput. Aided Mol. Des.* **2018**, *32*, 187–198. [CrossRef]
279. Mestres, J.; Knegtel, R.M.A. Similarity versus docking in 3D virtual screening. *Perspect. Drug Discov. Des.* **2000**, *20*, 191–207. [CrossRef]
280. Kruger, D.M.; Evers, A. Comparison of structure- and ligand-based virtual screening protocols considering hit list complementarity and enrichment factors. *ChemMedChem* **2010**, *5*, 148–158. [CrossRef]

281. Billones, J.B.; Carrillo, M.C.; Organo, V.G.; Macalino, S.J.; Sy, J.B.; Emnacen, I.A.; Clavio, N.A.; Concepcion, G.P. Toward antituberculosis drugs: In silico screening of synthetic compounds against *Mycobacterium tuberculosis*l,d-transpeptidase 2. *Drug Des. Devel Ther.* **2016**, *10*, 1147–1157. [CrossRef]
282. Fakhar, Z.; Govender, T.; Maguire, G.E.M.; Lamichhane, G.; Walker, R.C.; Kruger, H.G.; Honarparvar, B. Differential flap dynamics in l,d-transpeptidase2 from *Mycobacterium tuberculosis* revealed by molecular dynamics. *Mol. Biosyst.* **2017**, *13*, 1223–1234. [CrossRef]
283. Sandhu, P.; Akhter, Y. The drug binding sites and transport mechanism of the RND pumps from *Mycobacterium tuberculosis*: Insights from molecular dynamics simulations. *Arch. Biochem. Biophys.* **2016**, *592*, 38–49. [CrossRef]
284. Shah, P.; Mistry, J.; Reche, P.A.; Gatherer, D.; Flower, D.R. In silico design of *Mycobacterium tuberculosis* epitope ensemble vaccines. *Mol. Immunol.* **2018**, *97*, 56–62. [CrossRef]
285. Li, D.; Chi, B.; Wang, W.-W.; Gao, J.-M.; Wan, J. Exploring the possible binding mode of trisubstituted benzimidazoles analogues in silico for novel drug designtargeting Mtb FtsZ. *Med. Chem. Res.* **2017**, *26*, 153–169. [CrossRef]
286. Spitzer, R.; Jain, A.N. Surflex-Dock: Docking benchmarks and real-world application. *J. Comput. Aided Mol. Des.* **2012**, *26*, 687–699. [CrossRef]
287. Villoutreix, B.O.; Eudes, R.; Miteva, M.A. Structure-based virtual ligand screening: Recent success stories. *Comb. Chem. High Throughput Screen.* **2009**, *12*, 1000–1016. [CrossRef]
288. Talele, T.T.; Khedkar, S.A.; Rigby, A.C. Successful applications of computer aided drug discovery: Moving drugs from concept to the clinic. *Curr. Top. Med. Chem.* **2010**, *10*, 127–141. [CrossRef]
289. Clark, D.E. What has virtual screening ever done for drug discovery? *Expert Opin. Drug Discov.* **2008**, *3*, 841–851. [CrossRef]
290. Scior, T.; Bender, A.; Tresadern, G.; Medina-Franco, J.L.; Martinez-Mayorga, K.; Langer, T.; Cuanalo-Contreras, K.; Agrafiotis, D.K. Recognizing pitfalls in virtual screening: A critical review. *J. Chem. Inf. Model.* **2012**, *52*, 867–881. [CrossRef]
291. Baig, M.H.; Ahmad, K.; Roy, S.; Ashraf, J.M.; Adil, M.; Siddiqui, M.H.; Khan, S.; Kamal, M.A.; Provaznik, I.; Choi, I. Computer Aided Drug Design: Success and Limitations. *Curr. Pharm. Des.* **2016**, *22*, 572–581. [CrossRef]
292. Coupez, B.; Lewis, R.A. Docking and scoring—Theoretically easy, practically impossible? *Curr. Med. Chem.* **2006**, *13*, 2995–3003.
293. Geppert, H.; Vogt, M.; Bajorath, J. Current trends in ligand-based virtual screening: Molecular representations, data mining methods, new application areas, and performance evaluation. *J. Chem. Inf. Model.* **2010**, *50*, 205–216. [CrossRef]
294. Jain, A.N.; Nicholls, A. Recommendations for evaluation of computational methods. *J. Comput. Aided Mol. Des.* **2008**, *22*, 133–139. [CrossRef]
295. Lindorff-Larsen, K.; Maragakis, P.; Piana, S.; Shaw, D.E. Picosecond to Millisecond Structural Dynamics in Human Ubiquitin. *J. Phys. Chem. B* **2016**, *120*, 8313–8320. [CrossRef] [PubMed]
296. Noe, F. Beating the millisecond barrier in molecular dynamics simulations. *Biophys. J.* **2015**, *108*, 228–229. [CrossRef] [PubMed]
297. Shi, J.; Nobrega, R.P.; Schwantes, C.; Kathuria, S.V.; Bilsel, O.; Matthews, C.R.; Lane, T.J.; Pande, V.S. Atomistic structural ensemble refinement reveals non-native structure stabilizes a sub-millisecond folding intermediate of CheY. *Sci. Rep.* **2017**, *7*, 44116. [CrossRef]
298. Fujita, T. Recent Success Stories Leading to Commercializable Bioactive Compounds with the Aid of Traditional QSAR Procedures. *QSAR* **1997**, *16*, 107–112. [CrossRef]
299. Gao, Q.; Yang, L.; Zhu, Y. Pharmacophore based drug design approach as a practical process in drug discovery. *Curr. Comput. Aided Drug Des.* **2010**, *6*, 37–49. [CrossRef]
300. Sardari, S.; Dezfulian, M. Cheminformatics in anti-infective agents discovery. *Mini Rev. Med. Chem.* **2007**, *7*, 181–189. [CrossRef]
301. Topol, E.J. High-performance medicine: The convergence of human and artificial intelligence. *Nat. Med.* **2019**, *25*, 44–56. [CrossRef]

2

Pangenome Analysis of *Mycobacterium tuberculosis* Reveals Core-Drug Targets and Screening of Promising Lead Compounds for Drug Discovery

Hamza Arshad Dar [1], Tahreem Zaheer [1], Nimat Ullah [1], Syeda Marriam Bakhtiar [2], Tianyu Zhang [3], Muhammad Yasir [4,5], Esam I. Azhar [4,5,*] and Amjad Ali [1,*]

1 Atta-ur-Rahman School of Applied Biosciences, National University of Sciences and Technology, Islamabad 44000, Pakistan; darhamza000@gmail.com (H.A.D.); zaheertahreem@gmail.com (T.Z.); nimatscholar@gmail.com (N.U.)

2 Department of Bioinformatics and Biosciences, Capital University of Science and Technology Islamabad expressway, Kahuta Road, Zone-V, Islamabad 44000, Pakistan; marriam@cust.edu.pk

3 State Key Laboratory of Respiratory Disease, Guangzhou Institutes of Biomedicine and Health (GIBH), Chinese Academy of Sciences, Guangzhou 510530, China; zhang_tianyu@gibh.ac.cn

4 Special Infectious Agents Unit, King Fahd Medical Research Center, King Abdulaziz University, Jeddah 21589, Saudi Arabia; yamuhammad@kau.edu.sa

5 Medical Laboratory Technology Department, Faculty of Applied Medical Sciences, King Abdulaziz University, Jeddah 21589, Saudi Arabia

* Correspondence: eazhar@kau.edu.sa (E.I.A.); amjad.ali@asab.nust.edu.pk (A.A.).

Abstract: Tuberculosis, caused by *Mycobacterium tuberculosis* (*M. tuberculosis*), is one of the leading causes of human deaths globally according to the WHO TB 2019 report. The continuous rise in multi- and extensive-drug resistance in *M. tuberculosis* broadens the challenges to control tuberculosis. The availability of a large number of completely sequenced genomes of *M. tuberculosis* has provided an opportunity to explore the pangenome of the species along with the pan-phylogeny and to identify potential novel drug targets leading to drug discovery. We attempt to calculate the pangenome of *M. tuberculosis* that comprises a total of 150 complete genomes and performed the phylo-genomic classification and analysis. Further, the conserved core genome (1251 proteins) is subjected to various sequential filters (non-human homology, essentiality, virulence, physicochemical parameters, and pathway analysis) resulted in identification of eight putative broad-spectrum drug targets. Upon molecular docking analyses of these targets with ligands available at the DrugBank database shortlisted a total of five promising ligands with projected inhibitory potential; namely, 2′deoxy-thymidine-5′-diphospho-alpha-D-glucose, uridine diphosphate glucose, 2′-deoxy-thymidine-beta-L-rhamnose, thymidine-5′-triphosphate, and citicoline. We are confident that with further lead optimization and experimental validation, these lead compounds may provide a sound basis to develop safe and effective drugs against tuberculosis disease in humans.

Keywords: *Mycobacterium tuberculosis*; pangenome; drug targets; molecular docking; lead compounds; drug discovery; tuberculosis

1. Introduction

According to the 2019 global World Health Organization (WHO) report, tuberculosis (TB) is among the top ten causes of death and the leading cause of a single infectious agent (above HIV/AIDS) [1]. In 2018, this disease was responsible for 1.2 million deaths among HIV-negative people and an additional 251,000 deaths among HIV-positive people. The causative agent of human TB is *Mycobacterium tuberculosis* (*M. tuberculosis*).

TB is majorly an airborne disease where *M. tuberculosis* establishes infection inside the human body by overcoming the immune responses directed by the host against the foreign pathogen. Once inside, the bacteria infiltrate the host macrophages and persist inside them for years thus causing a chronic infection that reflects the failure of host immunity [2]. The increased occurrence of multidrug resistant (MDR) and extensively drug-resistant (XDR) strains of *M. tuberculosis* has been attributed to spontaneous mutations in the bacterial genome, followed by the emergence of these mutant strains at the expense of wild type strains [3]. This, in turn, has led to the loss of effectiveness of standard anti-TB drugs isoniazid and rifampicin.

The availability of the first *M. tuberculosis* genome sequence in 1998 along with further developments in the genomics and associated disciplines has enabled us to understand the importance of many proteins encoded in its genome [4,5]. Especially, the concept of pangenome can now be explored to obtain the core genome, i.e., genes present in all the strains of the dataset [6]. These genes can be exploited to design broad-spectrum therapeutics against the pathogenic species.

Various protocols in bioinformatics have helped scientists to process biological data of pathogens in order to prioritize drug targets, while the parallel developments in the cheminformatics help researchers access ligand databases such as the DrugBank and perform virtual screening for in silico-aided drug discovery [7,8]. Utilizing these useful tools, scientists have endeavored to identify lead compounds for tuberculosis [9,10]. Therefore, in this study, we used the integrative approach of pangenome analyses, subtractive genomics, and bioinformatics to prioritize potential drug targets in the *M. tuberculosis* genome. Further, we explored the structural association of these potential targets with FDA-approved drugs using molecular docking to shortlist promising lead molecules to aid drug development against TB.

Developing a new drug through conventional methods takes at least ten years of comprehensive research and huge funding; Nevertheless, the inclusion of computer-aided analyses at the initial stages can decrease the associated time and costs [11,12]. In silico drug screening serves as a valuable method to shortlist/prioritize only the most relevant compounds that could be checked later through experimental studies, and hence remove biomolecules that do not meet the required specifications to optimize the overall research in drug discovery [13]. Instead of focusing our attention on one drug target, we intended to scrutinize all high-ranked drug targets obtained computationally. Subject to experimental validation, this research work will provide a sound basis for developing novel therapeutics against the most troublesome bacterial pathogen *M. tuberculosis*.

2. Results and Discussion

2.1. Pangenome and Pan-Phylogeny Analysis of Mycobacterium tuberculosis Genomes

A total of 150 complete genomes and associated proteomes of *M. tuberculosis* were downloaded from the NCBI. Their information such as the accession number, strain name, and genome statistics are provided in Supplementary Table S1. The metadata associated with these bacterial strains such as the isolation source and the country of isolation is provided in Supplementary Table S2. Pangenome analysis of 150 *M. tuberculosis* complete genomes revealed that there were 5009 gene families in total (pangenome), among them, 1251 proteins were common (core genome) in all the studied genomes. The ratio of the core and pangenome size was found to be 0.25, thus the core forms 25% of the pangenome. This signifies the low level of genetic diversity in the *M. tuberculosis* strains. This trend is also visible in the pan-core genome plot, which projects that the global gene repertoire of this species is difficult to alter considerably in the future (Figure 1).

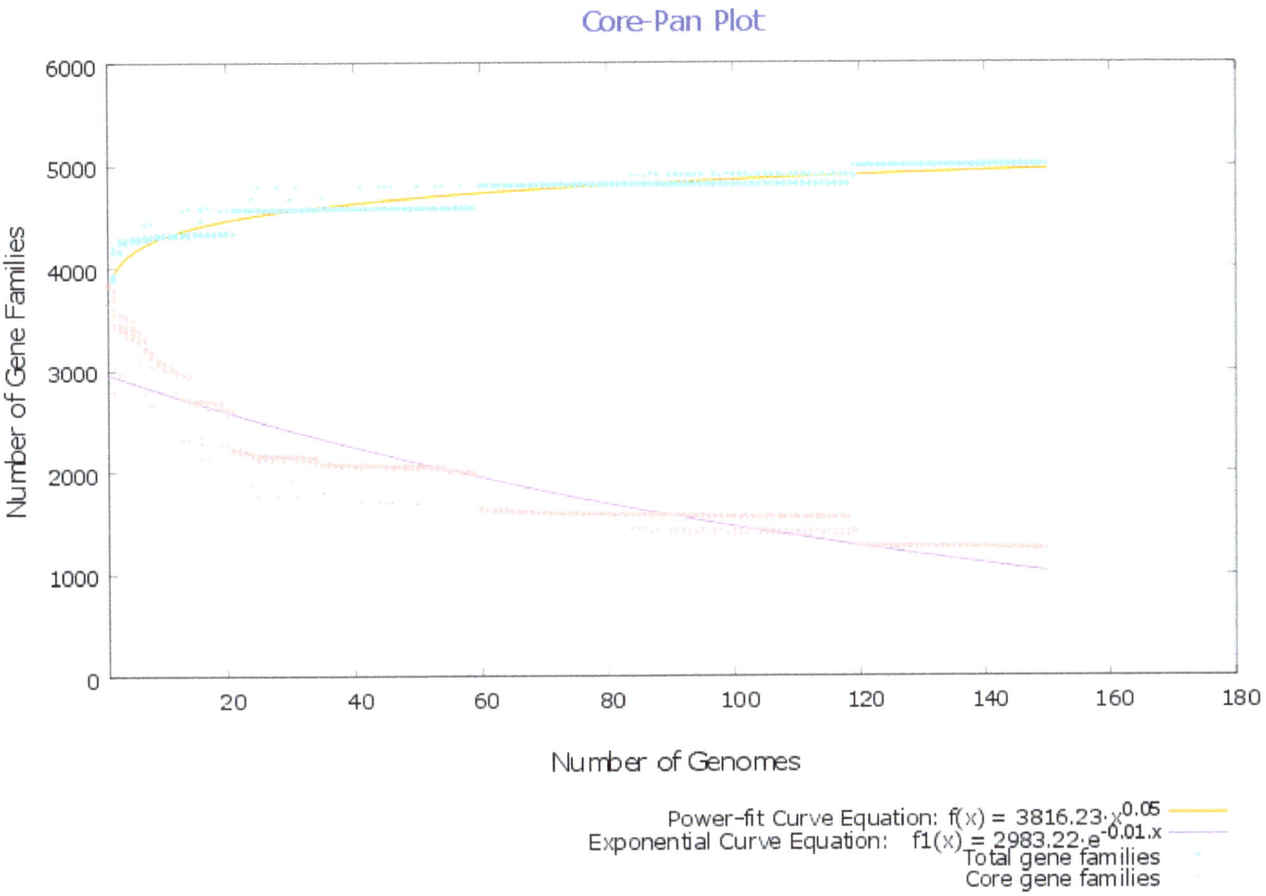

Figure 1. Pan-core plot of 150 *Mycobacterium tuberculosis* genomes. X-axis shows the number of genomes while the y-axis represents the number of gene families. With the addition of every genome, the pangenome size increased while the core genome size declined. The pangenome curve (shown in brown) has almost flattened, i.e., reached plateau. This suggests that the global gene repertoire of this species is unlikely to change significantly in the future and the pangenome is almost closed.

According to pangenome calculations, the b value of 0.0542 in the power-law regression model is indicative of a nearly close pangenome for *M. tuberculosis*. The pan-phylogeny based phylogenetic tree along with geographical source information is provided in Figure 2.

Each genome on average contained a total of 4102 protein-encoding genes. The core genome size (1251) thus accounted for 30.5% of the average genome size. Similarly, the minimum number of protein-encoding genes (3622) was present in strain RGTB423 while the maximum number of protein-encoding genes (4599) was present in strain 2279.

The level of conservation in the *M. tuberculosis* genomes is believed to be very high, with limited genetic variability between/across its various strains. Our genome-level analysis also indicates that the pangenome of this species is almost closed, with minimum variations. Multiple studies have corroborated this claim [14–16]. This is expected, as the lifestyle of this bacterium and its restricted niche makes it difficult to alter its gene pool [17]. Due to these unique conditions and their dependence on the host, it is suggested that there is less flexibility in its genome to accommodate more genes into the global gene repertoire. Hence, considering all this information now is the perfect opportunity to design and develop effective broad-spectrum therapeutics against this deadly human pathogen and to control the further spread of tuberculosis.

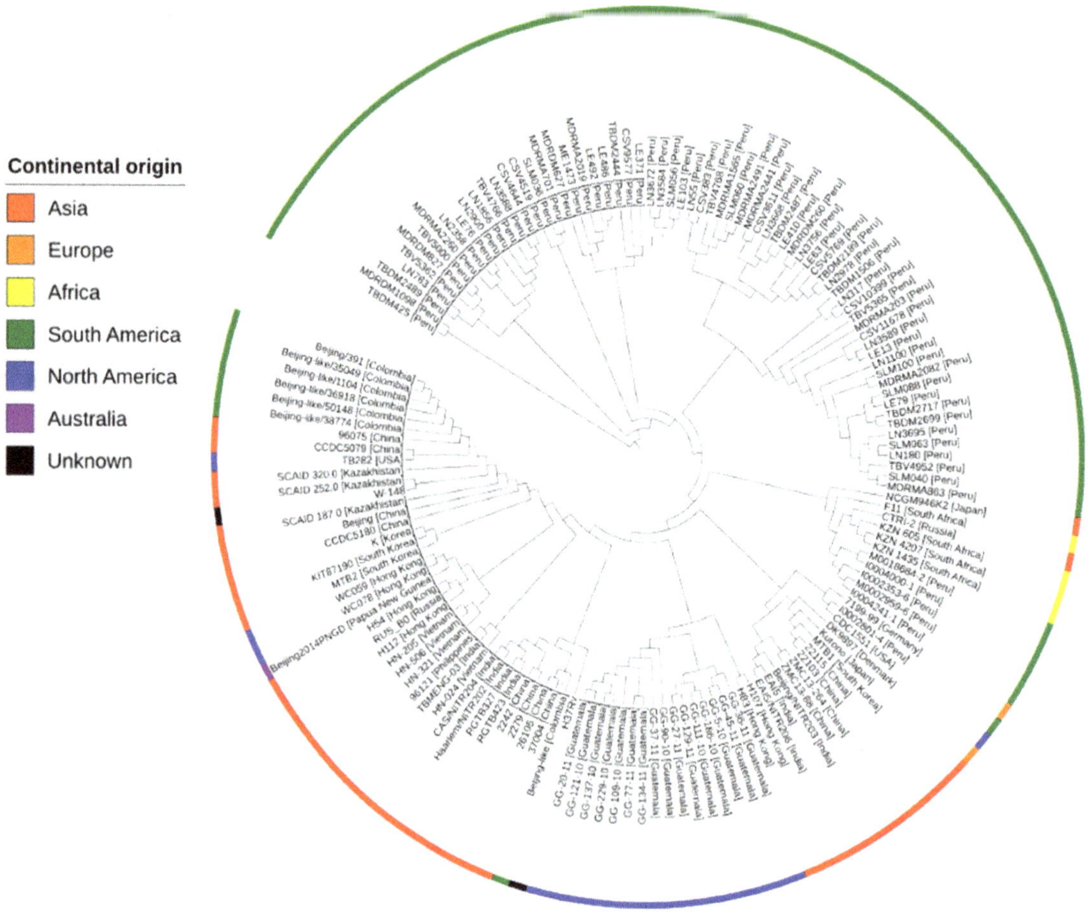

Figure 2. Pan-phylogeny tree of 150 complete genomes of *Mycobacterium tuberculosis*. Colored strips show the continental origin of strains. Overall, the strains originating from different geographical regions of the World clustered into different clades. This pan-phylogeny has been constructed based on accessory gene presence/absence data in different strains.

2.2. Subtractive Proteomics Revealed Putative *Mycobacterium tuberculosis* Drug Targets

Differential genome analysis was conducted on the core proteins of *M. tuberculosis* for the identification of therapeutic targets. Targets found to be human homologs could adversely affect the host metabolism, therefore, all those proteins were excluded in the first step that were identified as human homologs. The Rv numbers (gene identifiers or virulent strain of *Mycobacterium tuberculosis*) and the gene annotation were also conducted on these core proteins; the core genomes-associated data is provided in Supplementary Table S3. A total of 1185 proteins were identified as non-human homologous (Supplementary File S1) and were further screened based on their essentiality. Among them, 377 proteins were characterized as essential proteins and were considered crucial for pathogen survival (Supplementary File S2). If essential proteins are also functionally characterized as virulent, they are especially of vital significance to unveil novel therapeutic targets as these proteins help bacteria to modulate or degrade host defense mechanisms and may contribute to pathogenesis [18]. Therefore, the essential proteins were further screened to identify genes associated with pathogenicity. Among 377 essential proteins, VFDB and MvirDB identified a total of 93 virulence-related proteins involved in *M. tuberculosis* pathogenicity (Supplementary File S3). Since all the 93 proteins are non-human homologs and essential proteins associated with virulence, they represent an attractive dataset that could be explored for future vaccine production and drug design to tackle tuberculosis disease. However, for the purpose of this study, we further mined this large dataset to shortlist a few potential drug targets in order to facilitate the drug design and development against *M. tuberculosis*.

A total of 55 proteins were obtained after applying physiochemical checks, i.e., low molecular weights, a high value of the aliphatic index and negative GRAVY score (Supplementary File S4). Out of these, only eight proteins were identified by comparative pathway analysis to be involved in the unique bacterial metabolic pathway/s and were positively selected as *M. tuberculosis* drug targets to avoid targeting any human pathway upon drug therapy (Table 1).

Table 1. Metabolic pathway analysis of potential drug targets.

Protein Name	Rv Locus Number	KEGG Orthology	Metabolic Pathway(s)
dTDP-4-dehydrorhamnose reductase	Rv3266c	K00067	ko00521 Streptomycin biosynthesis ko00523 Polyketide sugar unit biosynthesis ko00541 *O*-Antigen nucleotide sugar biosynthesis ko01100 Metabolic pathways ko01110 Biosynthesis of secondary metabolites
glucose-1-phosphate thymidylyltransferase	Rv0334	K00973	ko00521 Streptomycin biosynthesis ko00523 Polyketide sugar unit biosynthesis ko00525 Acarbose and validamycin biosynthesis ko00541 O-Antigen nucleotide sugar biosynthesis ko01100 Metabolic pathways ko01110 Biosynthesis of secondary metabolites
two-component system regulator trcR	Rv1033c	K07672	ko02020 Two-component system
two-component system regulator mtrA	Rv3246c	K07670	ko02020 Two-component system
two-component system regulator regX3	Rv0491	K07776	ko02020 Two-component system
two-component system regulator kdpE	Rv1027c	K07667	ko02020 Two-component system ko02024 Quorum sensing
two-component system regulator devR	Rv3133c	K07695	ko02020 Two-component system
dTDP-4-dehydrorhamnose 3,5-epimerase	Rv3465	K01790	ko00521 Streptomycin biosynthesis ko00523 Polyketide sugar unit biosynthesis ko00541 O-Antigen nucleotide sugar biosynthesis ko01100 Metabolic pathways ko01110 Biosynthesis of secondary metabolites

Finally, a total of seven prioritized proteins were found to have similarity with targets associated with FDA-approved drugs and thus are likely druggable. These seven proteins, and their corresponding ligands, are tabulated in Table 2.

Table 2. The Autodock vina score of all drug targets with their ligands from the DrugBank database. The binding energies are indicated by a bold black color in the case of top interactions.

Target	Rv Locus Number	Ligand	Binding Energy
Glucose-1-phosphate thymidylyltransferase	Rv0334	2′-Deoxy-Thymidine-Beta-L-Rhamnose	−9.1
		2′deoxy-Thymidine-5′-Diphospho-Alpha-D-Glucose	−10.1
		Alpha-D-Glucose-1-Phosphate	−5.8
		Citicoline	−8.4
		Citric acid	−5.7
		Thymidine-5′-Triphosphate	−8.9
		Thymidine	−7.1
		Thymidine monophosphate	−7.7
		Uridine diphosphate glucose	−9.8
DNA-binding response regulator	Rv1027c	Phosphoaspartate	−5.2
		Guanosine-5′-Monophosphate	−7.9
		AlphaBeta-Methyleneadenosine-5′-Triphosphate	−7.3
		Adenosine-5′-Rp-Alpha-Thio-Triphosphate	−6.8
		2-Hydroxyestradiol	−7.9
dTDP-4-dehydrorhamnose 3,5-epimerase	Rv3465	2′deoxy-Thymidine-5′-Diphospho-Alpha-D-Glucose	−7.2
		3′-*O*-Acetylthymidine-5′-Diphosphate	−7.1
		D-tartaric acid	−4.6
		SS-(2-Hydroxyethyl)Thiocysteine	−4.6
		Thymidine_monophosphate	−6.8
		Thymidine-5′-diphospho-beta-D-xylose	−6.7

Table 2. *Cont.*

Target	Rv Locus Number	Ligand	Binding Energy
DNA-binding response regulator TrcR	Rv1033c	S-Methyl Phosphocysteine	−4.6
		Phosphoaspartate	−4.8
		Guanosine-5′-Monophosphate	−7.2
		Glycerine	−4
		AlphaBeta-Methyleneadenosine-5′-Triphosphate	−7.4
		Adenosine-5′-Rp-Alpha-Thio-Triphosphate	−7.6
		3-Aminosuccinimide	−4.5
		2-Hydroxyestradiol	−7.1
DNA-binding response regulator RegX3	Rv0491	2-Hydroxyestradiol	−7.1
		3-Aminosuccinimide	−4.4
		Adenosine-5′-Rp-Alpha-Thio-Triphosphate	−6.7
		AlphaBeta-Methyleneadenosine-5′-Triphosphate	−6.6
		Glycerine	−3.8

However, one prioritized target (two-component transcriptional regulatory protein DevR) did not show similarity to any drug target in the DrugBank database thus it is potentially a novel drug target worthy of experimental testing. Virtual screening may be performed with ligands from other ligand databases in order to find potent inhibitors of this protein. Literature studies were conducted on the seven proteins from Table 2 to understand their relevance as a drug target.

Among them, *trcR* has a crucial role in intracellular survival of *M. tuberculosis* and also in the regulation of Rv1057 expression, i.e., the β-propeller gene activated by the envelope stress [19]. In another study by Haydel et al.; they demonstrated that *trcR* and *trcS* two-component system genes are transcribed in broth-grown *M. tuberculosis* validated through reverse transcription PCR analysis. Moreover, through the SCOTS technique the expression of these genes are observed in liquid (broth) medium and after 18 h of *M. tuberculosis* growth in cultured human primary macrophages [20]. Nevertheless, the stimulatory signal for the TrcR-TrcS system is poorly understood and requires further research. Recently, another study, based on the drug target score, also ranked TrcR as the second-best therapeutic target in *M. tuberculosis* [21]. We believe that future studies are also needed to investigate this matter.

The dTDP-4-dehydrorhamnose reductase, another protein classified as a drug target by our study, is already known to be a high-confidence drug target [22]. This protein plays an important role in cell wall synthesis. Targeting the cell wall of *M. tuberculosis* through inhibitors is a good strategy, as has been recognized by earlier studies [23,24].

Similarly, *mtrA* (in Table 1) plays an important role in many crucial processes such as cell wall homeostasis and bacterial growth. It also has a role in cell division, DNA replication, and controls susceptibility of *M. tuberculosis* to the first line antimycobacterial drugs [25]. This signifies the necessity of *mtrA* for the growth of *M. tuberculosis*.

Another prioritized drug target RegX3 (in Table 1) has a role in aerobic respiration, virulence and phosphate absorption [26]. It is also required for optimal growth of *M. tuberculosis* in nutrient rich medium [27]. Moreover, RegX3 directly interacts with exs-5, another essential gene for the growth process. It also causes an increase in the production of membrane vesicles in *M. tuberculosis* [28].

The *kdpE* participates in the two-component system pathway and is involved in transcriptional regulation of Kdp-ATPase [29]. *KdpE* also has a role in the regulation of key factors involved in stress tolerance and energy metabolism [30,31]. Moreover, it is also notorious for its role in virulence caused by *M. tuberculosis*, *Pseudomonas aeruginosa*, *Salmonella enterica*, and *Staphylococcus aureus* [29,32–35]. Considering the situation, *kdpE* can be considered as a broad-spectrum therapeutic target for multiple pathogens.

The present study also prioritized drug target glucose-1-phosphate thymidylyltransferase. The protein is involved in three metabolic pathways namely, polyketide sugar unit biosynthesis, streptomycin biosynthesis, and the nucleotide sugars metabolism pathway [36–38]. All these pathways are crucial for survival of *M. tuberculosis* and elaborate on the relevance of glucose-1-phosphate thymidylyltransferase as a drug target. Additionally, the dTDP-4-dehydrorhamnose 3,5-epimerase protein obtained by our study is known to be a potential drug target in the rhamnose pathway [39].

2.3. Docking Analyses of Drug Targets Revealed Potential Lead Compounds for Drug Discovery

The Autodock vina docking scores of ligands with drug targets are elaborated in Table 2. Among all the drug–ligand interaction analyses, 2′deoxy-thymidine-5′-diphospho-alpha-D-glucose was found to have the lowest binding energy (−10.1 kcal/mol) with glucose-1-phosphate thymidylyltransferase (Figure 3).

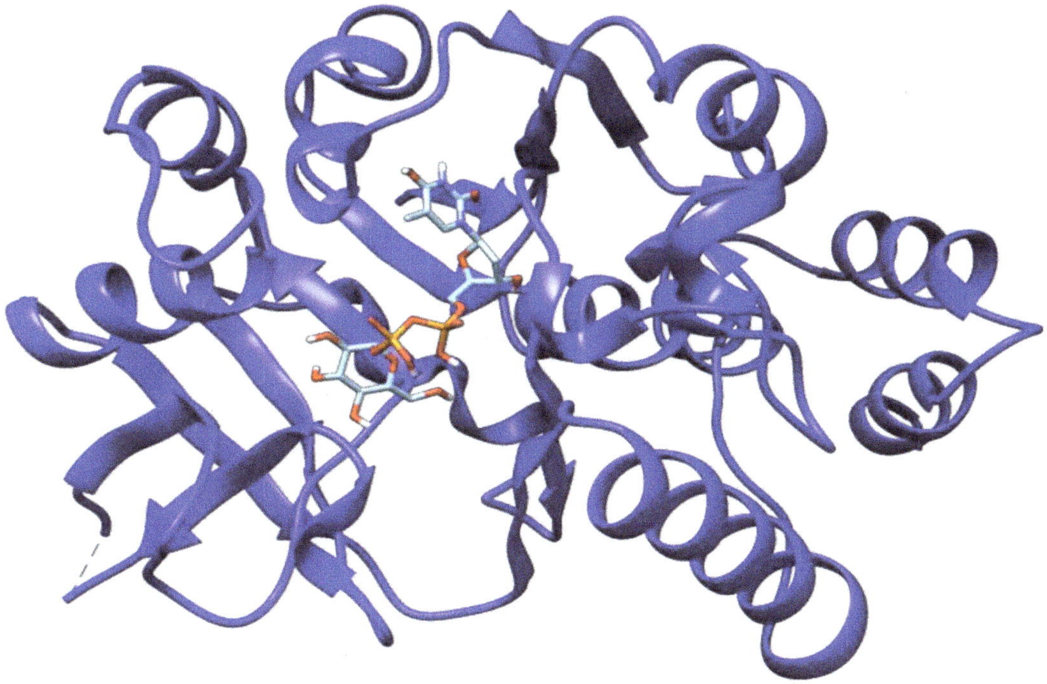

Figure 3. The docked complex of 2′deoxy-thymidine-5′-diphospho-alpha-D-glucose and glucose-1-phosphate thymidylyltransferase.

Interestingly, 2′deoxy-thymidine-5′-diphospho-alpha-D-glucose was found to associate with another prioritized drug target protein of this study DNA response regulator, however, the binding energy was somewhat higher (−7.2 kcal/mol) in that case. Nevertheless, our docking analyses proposed the 2′deoxy-thymidine-5′-diphospho-alpha-D-glucose compound as a high-ranked lead compound to develop a drug against tuberculosis.

The second high-ranked ligand in our study is uridine diphosphate glucose. This compound showed a binding energy of −9.8 kcal/mol with glucose-1-phosphate thymidylyltransferase (Figure 4), and thus may also represent a good target for lead optimization. Meanwhile, 2′-deoxy-thymidine-beta-L-rhamnose ligand exhibited docked energy of −9.1 kcal/mol with glucose-1-phosphate thymidylyltransferase (Figure 5).

This ligand also interacted with another prioritized protein of our study dTDP-4-dehydrorhamnose reductase with the binding energy of −8.3 kcal/mol. Another high-ranked ligand thymidine-5′-triphosphate ligand was found to have −8.9 kcal/mol binding energy with glucose-1-phosphate thymidylyltransferase (Figure 6) while citicoline, on the other hand, showed −8.4 kcal/mol binding energy with this same drug target (Figure 7).

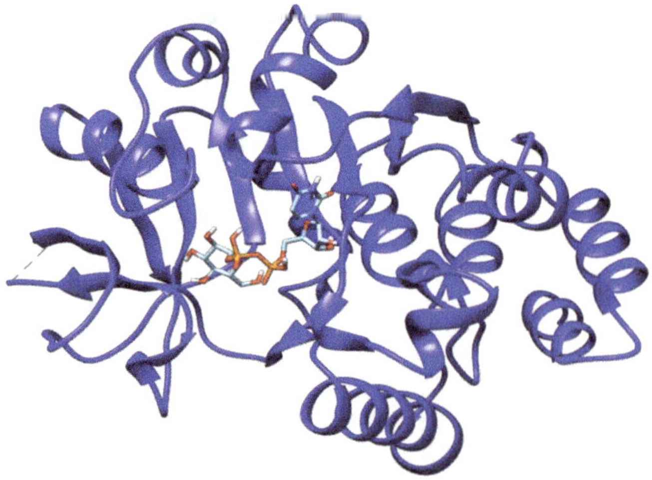

Figure 4. The docked complex of uridine diphosphate glucose and glucose-1-phosphate thymidylyltransferase.

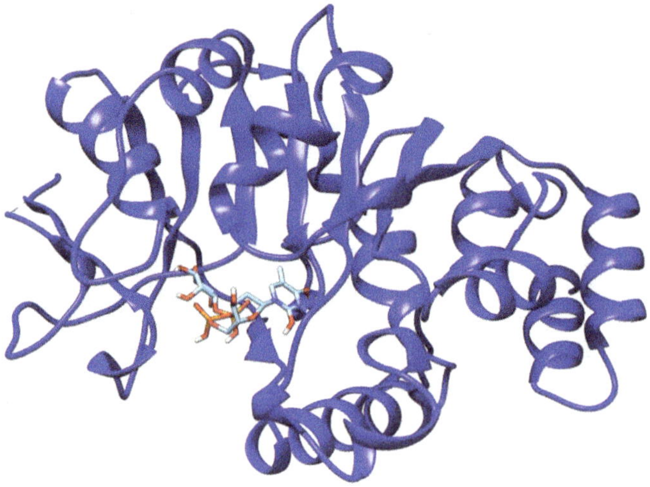

Figure 5. The docked complex of 2′-deoxy-thymidine-beta-L-rhamnose and glucose-1-phosphate thymidylyltransferase.

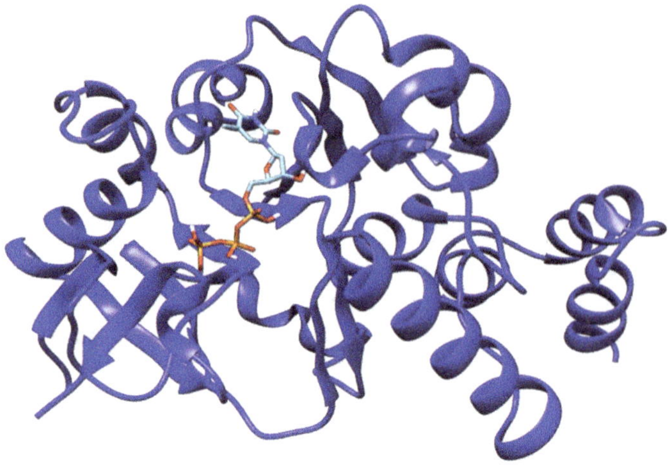

Figure 6. The docked complex of thymidine-5′-triphosphate and glucose-1-phosphate thymidylyltransferase.

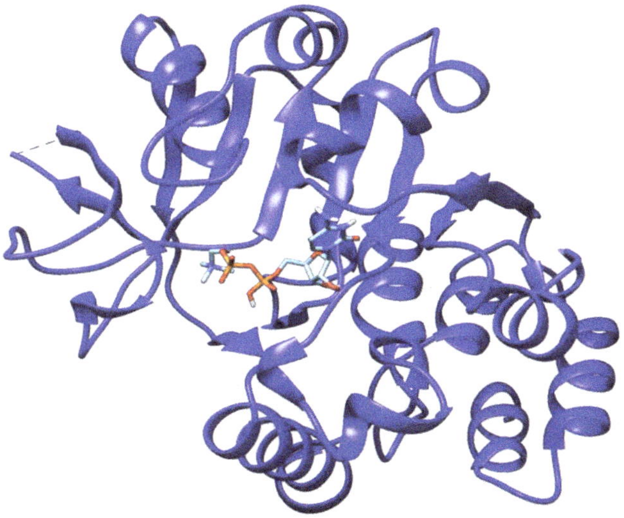

Figure 7. The docked complex of citicoline and glucose-1-phosphate thymidylyltransferase.

Thus, overall, this study shortlisted five top-ranked ligands with good binding affinity to drug targets and thus may guide drug development studies to counter *M. tuberculosis*. These ligands are 2′deoxy-thymidine-5′-diphospho-alpha-D-glucose, uridine diphosphate glucose, 2′-deoxy-thymidine-beta-L-rhamnose, thymidine-5′-triphosphate, and citicoline, which have good binding affinity with metabolic pathway proteins especially glucose-1-phosphate thymidylyltransferase. The protein is involved in three metabolic pathways namely, polyketide sugar unit biosynthesis, streptomycin biosynthesis, and nucleotide sugars metabolism pathway [36–38]. All these pathways are crucial for survival of *M. tuberculosis* and shortlisted repurposed drugs have higher affinity with the enzyme, i.e., glucose-1-phosphate thymidylyltransferase. Moreover, these drugs have a tendency to bind with dTDP-4-dehydrorhamnose 3,5-epimerase that is a potential drug target in rhamnose pathway [39]. These findings may provide a basis for the development of effective therapeutics against tuberculosis and/or replace currently available drugs to treat this deadly pathogen, however, experimental validation is needed to confirm these results.

3. Materials and Methods

The methodology adopted in this study was visualized in Figure 8. The different steps were elaborated below.

A total of 150 complete genome sequences of *Mycobacterium tuberculosis* were retrieved from the NCBI GenBank database and pangenome analysis was conducted to identify the genes shared by all the strains of our dataset (i.e., the core genome). The core genome was then subjected to various sequential filters of subtractive genomics (non-homology to humans, bacterial essentiality and virulence, physiochemical checks, comparative pathway analysis, and druggability analysis) to select potential drug targets. Finally, these proteins were subjected to molecular docking with ligands from the DrugBank database to identify potential lead compounds that could be useful to develop a drug against tuberculosis.

3.1. Collection of Genomic Data

The complete genome sequences off 150 *M. tuberculosis* strains and their associated proteomes were retrieved from the GenBank database (https://www.ncbi.nlm.nih.gov/genbank/) available at the National Center for Biotechnology Information (NCBI). These strains had been earlier isolated from all the geographical regions of the World.

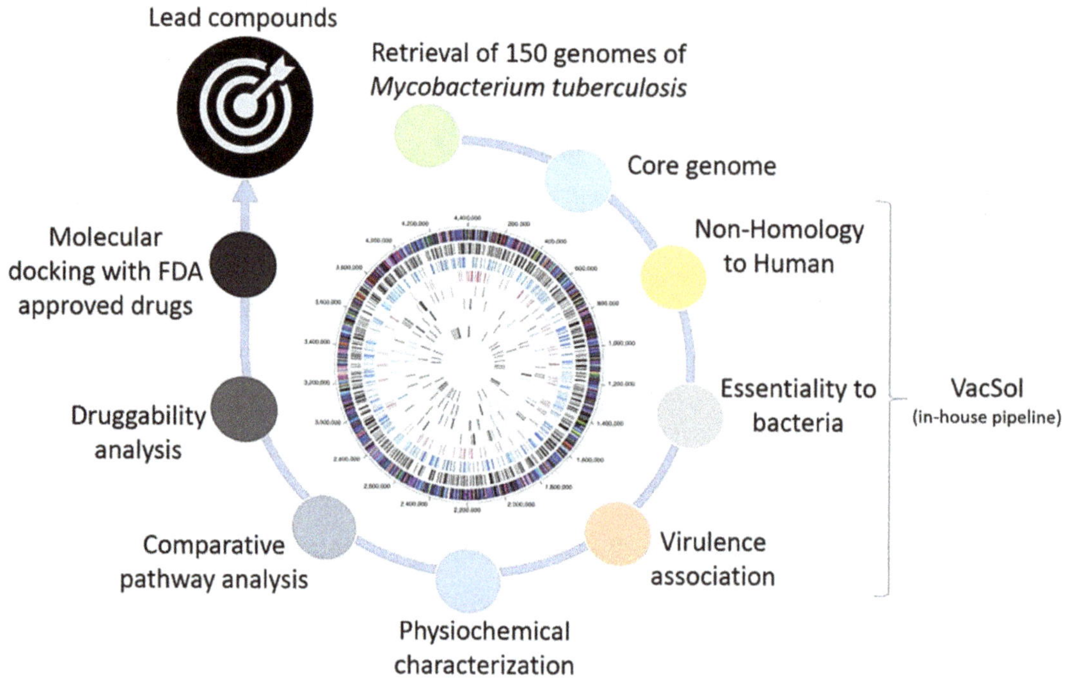

Figure 8. The methodology adopted in the study to find lead compounds (drugs) against *Mycobacterium tuberculosis*.

3.2. Pangenome Analysis of Mycobacterium tuberculosis Strains

Pangenome analysis was conducted on the genomes using the Bacterial Pan Genome Analysis (BPGA) tool to obtain highly conserved proteins of *M. tuberculosis* [40]. For this, we used the default threshold of 50% identity to generate orthologous protein clusters by the USEARCH algorithm [41]. BPGA calculates pan and core genome/proteome size by randomly considering 20 permutations and sequentially stating median values after the addition of each genome. Graphically, the core and pan-genome curves are generated by comparing the total number of common and unique gene families against the total number of genomes, respectively. The output also shows the number of new genes with the addition of every genome. The pan phylogeny was generated using the pan-matrix data and the associated pangenome tree was constructed using the neighbor-joining method with a default combination value of 20 iterations. Protein sequences associated with the core genome were retrieved and subjected to further screening steps to identify potential therapeutic targets.

3.3. Identification of Non-Host Homologous, Essential, and Virulence-Associated Proteins

To aid the preliminary identification of novel therapeutic targets in the core genome/proteome, we used an in-house pipeline VacSol for non-homology, essentiality, and virulence screening steps [42]. To avoid harmful responses in humans due to drug therapy, the drug targets must be non-homologous to human proteins, so for the identification of non-host homologous targets, the NCBI BLASTp tool (E-value 1×10^{-3}) was used to compare the core genome with the human genome [43]. From this non-host homologous conserved proteome, essential genes were identified using BLASTp against the Database of Essential Genes (DEG) at an E-value <0.0001 and bit score >100 [44]. The DEG comprises experimentally validated data collected from archaea, bacteria, and eukaryotes, including currently reported essential genomic elements such as genes that are required for cellular life. We subjected the selected proteins to BLASTp search against the Virulence Factor Database (VFDB) and the Microbial Virulence database (MvirDB) to identify potential virulence-associated factors [45,46]. The VFDB is a comprehensive online database that contains information about virulence factors of bacterial pathogens. Virulence factors are known gene products that enable a microorganism to establish itself within a host and thus enhance its disease-inducing potential [47]. MvirDB is another integrated online database comprising publicly available, organized sequences related to known virulence factors, toxins, and antibiotic resistance genes [46].

3.4. *Identification of Putative Mycobacterium tuberculosis Drug Targets*

To identify potential drug targets, the non-human homolog, essential, and virulence-associated core proteins of *M. tuberculosis* were further filtered based on physicochemical parameters such as molecular weight, pI (isoelectric point), grand average of hydropathicity (GRAVY) value, and aliphatic index using the ProtParam tool [48]. Low molecular weight proteins are considered good drug targets, as they are accessible to drugs [49]. A higher value of the aliphatic index of proteins indicates thermostability whereas the negative GRAVY (grand average of hydropathicity) value indicates the hydrophilic nature of putative drug targets [50]. After physicochemical filters, comparative pathway analysis of filtered proteins was performed using the KEGG Automatic Annotation Server (KAAS) version 2.1 to identify the proteins associated with pathogen-specific pathways to enable specific targeting of the pathogen [51].

Finally, druggability assessment of the shortlisted proteins was performed using BLASTp against the DrugBank database at default settings [52]. The druggability of potential targets is also a crucial screening step that evaluates the potential of prioritized targets to be modulated by a drug or drug-like entity [50]. The potential targets should bind to a drug or drug-like compound with high affinity. However, this was not considered an inclusion criterion as novel drug targets may not display homology to targets associated with FDA approved drugs and show specific affinity to other drugs from natural products [53].

3.5. *Molecular Docking of Putative Drug Targets with Drugs*

The sequences of drug targets were checked for the availability of crystal structures, if any, from the RCSB Protein DataBank [54]. Structural file PDB was downloaded, and all the attached ligands were removed from the crystal structure. The drug targets having no associated crystal structure available in the database were modeled using the i-TASSER server [55,56]. Structure with the highest C-Score was selected in each case as these models are of good quality and stability. Using the PyRx-incorporated Autodock vina tool, the structures of drug targets were subjected to molecular docking with the FDA-approved drugs identified earlier in the druggability analysis [57,58]. Blind docking was conducted by adjusting the grid-box in order to cover the whole protein space, and the default value of exhaustiveness (8) was selected. Both ligands and their targets were prepared in the PDBQT format as per requirements and molecular docking analysis was performed. Docked complexes with the lowest binding energies were comparatively analyzed to identify those ligands that associated strongly with drug targets. These ligands were thus shortlisted as lead compounds for developing a potent drug against tuberculosis.

Supplementary Materials: File S1: The core proteins of 150 *Mycobacterium tuberculosis* genomes found to be non-homologous to the human genome given in the FASTA format. File S2: The essential and non-human homolog core proteins identified in genomes under study given in the FASTA format. File S3: Projected virulence-associated proteins from the non-homologous essential core proteins given in the FASTA format. File S4: Protein targets found to have appropriate physiochemical parameters provided. Table S1: Information about 150 complete genome sequences of *Mycobacterium tuberculosis* such as strain name, biosample, bioproject, and genome statistics are provided. Table S2: The metadata associated with these bacterial strains such as isolation source and the country of isolation is provided. Table S3: The annotation of core gene targets and their Rv numbers.

Author Contributions: Conceptualization, H.A.D. and T.Z. (Tahreem Zaheer); Data curation, N.U. and S.M.B.; Formal analysis, T.Z. (Tahreem Zaheer) and S.M.B.; Investigation, T.Z. (Tianyu Zhang) and M.Y.; Methodology, H.A.D.; Project administration, A.A. and E.I.A.; Software, H.A.D. and N.U.; Supervision, A.A.; Validation, H.A.D, T.Z. (Tahreem Zaheer); N.U. and S.M.B.; Visualization, M.Y.; Writing—original draft, H.A.D. and T.Z. (Tahreem Zaheer); Writing—review and editing, E.I.A. and T.Z. (Tianyu Zhang) All authors have read and agreed to the published version of the manuscript.

References

1. World Health Organization. *Global Tuberculosis Report 2019*; World Health Organization: Geneva, Switzerland, 2019.
2. Gengenbacher, M.; Kaufmann, S.H.E. *Mycobacterium tuberculosis*: Success through dormancy. *FEMS Microbiol. Rev.* **2012**, *36*, 514–532. [CrossRef]
3. Gandhi, N.R.; Nunn, P.; Dheda, K.; Schaaf, H.S.; Zignol, M.; Van Soolingen, D. Multidrug-resistant and extensively drug-resistant tuberculosis: A threat to global control of tuberculosis. *Lancet* **2010**, *375*, 1830–1843. [CrossRef]
4. Brindha, S.; Vincent, S.; Velmurugan, D.; Ananthakrishnan, D.; Sundaramurthi, J.C.; Gnanadoss, J.J. Bioinformatics approach to prioritize known drugs towards repurposing for tuberculosis. *Med. Hypotheses* **2017**, *103*, 39–45. [CrossRef]
5. Cole, S.; Brosch, R.; Parkhill, J.; Garnier, T.; Churcher, C.; Harris, D. Deciphering the biology of Mycobacterium tuberculosis from the complete genome sequence. *Nature* **1998**, *393*, 537. [CrossRef]
6. Vernikos, G.; Medini, D.; Riley, D.R.; Tettelin, H. Ten years of pan-genome analyses. *Curr. Opin. Microbiol.* **2015**, *23*, 148–154. [CrossRef]
7. Sundaramurthi, J.C.; Brindha, S.; Reddy, T.B.K.; Hanna, L.E. Informatics resources for tuberculosis—Towards drug discovery. *Tuberculosis* **2012**, *92*, 133–138. [CrossRef]
8. Ekins, S.; Freundlich, J.S.; Choi, I.; Sarker, M.; Talcott, C. Computational databases, pathway and cheminformatics tools for tuberculosis drug discovery. *Trends Microbiol.* **2011**, *19*, 65–74. [CrossRef]
9. Karunakar, P.; Girija, C.R.; Krishnamurthy, V.; Krishna, V.; Shivakumar, K.V. In Silico antitubercular activity analysis of benzofuran and naphthofuran derivatives. *Tuberc. Res. Treat.* **2014**, *2014*. [CrossRef]
10. Perryman, A.L.; Yu, W.; Wang, X.; Ekins, S.; Forli, S.; Li, S.-G. A virtual screen discovers novel, fragment-sized inhibitors of *Mycobacterium tuberculosis* InhA. *J. Chem. Inf. Model* **2015**, *55*, 645–659. [CrossRef]
11. Timo, G.O.; Reis, R.; de Melo, A.F.; Costa, T.V.L.; de Magalhães, P.O.; Homem-de-Mello, M. Predictive power of in Silico approach to evaluate chemicals against *M. tuberculosis*: A systematic review. *Pharmaceuticals* **2019**, *12*, 135. [CrossRef]
12. Langer, T.; Wolber, G. Pharmacophore definition and 3D searches. *Drug Discov. Today Technol.* **2004**, *1*, 203–207. [CrossRef] [PubMed]
13. Sliwoski, G.; Kothiwale, S.; Meiler, J.; Lowe, E.W. Computational methods in drug discovery. *Pharmacol Rev.* **2014**, *66*, 334–395. [CrossRef] [PubMed]
14. Comas, I.; Chakravartti, J.; Small, P.M.; Galagan, J.; Niemann, S.; Kremer, K. Human T cell epitopes of *Mycobacterium tuberculosis* are evolutionarily hyperconserved. *Nat. Genet.* **2010**, *42*, 498. [CrossRef] [PubMed]
15. Kavvas, E.S.; Catoiu, E.; Mih, N.; Yurkovich, J.T.; Seif, Y.; Dillon, N. Machine learning and structural analysis of *Mycobacterium tuberculosis* pan-genome identifies genetic signatures of antibiotic resistance. *Nat. Commun.* **2018**, *9*, 4306. [CrossRef]
16. Cubillos-Ruiz, A.; Morales, J.; Zambrano, M.M. Analysis of the genetic variation in *Mycobacterium tuberculosis* strains by multiple genome alignments. *BMC Res. Notes* **2008**, *1*, 110. [CrossRef]
17. Medini, D.; Donati, C.; Tettelin, H.; Masignani, V.; Rappuoli, R. The microbial pan-genome. *Curr. Opin. Genet. Dev.* **2005**, *15*, 589–594. [CrossRef]
18. Naz, A.; Awan, F.M.; Obaid, A.; Muhammad, S.A.; Paracha, R.Z.; Ahmad, J. Identification of putative vaccine candidates against *Helicobacter pylori* exploiting exoproteome and secretome: A reverse vaccinology based approach. *Infect. Genet. Evol.* **2015**, *32*, 280–291. [CrossRef]
19. Pang, X.; Cao, G.; Neuenschwander, P.F.; Haydel, S.E.; Hou, G.; Howard, S.T. The β-propeller gene Rv1057 of *Mycobacterium tuberculosis* has a complex promoter directly regulated by both the MprAB and TrcRS two-component systems. *Tuberculosis* **2011**. [CrossRef]
20. Haydel, S.E.; Benjamin, W.H.; Dunlap, N.E.; Clark-Curtiss, J.E. Expression, autoregulation, and DNA binding properties of the *Mycobacterium tuberculosis* TrcR response regulator. *J. Bacteriol.* **2002**. [CrossRef]
21. Chakraborty, A.K.; Sarkar, I.; Sen, A. Herbal medicine meets bioinformatics for remedy of tuberculosis by *Mycobacterium tuberculosis* RGTB423. *Int. J. Data Min. Bioinform.* **2019**. [CrossRef]
22. Raman, K.; Yeturu, K.; Chandra, N. targetTB: A target identification pipeline for *Mycobacterium tuberculosis* through an interactome, reactome and genome-scale structural analysis. *BMC Syst. Biol.* **2008**, *2*, 109. [CrossRef]

23. Ma, Y.; Stern, R.J.; Scherman, M.S.; Vissa, V.D.; Yan, W.; Jones, V.C. Drug targeting *Mycobacterium tuberculosis* cell wall synthesis: Genetics of dTDP-rhamnose synthetic enzymes and development of a microtiter plate-based screen for inhibitors of conversion of dTDP-glucose to dTDP-rhamnose. *Antimicrob. Agents Chemother.* **2001**, *45*, 1407–1416. [CrossRef]
24. Barry, C.E., III. New horizons in the treatment of tuberculosis. *Biochem. Pharmacol.* **1997**, *54*, 1165–1172. [CrossRef]
25. Gorla, P.; Plocinska, R.; Sarva, K.; Satsangi, A.T.; Pandeeti, E.; Donnelly, R. MtrA response regulator controls cell division and cell wall metabolism and affects susceptibility of mycobacteria to the first line antituberculosis drugs. *Front. Microbiol.* **2018**. [CrossRef]
26. Li, X.; Lv, X.; Lin, Y.; Zhen, J.; Ruan, C.; Duan, W. Role of two-component regulatory systems in intracellular survival of *Mycobacterium tuberculosis*. *J. Cell Biochem.* **2019**, *120*, 12197–12207. [CrossRef]
27. Rifat, D.; Belchis, D.A.; Karakousis, P.C. SenX3-independent contribution of *regX3* to *Mycobacterium tuberculosis virulence*. *BMC Microbiol.* **2014**. [CrossRef]
28. White, D.W.; Elliott, S.R.; Odean, E.; Bemis, L.T.; Tischler, A.D. *Mycobacterium tuberculosis* Pst/SenX3-RegX3 regulates membrane vesicle production independently of ESX-5 activity. *MBio* **2018**, *9*. [CrossRef]
29. Freeman, Z.N.; Dorus, S.; Waterfield, N.R. The KdpD/KdpE two-component system: Integrating K+ homeostasis and virulence. *PLoS Pathog.* **2013**, *9*, e1003201. [CrossRef]
30. Njoroge, J.W.; Gruber, C.; Sperandio, V. The interacting Cra and KdpE regulators are involved in the expression of multiple virulence factors in enterohemorrhagic Escherichia coli. *J. Bacteriol.* **2013**, *195*, 2499–2508. [CrossRef]
31. Parker, C.T.; Russell, R.; Njoroge, J.W.; Jimenez, A.G.; Taussig, R.; Sperandio, V. Genetic and mechanistic analyses of the periplasmic domain of the enterohemorrhagic *Escherichia coli* QseC histidine sensor kinase. *J. Bacteriol.* **2017**, *199*. [CrossRef]
32. Parish, T.; Smith, D.A.; Kendall, S.; Casali, N.; Bancroft, G.J.; Stoker, N.G. Deletion of two-component regulatory systems increases the virulence of *Mycobacterium tuberculosis*. *Infect. Immun.* **2003**, *71*, 1134–1140. [CrossRef]
33. Alegado, R.A.; Chin, C.-Y.; Monack, D.M.; Tan, M.-W. The two-component sensor kinase KdpD is required for *Salmonella typhimurium* colonization of Caenorhabditis elegans and survival in macrophages. *Cell Microbiol.* **2011**, *13*, 1618–1637. [CrossRef]
34. Xue, T.; You, Y.; Hong, D.; Sun, H.; Sun, B. The *Staphylococcus aureus* KdpDE two-component system couples extracellular K+ sensing and Agr signaling to infection programming. *Infect. Immun.* **2011**, *79*, 2154–2167. [CrossRef]
35. Feinbaum, R.L.; Urbach, J.M.; Liberati, N.T.; Djonovic, S.; Adonizio, A.; Carvunis, A.-R. Genome-wide identification of Pseudomonas aeruginosa virulence-related genes using a Caenorhabditis elegans infection model. *PLoS Pathog.* **2012**, *8*, e1002813. [CrossRef]
36. Kornfeld, S.; Glaser, L. The enzymic synthesis of thymidine-linked sugars. I. Thymidine diphosphate glucose. *J. Biol. Chem.* **1961**, *56*, 184–185.
37. Brown, H.A.; Thoden, J.B.; Tipton, P.A.; Holden, H.M. The structure of glucose-1-phosphate thymidylyltransferase from *Mycobacterium tuberculosis* reveals the location of an essential magnesium ion in the RmlA-type enzymes. *Protein Sci.* **2018**. [CrossRef] [PubMed]
38. Qu, H.; Xin, Y.; Dong, X.; Ma, Y. An rmlA gene encoding D-glucose-1-phosphate thymidylyltransferase is essential for mycobacterial growth. *FEMS Microbiol. Lett.* **2007**. [CrossRef]
39. Kantardjieff, K.A.; Kim, C.-Y.; Naranjo, C.; Waldo, G.S.; Lekin, T.; Segelke, B.W. *Mycobacterium tuberculosis* RmlC epimerase (Rv3465): A promising drug-target structure in the rhamnose pathway. *Acta Crystallogr. Sect. D Biol. Crystallogr.* **2004**, *60*, 895–902. [CrossRef] [PubMed]
40. Chaudhari, N.M.; Gupta, V.K.; Dutta, C. BPGA- an ultra-fast pan-genome analysis pipeline. *Sci. Rep.* **2016**, *6*, 24373. [CrossRef]
41. Edgar, R.C. Search and clustering orders of magnitude faster than BLAST. *Bioinformatics* **2010**, *26*, 2460–2461. [CrossRef]
42. Rizwan, M.; Naz, A.; Ahmad, J.; Naz, K.; Obaid, A.; Parveen, T. VacSol: A high throughput in silico pipeline to predict potential therapeutic targets in prokaryotic pathogens using subtractive reverse vaccinology. *BMC Bioinform.* **2017**, *18*, 106. [CrossRef] [PubMed]

43. Nazir, Z.; Afridi, S.G.; Shah, M.; Shams, S.; Khan, A. Reverse vaccinology and subtractive genomics-based putative vaccine targets identification for *Burkholderia pseudomallei* Bp1651. *Microb. Pathog.* **2018**, *125*, 219–229.
44. Luo, H.; Lin, Y.; Gao, F.; Zhang, C.-T.; Zhang, R. DEG 10, an update of the database of essential genes that includes both protein-coding genes and noncoding genomic elements. *Nucleic Acids Res.* **2014**, *42*, D574–D580. [CrossRef] [PubMed]
45. Chen, L.; Yang, J.; Yu, J.; Yao, Z.; Sun, L.; Shen, Y. VFDB: A reference database for bacterial virulence factors. *Nucleic Acids Res.* **2005**, *33*, D325–D328. [CrossRef] [PubMed]
46. Zhou, C.E.; Smith, J.; Lam, M.; Zemla, A.; Dyer, M.D.; Slezak, T. MvirDB—A microbial database of protein toxins, virulence factors and antibiotic resistance genes for bio-defence applications. *Nucleic Acids Res.* **2007**, *35*, D391–D394. [CrossRef] [PubMed]
47. Peterson, J.W. Bacterial pathogenesis. In *Medical Microbiology*, 4th ed.; University of Texas Medical Branch at Galveston: Galveston, TX, USA, 1996.
48. Gasteiger, E.; Hoogland, C.; Gattiker, A.; Wilkins, M.R.; Appel, R.D.; Bairoch, A. Protein identification and analysis tools on the ExPASy server. In *The Proteomics Protocols Handbook*; Springer: Berlin/Heidelberg, Germany, 2005; pp. 571–607.
49. Chawley, P.; Samal, H.B.; Prava, J.; Suar, M.; Mahapatra, R.K. Comparative genomics study for identification of drug and vaccine targets in Vibrio cholerae: MurA ligase as a case study. *Genomics* **2014**, *103*, 83–93. [CrossRef]
50. Azam, S.S.; Shamim, A. An insight into the exploration of druggable genome of *Streptococcus gordonii* for the identification of novel therapeutic candidates. *Genomics* **2014**, *104*, 203–214. [CrossRef] [PubMed]
51. Moriya, Y.; Itoh, M.; Okuda, S.; Yoshizawa, A.C.; Kanehisa, M. KAAS: An automatic genome annotation and pathway reconstruction server. *Nucleic Acids Res.* **2007**, *35*, W182–W185. [CrossRef]
52. Wishart, D.S.; Feunang, Y.D.; Guo, A.C.; Lo, E.J.; Marcu, A.; Grant, J.R. DrugBank 5.0: A major update to the DrugBank database for 2018. *Nucleic Acids Res.* **2017**, *46*, D1074–D1082. [CrossRef]
53. Mondal, S.I.; Ferdous, S.; Jewel, N.A.; Akter, A.; Mahmud, Z.; Islam, M.M. Identification of potential drug targets by subtractive genome analysis of *Escherichia coli* O157: H7: An in silico approach. *Adv. Appl. Bioinforma. Chem. AABC* **2015**, *8*, 49. [CrossRef]
54. Berman, H.M.; Westbrook, J.; Feng, Z.; Gilliland, G.; Bhat, T.N.; Weissig, H. The protein data bank. *Nucleic Acids Res.* **2000**, *28*, 235–242. [CrossRef] [PubMed]
55. Roy, A.; Kucukural, A.; Zhang, Y. I-TASSER: A unified platform for automated protein structure and function prediction. *Nat. Protoc.* **2010**, *5*, 725. [CrossRef] [PubMed]
56. Zhang, Y. I-TASSER server for protein 3D structure prediction. *BMC Bioinform.* **2008**, *9*, 40. [CrossRef] [PubMed]
57. Dallakyan, S.; Olson, A.J. Small-molecule library screening by docking with PyRx. In *Chemical Biology*; Humana Press: New York, NY, USA, 2015; pp. 243–250.
58. Trott, O.; Olson, A.J. AutoDock Vina: Improving the speed and accuracy of docking with a new scoring function, efficient optimization, and multithreading. *J. Comput. Chem.* **2010**, *31*, 455–461. [CrossRef]

3

Oxidative Phosphorylation—An Update on a New, Essential Target Space for Drug Discovery in *Mycobacterium tuberculosis*

Caroline Shi-Yan Foo [1], Kevin Pethe [2,*] and Andréanne Lupien [3,4,*]

1 Laboratory of Virology and Chemotherapy, Rega Institute, Leuven 3000, Belgium; caroline.foo@kuleuven.be
2 Lee Kong Chian School of Medicine and School of Biological Sciences, Nanyang Technological University, Singapore 636921, Singapore
3 Infectious Diseases and Immunity in Global Health Program, Research Institute of the McGill University Health Centre, Montreal, QC H4A 3J1, Canada
4 McGill International TB Centre, Montreal, QC H4A 3J1, Canada
* Correspondence: kevin.pethe@ntu.edu.sg (K.P.); andreanne.lupien@mail.mcgill.ca (A.L.)

Abstract: New drugs with new mechanisms of action are urgently required to tackle the global tuberculosis epidemic. Following the FDA-approval of the ATP synthase inhibitor bedaquiline (Sirturo®), energy metabolism has become the subject of intense focus as a novel pathway to exploit for tuberculosis drug development. This enthusiasm stems from the fact that oxidative phosphorylation (OxPhos) and the maintenance of the transmembrane electrochemical gradient are essential for the viability of replicating and non-replicating *Mycobacterium tuberculosis* (*M. tb*), the etiological agent of human tuberculosis (TB). Therefore, new drugs targeting this pathway have the potential to shorten TB treatment, which is one of the major goals of TB drug discovery. This review summarises the latest and key findings regarding the OxPhos pathway in *M. tb* and provides an overview of the inhibitors targeting various components. We also discuss the potential of new regimens containing these inhibitors, the flexibility of this pathway and, consequently, the complexity in targeting it. Lastly, we discuss opportunities and future directions of this drug target space.

Keywords: *Mycobacterium tuberculosis*; energy metabolism; electron transport chain; oxidative phosphorylation; tuberculosis; drug discovery; bedaquiline; Q203

---

1. Introduction

Tuberculosis (TB) continues to have a significant global burden by remaining one of the top ten killers worldwide and the leading cause of death due to a single infectious agent [1]. The causative agent, *Mycobacterium tuberculosis* (*M. tb*), has evolved to adapt to a range of environmental stresses encountered during infection, giving rise to sub-populations of bacteria in heterogenous metabolic states, from actively replicating, to slow-growing, and dormant, non-replicating bacteria [2]. Conventional anti-TB drugs primarily target processes required for cell growth and replication, and are less efficacious against non-replicating bacteria, resulting in lengthy treatments in both drug-susceptible (DS-TB) and drug-resistant TB (DR-TB) cases [1,3]. In addition, current treatments for DR-TB are associated with low cure rates and toxicity [4–6]. Therefore, the successful elimination of the disease requires the development of new anti-TB drugs ideally active against non-replicating bacterial subpopulations and drug-resistant strains.

A new target space that has garnered increasing interest is energy metabolism, and in particular, the oxidative phosphorylation (OxPhos) pathway. The first clinical validation of this pathway as a mycobacterial drug target occurred in 2012, with the FDA approval of bedaquiline (BDQ) for treating

DR-TB by targeting the mycobacterial F_1F_0 ATP synthase [7]. This has been followed by the regulatory approvals of nitroimidazoles delamanid (Deltyba; DEL) and pretomanid (PA-824) [8,9], with the demonstration of PA-824 killing non-replicating *M. tb* by inhibition of the respiratory cytochromes through the release of nitric oxide (NO) [10]. Additionally, Telacebec (Q203), which is currently in Phase 2 clinical trials, targets the primary terminal oxidase cytochrome bcc-aa3 complex (Cyt-bcc-aa3) of *M. tb* [11,12]. Altogether, this highlights the vulnerability of energy metabolism in this pathogen and the sensitivity of components of the OxPhos pathway to specific chemical inhibition. Despite the high degree of conservation of this pathway between prokaryotes and eukaryotes, the ability to specifically target mycobacterial components without affecting the human mitochondrial counterparts has alleviated safety concerns, opening up a new and attractive target space for drug discovery.

From a biological viewpoint, this pathway is promising as a drug target space for several reasons. Whereas substrate-level phosphorylation can provide a sufficient amount of energy for replication in many bacteria, *M. tb* is dependent on the more energetically-efficient OxPhos to sustain growth [13–15]. This is probably linked to the absence of a NADH-dependent lactate dehydrogenase in mycobacteria, which would limit efficient fermentation [16,17]. During the OxPhos process, electrons are transferred from electron donors of central metabolism to oxygen through the electron transport chain (ETC). The energy released in this transfer is conserved by the proton-pumping components of the ETC, generating an electrochemical gradient in the form of a proton motive force (PMF).

This stored energy is then mined through the ATP synthase as protons flow back down the gradient to yield ATP. Since a sustained PMF and ATP replenishment are essential even for the viability of non-replicating *M. tb* [18–21], it is believed that inhibition of the OxPhos pathway is an effective strategy to eradicate non-replicating subpopulations, thereby shortening future treatment durations. Moreover, since drug efflux pumps are energy-dependent in actively transporting drugs out of the bacterial cell, perturbation of the PMF and ATP levels may interfere with their function as well [13]. It has been demonstrated that efflux pump activities play a significant role in drug susceptibility of *M. tb* [22–27] and, therefore, perturbation of the OxPhos pathway may indirectly aid in overcoming issues of efflux-pump mediated drug resistance.

In light of these significant interests in targeting energy metabolism in mycobacteria, this review aims to (1) summarise key findings of the main components comprising the OxPhos pathway of *M. tb*, (2) provide an overview of validated inhibitors of this pathway which are either in the discovery stage, in clinical development, or have been approved, (3) discuss the potential of new regimens containing these inhibitors, (4) highlight possible concerns in targeting this pathway, and (5) discuss future opportunities and directions for drug development in this space.

2. Main Components of the OxPhos Pathway in *M. tb*

The ETC of *M. tb* comprises nine primary dehydrogenases, which fuel the respiratory chain as electron donors, and four-terminal oxidoreductases, which catalyse the transfer of electrons to terminal electron acceptors such as oxygen [14]. The lipoquinone, menaquinone (MK), serves as the intermediary electron carrier between the primary dehydrogenases and terminal oxidoreductases. In the following section, we summarise the main components of the pathway against which inhibitors have been discovered and those which are potentially suitable drug targets. In particular, this includes the NADH dehydrogenases, succinate dehydrogenase, the MK biosynthesis pathway, the two terminal oxidases, ATP synthase and the PMF (Figure 1).

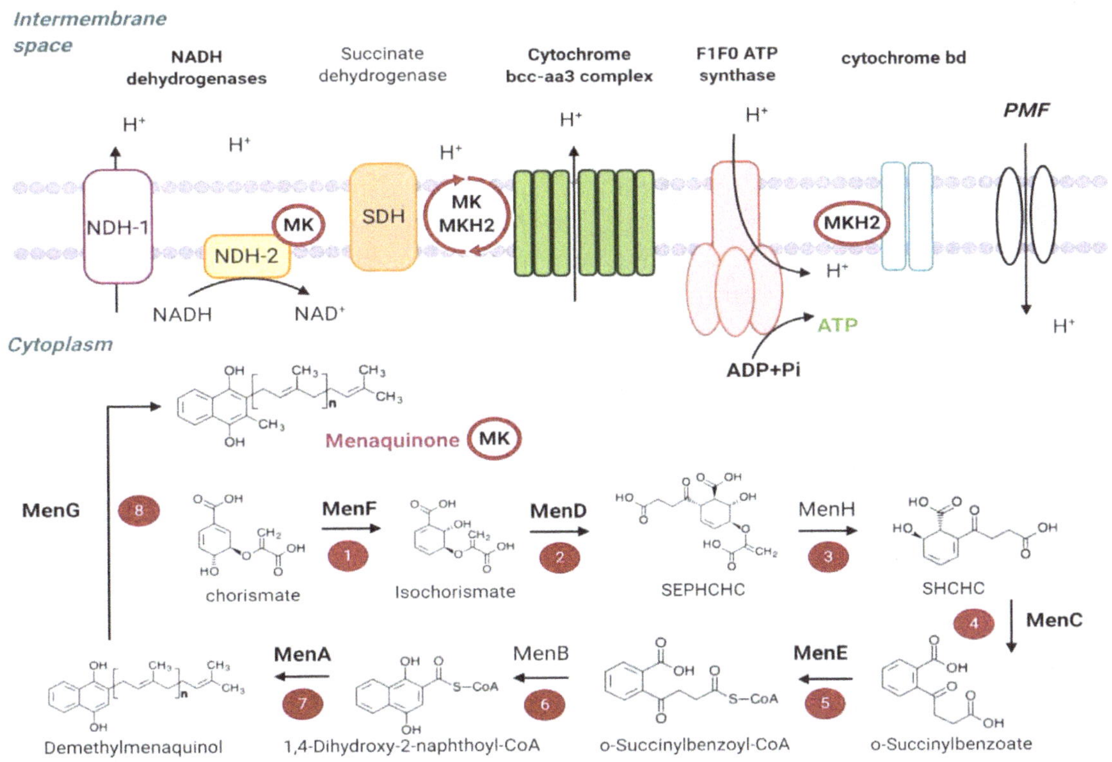

Figure 1. Schematic representation of the *Mycobacterium tuberculosis* (*M. tb*) electron transport chain (ETC) and menaquinone (MK) biosynthesis pathway. Electrons provided by NADH are fuelled to the ETC by the NADH dehydrogenases (mainly NDH-2 in *M. tb*), leading to the reduction of menaquinone (MKH2). MK is the sole carrier of electrons across the ETC and eight main enzymes are involved in its biosynthesis. The succinate dehydrogenases Sdh1 and Sdh2 also contribute to the reduction of the menaquinone pool. Electrons from the menaquinone pool are then transferred to one of the terminal oxidases, the proton-pumping Cyt-bcc-aa3 or the Cyt-bd oxidase, both of which catalyse the reduction of oxygen to water. Along the respiratory chain, protons are pumped across the membrane, which generate the proton motive force (PMF) that is then used by the F_1F_0 ATP synthase to produce ATP.

2.1. NADH Dehydrogenases

M. tb possesses three membrane-bound NADH dehydrogenases that are capable of transferring electrons to MK with the oxidation of NADH to NAD+. There is a proton-translocating type I NADH dehydrogenase (NDH-1) and two non-proton-translocating type II NADH dehydrogenases (NDH-2) [28]. NDH-2 has been chemically validated as a drug target in *M. tb* [28–30]. Unlike NDH-1, it is absent in the mammalian genome, which is an advantage to develop specific inhibitors. NDH-1 is encoded by the nuo operon, NuoA-NuoN, (rv3145-rv3158) and the two NDH-2 are identified as Ndh (encoded by ndh = rv1854c) and NdhA (encoded by ndhA = rv0392c) [17,28]. High-throughput transposon mutagenesis studies suggested that NDH-1 and NdhA are dispensable for growth, whereas Ndh is essential in vitro and in vivo [31–33]. However, recent studies have clarified the redundancy and essentiality of the NADH dehydrogenases. Detailed gene-deletion and gene-silencing studies of nuo, ndh, and ndhA performed by Vilcheze et al., established that individually, none of the NADH dehydrogenases are essential in vitro or in vivo [34]. Beites et al. further demonstrated that NDH-2 enzymes are jointly essential for growth in the presence of long-chain fatty acids, but are dispensable for growth on some carbon sources such as glycerol [35]. Moreover, a strain deficient for NDH-2 activity is only mildly attenuated in mice [35]. Both studies agree that while *M. tb* requires at least one non-proton-pumping NDH-2 enzyme for growth, chemically targeting NDH-2 alone will likely be inefficacious, but is conceivable as part of a rational drug combination.

2.2. *Succinate Dehydrogenase*

Succinate dehydrogenase (SDH), also known as complex II of the ETC, couples the oxidation of succinate to fumarate with the reduction of MK to menaquinol (MKH2) in *M. tb* [36]. This complex directly connects the tricarboxylic acid cycle and the OxPhos pathway, thereby playing a critical role in bacterial carbon metabolism and respiration [37]. Despite its significance, there has been a general reluctance to develop inhibitors against this complex due to the presence of a mammalian counterpart and the presence of two isotypes [38]. *M. tb* possesses two canonical SDH enzymes, Sdh1 and Sdh2, and an additional reversible fumarate reductase that can catalyse the reaction in both directions [39]. Independent transposon-site hybridization screens in *M. tb* suggest that Sdh1 is essential for optimal growth under aerobic conditions [32], whereas Sdh2 seems to play a more significant role in the growth arrest and dormancy of *M. tb* during its transition from aerobic to hypoxic conditions [40].

SDH enzymes also appear to function as an important regulator of respiration in *M. tb*. The deletion of sdh1 results in perturbation of respiration, leading to an increased rate of oxygen consumption which prevented recovery of *M. tb* from the stationary phase [41]. While the functional redundancy of these enzymes remains to be fully clarified, it is established that the SDH enzymes in *M. tb* are phylogenetically and biochemically distinct from each other, as well as from the mammalian complex [14,42,43]. On this basis, it would be theoretically possible to selectively inhibit the mycobacterial SDHs without off-target effects, although functional redundancy and structural differences between the mycobacterial SDHs would pose a challenge.

2.3. *Menaquinone (MK) Biosynthesis*

As the sole lipoquinone in mycobacteria, MK has a central and essential role in OxPhos [44,45]. Its biosynthetic pathway is a highly attractive drug target space as it is absent in humans, and has been demonstrated to be critical for maintaining mycobacterial survival under aerobic and anaerobic conditions [46]. In *M. tb*, the biosynthesis of MK mirrors that of *Escherichia coli*, in which the pathway has been better characterised [45]. Eight enzymes (MenF, MenD, MenH, MenC, MenE, MenB, MenA and MenG) are involved in the pathway, with MenF catalysing the first committed step of the conversion of chorismate [14]. Not all of the genes encoding for the MK synthesis pathway seem to be essential. Through initial transposon studies and confirmation by high-resolution phenotypic profiling experiments, most MK biosynthesis enzymes have been reported to be essential via transposon mutagenesis in H37Rv for *M. tb* growth, except for MenF, whose deletion resulted in a growth defect in *M. tb* [31–33].

Small molecules inhibiting MenD, MenE, MenB, MenA and MenG, and have been reported [47–51]. MenD is a thiamine diphosphate-dependent enzyme which catalyses the second step of MK biosynthesis. It uses 2-oxoglutarate and isochorismate for the synthesis of 2-Succinyl-5-enolpyruvyl-6-hydroxy-3-cyclohexene-1-carboxylate (SEPHCHC). MenE encodes for an o-succinylbenzoate-CoA ligase that converts o-succinylbenzoate (OSB) to OSB-CoA, and is the fifth step of MK biosynthesis in *M. tb*. It is responsible for the addition of a CoA group via an OSB-AMP intermediate [50]. MenB encodes for a 1,4-dihydroxy-2-naphthoyl-CoA (DHNA-CoA) synthase that catalyses the formation of DHNA-CoA from o-succinylbenzoate-CoA and is the sixth step of the MK biosynthesis [52]. MenA encodes for a DHNA-octaprenyltransferase, which is involved in the seventh step of the MK biosynthesis. It catalyses the conversion of 1,4-dihydroxy-2-naphthoate (DHNA) to demethylmenaquinone (DMK), and uses a variety of allylic isoprenyl diphosphates as substrates, requiring at least three isoprene units [46,49]. Bacterial MenA was reported to be homologous to the eukaryotic UbiA [53]. Additionally known as UbiE, MenG (rv0558) catalyses the methylation of DMK-9 using S-adenosylmethionine to form MK [54]. This reaction is the last step of MK biosynthesis in *M. tb*. That these enzymes of the MK biosynthesis pathway can be pharmacologically inhibited demonstrate their essentiality and highlight their potential as drug targets.

2.4. Terminal Oxidases

MKH2 is reoxidised with the transfer of electrons to branched routes of terminal respiratory oxidases or reductases. In *M. tb*, there are two terminal oxidases present which catalyse the four-electron reduction of oxygen to water, namely the proton-pumping Cyt-bcc-aa3 supercomplex and an alternative cytochrome bd oxidase (Cyt-bd) [39].

Cytochromes bcc and aa3 (also known as complexes III and IV) are encoded by qcrCAB and ctaB, ctaC, ctaD, ctaE, respectively, and form a supercomplex of Cyt-bcc-aa3 in mycobacteria [55–57]. As this complex is proton-pumping, it is energetically more favourable for optimum growth and seems to act as the primary respiratory route in *M. tb* under aerobic conditions [15]. Through inducible repression and genetic deletion, elegant studies revealed that, while the Cyt-bcc-aa3 complex is required for optimal *M. tb* growth rates in vitro and in mice, it is not strictly essential for growth nor persistence as long as the alternate Cyt-bd oxidase is expressed [35].

Following the first purification and initial characterisation of a hybrid respiratory complex consisting of *M. tb* cytochrome bcc and *Mycobacterium smegmatis* (*M. smeg*) cytochrome aa3 [56], the crystal structure of the Cyt-bcc-aa3 supercomplex of *M. smeg* has been recently solved by cryo-EM by two independent groups to a resolution of 3.3–3.5 Å [57,58]. This has enabled the full visualization of the supercomplex with its associated subunits, including cytochrome bcc subunits QcrC, QcrA (the Rieske iron-sulphur protein) and QcrB in a dimeric form with their respective prosthetic groups [57,58]. These studies shed light on the direct internal transfer of electrons from MKH2 to oxygen without the need for a separate cytochrome c electron shuttle as in other respiratory systems, and identifies novel subunits that contribute to the stability of the supercomplex, including an enzymatically active superoxide dismutase (SOD1). The presence of SOD1 in the bcc-aa3 supercomplex suggests the need for efficient ROS detoxification at a site dealing with a high amount of oxygen. Altogether, the structural information obtained from these studies is possibly relevant for further rationale-based TB drug discovery studies for inhibitors of this complex due to the high degree of sequence similarity of the quinol oxidation (Qp) site between *M. tb* and *M. smeg*, the site of inhibition of the TB drug candidate Q203 and other known QcrB inhibitors discovered thus far.

The bacterial-specific Cyt-bd is less characterised in *M. tb* [59]. The pathogen harbours genes encoding the two main subunits, CydA and CydB, and a putative ABC transporter CydDC, which has been proposed to be important for the assembly of the cytochrome in *E. coli* [60–63]. Genetic inactivation of the Cyt-bd-encoding genes in *M. tb* presented no loss of bacterial fitness and did not significantly impact ATP homeostasis under standard aerobic growth conditions, nor did it affect growth and persistence of *M. tb* in mice [35,64,65]. To date, two structures of the Cyt-bd have been reported in *Geobacillus thermodenitrificans* and *E. coli* [66,67], and these studies have highlighted the structural diversity within this family of enzymes. Given the low sequence homology of mycobacterial Cyt-bd to that of *G. thermodenitrificans* and *E. coli* [68], further structural studies of these enzymes in mycobacteria would be necessary to aid in drug development against the *M. tb* Cyt-bd oxidase. While structural and biochemical information are currently lacking for the *M. tb* Cyt-bd, similarities can be drawn with the *E. coli* homologue, which exhibits a very high affinity to oxygen and is non-proton-pumping, making it less efficient energetically compared to proton-pumping oxidases [69–71]. These characteristics would indicate a role of this terminal oxidase in bacterial survival in environments of low oxygen tension and protection against oxidative stress, even though it appears to function efficiently under normoxic conditions as well [65]. The upregulation of the cydAB operon has been reported for *M. tb* under hypoxia and in the presence of NO, as well as during the chronic phase of infection in mice [72–74], and when the function of the Cyt-bcc-aa3 is compromised [32,59–61,75–77].

2.5. ATP Synthase

M. tb possesses a F_1F_0 ATP synthase consisting of two functional domains, a membrane-embedded F0 unit and an external F1 domain, which is linked by central and periphery stalks on which F0 rotates [78]. This rotation is powered by a flow of protons down the electrochemical gradient of the PMF, and drives a cycle of conformational changes in the catalytic F1 domain, resulting in successive ADP binding and entrapment, ADP phosphorylation to form ATP and ATP release [79]. Conventionally, the ATP synthase is also capable of ATPase activity when intracellular ATP levels are high and the PMF is low, hydrolysing ATP while pumping protons across the cytoplasm to re-energise the PMF [80]. In mycobacteria however, the ATP synthase has been characteristically observed to have suppressed ATP hydrolysis activity, which has been postulated to be an adaptation to conserving ATP under low oxygen tensions [39,78,81,82].

In *M. tb*, the F_1F_0 ATP synthase is encoded by the atpBEFHAGDC operon and is essential for the viability of replicating and non-growing *M. tb* [31–33,83], highlighting its critical role in ATP production and in maintaining a respiratory electron flow in all metabolic states [84]. Even though intracellular ATP levels in non-replicating *M. tb* are significantly reduced compared to replicating bacilli, basal levels of ATP are still maintained in non-replicating states [19,21]. The essentiality of the ATP synthase in these conditions is underlined by the fact that its pharmacological inhibition by BDQ, a specific ATP synthase inhibitor, kills hypoxic, non-replicating *M. tb* [83].

Interestingly, the mycobacterial ATP synthase is deprived of efficient ATP hydrolysis activity [82]. As a step towards uncovering the molecular basis of the extreme latency of ATP hydrolysis, a crystal structure of the *M. smeg* catalytic F1 domain revealed similarities with the *Caldalkalibacillus thermarum* F1-ATPase, which also hydrolyses ATP poorly [85]. This is likely due to an arrest in the catalytic rotary cycle of the F1 component, resulting in the inability to release products of ATP hydrolysis. The ε-subunit of the F1 module of *M. tb*, whose structure has been recently solved by nuclear magnetic resonance (NMR), has been implicated in the regulation of ATP hydrolysis. The removal of its C-terminal resulted in an increased ATP hydrolysis rate and decreased ATP synthesis [86]. Furthermore, Saw et al., demonstrated that this site is amenable to chemical inhibition in *M. smeg* by epigallocatechin gallate, the most abundant catechin in green tea [87]. Other subunits involved in the regulation of ATP hydrolysis include the γ- and α- subunits of the F1 module [88,89]. Altogether, these advances in the understanding of the F_1F_0 ATP synthase aid in identifying new, specific inhibitors that either block *de novo* ATP synthesis and/or activate ATP hydrolysis, with the aim of depleting the residual pool of ATP in *M. tb*.

2.6. Proton Motive Force (PMF)

As in all other bacteria, an energised cell membrane is essential for the viability and growth of *M. tb* in all metabolic states [19]. The generation and maintenance of a PMF, consisting of an electrical potential due to charge separation across the membrane and a chemical potential of protons, is, therefore, vital and occurs mainly through the proton-pumping components of the ETC [14]. A PMF of about - 110 mV has been measured both in aerobic, replicating and in hypoxic, non-growing *M. tb*, indicating that even in a non-growing state, the bacteria maintain a similarly energized membrane [19]. This PMF is less than the typical PMF range of −180 to −200 mV observed in other bacteria, a difference which has been postulated to be an adaptation to host physiological environments of low nutrient levels and/or terminal electron acceptors [39,78,90].

3. Overview of the Inhibitors Targeting the OxPhos Pathway

3.1. NADH Dehydrogenases

NADH dehydrogenases play a major role in maintaining mycobacterial respiratory chain energization by using MK as an electron carrier. NDH-1 is non-essential for mycobacterial growth and for persistence [19,34]. Therefore, no drug development is currently in progress for inhibitors of mycobacterial NDH-1 [39]. NDH-2 is widespread in bacteria and the mitochondria of fungi, plants and some protists. In some organisms, more than one copy is present [91]. Notably, NDH-2 (Ndh and NdhA) are absent in mammalian genomes, suggesting a potential leading target for anti-mycobacterial drug development.

Several inhibitors have been found to target NDH-2 in mycobacteria, including the phenothiazines, quinolinyl pyrimidines and 2-mercapto-quinazolinones (Table 1). It is also thought that NDH-2 plays a role in the reduction of the anti-leprosy drug clofazimine (CFZ), leading to the production of reactive oxygen species (ROS) and, consequently, its bactericidal activity against *M. tb* [92]. However, CFZ is still potent against a *M. tb* Δndh-2 mutant strain, indicating that CFZ does not require activation by NDH-2 to exert its anti-mycobacterial potency [35]. Further studies will be needed to understand the mechanism of action of CFZ against mycobacteria. The CFZ analogue TBI-166 is more potent than CFZ against *M. tb in vitro*, and it is at least as potent as CFZ in acute and chronic murine models of TB while being potentially associated with less skin discoloration [93]. A study by Beites et al. demonstrated that the inactivation of both NDH-2 (Δndh-2) can be achieved in the absence of fatty acids in the growth media. Interestingly, rotenone, an inhibitor of NDH-1, has bactericidal activity against Δndh-2, which suggests that NDH-1 and NDH-2 have a redundant role in *M. tb* [35].

The phenothiazines, a class of antipsychotic drugs, including thioridazine, chlorpromazine and trifluoperazine, have been widely studied against *M. tb*. They have activity in vitro against *M. tb* with minimum inhibitory concentration (MIC) of thioridazine, chlorpromazine and trifluoperazine ranging between 5 to 32 μg/mL [94–98]. However, their limited potency coupled with an unfavourable toxicological profile preclude clinical use for TB treatment [99]. However, phenothiazines accumulate in macrophages and are particularly potent against intracellular *M. tb* [100,101]. Current efforts aim at developing new phenothiazine derivatives with improved activity against *M. tb* and reduced toxicity [102–105].

Another class of NDH-2 inhibitors is the quinolinyl pyrimidines [106]. This class of compounds was identified during an NDH-2 target-based high-throughput screening of more than 100 000 compounds. The series showed a good inhibitory range against *M. tb* in vitro, with MIC_{50} below 1 μg/mL [106]. In contrast to the phenothiazines, the quinolinyl pyrimidines series is not hemolytic.

CBR-1825 and CBR-4032 are two representatives compounds of the thioquinazoline (TQZ) and tetrahydroindazole scaffolds, respectively, that were identified in a high-throughput screen of over 800 000 compounds in mycobacterial inverted membrane vesicles (IMVs) [29]. The assay was designed to identify small-molecules interfering with ATP production. CBR-1825 and CBR-4032 had an MIC_{50} of 0.43 μM and 6.6 μM, respectively, when tested, and no apparent cytotoxicity [29]. Both compounds are bactericidal against *M. tb* in vitro and seem to perturb NADH turnover. Sequencing of three escape mutants resistant to TQZ revealed a non-synonymous mutation in the promoter region of ndhA (rv0392c), suggesting that these compounds target NDH-2.

A 2-mercapto-quinazolinones cluster of hits (1, 2, and 3) was identified in a screening of a commercial diversity library [30]. Compound 1 potently inhibiting *M. tb* growth in vitro in the low micromolar range without cytotoxicity against HepG2 cells [30]. Bioenergetic analyses conducted in cells in which the membrane potential was uncoupled from ATP production revealed a decrease in oxygen consumption rates (OCR) in response to the inhibitor, while IMVs showed mercapto-quinazolinone-dependent inhibition of ATP production when NADH was the primary electron donor of the respiratory chain. Enzyme kinetic studies further demonstrated non-competitive inhibition of recombinant *M. tb* Ndh protein [30]. Resistance to the compounds in *M. tb* was conferred by promoter mutations in ndhA. Interestingly, hypersusceptibility to this class of compounds was observed when ndhA was deleted, suggesting that NDH-1 and other electron donors cannot compensate for the inhibition of NDH-2 by 2-mercapto-quinazolinones [30]. Chemical optimisation is required to improve the pharmacokinetics (PK) properties of this interesting series [30].

Quinolinequinones (QQ) exert mycobactericidal activity through NDH-2 inhibition. Interestingly, QQ prevent the emergence of persistent cells in a time- and dose-dependant manner in *Mycobacterium bovis* BCG in vitro [107]. This scaffold is known for its anti-cancer and anti-inflammatory properties, and can be modified to give rise to derivatives with anti-mycobacterial activity [108–110]. Mulchin BJ et al. synthesised a range of 6,7-substituted-5,8-quinolinequinones, and their anti-mycobacterial activities were assessed against *M. bovis* BCG, in addition to their anti-tumour and anti-inflammatory properties [111]. Several compounds containing amine and halogen functionality exhibited tuberculostatic activity in the range 3–12.5 μg/mL [111]. The derivative QQ8c stimulated NADH oxidation in *M. tb* and *M. smeg* IMVs. Ndh overexpression enhanced the stimulation of NADH oxidation [107]. This increase in NDH-2 catalytic activity has been associated with the production of lethal concentrations of ROS. Recently, Santoso et al. synthesised a library of 32 new QQ derivatives, with one derivative (16b) showing enhanced in vitro activity against *M. tb* [112]. Activation of NADH-dependent oxygen consumption in *M. smeg* IMVs in the presence of 16b suggests that this new inhibitor has the same anti-mycobacterial mechanism of action than QQ8c [112].

Table 1. Structures of the NADH dehydrogenase inhibitors discussed in this review.

Chemical Class	Represented by	Structure	References
Riminophenazines	Clofazimine	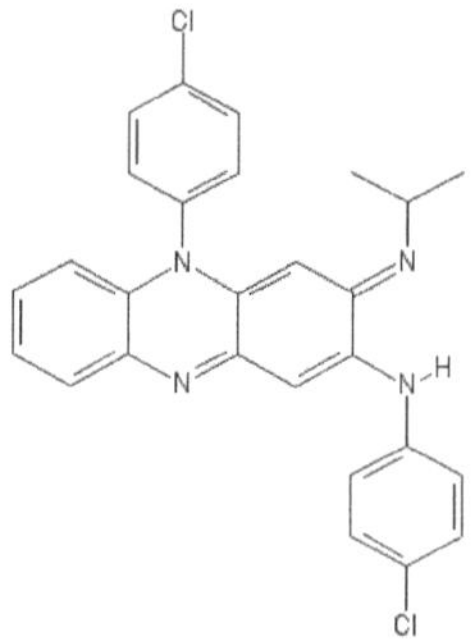	[113]
	TBI-166	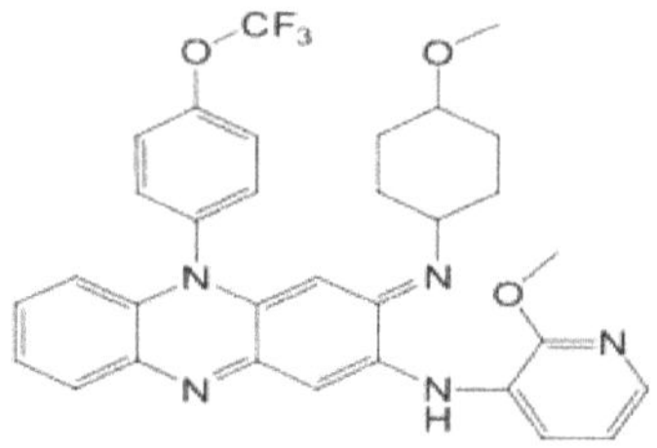	[114]
Phenothiazines	Chlorpromazine	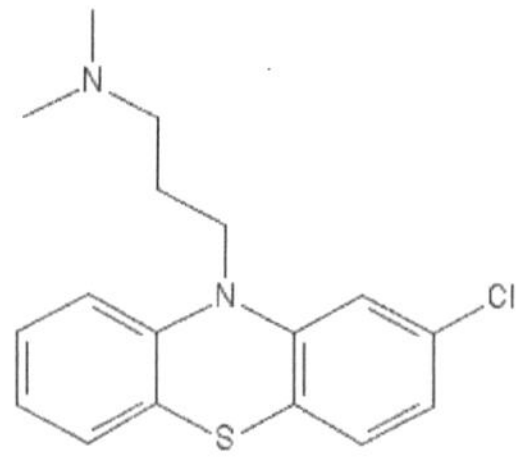	[99]
	Thioridazine	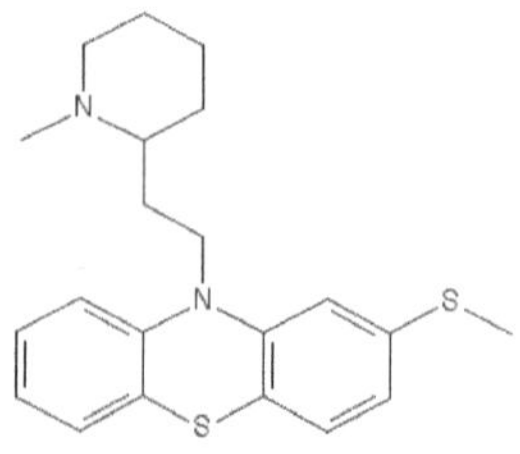	
	Trifluoperazine	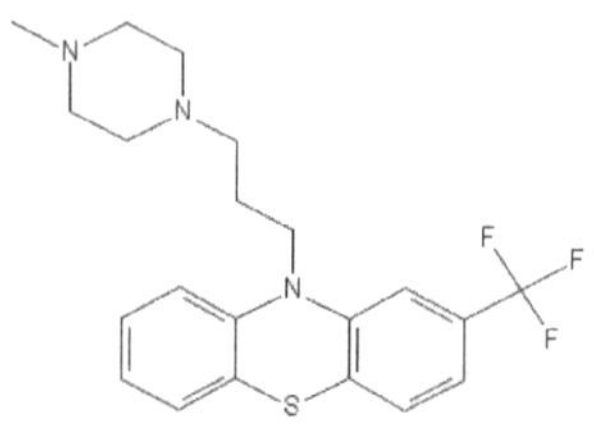	

Table 1. *Cont.*

Chemical Class	Represented by	Structure	References
Quinolinyl pyrimidines	13a	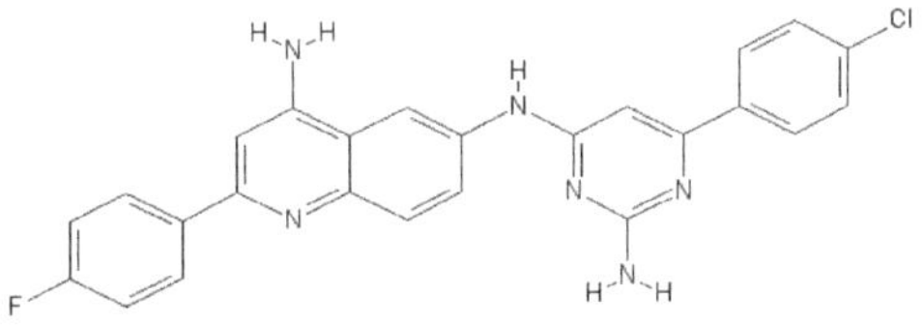	[106]
Thioquinazoline	CBR-1825	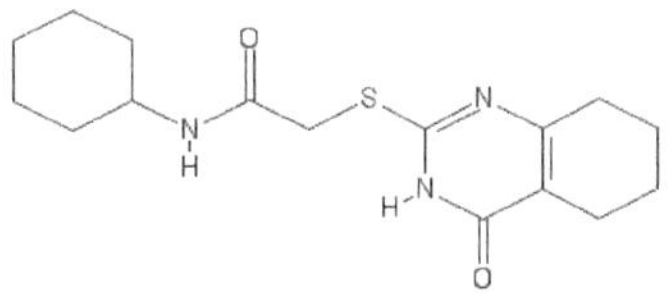	[29]
Tetrahydroindazole	CBR-4032	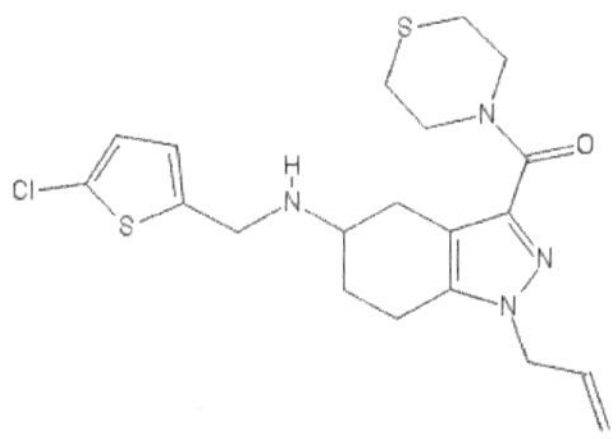	[29]
2-mercapto-quinazolinone	1	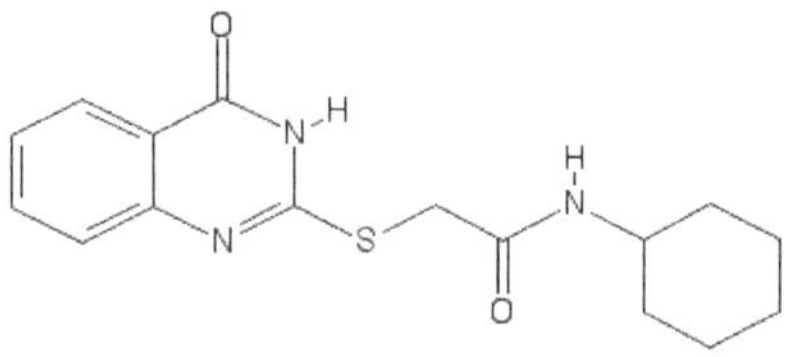	[30]
Quinolinequinones	QQ8c	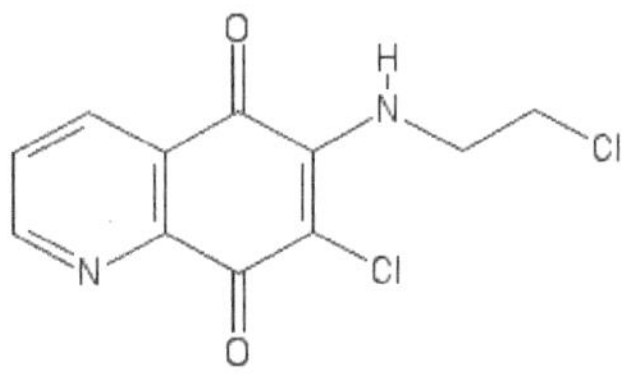	[107,111]
	16b	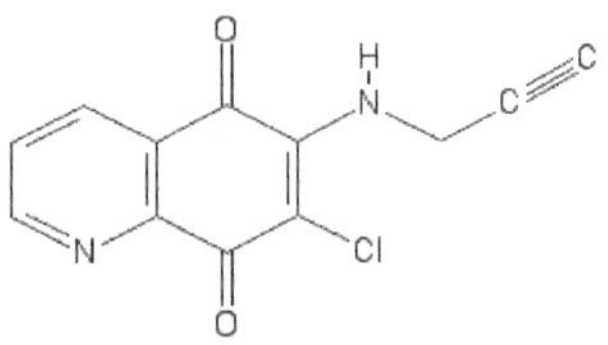	[112]

3.2. *Menaquinone (MK) Biosynthesis*

The essentiality of this pathway makes it an attractive target for anti-TB drug development. To date, chemical inhibitors of MenA, MenB, MenG, MenD and MenE have proven efficacious in inhibiting *M. tb* growth. Inhibitors of the MK biosynthesis discussed in this review are listed in Table 2.

Table 2. Menaquinone (MK) biosynthesis inhibitors discussed in this review.

Chemical Class	Represented by	Structure	Ref
	MenD inhibitors		
methyl succinylphosphonate	2	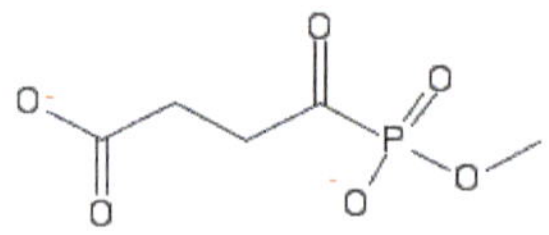	[115]
succinylphosphonate	1	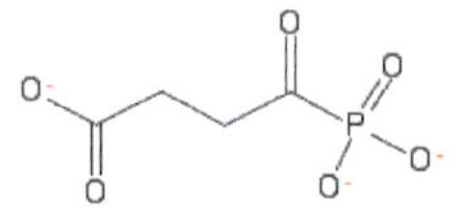	[115]
	MenE inhibitors		
vinyl sulphonamide MeOSB-AVSN	3	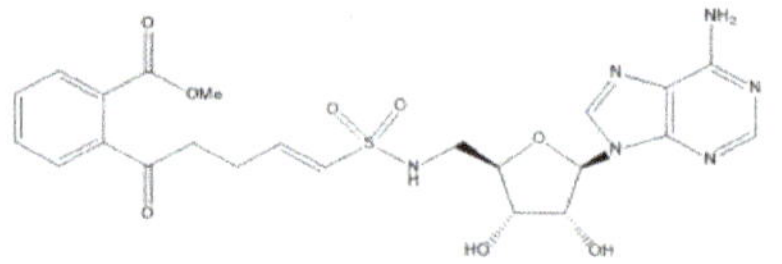	[50]
	MenA inhibitors		
benzophenone O-methyl oxime derivatives	(R)-13	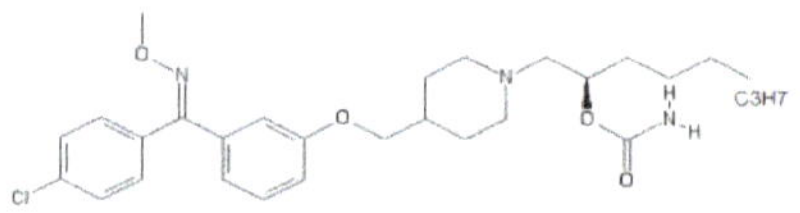	[49]
4-bromophenyl)[2-fluoro-4-[[6-(methyl-2-propenylamino) hexyl]oxy]phenyl]-methanone	Ro-48-8071	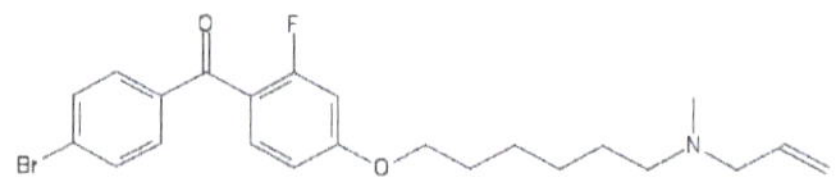	[46]
aminoalkoxydiphenylmethane	CSU-20	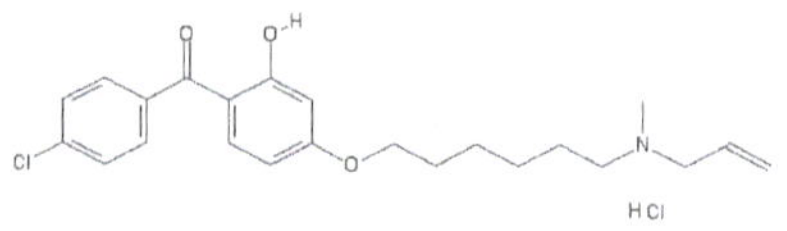	[46,116]
bicyclic inhibitors	NM-4	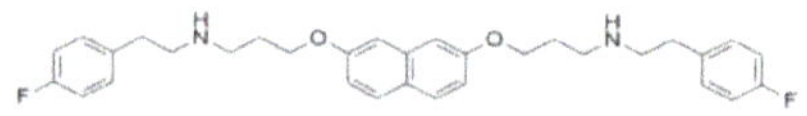	[117]
	MenG inhibitors		
diphenylborinic acid quinoline esters	4b	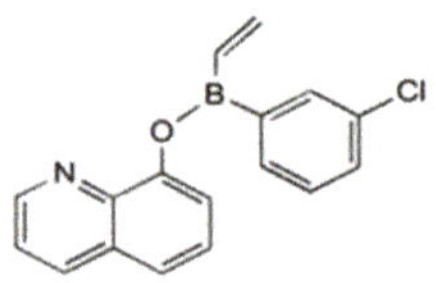	[118]
biphenyl amide	DG70	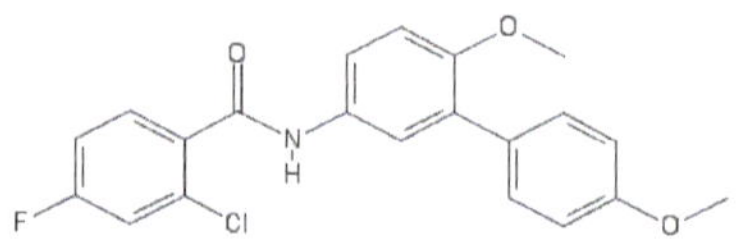	[51]

3.2.1. MenD

Studies by Fang et al. identified two compounds, methyl succinylphosphonate (2) and succinylphosphonate (1), that inhibit *M. tb* MenD at a Ki of 0.7 and 16 μM, respectively [115]. These inhibitors are structural analogues of the substrate 2-oxoglutarate and bind covalently to MenD. The resolution of the three-dimensional structure of *M. tb* MenD by NMR will support target-based drug design [119].

3.2.2. MenE

Due to the instability of OSB, efforts to create MenE inhibitors were mainly focused on the inhibition of the assembly of the OSB-AMP intermediate. Lu et al. identified three potential MenE inhibitors using the OSB as a scaffold [50,120]. In these inhibitors, the AMP moiety was replaced with a bioisosteres sulphamate, a sulphamide, and a vinyl sulphonamide group [120]. The vinyl sulphonamide compound was the most potent with IC_{50} of 5.7 μM against the purified *M. tb* MenE enzyme [50].

3.2.3. MenA

Several inhibitors have been identified to target MenA. Aurachin RE is a natural product from *Rhodococcus erythropolis* JCM6824, and harbours potent activity against a wide range of Gram-positive and Gram-negative bacteria, including *Corynebacterium glutamicum* [121]. Using the aurachin RE scaffold, Debnath et al. synthesised a series of more than 400 derivatives that were assessed for their ability to specifically inhibit the *M. tb* MenA enzyme [49]. Compounds with IC_{50} lower than 20 μM against *M. tb* and *M. smeg*, and without activity against *Staphylococcus aureus* MenA enzyme, were identified [49]. The lead compound of this series, (R)-13, had a MIC of 2.3 μg/mL against *M. tb*. The compound is also bactericidal against hypoxic, non-replicating mycobacteria, suggesting a high MK turnover rate during persistence.

Ro 48-8071, a (4-bromophenyl)[2-fluoro-4-[[6-(methyl-2-propenylamino)hexyl]oxy] phenyl]-methanone developed by Hoffman La Roche Inc is a known inhibitor of oxidosqualene cyclase, which is involved in cholesterol biosynthesis in mammalians. It is effective against *M. tb*, *M. bovis* BCG and *M. smeg* [46,53]. The target of Ro 48-8071 was inferred from metabolic labelling experiment in *M. bovis BCG* [46]. The synthesis of a neutral, apolar liquid, which was biochemically identified as MK through the incorporation of radiolabelled isoprenoid precursors and methionine, was inhibited in the presence of Ro 48-8071 [46]. Moreover, when *M. smeg* was treated with Ro 48-8071, a reduction of 2.5–3.3-fold in the concentrations of DMK-9 and MK-9 was observed, suggesting that the compound inhibits the late steps of MK biosynthesis in mycobacteria. Ro 48-8071 decreased the oxygen consumption in *M. smeg* and *M. tb*, a phenotype that was rescued by MK supplementation. To validate MenA as the direct target of Ro 48-8071, MenA activity was assessed in membranes prepared from a recombinant *E.coli* strain expressing the *M. tb* MenA [46]. An eight-fold decrease in MenA activity was observed upon treatment with Ro 48-8071, indicating that MenA is the target of this inhibitor. Structure-activity relationship (SAR) studies led to the derivative CSU-20 which has improved MIC against *M. tb* and was bactericidal against hypoxic, non-replicating mycobacteria [46]. Dhiman et al. showed that Ro 48-8071 has dual activity against MenA by behaving as a non-competitive inhibitor of the substrate DHNA, but also as a competitive inhibitor of isoprenyl diphosphate [122].

The bicyclic long-chain fatty acids 7-methoxy-2-naphthol-based inhibitors also target MenA [117,123,124]. Berube et al. tested four compounds of this series (NM-1 to NM-4) for their ability to inhibit MenA and *M. tb* growth. The most active compound, NM-4, had an MIC_{90} of 4.5 μM and was bactericidal against replicating and non-replicating *M. tb* [117]. NM-4 was synergistic with BDQ, CFZ and imidazopyridine ND-10885 in vitro against *M. tb*, with culture sterilisation observed after 21 days of incubation. This new lead is non-cytotoxic, specific for Gram-positive bacteria, and amenable to chemical optimisation, properties that could be exploited to optimise the chemical series [124]. Further characterisation work on the PK/PD properties and in vivo activity remains to be undertaken.

3.2.4. MenG

Benkovic et al. identified inhibitors of CcrM, an essential DNA methyltransferase in the α-proteobacteria *Caulobacter crescentus*, which were later demonstrated to inhibit MenH in *B. subtilis*-an orthologue of *M. tb* MenG [118]. The derivative compound 12a, a diphenylborinic acid quinoline ester, was the most active MenH inhibitor in *Bacillus subtillis*. In *M. tb*, the MICs of the derivatives range from 0.31 to 0.64 μg/mL, and to our knowledge, no further SAR and target validation studies have been performed.

Another chemical class of MenG inhibitors, the biphenyl amides, were also identified in a whole-cell screen targeting the mycobacterial respiratory pathway. 168 small molecules with anti-TB activity from GlaxoSmithKline were screened against a *M. bovis* BCG strain containing a mWasabi reporter fused to the putative promoter of cydAB, a reporter system used to identify drugs targeting respiration [51,125]. The compound GSK1733953A, also known as DG70, induced the expression of the reporter strain compared to untreated control. This bactericidal compound showed specific activity against drug-susceptible and drug-resistant *M. tb*. DG70 was bactericidal against nutrient-starved *M. tb*, which mimics a sub-population that is particularly difficult to kill [51]. MK-4 supplementation rescued the bactericidal potency of DG70, implying that the MK biosynthesis pathway is involved in the mechanism of action of this compound. Resistant mutants selected in *M. tb* H37Rv with DG70 harboured mutations V20A, F118L, W75A, and S188A in MenG, leading to high-level resistance to DG70. DG70 was also shown to block *de novo* biosynthesis of MK, highlighting its role as an inhibitor of MenG. Interestingly, this compound showed synergism with BDQ, isoniazid (INH) and rifampicin (RIF) in time-kill assays, suggesting that MenG inhibitors could be part of a potent drug combination [51].

3.3. Inhibitors of the Cyt-bcc-aa3 Complex

A number of chemically-diverse and distinct scaffolds target the *M. tb* cytochrome bcc oxidase by binding at the Qp site of the QcrB subunit, otherwise known as the stigmatellin pocket. The Qp site is one of two quinol catalytic sites on QcrB. The promiscuous nature of this target has been attributed to its localization in the bacterial membrane, as with other membrane-associated targets [54,68]. In this section, we provide an overview of chemical classes reported to inhibit the Cyt-bcc-aa3 terminal oxidase (Table 3).

Table 3. Inhibitors of the Cyt-bcc-aa3 complex and the bd oxidase discussed in this review.

Chemical Class	Represented by	Structure	Ref
	Cytochrome bcc inhibitors		
Imidazopyridines	Q203 (Telacebec)	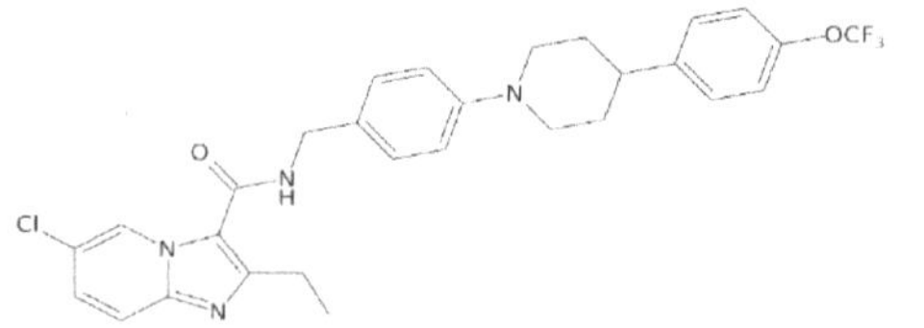	[12]
Imidazo[2,1-b]thiazole-5-carboxamide	ND-11543	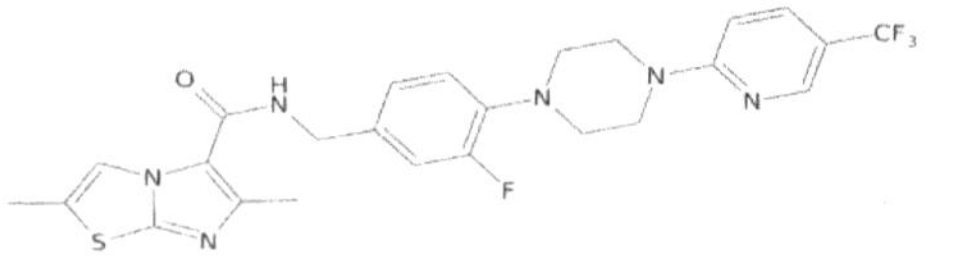	[126]
Imidazopyridine ethers	19e	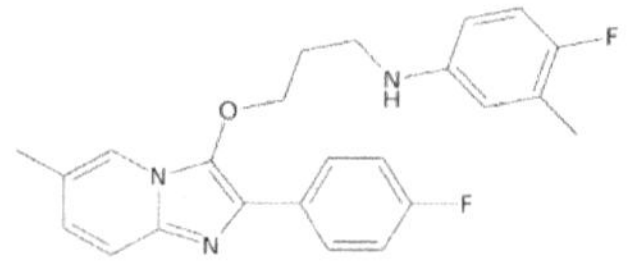	[127]
Pyrazolo[1,5-a]pyridine-3-carboxamide	TB47	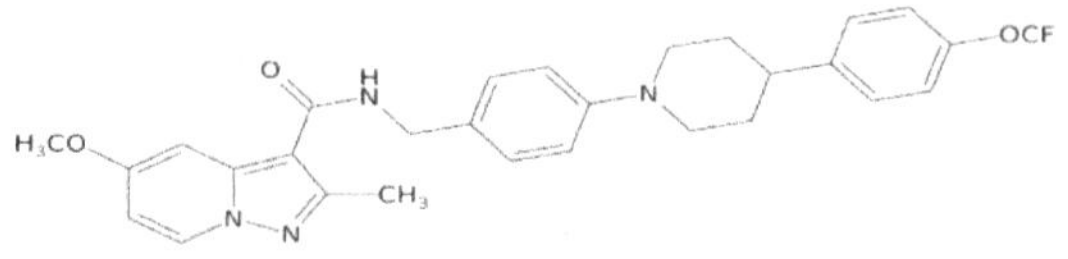	[128]

Table 3. *Cont.*

Chemical Class	Represented by	Structure	Ref
Lansoprazole sulphide (LPZS)		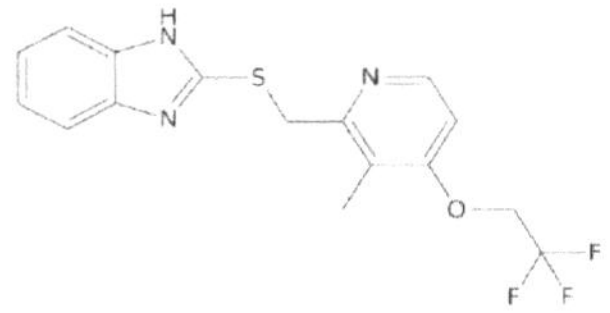	[129]
Phenoxyalkylbenzimidazole	54	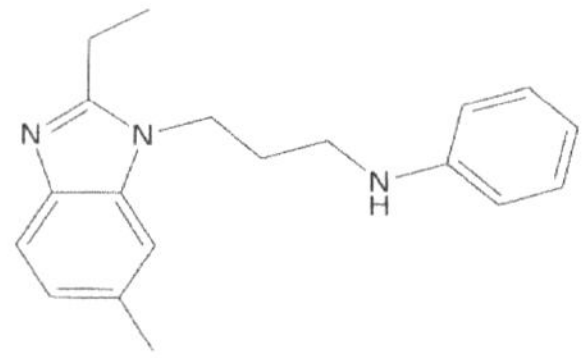	[130]
Pyrrolo[3,4-c]pyridine(2H)-dione	5h	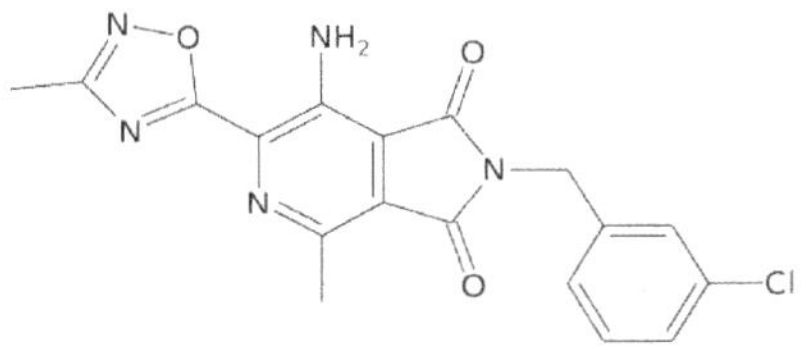	[131]
2-(quinolin-4-yloxy)acetamides	5s	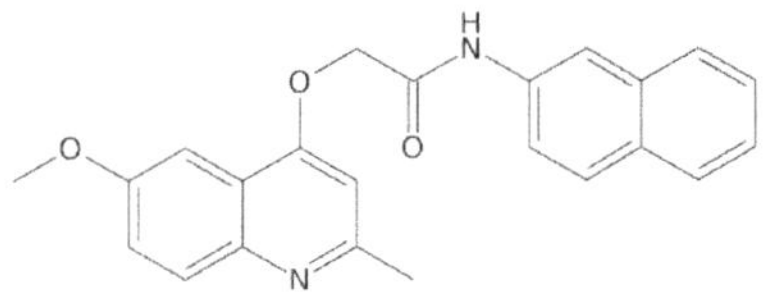	[132]
	12 n	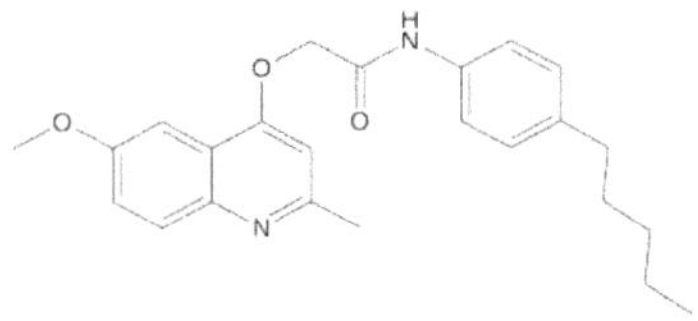	[133]
Arylvinylpiperazine amides	AX-35	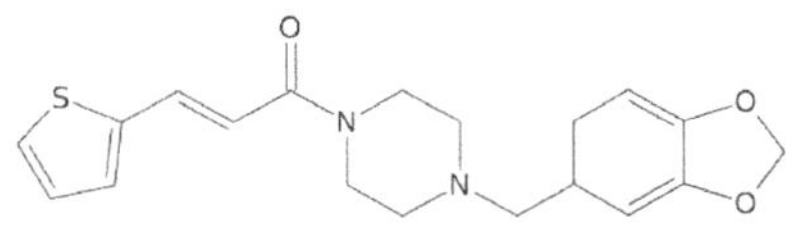	[76]
Morpholino thiophenes	37	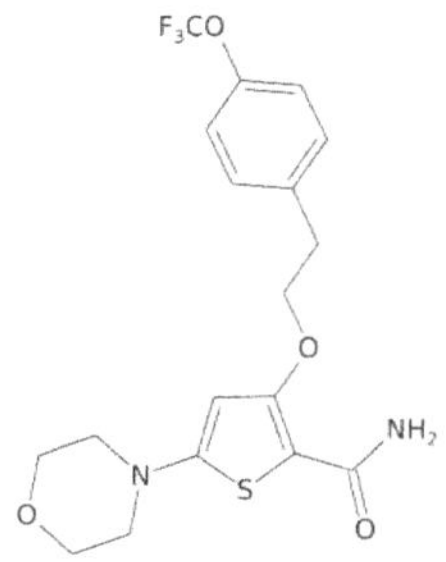	[134]
4-Amino-thieno[2,3-d]pyrimidines	CWHM-1023	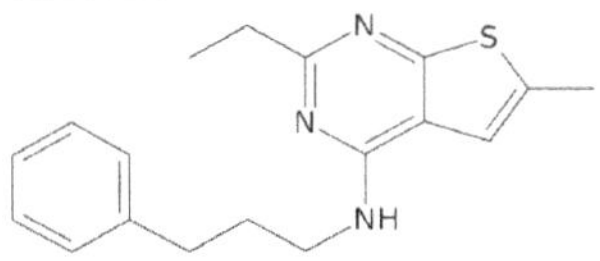	[135]

Table 3. *Cont.*

Chemical Class	Represented by	Structure	Ref
2-Ethylthio-4-methylaminoquinazolines	11726148	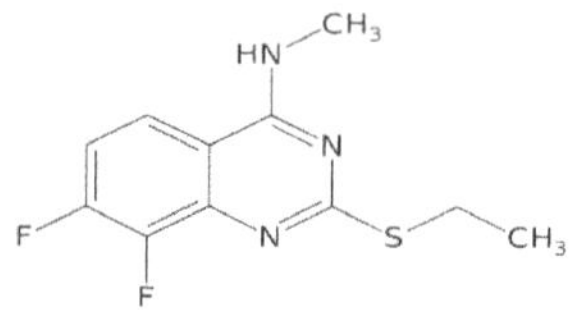	[77]
Cyt-bd inhibitor			
Aurachin D		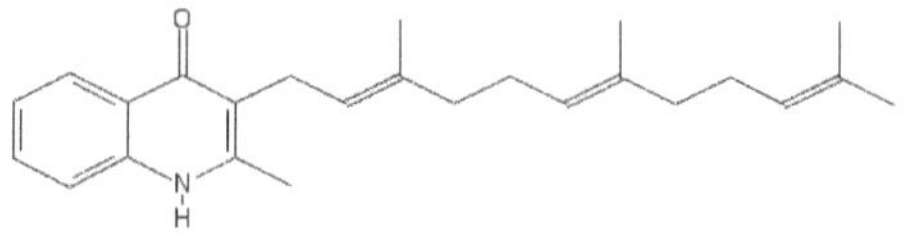	[136]

Several promising hits belonging to the chemical class of imidazopyridines (IPs) have been identified in independent screening programs [12,75,137–139]. Extensive efforts have been undertaken to optimise and to explore the SAR of this scaffold [126,140–143]. To date, the most advanced QcrB inhibitor is Q203, an IP derivative in Phase 2 clinical trials. The drug candidate was initially discovered in a phenotypic high-content screen in *M. tb*-infected macrophages and further optimised to achieve an MIC_{50} of 2.7 nM against *M. tb* H37Rv in vitro. Its activity is comparable to that of BDQ and INH in a mouse model of chronic TB infection [12]. In addition to its potency, the positive results from the Phase 1 and Phase 2a early bactericidal activity clinical trial indicate its safety and tolerability in TB patients, emphasizing the specificity of bacterial inhibition without affecting the human counterpart [144]. Resistant mutants generated to Q203 revealed amino acid mutations T313A or T313I in QcrB [12]. This interaction between Q203 and QcrB has recently been biochemically demonstrated by in-cell NMR using whole *M. smeg* cells expressing the *M. tb* QcrCAB complex and a Q203 derivative, indicating target engagement at the Qp site of QcrB [145]. While bacteriostatic on its own in *M. tb*, Q203 becomes highly bactericidal when the alternate Cyt-bd oxidase is absent, as demonstrated in *M. tb*-infected macrophages and in a mouse model of acute TB infection [65,146]. Q203 is also highly bactericidal and potent against *Mycobacterium ulcerans*, reducing bacterial load in a mouse footpad infection model of Buruli ulcer by 99.99% at a dose of 0.5 mg/kg administered three times per week for four weeks [147]. This highlights additional opportunities for repurposing QcrB inhibitors against other organisms that do not harbour functional alternative terminal oxidases, such as *M. ulcerans* and *Mycobacterium leprae*.

Extended SAR studies of IPs imidazopyridine carboxamides led to the novel scaffold imidazothiazole carboxamides (ITA), of which analogues have nanomolar potency (MIC < 10 nM) against replicating and drug-resistant *M. tb* [143]. Derivatives of this class also demonstrate intracellular activity in macrophages and in vivo [143]. Additionally, cross-resistance studies with strains harbouring QcrB mutations and dose-response studies in a *M. tb* strain without Cyt-bd oxidase indicate that these compounds target QcrB [143]. This series is promising for its tolerability and good oral bioavailability in mice [126].

Imidazopyridine ethers (IPEs) were identified from a biochemical screen of AstraZeneca's corporate compound collection aimed at identifying inhibitors of ATP homeostasis [127]. The extent of ATP synthesis inhibition, as measured in IMV of *M. smeg*, correlated well with anti-tubercular potency in *M. tb*, with a MIC of 0.03 μM for some optimised derivatives [127]. While generating resistant mutants to the series was unsuccessful, target site deconvolution through a series of biochemical tests and cell-based assays indicated that these chemical entities target the Cyt-bcc-aa3 complex. These series have been deprioritised by the group due to their poor solubility and poor PK profile [127].

Structurally similar to the IPs, the pyrazolopyridine carboxamide series were designed as novel anti-tubercular agents through a scaffold hopping strategy [148,149]. The lead compound, TB-47, is currently in early-stage development. It has activity against replicating *M. tb* in vitro with MICs of 0.016 to 0.5 μg/mL when tested against a panel of *M. tb* drug-susceptible and drug-resistant clinical isolates, and a high-selective index. Furthermore, TB-47 is well-tolerated and has good oral bioavailability in rats. While it did not display bactericidal activity alone in mouse models of acute and chronic TB infection, TB-47 potentiated the activity of pyrazinamide (PZA) and RIF during an acute TB infection in mice [128]. The authors speculated that alteration of the NADH/NAD^+ ratio triggered by QcrB inhibition sensitized the bacteria to the front-line drugs. While this hypothesis is interesting, it remains to be further explored since no positive interactions between RIF and the QcrB inhibitor Q203 in vitro have been observed [150]. Resistant mutants to TB-47 were generated in a *M. smeg* strain with a deletion of Cyt-bd oxidase, and whole-genome sequencing of the isolates revealed mutation H190Y in QcrB of *M. smeg* [128]. This residue, equivalent to H195 in *M. tb*, is located in the cd2 loop of QcrB, which is thought to interact with the Qp site [128].

A host cell-based screen of FDA-approved drugs of the Prestwick chemical library for compounds that protect lung fibroblasts from *M. tb*-induced cytotoxicity identified the gastric proton-pump inhibitor, lansoprazole (LPZ, Prevacid), as a potent hit compound [129]. LPZ is a prodrug that requires the host cell environment for conversion into lansoprazole sulphide (LPZS). Oral administration of LPZS significantly reduced bacterial burden during an acute TB infection in mice, and the compound lacks cytotoxicity, being well-tolerated in mice at a dose of 300 mg/kg. Whole-genome sequencing of resistant mutants generated to LPZS revealed mutation L176P in QcrB, and cross-resistance studies with imidazopyridine amide compounds and the T313A mutant strain indicated a distinct binding mode [129]. A follow-up study demonstrated that when LPZ is administered orally or intraperitoneally (i.p.) to rats, conversion to the active metabolite LPZS is undetectable in plasma and lung tissue, whereas LPZS was highly stable after i.p. administration [151]. In spite of this, LPZ intake has been found to significantly protect against TB incidence in individuals based on a cohort study conducted using the United Kingdom Clinical Practice Research Datalink [152].

The phenoxyalkylbenzimidazole (PAB) series, with an excellent growth-inhibitory potency and low cytotoxicity, is another promising QcrB inhibitor [130,153]. The lead compound, 54, demonstrated good efficacy against intracellular *M. tb*. Resistant mutants to PAB isolated in *M. tb* revealed mutations in qcrB and rv1339, a gene of unknown function. Through additional cross-resistance studies, QcrB was implicated as the main target [130]. The mutations identified in QcrB were A179P, M342T, W312C, and W312G, residues of the Qp binding site. Interestingly, while PAB compounds are bacteriostatic against actively growing *M. tb*, as with other QcrB inhibitors such as Q203 and LPZS, they are bactericidal against *M. tb* grown under conditions of nutrient starvation, in contrast to the lack of activity of other QcrB inhibitors in non-replicating models [129]. This discrepancy may be due to a potential involvement of a secondary target of PAB, for instance, rv1339, the second gene in which mutations were identified from resistant mutants.

The screening of a library of small polar molecules in a distinctive chemical space conducted at the Novartis Institute for Tropical Diseases led to the identification of hit compound pyrrolo[3,4-c]pyridine-1,3(2H)-dione, which was further optimised to increase its stability by replacing the ester moiety with a methyl oxadiazole bioisostere [131]. Lead compound 5h has an MIC_{90} below 0.156 μM in replicating *M. tb*, and is non-cytotoxic. The high clearance and poor plasma exposure of 5h in mouse PK studies could be improved by co-dosing with a pan-CYP inhibitor, such that a compound concentration above that of the MIC could be achieved in the blood for 6 h at a dose of 20 mg/kg. While attempts at isolating resistant mutants to this novel chemical class were unsuccessful, *M. tb* with a Cyt-bd oxidase deletion was hypersusceptible to the analogues. Moreover, the presence of mutation A317T in QcrB in this strain rendered *M. tb* resistant to the compounds, thus implicating QcrB in the mechanism of action of this class. Further studies on the pyrrolo[3,4-c]pyridine-1,3(2H)-diones will be aimed at improving their plasma concentration in vivo.

In 2013, GlaxoSmithKline published the results of a large phenotypic screening campaign against *M. bovis* BCG and *M. tb*, in which 177 hits belonging to several structurally distinct groups were identified [125]. To date, these chemical starting points have led to the discovery of two new classes of QcrB inhibitors, the 2-quinolin-4-yloxyacetamides (QOA) and the arylvinylpiperazine amides. Several

SAR studies of the QOAs have been reported and are in agreement regarding the potency of this chemical entity against *M. tb*, the lack of toxicity in a zebrafish model and the narrow-spectrum activity specific for *M. tb* [132,154,155]. Independent work through cross-resistance studies and isolation of resistance mutants harbouring the mutation T313A in QcrB confirmed cytochrome bcc as the target of QOAs [155,156]. The solubility and stability of this series, as well as their in vivo potency, remain to be addressed [133,154]. The arylvinylpiperazine amides were generated through lead optimisation and SAR studies conducted with GW861072X from the GSK screen, which was an attractive starting point for its structural simplicity and potent activity against *M. bovis* and *M. tb* [76]. The most potent analogues have improved MICs compared to the parent scaffold, displaying low cytotoxicity and activity against intracellular *M. tb*. The lead compound, AX-35 and two other analogues, AX-37 and AX-39, were also active in an acute TB infection model in mice. While isolation of *M. tb*-resistant mutants on agar proved unsuccessful, continual and increasing exposure of *M. tb* to AX-35 over several passages in liquid culture resulted in the selection of resistant clones harbouring the mutations S182P, M342V and M342I in QcrB. Cross-resistance studies provided insight on residues which were important for the binding of the compound to QcrB, indicating a slightly different interaction with the quinol binding pocket than Q203 and LPZS. Improving the metabolic stability of this series would likely improve the in vivo activity in mice, although these compounds appear to be more stable in human microsomes.

The morpholino-thiophenes were identified from the Lilly corporate library that was screened in an aerobic whole-cell phenotypic setting against *M. tb*. The series was extensively profiled and optimised, with the lead of this series having an MIC_{90} of 0.24 μM against *M. tb*, a high-selective index and improved microsomal stability [134]. In an acute model of TB infection, the lead compound reduced the bacterial burden by 0.8 log CFUs in mouse lungs. Cross-resistance studies of the compounds to *M. tb* strains harbouring QcrB T313I and M342T mutations indicated that the compounds interact with the quinol binding site of QcrB.

4-amino-thieno[2,3-d] pyrimidines were found to inhibit the growth of *M. smeg* in a screen of small-molecule nucleotide mimetics from ChemBridge Corporation. The most potent compound of the series, CWHM-1023, had an IC_{50} of 0.083 μM against *M. tb* [135]. Resistant mutants raised to CWHM-1023 in *M. tb* had mutations A178T, A178V, V338G, G175S or G315S in QcrB, and this target was further confirmed by the increased susceptibility of a *M. tb* strain lacking Cyt-bd oxidase to the compounds.

The most recent class of Cyt-bcc-aa3 inhibitors identified are the quinazoline derivatives, 2-ethylthio-4-methylaminoquinazolines [77]. The most potent derivatives have activity against in vitro and intracellular *M. tb* in the micromolar range, and have low cytotoxicity in human hepatocytes. The lead compound 11726148 has a low clearance in human microsomes and was active in an acute TB infection model. Whole-genome sequencing of *M. tb* resistant mutants to the quinazoline derivatives revealed mutations Trp312Gly and Gly175Ser in QcrB. Interestingly, one escape mutant has a SNP in qcrA leading to the substitution of Leu356Val in QcrA, the Rieske iron-sulphur protein of the Cyt-bcc-aa3. Mapping of the mutated residues on a model of the *M. smeg* Cyt-bcc-aa3 complex [58] indicated that all of the mutated residues, including Leu356Val in QcrA, map to the Qp site of QcrB. This is in line with the Q-cycle model, in which quinol oxidation occurs at the interface of cytochrome b and the 2Fe-2S cluster domain of the Rieske protein, which make up the catalytic Qp site [57,157]. Cross-resistance studies confirmed the target of QcrB, and also reveal the role of Leu356Val in QcrA in its interaction with other QcrB inhibitors, namely Q203, AX-35, and LPZS. With the implication of QcrA in the pharmacological inhibition of Cyt-bcc-aa3, novel inhibitors can be generated which target both QcrB and QcrA subunits using structure-assisted drug-design to decrease the likelihood of resistance to QcrB inhibitors. Within this novel class, lead compound 11726148 appears the most amenable for further optimisation, as its phenyl moiety can be changed on different heterocycles to improve pharmacological properties.

The Qp site of the Cyt-bcc-aa3 complex is particularly susceptible to chemical inhibition, as evident from the multitude of structurally diverse and distinct compounds detailed above. It has been consistently observed across several of the studies that characteristic consequences of cytochrome bcc inhibition include a general depletion of intracellular bacterial ATP levels, an upregulation of Cyt-bd oxidase, and an increase in OCR and bacterial respiration due to Cyt-bd [12,76,77,128–130,134,135,155, 158]. This compensation by the alternate terminal oxidase leads to an incomplete respiratory shutdown in *M. tb*, resulting in the bacteriostatic nature of cytochrome bcc inhibitors alone. However, with the deletion of Cyt-bd, mycobacterial respiration is effectively blocked, and cytochrome bcc inhibitors become bactericidal [65,76,77]. Taken altogether, these concerted efforts have generated a potential pool of backup cytochrome bcc inhibitors as Q203 continues in clinical trials. Additionally, these findings have highlighted the extreme vulnerability of *M. tb* without both of its terminal oxidases, and the immense potential of both respiratory branches as drug targets.

3.4. Inhibitors of Cyt-bd Oxidase

Aurachin D is a quinone analogue of the aurachin class that inhibits Cyt-bd oxidase of *E. coli* [136] (Table 3). When tested against membrane vesicles of *M. smeg*, aurachin D demonstrated dose-dependent inhibition of oxygen consumption of up to 50% [159]. Oxygen consumption was further inhibited by 90% in membrane vesicles without QcrCAB, indicating the likelihood of aurachin D targeting Cyt-bd in mycobacteria as well. On its own, aurachin D did not display activity against replicating *M. smeg* nor *M. tb* [159,160]. In spite of the lack of observable activity alone, aurachin D in combination with Q203 resulted in a ~10-fold decrease of the MIC of Q203 against *M. tb*, as well as enhanced bactericidal killing of *M. tb* by >2 log10 CFUs, demonstrating that aurachin D does indeed potentiate the activity of Q203 [160]. However, it remains to be demonstrated that aurachin D is a specific Cyt-bd inhibitor in mycobacteria as given its structural relation with MK, it may interfere with other respiratory complexes. This is particularly important since it was recently demonstrated that small-molecules are able to enhance the bactericidal potency of QcrB inhibitors without targeting the Cyt-bd [161].

It was shown that genetically inactivating both terminal oxidases completely abolished the in vitro growth of *M. tb* [35]. This also dramatically impacted bacterial fitness in vivo in mice, with a strain having a knockdown of Cyt-bcc-aa3 and a knockout of Cyt-bd being unable to establish an initial infection [35]. Even if an initial infection could be first achieved by regulating the expression of one of the terminal oxidases, the absence of both terminal oxidases led to severe persistence defects, with a decrease of five orders of magnitude in bacterial load in 35 days [35]. These findings are consistent with previous reports, whereby the joint inactivation, either pharmacologically or genetically, of both cytochrome bcc and bd oxidases resulted in bactericidal effects on *M. tb* in vitro and in vivo [65,76,77,160]. Exploiting the synthetic lethal interaction between these two terminal oxidases is an extremely attractive approach to eradicate *M. tb*. Inhibitors of this alternate terminal oxidase may have been missed in previous screens, which may be due to the fact that many screens have been performed under conditions in which the Cyt-bd is non-essential. In light of this, screening under stressed conditions may lead to the identification of Cyt-bd inhibitors amenable to chemical optimisation.

3.5. Inhibitors of the F_1F_0 ATP Synthase

The F_1F_0 ATP synthase is a clinically-validated drug target in *M. tb*, since the approval of BDQ by the US FDA for the treatment of multi-drug resistant TB. The mechanism of action of BDQ has been extensively studied in mycobacteria [20,83,162–164]. Briefly, BDQ binds to the c-subunit and the ε-subunit of the ATP synthase by mimicking key residues in the proton transfer chain and blocking the rotary movement of the c-subunit during the catalysis of ATP [165,166], disrupting a fundamental process for bacterial survival in both actively growing and non-growing states [20,162]. The inhibition of the ATP synthase leads to ATP depletion and also dissipation of the membrane potential, as BDQ was shown to have uncoupling properties mediated by the H+/K+ antiporter [167]. Unfortunately, drug resistance to BDQ has already emerged in MDR-TB patients, with several mechanisms of resistance having been reported [27,168–170]. Predominantly, mutations in atpE, the transcriptional repressor of the MmpL5-MmpS5, and the coding region of this efflux pump have been identified in humans [170–173]. In light of the emergence of resistance and the cardiotoxicity (QT prolongation) associated with BDQ treatment [174], efforts are currently ongoing to develop optimised diarylquinoline analogues (Table 4). The development of BDQ analogues 3,5-dialkoxypyridines is particularly interesting [175–180]. The preclinical candidate of this series, TBAJ-876, is less cardiotoxic than BDQ and 10 times more potent [180]. Through the isolation of resistant mutants and NMR studies, TBAJ-876 was shown to target the c- and ε-subunits of the ATP synthase at the same binding site as BDQ, indicating that this new analogue retains the mechanism of action of BDQ [180]. Kumar et al. screened a set of 700 compounds from the CSIR-IIIM repository for inhibition of mycobacterial ATP synthase activity using IMVs of *M. smeg*, leading to the identification of two compounds, the thiazolidine 5228485 and the cyclohexanediones 5220632. Both compounds inhibited ATP synthesis in IMVs and had MICs in the low micromolar range [181]. These bactericidal compounds were active against drug-resistant *M. tb* strains and non-replicating *M. tb* without apparent cytotoxicity [181]. Mutants selected against each compound were cross-resistant to BDQ, although resistance studies additionally suggest that these compounds may inhibit a secondary target besides the ATP synthase [181]. Further SAR and mechanistic studies are needed to fully understand the mechanism of action and for the development of these two new classes of ATP synthase inhibitors.

Table 4. Inhibitors of the ATP synthase discussed in this review.

Chemical Class	Represented by	Structure	Ref
Diarylquinoline	BDQ	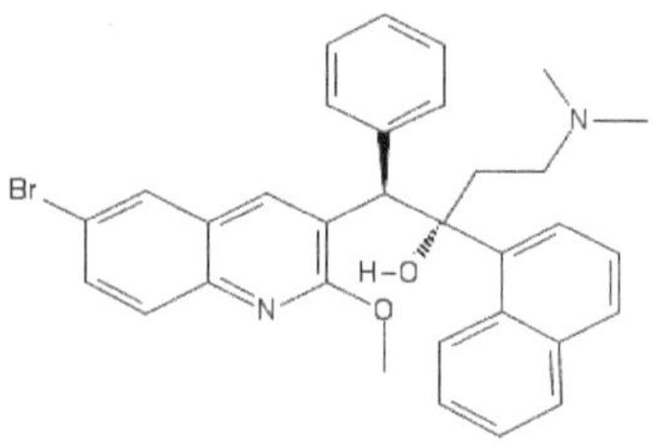	[83]
	TBAJ-587	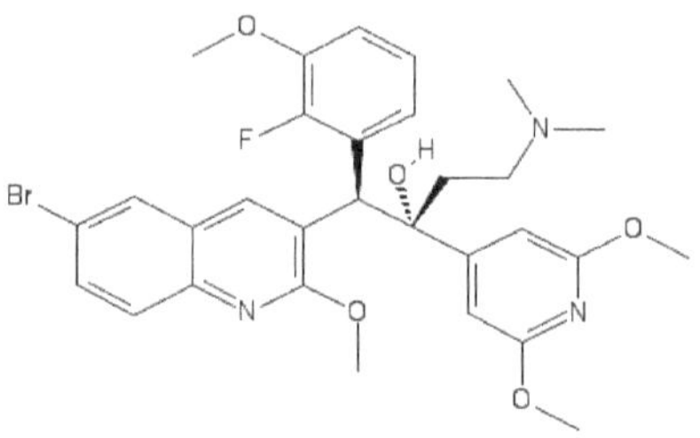	[175–177]
	TBAJ-876	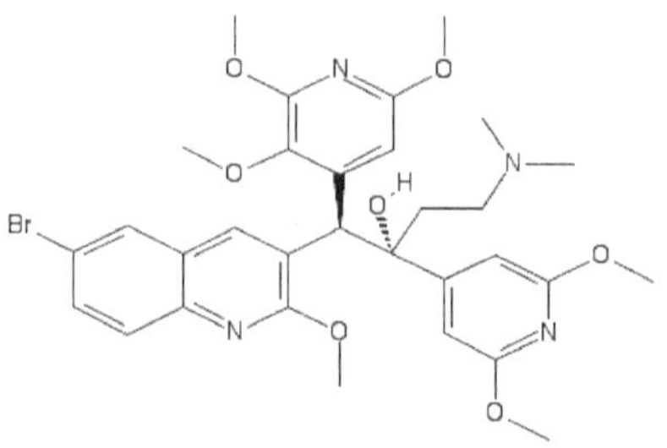	[175–177]
Thiazolidines	5228485	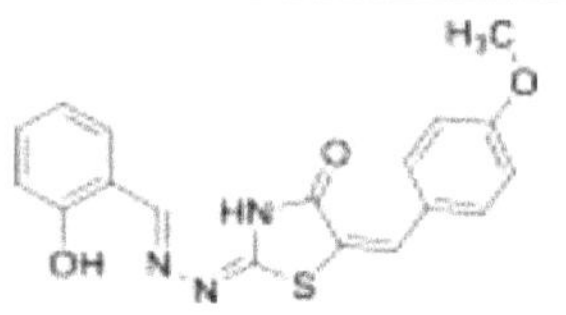	[181]

Table 4. *Cont.*

Chemical Class	Represented by	Structure	Ref
Cyclohexanediones	5220632	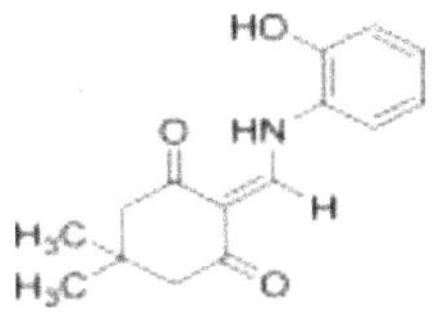	[181]
Squaramides	31f	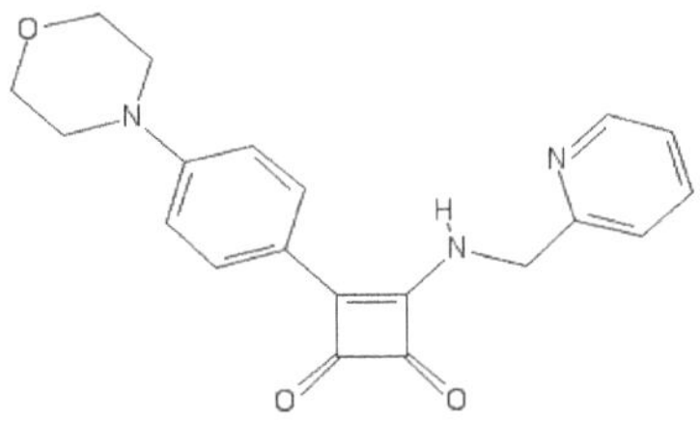	[127]

Squaramides were identified in the same screen as imidazo[1,2-a]pyridine ethers (IPE) (see section inhibitors of the Cyt-bcc-aa3) [127], with both compounds identified as inhibitors of ATP synthesis. Isolation of mutants resistant to squaramides revealed the presence of mutations in the α- and c- subunits of the ATP synthase. Interestingly, these mutants showed no cross-resistance to BDQ, suggesting a different mode of interaction with the ATP synthase than BDQ. Docking analysis of the most potent squaramide derivative, 31f (MIC *M. tb* 0.8 μM), showed that squaramides bind at the interface of the α and c -subunits of the ATP synthase. Compound 31f shows good accumulation in the serum in mice at a concentration above the MIC for over 15 h when administered with 100 mg/kg ABT, and was bacteriostatic in an acute model of TB. Further optimisation of the PK properties and in vivo safety is needed to advance this compound as a potential pre-clinical candidate for TB.

3.6. PMF

A wide range of compounds currently exists that target the PMF in bacteria, including rotenone which inhibits major proton pumps and protonophores (e.g., carbonyl cyanide m-chlorophenyl hydrazone, also known as CCCP), which translocate protons across the cell membranes [14] (Table 5). More specifically to mycobacteria, pyrazinoic acid, the active form of the first-line TB drug PZA, was demonstrated to decrease PMF and ATP levels in *M. bovis* BCG [182]. Several other compounds active against *M. tb* including SQ109, BDQ and CFZ were also found to be multi-targeting by behaving as uncouplers in addition to targeting enzymes [183]. While such an intrinsic and critical characteristic of the ETC is highly attractive therapeutically, such an approach would necessitate identifying compounds that are specific to the perturbation of mycobacterial PMF.

Recently, 2-aminoimidazoles (2-AI), a class of molecules with anti-biofilm activity, was shown to revert drug tolerance in an in vitro *M. tb* biofilm model [184]. This class of compounds potentiate the activity of β-lactams by altering protein secretion and lipid export, suggesting that 2-AI may perturb membrane energization [185]. Derivative 2B8 rapidly depolarized the membrane potential of live *M. smeg*, and collapsed the ΔpH generated by *M. smeg* IMVs energized with NADH, similar to CCCP and other mycobacterial uncouplers. In addition, a decrease in the OCR and intracellular ATP levels were observed in *M. tb* upon exposure to 2B8. Taken together, the perturbations of 2B8 on the PMF, OCR and ATP synthesis validates its uncoupling activity in mycobacteria [184].

Table 5. Inhibitors of the mycobacterial proton motive force (PMF) discuss in this review.

Chemical Class	Represented by	Structure	Ref
Ethylenediamine	SQ109	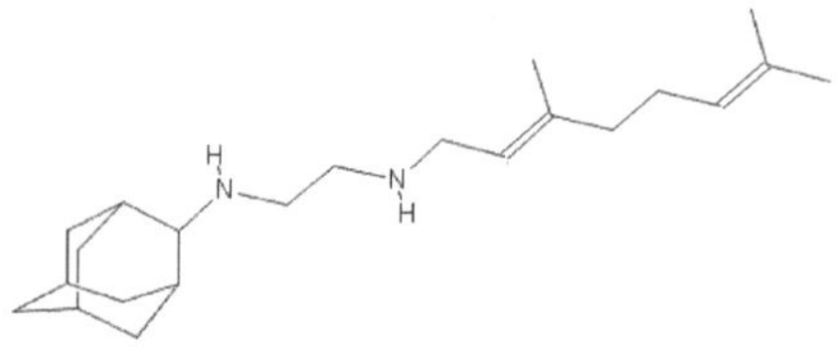	[186,187]
Pyrazinamide		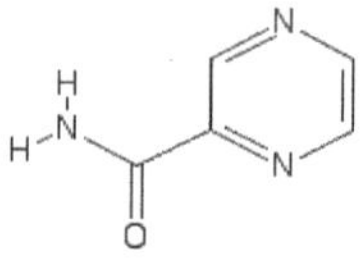	[188]
2-Aminoimidazoles	2B8	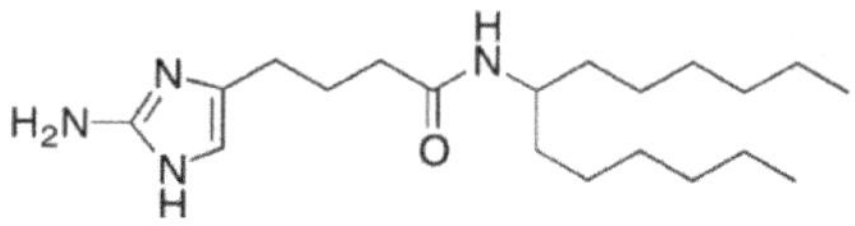	[184]

3.7. Respiratory Poisoning

NO is a key component of the innate immune response against intracellular pathogens like *M. tb* [189]. Two drugs, PA-824 and DEL (OPC-67683), were shown to release NO when activated by the deazaflavin-dependant nitroreductase Ddn (rv3547) of *M. tb* [10,190]. PA-824 and DEL are bicyclic nitroimidazoles that are approved for the treatment of DR-TB as part of a drug combination. Both drugs kill replicating and non-replicating *M. tb*. Under aerobic conditions, PA-824 and DEL inhibit mycolic acid synthesis [191,192], whereas, under anaerobic conditions, Singh et al. identified that the release of NO correlated with the formation of des-nitroimidazole metabolites, leading to the antimicrobial activity of PA-824 [10]. Transcriptomic analysis of *M. tb* treated with DEL and PA-824 revealed that respiratory poisoning by NO is fundamental for the activity of the drug in mycobacteria [193]. The transcriptomic profile of bacteria exposed to DEL and PA-824 is similar to potassium cyanide, a cytochrome c oxidase-specific inhibitor, which suggests that NO poisoning in *M. tb* may lead to the inhibition of the terminal oxidases [190].

4. Combinations Including ETC Inhibitors

TB treatment relies on the combination of several antibacterial agents. New regimens for TB need to be (1) effective against DS- and DR-TB, (2) contain drugs with new mechanisms of action, (3) are suitable for oral administration, and (4) do not interfere with drugs used to treat chronic conditions or chronic infections [194]. An effective regimen should combine drugs that preserve or even potentiate their activity (additivity or synergism) when given as a regimen. Due to their ability to perturb the energy metabolism of replicating and non-replicating *M. tb*, including drugs that target the ETC may shorten treatments against DS- and DR-TB. The recent approval of the BPaL regimen (BDQ-PA824-Linezolid; Nix-TB trial) for DR-TB highlights that inhibiting components of the ETC is key in developing new regimens against *M. tb*, even though the relative contribution of each drug to the sterilizing potency of the BPaL regimen remains to be further investigated in humans.

Several inhibitors in lead optimisation were tested in combination with other anti-TB drugs. PAB, a Cyt-bcc oxidase inhibitor, resulted in the synergistic killing of *M. tb* under both replicating and non-replicating conditions when combined with CFZ [195]. PABs in combination with BDQ demonstrated antagonism at early time points, particularly under non-replicating conditions. However, this antagonistic effect disappeared within three weeks, with PAB-BDQ combinations becoming highly bactericidal [195]. The specificity of the PAB series needs to be further studied since it kills nutrient-starved *M. tb* while remaining bacteriostatic against replicating mycobacteria, a property not shared with other specific Cyt-bcc inhibitors [130,153]. A MenA inhibitor, NM-4, was synergistic even at low doses together with sub-bactericidal concentrations of BDQ, CFZ, and the QcrB inhibitor ND-10885 [196], causing enhanced and efficient killing of *M. tb* in a time-kill curve assay [117]. These preliminary results underline the need to assess the efficacy of candidates in combination for TB therapy in an early stage of development.

Several ETC inhibitors are currently in ongoing pre-clinical and clinical trials to assess their efficacy against TB as part of new regimens [11]. These include BDQ, TBAJ-587 and TBAJ-876 (ATP synthase inhibitors), the first-line anti-TB drug PZA and SQ109 (inhibitors of the PMF), CFZ and its analogue TBI-166, and Q203 (inhibitor of Cyt-bcc-aa3 oxidase) [11]. SQ109 was reported to enhance the activity of anti-tuberculosis drugs INH, RIF and BDQ, and to shorten the time required to cure *M. tb*-infected mice [197]. Additionally, several inhibitors of the ETC compounds have a multi-target activity against the bacilli. The uncoupling effects of SQ109, PZA, BDQ, and CFZ suggest that these inhibitors may have a critical role due to their multi-targeting activity and should be taken into consideration for the further development of regimens against *M. tb*, particularly against DR-TB [183]. Assessing the in vitro or in vivo combinatory effects with repurposed or approved drugs for the treatment of TB has been another fruitful avenue to find new potential regimens comprising drug candidates that target the ETC. An example is TBI-166, an analogue of clofazimine with excellent potency alone or in combination with BDQ, PZA and linezolid in vitro and in vivo [198].

Q203 and BDQ were the first-in-class, orally-available representatives of the Cyt-bcc-aa3 and ATP synthase inhibitors, respectively. Q203 is currently in Phase 2b clinical trials and demonstrated potency in a 14-day, proof-of-concept design study of early bactericidal activity. It was safe and well-tolerated throughout the different dose strengths (100, 200 and 300 mg). Preliminary studies in vivo using a mouse footpad infection model of Buruli ulcer (*M. ulcerans*) showed that the addition of Q203 to the two-drug regimen of RIF and CFZ, or the three-drug regimen rifamycin, CFZ, and BDQ can decrease the treatment duration from four to two weeks, without any relapse after 12 weeks from the completion of treatment [199]. A similar approach could be developed to find an effective Q203-based regimen against *M. tb* with the addition of a chemical inhibitor of the Cyt-bd. Nonetheless, the plasticity and the possible re-routing of the mycobacterial ETC through chemical inhibition can be used against mycobacteria to conceive an effective regimen. Bioenergetics and *ex vivo* efficacy studies revealed that a combination of BDQ, CFZ and Q203 killed *M. tb* synergistically, with BDQ and Q203 potentiating CFZ's ROS production [158]. These results suggest that the potentiation of Q203 can be achieved without a Cyt-bd oxidase inhibitor as well.

With the number of BDQ-containing regimens undergoing clinical trials, BDQ seems a drug of choice for further development of TB therapy. Several Phase 1 and 2 clinical trials which include BDQ are currently in progress [194]. However, the emergence of resistance and its high cardiotoxicity may jeopardize the potency of this antitubercular drug. The development of new ATP synthase inhibitors that harbour less cardiotoxicity and are potentially less prone to the development of resistance, such as TBAJ-876 and TBAJ-587, will most likely lead to the development of new regimens including these second generation of diaryquinolines [179,180].

5. Conclusions and Perspectives

This review has highlighted the current efforts made to find new inhibitors against components of the ETC. To date, tackling the mycobacterial OxPhos pathway has been a prolific avenue in finding new inhibitors against *M. tb*, as well as other mycobacteria such as *M. ulcerans*. Deciphering the role of each new scaffold targeting ETC components will enable a further understanding of this pivotal pathway in *M. tb* survival and metabolism. Several components are still poorly exploited as potential targets for chemical inhibition, either due to their homology to eukaryotic components or their regulation as a specific bacterial response to the environment/stress (e.g., Cyt-bd). Redundancy of several components of the ETC further complicates the establishment of a background regimen comprising of ETC inhibitors. A deeper understanding of the intricately-linked energy metabolism processes would be required to target the various metabolic pathways which *M. tb* can reroute to, such that a successful regimen can be developed. Most screens to identify inhibitors of the OxPhos have been conducted using whole-cell assays, target-based assays or phenotypic screening using ATP as a readout. However, these screening methods may not be suitable for the identification of inhibitors of some components such as the Cyt-bd, which are conditionally essential under specific conditions. Therefore, a better understanding of the modulation of the ETC under the host physiological conditions encountered by *M. tb* would be of great interest for further development of energy metabolism inhibitors. Lastly, ETC inhibitors have the potential to revolutionise future TB treatments by contributing to efficacious regimens which are simpler and shorter, as evident from BDQ's role in the novel, three-drug, all-oral BPaL regimen.

Author Contributions: Conceptualization, C.S.-Y.F., K.P. and A.L.; writing—original draft preparation, C.S.-Y.F., K.P. and A.L.; writing—review and editing, C.S.-Y.F., K.P. and A.L.; visualization, C.S.-Y.F. and A.L.; project administration, K.P. and A.L.; funding acquisition, K.P. All authors have read and agreed to the published version of the manuscript.

Acknowledgments: We would like to thank Marcel Behr and Jean-Yves Dubé for their contributions to the revision of the manuscript.

References

1. WHO | Global Tuberculosis Report 2019. Available online: http://www.who.int/tb/publications/global_report/en/ (accessed on 17 February 2020).
2. McKinney, J.D. In vivo veritas: The search for TB drug targets goes live. *Nat. Med.* **2000**, *6*, 1330–1333. [CrossRef] [PubMed]
3. WHO | WHO Consolidated Guidelines on Drug-Resistant Tuberculosis Treatment. Available online: http://www.who.int/tb/publications/2019/consolidated-guidelines-drug-resistant-TB-treatment/en/ (accessed on 17 February 2020).
4. Sotgiu, G.; Centis, R.; D'ambrosio, L.; Migliori, G.B. Tuberculosis treatment and drug regimens. *Cold Spring Harb. Perspect. Med.* **2015**, *5*, a017822. [CrossRef] [PubMed]
5. Borisov, S.; Danila, E.; Maryandyshev, A.; Dalcolmo, M.; Miliauskas, S.; Kuksa, L.; Manga, S.; Skrahina, A.; Diktanas, S.; Codecasa, L.R.; et al. Surveillance of adverse events in the treatment of drug-resistant tuberculosis: First global report. *Eur. Respir. J.* **2019**, *54*, 1901522. [CrossRef] [PubMed]
6. Akkerman, O.; Aleksa, A.; Alffenaar, J.-W.; Al-Marzouqi, N.H.; Arias-Guillén, M.; Belilovski, E.; Bernal, E.; Boeree, M.J.; Borisov, S.E.; Bruchfeld, J.; et al. Surveillance of adverse events in the treatment of drug-resistant tuberculosis: A global feasibility study. *Int. J. Infect. Dis.* **2019**, *83*, 72–76. [CrossRef]
7. Janssen Therapeutics, Division of Janssen Products, LP. (2019) Sirturo ®: HIGHLIGHTS OF PRESCRIBING INFORMATION. Available online: https://www.accessdata.fda.gov/drugsatfda_docs/label/2019/204384s010lbl.pdf (accessed on 26 March 2020).
8. European Medicines Agency-Find Medicine-Deltyba. Available online: http://www.ema.europa.eu/ema/index.jsp?curl=pages/medicines/human/medicines/002552/human_med_001699.jsp&mid=WC0b01ac058001d124 (accessed on 31 May 2018).
9. U.S. Food and Drug Administration FDA Approves New Drug for Treatment-Resistant Forms of Tuberculosis that Affects the Lungs. Available online: http://www.fda.gov/news-events/press-announcements/fda-approves-new-drug-treatment-resistant-forms-tuberculosis-affects-lungs (accessed on 31 January 2020).
10. Singh, R.; Manjunatha, U.; Boshoff, H.I.M.; Ha, Y.H.; Niyomrattanakit, P.; Ledwidge, R.; Dowd, C.S.; Lee, I.Y.; Kim, P.; Zhang, L.; et al. PA-824 kills nonreplicating Mycobacterium tuberculosis by intracellular NO release. *Science* **2008**, *322*, 1392–1395. [CrossRef]
11. Pipeline | Working Group for New TB Drugs. Available online: https://www.newtbdrugs.org/pipeline/clinical (accessed on 17 February 2020).

12. Pethe, K.; Bifani, P.; Jang, J.; Kang, S.; Park, S.; Ahn, S.; Jiricek, J.; Jung, J.; Jeon, H.K.; Cechetto, J.; et al. Discovery of Q203, a potent clinical candidate for the treatment of tuberculosis. *Nat. Med.* **2013**, *19*, 1157–1160. [CrossRef]
13. Bald, D.; Villellas, C.; Lu, P.; Koul, A. Targeting energy metabolism in mycobacterium tuberculosis, a new paradigm in antimycobacterial drug discovery. *mBio* **2017**, *8*, e00272-17. [CrossRef]
14. Cook, G.M.; Hards, K.; Dunn, E.; Heikal, A.; Nakatani, Y.; Greening, C.; Crick, D.C.; Fontes, F.L.; Pethe, K.; Hasenoehrl, E.; et al. Oxidative phosphorylation as a target space for tuberculosis: Success, caution, and future directions. *Microbiol. Spectr.* **2017**, *5*. [CrossRef]
15. Matsoso, L.G.; Kana, B.D.; Crellin, P.K.; Lea-Smith, D.J.; Pelosi, A.; Powell, D.; Dawes, S.S.; Rubin, H.; Coppel, R.L.; Mizrahi, V. Function of the cytochrome bc1-aa3 branch of the respiratory network in mycobacteria and network adaptation occurring in response to its disruption. *J. Bacteriol.* **2005**, *187*, 6300–6308. [CrossRef]
16. Billig, S.; Schneefeld, M.; Huber, C.; Grassl, G.A.; Eisenreich, W.; Bange, F.-C. Lactate oxidation facilitates growth of Mycobacterium tuberculosis in human macrophages. *Sci. Rep.* **2017**, *7*, 6484. [CrossRef] [PubMed]
17. Cole, S.T.; Brosch, R. Deciphering the biology of Mycobacterium tuberculosis from the complete genome sequence. *Trends Biochem. Sci.* **1997**, *22*, 28–31.
18. Boshoff, H.I.M.; Barry 3rd, C.E. Tuberculosis—Metabolism and respiration in the absence of growth. *Nat. Rev. Microbiol.* **2005**, *3*, 70–80. [CrossRef] [PubMed]
19. Rao, S.P.S.; Alonso, S.; Rand, L.; Dick, T.; Pethe, K. The protonmotive force is required for maintaining ATP homeostasis and viability of hypoxic, nonreplicating mycobacterium tuberculosis. *Proc. Natl. Acad. Sci. USA* **2008**, *105*, 11945–11950. [CrossRef] [PubMed]
20. Koul, A.; Vranckx, L.; Dendouga, N.; Balemans, W.; den Wyngaert, I.V.; Vergauwen, K.; Göhlmann, H.W.H.; Willebrords, R.; Poncelet, A.; Guillemont, J.; et al. Diarylquinolines are bactericidal for dormant mycobacteria as a result of disturbed ATP homeostasis. *J. Biol. Chem.* **2008**, *283*, 25273–25280. [CrossRef] [PubMed]
21. Gengenbacher, M.; Rao, S.P.S.; Pethe, K.; Dick, T. Nutrient-starved, non-replicating Mycobacterium tuberculosis requires respiration, ATP synthase and isocitrate lyase for maintenance of ATP homeostasis and viability. *Microbiol. Read. Engl.* **2010**, *156*, 81–87. [CrossRef] [PubMed]
22. Adams, K.N.; Takaki, K.; Connolly, L.E.; Wiedenhoft, H.; Winglee, K.; Humbert, O.; Edelstein, P.H.; Cosma, C.L.; Ramakrishnan, L. Drug tolerance in replicating mycobacteria mediated by a macrophage-induced efflux mechanism. *Cell* **2011**, *145*, 39–53. [CrossRef]
23. Machado, D.; Couto, I.; Perdigão, J.; Rodrigues, L.; Portugal, I.; Baptista, P.; Veigas, B.; Amaral, L.; Viveiros, M. Contribution of efflux to the emergence of isoniazid and multidrug resistance in Mycobacterium tuberculosis. *PLoS ONE* **2012**, *7*, e34538. [CrossRef]
24. Adams, K.N.; Szumowski, J.D.; Ramakrishnan, L. Verapamil, and its metabolite norverapamil, inhibit macrophage-induced, bacterial efflux pump-mediated tolerance to multiple anti-tubercular drugs. *J. Infect. Dis.* **2014**, *210*, 456–466. [CrossRef]
25. Coelho, T.; Machado, D.; Couto, I.; Maschmann, R.; Ramos, D.; von Groll, A.; Rossetti, M.L.; Silva, P.A.; Viveiros, M. Enhancement of antibiotic activity by efflux inhibitors against multidrug resistant Mycobacterium tuberculosis clinical isolates from Brazil. *Front. Microbiol.* **2015**, *6*, 330. [CrossRef]
26. Li, G.; Zhang, J.; Guo, Q.; Jiang, Y.; Wei, J.; Zhao, L.; Zhao, X.; Lu, J.; Wan, K. Efflux pump gene expression in multidrug-resistant Mycobacterium tuberculosis clinical isolates. *PLoS ONE* **2015**, *10*, e0119013. [CrossRef] [PubMed]
27. Andries, K.; Villellas, C.; Coeck, N.; Thys, K.; Gevers, T.; Vranckx, L.; Lounis, N.; de Jong, B.C.; Koul, A. Acquired resistance of Mycobacterium tuberculosis to bedaquiline. *PLoS ONE* **2014**, *9*, e102135. [CrossRef] [PubMed]
28. Weinstein, E.A.; Yano, T.; Li, L.-S.; Avarbock, D.; Avarbock, A.; Helm, D.; McColm, A.A.; Duncan, K.; Lonsdale, J.T.; Rubin, H. Inhibitors of type II NADH:menaquinone oxidoreductase represent a class of antitubercular drugs. *Proc. Natl. Acad. Sci. USA* **2005**, *102*, 4548–4553. [CrossRef] [PubMed]
29. Harbut, M.B.; Yang, B.; Liu, R.; Yano, T.; Vilchèze, C.; Cheng, B.; Lockner, J.; Guo, H.; Yu, C.; Franzblau, S.G.; et al. Small molecules targeting mycobacterium tuberculosis Type II NADH dehydrogenase exhibit antimycobacterial activity. *Angew. Chem. Int. Ed. Engl.* **2018**, *57*, 3478–3482. [CrossRef] [PubMed]

30. Murugesan, D.; Ray, P.C.; Bayliss, T.; Prosser, G.A.; Harrison, J.R.; Green, K.; Soares de Melo, C.; Feng, T.-S.; Street, L.J.; Chibale, K.; et al. 2-Mercapto-Quinazolinones as inhibitors of Type II NADH Dehydrogenase and Mycobacterium tuberculosis: Structure-activity relationships, mechanism of action and absorption, distribution, metabolism, and excretion characterization. *ACS Infect. Dis.* **2018**, *4*, 954–969. [CrossRef] [PubMed]
31. Sassetti, C.M.; Boyd, D.H.; Rubin, E.J. Genes required for mycobacterial growth defined by high density mutagenesis. *Mol. Microbiol.* **2003**, *48*, 77–84. [CrossRef] [PubMed]
32. Griffin, J.E.; Gawronski, J.D.; Dejesus, M.A.; Ioerger, T.R.; Akerley, B.J.; Sassetti, C.M. High-resolution phenotypic profiling defines genes essential for mycobacterial growth and cholesterol catabolism. *PLoS Pathog.* **2011**, *7*, e1002251. [CrossRef]
33. DeJesus, M.A.; Gerrick, E.R.; Xu, W.; Park, S.W.; Long, J.E.; Boutte, C.C.; Rubin, E.J.; Schnappinger, D.; Ehrt, S.; Fortune, S.M.; et al. Comprehensive essentiality analysis of the mycobacterium tuberculosis genome via saturating transposon mutagenesis. *mBio* **2017**, *8*, e02133-16. [CrossRef]
34. Vilchèze, C.; Weinrick, B.; Leung, L.W.; Jacobs, W.R. Plasticity of Mycobacterium tuberculosis NADH dehydrogenases and their role in virulence. *Proc. Natl. Acad. Sci. USA* **2018**, *115*, 1599–1604. [CrossRef]
35. Beites, T.; O'Brien, K.; Tiwari, D.; Engelhart, C.A.; Walters, S.; Andrews, J.; Yang, H.-J.; Sutphen, M.L.; Weiner, D.M.; Dayao, E.K.; et al. Plasticity of the mycobacterium tuberculosis respiratory chain and its impact on tuberculosis drug development. *Nat. Commun.* **2019**, *10*, 4970. [CrossRef]
36. Maklashina, E.; Cecchini, G.; Dikanov, S.A. Defining a direction: Electron transfer and catalysis in Escherichia coli complex II enzymes. *Biochim. Biophys. Acta* **2013**, *1827*, 668–678. [CrossRef] [PubMed]
37. Hards, K.; Adolph, C.; Harold, L.K.; McNeil, M.B.; Cheung, C.-Y.; Jinich, A.; Rhee, K.Y.; Cook, G.M. Two for the price of one: Attacking the energetic-metabolic hub of mycobacteria to produce new chemotherapeutic agents. *Prog. Biophys. Mol. Biol.* **2019**, S0079610719302111. [CrossRef] [PubMed]
38. Rutter, J.; Winge, D.R.; Schiffman, J.D. Succinate dehydrogenase—Assembly, regulation and role in human disease. *Mitochondrion* **2010**, *10*, 393–401. [CrossRef] [PubMed]
39. Cook, G.M.; Hards, K.; Vilchèze, C.; Hartman, T.; Berney, M. Energetics of respiration and oxidative phosphorylation in mycobacteria. *Microbiol. Spectr.* **2014**, *2*, 389–409. [CrossRef] [PubMed]
40. Baek, S.-H.; Li, A.H.; Sassetti, C.M. Metabolic regulation of mycobacterial growth and antibiotic sensitivity. *PLoS Biol.* **2011**, *9*, e1001065. [CrossRef] [PubMed]
41. Hartman, T.; Weinrick, B.; Vilchèze, C.; Berney, M.; Tufariello, J.; Cook, G.M.; Jacobs, W.R.J., Jr. Succinate Dehydrogenase is the Regulator of Respiration in Mycobacterium tuberculosis. *PLoS Pathog.* **2014**, *10*, e1004510. [CrossRef]
42. Lemos, R.S.; Fernandes, A.S.; Pereira, M.M.; Gomes, C.M.; Teixeira, M. Quinol:fumarate oxidoreductases and succinate:quinone oxidoreductases: Phylogenetic relationships, metal centres and membrane attachment. *Biochim. Biophys. Acta* **2002**, *1553*, 158–170. [CrossRef]
43. Pecsi, I.; Hards, K.; Ekanayaka, N.; Berney, M.; Hartman, T.; Jacobs, W.R.; Cook, G.M. Essentiality of succinate dehydrogenase in mycobacterium smegmatis and its role in the generation of the membrane potential under hypoxia. *mBio* **2014**, *5*, e01093-14. [CrossRef]
44. Collins, M.D.; Jones, D. Distribution of isoprenoid quinone structural types in bacteria and their taxonomic implication. *Microbiol. Rev.* **1981**, *45*, 316–354. [CrossRef]
45. Meganathan, R. Biosynthesis of menaquinone (vitamin K2) and ubiquinone (coenzyme Q): A perspective on enzymatic mechanisms. In *Vitamins & Hormones*; Cofactor Biosynthesis; Academic Press: Cambridge, MA, USA, 2001; Volume 61, pp. 173–218.
46. Dhiman, R.K.; Mahapatra, S.; Slayden, R.A.; Boyne, M.E.; Lenaerts, A.; Hinshaw, J.C.; Angala, S.K.; Chatterjee, D.; Biswas, K.; Narayanasamy, P.; et al. Menaquinone synthesis is critical for maintaining mycobacterial viability during exponential growth and recovery from non-replicating persistence. *Mol. Microbiol.* **2009**, *72*, 85–97. [CrossRef]
47. Kurosu, M.; Crick, D. MenA is a promising drug target for developing novel lead molecules to combat mycobacterium tuberculosis. *Med. Chem.* **2009**, *5*, 197–207. [CrossRef] [PubMed]
48. Li, X.; Liu, N.; Zhang, H.; Knudson, S.E.; Li, H.-J.; Lai, C.-T.; Simmerling, C.; Slayden, R.A.; Tonge, P.J. CoA Adducts of 4-Oxo-4-phenylbut-2-enoates: Inhibitors of MenB from the M. tuberculosis Menaquinone Biosynthesis Pathway. *ACS Med. Chem. Lett.* **2011**, *2*, 818–823. [CrossRef] [PubMed]

49. Debnath, J.; Siricilla, S.; Wan, B.; Crick, D.C.; Lenaerts, A.J.; Franzblau, S.G.; Kurosu, M. Discovery of selective menaquinone biosynthesis inhibitors against Mycobacterium tuberculosis. *J. Med. Chem.* **2012**, *55*, 3739–3755. [CrossRef] [PubMed]
50. Lu, X.; Zhang, H.; Tonge, P.J.; Tan, D.S. Mechanism-based inhibitors of MenE, an acyl-CoA synthetase involved in bacterial menaquinone biosynthesis. *Bioorg. Med. Chem. Lett.* **2008**, *18*, 5963–5966. [CrossRef]
51. Sukheja, P.; Kumar, P.; Mittal, N.; Li, S.-G.; Singleton, E.; Russo, R.; Perryman, A.L.; Shrestha, R.; Awasthi, D.; Husain, S.; et al. A novel small-molecule inhibitor of the mycobacterium tuberculosis demethylmenaquinone methyltransferase meng is bactericidal to both growing and nutritionally deprived persister cells. *mBio* **2017**, *8*, e02022-16. [CrossRef]
52. Truglio, J.J.; Theis, K.; Feng, Y.; Gajda, R.; Machutta, C.; Tonge, P.J.; Kisker, C. Crystal structure of Mycobacterium tuberculosis MenB, a key enzyme in vitamin K2 biosynthesis. *J. Biol. Chem.* **2003**, *278*, 42352–42360. [CrossRef]
53. Morand, O.H.; Aebi, J.D.; Dehmlow, H.; Ji, Y.H.; Gains, N.; Lengsfeld, H.; Himber, J. Ro 48-8.071, a new 2,3-oxidosqualene:lanosterol cyclase inhibitor lowering plasma cholesterol in hamsters, squirrel monkeys, and minipigs: Comparison to simvastatin. *J. Lipid Res.* **1997**, *38*, 373–390.
54. Goldman, R.C. Why are membrane targets discovered by phenotypic screens and genome sequencing in Mycobacterium tuberculosis? *Tuberc. Edinb. Scotl.* **2013**, *93*, 569–588. [CrossRef]
55. Megehee, J.A.; Hosler, J.P.; Lundrigan, M.D. Evidence for a cytochrome bcc-aa3 interaction in the respiratory chain of Mycobacterium smegmatis. *Microbiol. Read. Engl.* **2006**, *152*, 823–829. [CrossRef]
56. Kim, M.-S.; Jang, J.; Ab Rahman, N.B.; Pethe, K.; Berry, E.A.; Huang, L.-S. Isolation and characterization of a hybrid respiratory supercomplex consisting of mycobacterium tuberculosis cytochrome bcc and mycobacterium smegmatis cytochrome aa3. *J. Biol. Chem.* **2015**, *290*, 14350–14360. [CrossRef]
57. Gong, H.; Li, J.; Xu, A.; Tang, Y.; Ji, W.; Gao, R.; Wang, S.; Yu, L.; Tian, C.; Li, J.; et al. An electron transfer path connects subunits of a mycobacterial respiratory supercomplex. *Science* **2018**, *362*, eaat8923. [CrossRef] [PubMed]
58. Wiseman, B.; Nitharwal, R.G.; Fedotovskaya, O.; Schäfer, J.; Guo, H.; Kuang, Q.; Benlekbir, S.; Sjöstrand, D.; Ädelroth, P.; Rubinstein, J.L.; et al. Structure of a functional obligate complex III 2 IV 2 respiratory supercomplex from Mycobacterium smegmatis. *Nat. Struct. Mol. Biol.* **2018**, *25*, 1128–1136. [CrossRef] [PubMed]
59. Borisov, V.B.; Gennis, R.B.; Hemp, J.; Verkhovsky, M.I. The cytochrome bd respiratory oxygen reductases. *Biochim. Biophys. Acta* **2011**, *1807*, 1398–1413. [CrossRef] [PubMed]
60. Allen, R.J.; Brenner, E.P.; VanOrsdel, C.E.; Hobson, J.J.; Hearn, D.J.; Hemm, M.R. Conservation analysis of the CydX protein yields insights into small protein identification and evolution. *BMC Genom.* **2014**, *15*, 946. [CrossRef] [PubMed]
61. Poole, R.K.; Hatch, L.; Cleeter, M.W.J.; Gibson, F.; Cox, G.B.; Wu, G. Cytochrome bd biosynthesis in Escherichia coli: The sequences of the cydC and cydD genes suggest that they encode the components of an ABC membrane transporter. *Mol. Microbiol.* **1993**, *10*, 421–430. [CrossRef]
62. Shepherd, M. The CydDC ABC transporter of Escherichia coli: New roles for a reductant efflux pump. *Biochem. Soc. Trans.* **2015**, *43*, 908–912. [CrossRef]
63. Mascolo, L.; Bald, D. Cytochrome bd in Mycobacterium tuberculosis: A respiratory chain protein involved in the defense against antibacterials. *Prog. Biophys. Mol. Biol.* **2019**. [CrossRef]
64. Berney, M.; Hartman, T.E.; Jacobs, W.R. A Mycobacterium tuberculosis Cytochrome bd Oxidase Mutant Is Hypersensitive to Bedaquiline. *mBio* **2014**, *5*, e01275-14. [CrossRef]
65. Kalia, N.P.; Hasenoehrl, E.J.; Rahman, N.B.A.; Koh, V.H.; Ang, M.L.T.; Sajorda, D.R.; Hards, K.; Grüber, G.; Alonso, S.; Cook, G.M.; et al. Exploiting the synthetic lethality between terminal respiratory oxidases to kill Mycobacterium tuberculosis and clear host infection. *Proc. Natl. Acad. Sci. USA* **2017**, *114*, 7426–7431. [CrossRef]
66. Safarian, S.; Rajendran, C.; Müller, H.; Preu, J.; Langer, J.D.; Ovchinnikov, S.; Hirose, T.; Kusumoto, T.; Sakamoto, J.; Michel, H. Structure of a bd oxidase indicates similar mechanisms for membrane-integrated oxygen reductases. *Science* **2016**, *352*, 583–586. [CrossRef]
67. Safarian, S.; Hahn, A.; Mills, D.J.; Radloff, M.; Eisinger, M.L.; Nikolaev, A.; Meier-Credo, J.; Melin, F.; Miyoshi, H.; Gennis, R.B.; et al. Active site rearrangement and structural divergence in prokaryotic respiratory oxidases. *Science* **2019**, *366*, 100–104. [CrossRef] [PubMed]

68. Lee, B.S.; Sviriaeva, E.; Pethe, K. Targeting the cytochrome oxidases for drug development in mycobacteria. *Prog. Biophys. Mol. Biol.* **2020**. [CrossRef] [PubMed]
69. D'mello, R.; Hill, S.; Poole, R.K. The cytochrome bd quinol oxidase in Escherichia coli has an extremely high oxygen affinity and two oxygen-binding haems: Implications for regulation of activity in vivo by oxygen inhibition. *Microbiology* **1996**, *142*, 755–763. [CrossRef] [PubMed]
70. Miller, M.J.; Gennis, R.B. The cytochrome d complex is a coupling site in the aerobic respiratory chain of Escherichia coli. *J. Biol. Chem.* **1985**, *260*, 14003–14008. [PubMed]
71. Jasaitis, A.; Borisov, V.B.; Belevich, N.P.; Morgan, J.E.; Konstantinov, A.A.; Verkhovsky, M.I. Electrogenic reactions of cytochrome bd. *Biochemistry* **2000**, *39*, 13800–13809. [CrossRef]
72. Gopinath, V.; Raghunandanan, S.; Gomez, R.L.; Jose, L.; Surendran, A.; Ramachandran, R.; Pushparajan, A.R.; Mundayoor, S.; Jaleel, A.; Kumar, R.A. Profiling the proteome of mycobacterium tuberculosis during dormancy and reactivation. *Mol. Cell. Proteom.* **2015**, *14*, 2160–2176. [CrossRef]
73. Cortes, T.; Schubert, O.T.; Banaei-Esfahani, A.; Collins, B.C.; Aebersold, R.; Young, D.B. Delayed effects of transcriptional responses in Mycobacterium tuberculosis exposed to nitric oxide suggest other mechanisms involved in survival. *Sci. Rep.* **2017**, *7*, 1–9. [CrossRef]
74. Shi, L.; Sohaskey, C.D.; Kana, B.D.; Dawes, S.; North, R.J.; Mizrahi, V.; Gennaro, M.L. Changes in energy metabolism of Mycobacterium tuberculosis in mouse lung and under in vitro conditions affecting aerobic respiration. *Proc. Natl. Acad. Sci. USA* **2005**, *102*, 15629–15634. [CrossRef]
75. Arora, K.; Ochoa-Montano, B.; Tsang, P.S.; Blundell, T.L.; Dawes, S.S.; Mizrahi, V.; Bayliss, T.; Mackenzie, C.J.; Cleghorn, L.A.T.; Ray, P.C.; et al. Respiratory flexibility in response to inhibition of cytochrome c oxidase in mycobacterium tuberculosis. *Antimicrob. Agents Chemother.* **2014**, *58*, 6962–6965. [CrossRef]
76. Foo, C.S.; Lupien, A.; Kienle, M.; Vocat, A.; Benjak, A.; Sommer, R.; Lamprecht, D.A.; Steyn, A.J.C.; Pethe, K.; Piton, J.; et al. Arylvinylpiperazine Amides, a New Class of Potent Inhibitors Targeting QcrB of Mycobacterium tuberculosis. *mBio* **2018**, *9*. [CrossRef]
77. Lupien, A.; Foo, C.S.-Y.; Savina, S.; Vocat, A.; Piton, J.; Monakhova, N.; Benjak, A.; Lamprecht, D.A.; Steyn, A.J.C.; Pethe, K.; et al. New 2-Ethylthio-4-methylaminoquinazoline derivatives inhibiting two subunits of cytochrome bc1 in Mycobacterium tuberculosis. *PLoS Pathog.* **2020**, *16*, e1008270. [CrossRef] [PubMed]
78. Lu, P.; Lill, H.; Bald, D. ATP synthase in mycobacteria: Special features and implications for a function as drug target. *Biochim. Biophys. Acta BBA-Bioenerg.* **2014**, *1837*, 1208–1218. [CrossRef] [PubMed]
79. Walker, J.E. The ATP synthase: The understood, the uncertain and the unknown. *Biochem. Soc. Trans.* **2013**, *41*, 1–16. [CrossRef] [PubMed]
80. von Ballmoos, C.; Cook, G.M.; Dimroth, P. Unique rotary atp synthase and its biological diversity. *Annu. Rev. Biophys.* **2008**, *37*, 43–64. [CrossRef]
81. Higashi, T.; Kalra, V.K.; Lee, S.H.; Bogin, E.; Brodie, A.F. Energy-transducing membrane-bound coupling factor-ATPase from Mycobacterium phlei. I. Purification, homogeneity, and properties. *J. Biol. Chem.* **1975**, *250*, 6541–6548.
82. Haagsma, A.C.; Driessen, N.N.; Hahn, M.-M.; Lill, H.; Bald, D. ATP synthase in slow- and fast-growing mycobacteria is active in ATP synthesis and blocked in ATP hydrolysis direction. *FEMS Microbiol. Lett.* **2010**, *313*, 68–74. [CrossRef]
83. Andries, K.; Verhasselt, P.; Guillemont, J.; Göhlmann, H.W.H.; Neefs, J.-M.; Winkler, H.; Gestel, J.V.; Timmerman, P.; Zhu, M.; Lee, E.; et al. A Diarylquinoline drug active on the ATP synthase of mycobacterium tuberculosis. *Science* **2005**, *307*, 223–227. [CrossRef]
84. Bald, D.; Koul, A. Respiratory ATP synthesis: The new generation of mycobacterial drug targets? *FEMS Microbiol. Lett.* **2010**, *308*, 1–7. [CrossRef]
85. Zhang, A.T.; Montgomery, M.G.; Leslie, A.G.W.; Cook, G.M.; Walker, J.E. The structure of the catalytic domain of the ATP synthase from Mycobacterium smegmatis is a target for developing antitubercular drugs. *Proc. Natl. Acad. Sci. USA* **2019**, *116*, 4206–4211. [CrossRef]
86. Joon, S.; Ragunathan, P.; Sundararaman, L.; Nartey, W.; Kundu, S.; Manimekalai, M.S.S.; Bogdanović, N.; Dick, T.; Grüber, G. The NMR solution structure of *Mycobacterium tuberculosis* F- ATP synthase subunit ε provides new insight into energy coupling inside the rotary engine. *FEBS J.* **2018**, *285*, 1111–1128. [CrossRef]

87. Saw, W.-G.; Wu, M.-L.; Ragunathan, P.; Biuković, G.; Lau, A.-M.; Shin, J.; Harikishore, A.; Cheung, C.-Y.; Hards, K.; Sarathy, J.P.; et al. Disrupting coupling within mycobacterial F-ATP synthases subunit ε causes dysregulated energy production and cell wall biosynthesis. *Sci. Rep.* **2019**, *9*, 1–15. [CrossRef] [PubMed]
88. Hotra, A.; Suter, M.; Biuković, G.; Ragunathan, P.; Kundu, S.; Dick, T.; Grüber, G. Deletion of a unique loop in the mycobacterial F-ATP synthase γ subunit sheds light on its inhibitory role in ATP hydrolysis-driven H+ pumping. *FEBS J.* **2016**, *283*, 1947–1961. [CrossRef] [PubMed]
89. Ragunathan, P.; Sielaff, H.; Sundararaman, L.; Biuković, G.; Manimekalai, M.S.S.; Singh, D.; Kundu, S.; Wohland, T.; Frasch, W.; Dick, T.; et al. The uniqueness of subunit α of mycobacterial F-ATP synthases: An evolutionary variant for niche adaptation. *J. Biol. Chem.* **2017**, *292*, 11262–11279. [CrossRef] [PubMed]
90. Kinoshita, N.; Unemoto, T.; Kobayashi, H. Proton motive force is not obligatory for growth of Escherichia coli. *J. Bacteriol.* **1984**, *160*, 1074–1077. [CrossRef] [PubMed]
91. Melo, A.M.P.; Bandeiras, T.M.; Teixeira, M. New insights into type II NAD (P) H:quinone oxidoreductases. *Microbiol. Mol. Biol. Rev.* **2004**, *68*, 603–616. [CrossRef]
92. Yano, T.; Kassovska-Bratinova, S.; Teh, J.S.; Winkler, J.; Sullivan, K.; Isaacs, A.; Schechter, N.M.; Rubin, H. Reduction of clofazimine by mycobacterial type 2 NADH: Quinone oxidoreductase: A pathway for the generation of bactericidal levels of reactive oxygen species. *J. Biol. Chem.* **2011**, *286*, 10276–10287. [CrossRef]
93. Xu, J.; Wang, B.; Fu, L.; Zhu, H.; Guo, S.; Huang, H.; Yin, D.; Zhang, Y.; Lu, Y. In vitro and in vivo activities of the Riminophenazine TBI-166 against Mycobacterium tuberculosis. *Antimicrob. Agents Chemother.* **2019**, *63*, e02155-18. [CrossRef]
94. Bourdon, J.L. Contribution to the study of the antibiotic properties of chlorpromazine or 4560 RP. *Ann. Inst. Pasteur* **1961**, *101*, 876–886.
95. Amaral, L.; Kristiansen, J.E.; Abebe, L.S.; Millett, W. Inhibition of the respiration of multi-drug resistant clinical isolates of Mycobacterium tuberculosis by thioridazine: Potential use for initial therapy of freshly diagnosed tuberculosis. *J. Antimicrob. Chemother.* **1996**, *38*, 1049–1053. [CrossRef]
96. Bettencourt, M.V.; Bosne-David, S.; Amaral, L. Comparative in vitro activity of phenothiazines against multidrug-resistant Mycobacterium tuberculosis. *Int. J. Antimicrob. Agents* **2000**, *16*, 69–71. [CrossRef]
97. Ratnakar, P.; Murthy, P.S. Antitubercular activity of trifluoperazine, a calmodulin antagonist. *FEMS Microbiol. Lett.* **1992**, *76*, 73–76. [CrossRef] [PubMed]
98. Gadre, D.V.; Talwar, V. In vitro susceptibility testing of Mycobacterium tuberculosis strains to trifluoperazine. *J. Chemother. Florence Italy* **1999**, *11*, 203–206. [CrossRef] [PubMed]
99. Amaral, L.; Kristiansen, J.E.; Viveiros, M.; Atouguia, J. Activity of phenothiazines against antibiotic-resistant Mycobacterium tuberculosis: A review supporting further studies that may elucidate the potential use of thioridazine as anti-tuberculosis therapy. *J. Antimicrob. Chemother.* **2001**, *47*, 505–511. [CrossRef] [PubMed]
100. Amaral, L.; Viveiros, M. Thioridazine: A non-antibiotic drug highly effective, in combination with first line anti-tuberculosis drugs, against any form of antibiotic resistance of mycobacterium tuberculosis due to its multi-mechanisms of action. *Antibiotics* **2017**, *6*, 3. [CrossRef]
101. Crowle, A.J.; Douvas, G.S.; May, M.H. Chlorpromazine: A drug potentially useful for treating mycobacterial infections. *Chemotherapy* **1992**, *38*, 410–419. [CrossRef]
102. Salie, S.; Hsu, N.-J.; Semenya, D.; Jardine, A.; Jacobs, M. Novel non-neuroleptic phenothiazines inhibit Mycobacterium tuberculosis replication. *J. Antimicrob. Chemother.* **2014**, *69*, 1551–1558. [CrossRef]
103. He, C.-X.; Meng, H.; Zhang, X.; Cui, H.-Q.; Yin, D.-L. Synthesis and bio-evaluation of phenothiazine derivatives as new anti-tuberculosis agents. *Chin. Chem. Lett.* **2015**, *26*, 951–954. [CrossRef]
104. Jardine, M.A.; Jacobs, M. Phenothiazine Derivatives and Their Use against Tuberculosis. WO2014080378A1, 30 May 2014.
105. Trivedi, A.R.; Siddiqui, A.B.; Shah, V.H. Design, synthesis, characterization and antitubercular activity of some 2-heterocycle-substituted phenothiazines. *Arkivoc* **2008**, *2008*, 210–217.
106. Shirude, P.S.; Paul, B.; Roy Choudhury, N.; Kedari, C.; Bandodkar, B.; Ugarkar, B.G. Quinolinyl Pyrimidines: Potent Inhibitors of NDH-2 as a Novel Class of Anti-TB Agents. *ACS Med. Chem. Lett.* **2012**, *3*, 736–740. [CrossRef]
107. Heikal, A.; Hards, K.; Cheung, C.-Y.; Menorca, A.; Timmer, M.S.M.; Stocker, B.L.; Cook, G.M. Activation of type II NADH dehydrogenase by quinolinequinones mediates antitubercular cell death. *J. Antimicrob. Chemother.* **2016**, *71*, 2840–2847. [CrossRef]

108. Bringmann, G.; Reichert, Y.; Kane, V.V. The total synthesis of streptonigrin and related antitumor antibiotic natural products. *Tetrahedron* **2004**, *60*, 3539–3574. [CrossRef]
109. Colucci, M.A.; Moody, C.J.; Couch, G.D. Natural and synthetic quinones and their reduction by the quinone reductase enzyme NQO1: From synthetic organic chemistry to compounds with anticancer potential. *Org. Biomol. Chem.* **2008**, *6*, 637–656. [CrossRef] [PubMed]
110. Pearce, A.N.; Chia, E.W.; Berridge, M.V.; Clark, G.R.; Harper, J.L.; Larsen, L.; Maas, E.W.; Page, M.J.; Perry, N.B.; Webb, V.L.; et al. Anti-inflammatory thiazine alkaloids isolated from the New Zealand ascidian Aplidium sp.: Inhibitors of the neutrophil respiratory burst in a model of gouty arthritis. *J. Nat. Prod.* **2007**, *70*, 936–940. [CrossRef] [PubMed]
111. Mulchin, B.J.; Newton, C.G.; Baty, J.W.; Grasso, C.H.; Martin, W.J.; Walton, M.C.; Dangerfield, E.M.; Plunkett, C.H.; Berridge, M.V.; Harper, J.L.; et al. The anti-cancer, anti-inflammatory and tuberculostatic activities of a series of 6,7-substituted-5,8-quinolinequinones. *Bioorg. Med. Chem.* **2010**, *18*, 3238–3251. [CrossRef]
112. Santoso, K.T.; Menorca, A.; Cheung, C.-Y.; Cook, G.M.; Stocker, B.L.; Timmer, M.S.M. The synthesis and evaluation of quinolinequinones as anti-mycobacterial agents. *Bioorg. Med. Chem.* **2019**, *27*, 3532–3545. [CrossRef]
113. Barry, V.C.; Belton, J.G.; Conalty, M.L.; Denneny, J.M.; Edward, D.W.; O'sullivan, J.F.; Twomey, D.; Winder, F. A new series of phenazines (rimino-compounds) with high antituberculosis activity. *Nature* **1957**, *179*, 1013–1015. [CrossRef]
114. Zhang, D.; Liu, Y.; Zhang, C.; Zhang, H.; Wang, B.; Xu, J.; Fu, L.; Yin, D.; Cooper, C.B.; Ma, Z.; et al. Synthesis and biological evaluation of novel 2-methoxypyridylamino-substituted riminophenazine derivatives as antituberculosis agents. *Molecules* **2014**, *19*, 4380–4394. [CrossRef]
115. Fang, M.; Toogood, R.D.; Macova, A.; Ho, K.; Franzblau, S.G.; McNeil, M.R.; Sanders, D.A.R.; Palmer, D.R.J. Succinylphosphonate esters are competitive inhibitors of mend that show active-site discrimination between homologous α-ketoglutarate-decarboxylating enzymes. *Biochemistry* **2010**, *49*, 2672–2679. [CrossRef]
116. Kurosu, M.; Narayanasamy, P.; Biswas, K.; Dhiman, R.; Crick, D.C. Discovery of 1,4-dihydroxy-2-naphthoate [corrected] prenyltransferase inhibitors: New drug leads for multidrug-resistant gram-positive pathogens. *J. Med. Chem.* **2007**, *50*, 3973–3975. [CrossRef]
117. Berube, B.J.; Russell, D.; Castro, L.; Choi, S.; Narayanasamy, P.; Parish, T. Novel mena inhibitors are bactericidal against mycobacterium tuberculosis and synergize with electron transport chain inhibitors. *Antimicrob. Agents Chemother.* **2019**, *63*, e02661-18. [CrossRef]
118. Benkovic, S.J.; Baker, S.J.; Alley, M.R.K.; Woo, Y.-H.; Zhang, Y.-K.; Akama, T.; Mao, W.; Baboval, J.; Rajagopalan, P.T.R.; Wall, M.; et al. Identification of borinic esters as inhibitors of bacterial cell growth and bacterial methyltransferases, CcrM and MenH. *J. Med. Chem.* **2005**, *48*, 7468–7476. [CrossRef] [PubMed]
119. Jirgis, E.N.M.; Bashiri, G.; Bulloch, E.M.M.; Johnston, J.M.; Baker, E.N. Structural views along the mycobacterium tuberculosis MenD reaction pathway illuminate key aspects of thiamin diphosphate-dependent enzyme mechanisms. *Structure* **2016**, *24*, 1167–1177. [CrossRef] [PubMed]
120. Lu, X.; Zhou, R.; Sharma, I.; Li, X.; Kumar, G.; Swaminathan, S.; Tonge, P.J.; Tan, D.S. Stable analogues of OSB-AMP: Potent inhibitors of MenE, the o-succinylbenzoate-CoA synthetase from bacterial menaquinone biosynthesis. *Chembiochem Eur. J. Chem. Biol.* **2012**, *13*, 129–136. [CrossRef] [PubMed]
121. Kitagawa, W.; Tamura, T. A Quinoline Antibiotic from Rhodococcus erythropolis JCM 6824. *J. Antibiot. (Tokyo)* **2008**, *61*, 680–682. [CrossRef]
122. Dhiman, R.K.; Pujari, V.; Kincaid, J.M.; Ikeh, M.A.; Parish, T.; Crick, D.C. Characterization of MenA (isoprenyl diphosphate:1,4-dihydroxy-2-naphthoate isoprenyltransferase) from Mycobacterium tuberculosis. *PLoS ONE* **2019**, *14*, e0214958. [CrossRef]
123. Choi, S.; Frandsen, J.; Narayanasamy, P. Novel long-chain compounds with both immunomodulatory and MenA inhibitory activities against Staphylococcus aureus and its biofilm. *Sci. Rep.* **2017**, *7*, 40077. [CrossRef]
124. Choi, S.; Larson, M.A.; Hinrichs, S.H.; Bartling, A.M.; Frandsen, J.; Narayanasamy, P. Discovery of bicyclic inhibitors against menaquinone biosynthesis. *Future Med. Chem.* **2016**, *8*, 11–16. [CrossRef]
125. Ballell, L.; Bates, R.H.; Young, R.J.; Alvarez-Gomez, D.; Alvarez-Ruiz, E.; Barroso, V.; Blanco, D.; Crespo, B.; Escribano, J.; González, R.; et al. Fueling open-source drug discovery: 177 small-molecule leads against tuberculosis. *ChemMedChem* **2013**, *8*, 313–321. [CrossRef]

126. Moraski, G.C.; Deboosère, N.; Marshall, K.L.; Weaver, H.A.; Vandeputte, A.; Hastings, C.; Woolhiser, L.; Lenaerts, A.J.; Brodin, P.; Miller, M.J. Intracellular and in vivo evaluation of imidazo[2,1-b]thiazole-5-carboxamide anti-tuberculosis compounds. *PLoS ONE* **2020**, *15*, e0227224. [CrossRef]
127. Tantry, S.J.; Markad, S.D.; Shinde, V.; Bhat, J.; Balakrishnan, G.; Gupta, A.K.; Ambady, A.; Raichurkar, A.; Kedari, C.; Sharma, S.; et al. Discovery of Imidazo[1,2-a]pyridine ethers and squaramides as selective and potent inhibitors of mycobacterial adenosine triphosphate (ATP) synthesis. *J. Med. Chem.* **2017**, *60*, 1379–1399. [CrossRef]
128. Lu, X.; Williams, Z.; Hards, K.; Tang, J.; Cheung, C.-Y.; Aung, H.L.; Wang, B.; Liu, Z.; Hu, X.; Lenaerts, A.; et al. Pyrazolo[1,5- a]pyridine inhibitor of the respiratory cytochrome bcc complex for the treatment of drug-resistant tuberculosis. *ACS Infect. Dis.* **2019**, *5*, 239–249. [CrossRef] [PubMed]
129. Rybniker, J.; Vocat, A.; Sala, C.; Busso, P.; Pojer, F.; Benjak, A.; Cole, S.T. Lansoprazole is an antituberculous prodrug targeting cytochrome bc1. *Nat. Commun.* **2015**, *6*, 7659. [CrossRef] [PubMed]
130. Chandrasekera, N.S.; Berube, B.J.; Shetye, G.; Chettiar, S.; O'Malley, T.; Manning, A.; Flint, L.; Awasthi, D.; Ioerger, T.R.; Sacchettini, J.; et al. Improved phenoxyalkylbenzimidazoles with activity against Mycobacterium tuberculosis appear to target QcrB. *ACS Infect. Dis.* **2017**, *3*, 898–916. [CrossRef] [PubMed]
131. van der Westhuyzen, R.; Winks, S.; Wilson, C.R.; Boyle, G.A.; Gessner, R.K.; Soares de Melo, C.; Taylor, D.; de Kock, C.; Njoroge, M.; Brunschwig, C.; et al. Pyrrolo[3,4-c]pyridine-1,3(2H)-diones: A novel antimycobacterial class targeting mycobacterial respiration. *J. Med. Chem.* **2015**, *58*, 9371–9381. [CrossRef] [PubMed]
132. Pissinate, K.; Villela, A.D.; Rodrigues-Junior, V.; Giacobbo, B.C.; Grams, E.S.; Abbadi, B.L.; Trindade, R.V.; Roesler Nery, L.; Bonan, C.D.; Back, D.F.; et al. 2-(Quinolin-4-yloxy)acetamides are active against drug-susceptible and drug-resistant mycobacterium tuberculosis strains. *ACS Med. Chem. Lett.* **2016**, *7*, 235–239. [CrossRef] [PubMed]
133. Giacobbo, B.C.; Pissinate, K.; Rodrigues-Junior, V.; Villela, A.D.; Grams, E.S.; Abbadi, B.L.; Subtil, F.T.; Sperotto, N.; Trindade, R.V.; Back, D.F.; et al. New insights into the SAR and drug combination synergy of 2-(quinolin-4-yloxy)acetamides against Mycobacterium tuberculosis. *Eur. J. Med. Chem.* **2017**, *126*, 491–501. [CrossRef]
134. Cleghorn, L.A.T.; Ray, P.C.; Odingo, J.; Kumar, A.; Wescott, H.; Korkegian, A.; Masquelin, T.; Lopez Moure, A.; Wilson, C.; Davis, S.; et al. Identification of morpholino thiophenes as novel mycobacterium tuberculosis inhibitors, targeting QcrB. *J. Med. Chem.* **2018**, *61*, 6592–6608. [CrossRef]
135. Harrison, G.A.; Bridwell, A.E.M.; Singh, M.; Jayaraman, K.; Weiss, L.A.; Kinsella, R.L.; Aneke, J.S.; Flentie, K.; Schene, M.E.; Gaggioli, M.; et al. Identification of 4-Amino-Thieno[2,3-d]Pyrimidines as QcrB Inhibitors in Mycobacterium tuberculosis. *mSphere* **2019**, *4*, e00606-19. [CrossRef]
136. Meunier, B.; Madgwick, S.A.; Reil, E.; Oettmeier, W.; Rich, P.R. New inhibitors of the quinol oxidation sites of bacterial cytochromes bo and bd. *Biochemistry* **1995**, *34*, 1076–1083. [CrossRef]
137. Moraski, G.C.; Markley, L.D.; Hipskind, P.A.; Boshoff, H.; Cho, S.; Franzblau, S.G.; Miller, M.J. Advent of Imidazo[1,2-a]pyridine-3-carboxamides with potent multi- and extended drug resistant antituberculosis activity. *ACS Med. Chem. Lett.* **2011**, *2*, 466–470. [CrossRef]
138. Abrahams, K.A.; Cox, J.A.G.; Spivey, V.L.; Loman, N.J.; Pallen, M.J.; Constantinidou, C.; Fernández, R.; Alemparte, C.; Remuiñán, M.J.; Barros, D.; et al. Identification of novel imidazo[1,2-a]pyridine inhibitors targeting M. tuberculosis QcrB. *PLoS ONE* **2012**, *7*, e52951. [CrossRef] [PubMed]
139. Mak, P.A.; Rao, S.P.S.; Ping Tan, M.; Lin, X.; Chyba, J.; Tay, J.; Ng, S.H.; Tan, B.H.; Cherian, J.; Duraiswamy, J.; et al. A high-throughput screen to identify inhibitors of atp homeostasis in non-replicating mycobacterium tuberculosis. *ACS Chem. Biol.* **2012**, *7*, 1190–1197. [CrossRef]
140. Moraski, G.C.; Markley, L.D.; Cramer, J.; Hipskind, P.A.; Boshoff, H.; Bailey, M.; Alling, T.; Ollinger, J.; Parish, T.; Miller, M.J. Advancement of Imidazo[1,2-a]pyridines with improved pharmacokinetics and nanomolar activity against mycobacterium tuberculosis. *ACS Med. Chem. Lett.* **2013**, *4*, 675–679. [CrossRef] [PubMed]
141. Moraski, G.C.; Oliver, A.G.; Markley, L.D.; Cho, S.; Franzblau, S.G.; Miller, M.J. Scaffold-switching: An exploration of 5,6-fused bicyclic heteroaromatics systems to afford antituberculosis activity akin to the imidazo[1,2-a]pyridine-3-carboxylates. *Bioorg. Med. Chem. Lett.* **2014**, *24*, 3493–3498. [CrossRef] [PubMed]

142. Kang, S.; Kim, R.Y.; Seo, M.J.; Lee, S.; Kim, Y.M.; Seo, M.; Seo, J.J.; Ko, Y.; Choi, I.; Jang, J.; et al. Lead optimization of a novel series of imidazo[1,2-a]pyridine amides leading to a clinical candidate (Q203) as a multi- and extensively-drug-resistant anti-tuberculosis agent. *J. Med. Chem.* **2014**, *57*, 5293–5305. [CrossRef] [PubMed]
143. Moraski, G.C.; Seeger, N.; Miller, P.A.; Oliver, A.G.; Boshoff, H.I.; Cho, S.; Mulugeta, S.; Anderson, J.R.; Franzblau, S.G.; Miller, M.J. Arrival of Imidazo[2,1-b]thiazole-5-carboxamides: Potent anti-tuberculosis agents that target QcrB. *ACS Infect. Dis.* **2016**, *2*, 393–398. [CrossRef] [PubMed]
144. Telacebec (Q203) | Working Group for New TB Drugs. Available online: https://www.newtbdrugs.org/pipeline/compound/telacebec-q203 (accessed on 3 February 2020).
145. Bouvier, G.; Simenel, C.; Jang, J.; Kalia, N.P.; Choi, I.; Nilges, M.; Pethe, K.; Izadi-Pruneyre, N. Target engagement and binding mode of an antituberculosis drug to its bacterial target deciphered in whole living cells by NMR. *Biochemistry* **2019**, *58*, 526–533. [CrossRef]
146. Moosa, A.; Lamprecht, D.A.; Arora, K.; Barry, C.E.; Boshoff, H.I.M.; Ioerger, T.R.; Steyn, A.J.C.; Mizrahi, V.; Warner, D.F. Susceptibility of mycobacterium tuberculosis cytochrome bd oxidase mutants to compounds targeting the terminal respiratory oxidase, cytochrome c. *Antimicrob. Agents Chemother.* **2017**, *61*, e01338-17. [CrossRef]
147. Scherr, N.; Bieri, R.; Thomas, S.S.; Chauffour, A.; Kalia, N.P.; Schneide, P.; Ruf, M.-T.; Lamelas, A.; Manimekalai, M.S.S.; Grüber, G.; et al. Targeting the Mycobacterium ulcerans cytochrome bc1:aa3 for the treatment of Buruli ulcer. *Nat. Commun.* **2018**, *9*, 5370. [CrossRef]
148. Tang, J.; Wang, B.; Wu, T.; Wan, J.; Tu, Z.; Njire, M.; Wan, B.; Franzblauc, S.G.; Zhang, T.; Lu, X.; et al. Design, synthesis, and biological evaluation of Pyrazolo[1,5-a]pyridine-3-carboxamides as novel antitubercular agents. *ACS Med. Chem. Lett.* **2015**, *6*, 814–818. [CrossRef]
149. Lu, X.; Tang, J.; Cui, S.; Wan, B.; Franzblauc, S.G.; Zhang, T.; Zhang, X.; Ding, K. Pyrazolo[1,5-a]pyridine-3-carboxamide hybrids: Design, synthesis and evaluation of anti-tubercular activity. *Eur. J. Med. Chem.* **2017**, *125*, 41–48. [CrossRef] [PubMed]
150. Lee, B.S.; Kalia, N.P.; Jin, X.E.F.; Hasenoehrl, E.J.; Berney, M.; Pethe, K. Inhibitors of energy metabolism interfere with antibiotic-induced death in mycobacteria. *J. Biol. Chem.* **2019**, *294*, 1936–1943. [CrossRef] [PubMed]
151. Mdanda, S.; Baijnath, S.; Shobo, A.; Singh, S.D.; Maguire, G.E.M.; Kruger, H.G.; Arvidsson, P.I.; Naicker, T.; Govender, T. Lansoprazole-sulfide, pharmacokinetics of this promising anti-tuberculous agent. *Biomed. Chromatogr.* **2017**, *31*, e4035. [CrossRef] [PubMed]
152. Yates, T.A.; Tomlinson, L.A.; Bhaskaran, K.; Langan, S.; Thomas, S.; Smeeth, L.; Douglas, I.J. Lansoprazole use and tuberculosis incidence in the United Kingdom Clinical Practice Research Datalink: A population based cohort. *PLoS Med.* **2017**, *14*, e1002457. [CrossRef]
153. Chandrasekera, N.S.; Alling, T.; Bailey, M.A.; Files, M.; Early, J.V.; Ollinger, J.; Ovechkina, Y.; Masquelin, T.; Desai, P.V.; Cramer, J.W.; et al. Identification of phenoxyalkylbenzimidazoles with antitubercular activity. *J. Med. Chem.* **2015**, *58*, 7273–7285. [CrossRef]
154. Pitta, E.; Rogacki, M.K.; Balabon, O.; Huss, S.; Cunningham, F.; Lopez-Roman, E.M.; Joossens, J.; Augustyns, K.; Ballell, L.; Bates, R.H.; et al. Searching for New Leads for Tuberculosis: Design, Synthesis, and Biological Evaluation of Novel 2-Quinolin-4-yloxyacetamides. *J. Med. Chem.* **2016**, *59*, 6709–6728. [CrossRef]
155. Phummarin, N.; Boshoff, H.I.; Tsang, P.S.; Dalton, J.; Wiles, S.; Barry 3rd, C.E.; Copp, B.R. SAR and identification of 2-(quinolin-4-yloxy)acetamides as Mycobacterium tuberculosis cytochrome bc 1 inhibitors. *Medchemcomm* **2016**, *7*, 2122–2127. [CrossRef]
156. Subtil, F.T.; Villela, A.D.; Abbadi, B.L.; Rodrigues-Junior, V.S.; Bizarro, C.V.; Timmers, L.F.S.M.; de Souza, O.N.; Pissinate, K.; Machado, P.; López-Gavín, A.; et al. Activity of 2-(quinolin-4-yloxy)acetamides in Mycobacterium tuberculosis clinical isolates and identification of their molecular target by whole-genome sequencing. *Int. J. Antimicrob. Agents* **2018**, *51*, 378–384. [CrossRef]
157. Berry, E.A.; Guergova-Kuras, M.; Huang, L.S.; Crofts, A.R. Structure and function of cytochrome bc complexes. *Annu. Rev. Biochem.* **2000**, *69*, 1005–1075. [CrossRef]
158. Lamprecht, D.A.; Finin, P.M.; Rahman, M.A.; Cumming, B.M.; Russell, S.L.; Jonnala, S.R.; Adamson, J.H.; Steyn, A.J.C. Turning the respiratory flexibility of *Mycobacterium tuberculosis* against itself. *Nat. Commun.* **2016**, *7*, 12393. [CrossRef]

159. Lu, P.; Heineke, M.H.; Koul, A.; Andries, K.; Cook, G.M.; Lill, H.; van Spanning, R.; Bald, D. The cytochrome bd-type quinol oxidase is important for survival of Mycobacterium smegmatis under peroxide and antibiotic-induced stress. *Sci. Rep.* **2015**, *5*, 10333. [CrossRef] [PubMed]
160. Lu, P.; Asseri, A.H.; Kremer, M.; Maaskant, J.; Ummels, R.; Lill, H.; Bald, D. The anti-mycobacterial activity of the cytochrome bcc inhibitor Q203 can be enhanced by small-molecule inhibition of cytochrome bd. *Sci. Rep.* **2018**, *8*, 2625. [CrossRef] [PubMed]
161. Flentie, K.; Harrison, G.A.; Tükenmez, H.; Livny, J.; Good, J.A.D.; Sarkar, S.; Zhu, D.X.; Kinsella, R.L.; Weiss, L.A.; Solomon, S.D.; et al. Chemical disarming of isoniazid resistance in Mycobacterium tuberculosis. *Proc. Natl. Acad. Sci. USA* **2019**, *116*, 10510–10517. [CrossRef] [PubMed]
162. Tran, S.L.; Cook, G.M. The F1Fo-ATP synthase of Mycobacterium smegmatis is essential for growth. *J. Bacteriol.* **2005**, *187*, 5023–5028. [CrossRef]
163. Koul, A.; Dendouga, N.; Vergauwen, K.; Molenberghs, B.; Vranckx, L.; Willebrords, R.; Ristic, Z.; Lill, H.; Dorange, I.; Guillemont, J.; et al. Diarylquinolines target subunit c of mycobacterial ATP synthase. *Nat. Chem. Biol.* **2007**, *3*, 323–324. [CrossRef]
164. Haagsma, A.C.; Podasca, I.; Koul, A.; Andries, K.; Guillemont, J.; Lill, H.; Bald, D. Probing the interaction of the diarylquinoline TMC207 with its target mycobacterial ATP synthase. *PLoS ONE* **2011**, *6*, e23575. [CrossRef]
165. Nesci, S.; Trombetti, F.; Algieri, C.; Pagliarani, A. A therapeutic role for the F1FO-ATP synthase. *SLAS Discov. Adv. Life Sci. R D* **2019**, *24*, 893–903. [CrossRef]
166. Preiss, L.; Langer, J.D.; Yildiz, Ö.; Eckhardt-Strelau, L.; Guillemont, J.E.G.; Koul, A.; Meier, T. Structure of the mycobacterial ATP synthase Fo rotor ring in complex with the anti-TB drug bedaquiline. *Sci. Adv.* **2015**, *1*, e1500106. [CrossRef]
167. Hards, K.; McMillan, D.G.G.; Schurig-Briccio, L.A.; Gennis, R.B.; Lill, H.; Bald, D.; Cook, G.M. Ionophoric effects of the antitubercular drug bedaquiline. *Proc. Natl. Acad. Sci. USA* **2018**, *115*, 7326–7331. [CrossRef]
168. Hartkoorn, R.C.; Uplekar, S.; Cole, S.T. Cross-resistance between clofazimine and bedaquiline through upregulation of MmpL5 in Mycobacterium tuberculosis. *Antimicrob. Agents Chemother.* **2014**, *58*, 2979–2981. [CrossRef]
169. Almeida, D.; Ioerger, T.; Tyagi, S.; Li, S.-Y.; Mdluli, K.; Andries, K.; Grosset, J.; Sacchettini, J.; Nuermberger, E. Mutations in pepQ confer low-level resistance to bedaquiline and clofazimine in mycobacterium tuberculosis. *Antimicrob. Agents Chemother.* **2016**, *60*, 4590–4599. [CrossRef] [PubMed]
170. Xu, J.; Wang, B.; Hu, M.; Huo, F.; Guo, S.; Jing, W.; Nuermberger, E.; Lu, Y. Primary clofazimine and bedaquiline resistance among isolates from patients with multidrug-resistant tuberculosis. *Antimicrob. Agents Chemother.* **2017**, *61*, e00239-17. [CrossRef] [PubMed]
171. Ghajavand, H.; Kargarpour Kamakoli, M.; Khanipour, S.; Pourazar Dizaji, S.; Masoumi, M.; Rahimi Jamnani, F.; Fateh, A.; Siadat, S.D.; Vaziri, F. High prevalence of bedaquiline resistance in treatment-naive tuberculosis patients and verapamil effectiveness. *Antimicrob. Agents Chemother.* **2019**, *63*, e02530-18. [CrossRef] [PubMed]
172. Zimenkov, D.V.; Nosova, E.Y.; Kulagina, E.V.; Antonova, O.V.; Arslanbaeva, L.R.; Isakova, A.I.; Krylova, L.Y.; Peretokina, I.V.; Makarova, M.V.; Safonova, S.G.; et al. Examination of bedaquiline- and linezolid-resistant Mycobacterium tuberculosis isolates from the Moscow region. *J. Antimicrob. Chemother.* **2017**, *72*, 1901–1906. [CrossRef] [PubMed]
173. Villellas, C.; Coeck, N.; Meehan, C.J.; Lounis, N.; de Jong, B.; Rigouts, L.; Andries, K. Unexpected high prevalence of resistance-associated Rv0678 variants in MDR-TB patients without documented prior use of clofazimine or bedaquiline. *J. Antimicrob. Chemother.* **2017**, *72*, 684–690. [PubMed]
174. Guglielmetti, L.; Tiberi, S.; Burman, M.; Kunst, H.; Wejse, C.; Togonidze, T.; Bothamley, G.; Lange, C. QT prolongation and cardiac toxicity of new tuberculosis drugs in Europe: A tuberculosis network European trialsgroup (TBnet) study. *Eur. Respir. J.* **2018**, *52*, 1800537. [CrossRef]
175. Tong, A.S.T.; Choi, P.J.; Blaser, A.; Sutherland, H.S.; Tsang, S.K.Y.; Guillemont, J.; Motte, M.; Cooper, C.B.; Andries, K.; Van den Broeck, W.; et al. 6-Cyano analogues of bedaquiline as less lipophilic and potentially safer diarylquinolines for tuberculosis. *ACS Med. Chem. Lett.* **2017**, *8*, 1019–1024. [CrossRef]
176. Choi, P.J.; Sutherland, H.S.; Tong, A.S.T.; Blaser, A.; Franzblau, S.G.; Cooper, C.B.; Lotlikar, M.U.; Upton, A.M.; Guillemont, J.; Motte, M.; et al. Synthesis and evaluation of analogues of the tuberculosis drug bedaquiline containing heterocyclic B-ring units. *Bioorg. Med. Chem. Lett.* **2017**, *27*, 5190–5196. [CrossRef]

177. Sutherland, H.S.; Tong, A.S.T.; Choi, P.J.; Conole, D.; Blaser, A.; Franzblau, S.G.; Cooper, C.B.; Upton, A.M.; Lotlikar, M.U.; Denny, W.A.; et al. Structure-activity relationships for analogs of the tuberculosis drug bedaquiline with the naphthalene unit replaced by bicyclic heterocycles. *Bioorg. Med. Chem.* **2018**, *26*, 1797–1809. [CrossRef]
178. Blaser, A.; Sutherland, H.S.; Tong, A.S.T.; Choi, P.J.; Conole, D.; Franzblau, S.G.; Cooper, C.B.; Upton, A.M.; Lotlikar, M.; Denny, W.A.; et al. Structure-activity relationships for unit C pyridyl analogues of the tuberculosis drug bedaquiline. *Bioorg. Med. Chem.* **2019**, *27*, 1283–1291. [CrossRef]
179. Sutherland, H.S.; Tong, A.S.T.; Choi, P.J.; Blaser, A.; Conole, D.; Franzblau, S.G.; Lotlikar, M.U.; Cooper, C.B.; Upton, A.M.; Denny, W.A.; et al. 3,5-Dialkoxypyridine analogues of bedaquiline are potent antituberculosis agents with minimal inhibition of the hERG channel. *Bioorg. Med. Chem.* **2019**, *27*, 1292–1307. [CrossRef]
180. Sarathy, J.P.; Ragunathan, P.; Shin, J.; Cooper, C.B.; Upton, A.M.; Grüber, G.; Dick, T. TBAJ-876 retains bedaquiline's activity against subunits c and ε of mycobacterium tuberculosis F-ATP synthase. *Antimicrob. Agents Chemother.* **2019**, *63*, e01191-19. [CrossRef] [PubMed]
181. Kumar, S.; Mehra, R.; Sharma, S.; Bokolia, N.P.; Raina, D.; Nargotra, A.; Singh, P.P.; Khan, I.A. Screening of antitubercular compound library identifies novel ATP synthase inhibitors of mycobacterium tuberculosis. *Tuberc. Edinb. Scotl.* **2018**, *108*, 56–63. [CrossRef] [PubMed]
182. Lu, P.; Haagsma, A.C.; Pham, H.; Maaskant, J.J.; Mol, S.; Lill, H.; Bald, D. Pyrazinoic acid decreases the proton motive force, respiratory ATP synthesis activity, and cellular ATP levels. *Antimicrob. Agents Chemother.* **2011**, *55*, 5354–5357. [CrossRef] [PubMed]
183. Feng, X.; Zhu, W.; Schurig-Briccio, L.A.; Lindert, S.; Shoen, C.; Hitchings, R.; Li, J.; Wang, Y.; Baig, N.; Zhou, T.; et al. Antiinfectives targeting enzymes and the proton motive force. *Proc. Natl. Acad. Sci. USA* **2015**, *112*, E7073–E7082. [CrossRef] [PubMed]
184. Jeon, A.B.; Ackart, D.F.; Li, W.; Jackson, M.; Melander, R.J.; Melander, C.; Abramovitch, R.B.; Chicco, A.J.; Basaraba, R.J.; Obregón-Henao, A. 2-aminoimidazoles collapse mycobacterial proton motive force and block the electron transport chain. *Sci. Rep.* **2019**, *9*, 1513. [CrossRef] [PubMed]
185. Jeon, A.B.; Obregón-Henao, A.; Ackart, D.F.; Podell, B.K.; Belardinelli, J.M.; Jackson, M.; Nguyen, T.V.; Blackledge, M.S.; Melander, R.J.; Melander, C.; et al. 2-aminoimidazoles potentiate ß-lactam antimicrobial activity against Mycobacterium tuberculosis by reducing ß-lactamase secretion and increasing cell envelope permeability. *PLoS ONE* **2017**, *12*, e0180925. [CrossRef]
186. Protopopova, M.; Hanrahan, C.; Nikonenko, B.; Samala, R.; Chen, P.; Gearhart, J.; Einck, L.; Nacy, C.A. Identification of a new antitubercular drug candidate, SQ109, from a combinatorial library of 1,2-ethylenediamines. *J. Antimicrob. Chemother.* **2005**, *56*, 968–974. [CrossRef]
187. Li, K.; Schurig-Briccio, L.A.; Feng, X.; Upadhyay, A.; Pujari, V.; Lechartier, B.; Fontes, F.L.; Yang, H.; Rao, G.; Zhu, W.; et al. Multitarget drug discovery for tuberculosis and other infectious diseases. *J. Med. Chem.* **2014**, *57*, 3126–3139. [CrossRef]
188. Zhang, Y.; Wade, M.M.; Scorpio, A.; Zhang, H.; Sun, Z. Mode of action of pyrazinamide: Disruption of Mycobacterium tuberculosis membrane transport and energetics by pyrazinoic acid. *J. Antimicrob. Chemother.* **2003**, *52*, 790–795. [CrossRef]
189. Yang, C.-S.; Yuk, J.-M.; Jo, E.-K. The role of nitric oxide in mycobacterial infections. *Immune Netw.* **2009**, *9*, 46–52. [CrossRef]
190. Manjunatha, U.; Boshoff, H.I.; Barry, C.E. The mechanism of action of PA-824. *Commun. Integr. Biol.* **2009**, *2*, 215–218. [CrossRef] [PubMed]
191. Stover, C.K.; Warrener, P.; VanDevanter, D.R.; Sherman, D.R.; Arain, T.M.; Langhorne, M.H.; Anderson, S.W.; Towell, J.A.; Yuan, Y.; McMurray, D.N.; et al. A small-molecule nitroimidazopyran drug candidate for the treatment of tuberculosis. *Nature* **2000**, *405*, 962–966. [CrossRef]
192. Matsumoto, M.; Hashizume, H.; Tomishige, T.; Kawasaki, M.; Tsubouchi, H.; Sasaki, H.; Shimokawa, Y.; Komatsu, M. OPC-67683, a nitro-dihydro-imidazooxazole derivative with promising action against tuberculosis in vitro and in mice. *PLoS Med.* **2006**, *3*, e466. [CrossRef]
193. Van den Bossche, A.; Varet, H.; Sury, A.; Sismeiro, O.; Legendre, R.; Coppee, J.-Y.; Mathys, V.; Ceyssens, P.-J. Transcriptional profiling of a laboratory and clinical Mycobacterium tuberculosis strain suggests respiratory poisoning upon exposure to delamanid. *Tuberc. Edinb. Scotl.* **2019**, *117*, 18–23. [CrossRef] [PubMed]
194. Developing New TB Regimens. Available online: https://www.tballiance.org/rd/developing-new-regimens (accessed on 23 December 2019).

195. Berube, B.J.; Parish, T. Combinations of respiratory chain inhibitors have enhanced bactericidal activity against mycobacterium tuberculosis. *Antimicrob. Agents Chemother.* **2018**, *62*, e01677-17. [CrossRef] [PubMed]
196. Moraski, G.C.; Cheng, Y.; Cho, S.; Cramer, J.W.; Godfrey, A.; Masquelin, T.; Franzblau, S.G.; Miller, M.J.; Schorey, J. Imidazo[1,2-a]Pyridine-3-Carboxamides are active antimicrobial agents against mycobacterium avium infection in vivo. *Antimicrob. Agents Chemother.* **2016**, *60*, 5018–5022. [CrossRef]
197. Heinrich, N.; Dawson, R.; du Bois, J.; Narunsky, K.; Horwith, G.; Phipps, A.J.; Nacy, C.A.; Aarnoutse, R.E.; Boeree, M.J.; Gillespie, S.H.; et al. Early phase evaluation of SQ109 alone and in combination with rifampicin in pulmonary TB patients. *J. Antimicrob. Chemother.* **2015**, *70*, 1558–1566. [CrossRef]
198. Zhang, Y.; Zhu, H.; Fu, L.; Wang, B.; Guo, S.; Chen, X.; Liu, Z.; Huang, H.; Yang, T.; Lu, Y. Identifying regimens containing TBI-166, a new drug candidate against mycobacterium tuberculosis in vitro and in vivo. *Antimicrob. Agents Chemother.* **2019**, *63*, e02496-18. [CrossRef]
199. Converse, P.J.; Almeida, D.V.; Tyagi, S.; Xu, J.; Nuermberger, E.L. Shortening buruli ulcer treatment with combination therapy targeting the respiratory chain and exploiting mycobacterium ulcerans gene decay. *Antimicrob. Agents Chemother.* **2019**, *63*, e00426-19. [CrossRef]

4

Mycobacterial Cell Wall: A Source of Successful Targets for Old and New Drugs

Catherine Vilchèze

Einstein College of Medicine, 1301 Morris Park Avenue, the Bronx, New York, NY 10461, USA; catherine.vilcheze@einsteinmed.org

Abstract: Eighty years after the introduction of the first antituberculosis (TB) drug, the treatment of drug-susceptible TB remains very cumbersome, requiring the use of four drugs (isoniazid, rifampicin, ethambutol and pyrazinamide) for two months followed by four months on isoniazid and rifampicin. Two of the drugs used in this "short"-course, six-month chemotherapy, isoniazid and ethambutol, target the mycobacterial cell wall. Disruption of the cell wall structure can enhance the entry of other TB drugs, resulting in a more potent chemotherapy. More importantly, inhibition of cell wall components can lead to mycobacterial cell death. The complexity of the mycobacterial cell wall offers numerous opportunities to develop drugs to eradicate *Mycobacterium tuberculosis*, the causative agent of TB. In the past 20 years, researchers from industrial and academic laboratories have tested new molecules to find the best candidates that will change the face of TB treatment: drugs that will shorten TB treatment and be efficacious against active and latent, as well as drug-resistant TB. Two of these new TB drugs block components of the mycobacterial cell wall and have reached phase 3 clinical trial. This article reviews TB drugs targeting the mycobacterial cell wall in use clinically and those in clinical development.

Keywords: tuberculosis; discovery; mode of action; drug resistance; toxicity; target

1. Introduction

In 1882, when Robert Koch made his ground-breaking announcement that he had discovered, isolated and cultured the bacterium responsible for tuberculosis (TB), there were no curative options for people infected with TB. In Roman times, the personal physician of the emperor Marcus Aurelius (161–180) was prescribing sea trips, fresh air and milk to treat TB patients [1]. English, French and German physicians revisited this concept 17 centuries later. In 1840, the English physician George Bodington wrote an essay "On the treatment and cure of pulmonary consumption," where he recommended fresh, cold and open air, exercise, a healthy diet and wine to treat TB patients. He opposed the treatment popular at the time: confinement of TB patients and the use of drugs such as digitalis and antimony potassium tartrate [2]. The journal Lancet published a harsh review of this essay, describing it as "very crude ideas and unsupported assertions" [3], but later admitted that they had been wrong [4]. Other English physicians followed Bodington's ideas of fresh-air treatment for TB patients but were dismissed by the medical intelligentsia [5]. On the other side of the Channel, the French physician Amédée Latour prescribed sunshine, fresh air, exercise and rich food containing 1/8 oz of sea salt every morning to treat TB [6]. The German physician Hermann Brehmer advocated high altitude, fresh air, exercise and a rich diet with some alcohol for the treatment of TB patients [5]. He opened the first sanatorium in 1854 in Görbersdorf, Prussia, to implement his concept. Sanatoria were beneficial to TB patients with early stages of disease. Lower mortality rates were observed in sanatoria compared to TB patients treated at home [1,7]. Sanatoria would close one hundred years later with the introduction of the first multiantimycobacterial drug regimen to treat TB.

The first drug against the etiologic agent of TB, ***Mycobacterium tuberculosis***, was streptomycin, isolated from the soil bacterium ***Streptomyces griseus*** and shown to have activity against ***M. tuberculosis*** in 1944 [8,9]. Streptomycin was tested on a 21-year-old woman with advanced pulmonary TB and gave "impressive therapeutic effects" [10,11]. Unfortunately, resistance to streptomycin developed quickly [12,13]. In 1946, Jorgen Lehmann published the discovery of the antimycobacterial activity of para-aminosalicylic acid (PAS) in vitro, in guinea pigs and in TB patients [14]. The addition of PAS to streptomycin treatment drastically reduced the emergence of streptomycin-resistant strains in TB patients but did not abolish it [15]. It would take the introduction of a new TB drug, isoniazid (INH), in 1952 to achieve a successful treatment for TB [16].

INH is one of the most effective drugs against ***M. tuberculosis***, which is still used to this day to treat active and latent ***M. tuberculosis*** infections. INH is part of a four-drug regimen (INH, rifampicin (RIF), ethambutol (EMB) and pyrazinamide (PZA)) to treat drug-susceptible ***M. tuberculosis*** infection. While RIF targets the RNA polymerase RpoB and PZA's mechanism of action is still unclear, INH and EMB target the mycobacterial cell wall.

The ***M. tuberculosis*** cell wall has an intricate and unique structure composed of a thick peptidoglycan layer and an outer membrane made up mostly of various lipopolysaccharides and fatty acids with imbedded glycolipids and wax esters. This lipid-rich cell wall forms a low-permeability barrier that protects ***M. tuberculosis*** against most antibiotics. This is one of the many challenges facing TB drug development and the main reason drug target-based screening has been rather unsuccessful [17,18]. Bacteria require an intact cell membrane in order to survive; therefore, the biosynthesis of cell wall components could be considered a weakness to exploit with new and more potent drugs. The ever-expanding threat of drug resistance should motivate greater alacrity in developing these new therapies. Global drug surveillance data from the World Health Organization indicates that in 2018, half a million people were infected with rifampicin- or multidrug-resistant (MDR) TB, and 6% of them had extensively drug-resistant (XDR) TB [19]. While an MDR ***M. tuberculosis*** strain is "only" resistant to INH and RIF, an XDR strain is resistant to at least five TB drugs (INH, RIF and three second-line TB drugs). Treatment for drug-resistant TB is very long (minimum 20 months), requiring multiple drugs with potential severe adverse reactions. MDR TB treatment's success rate is approximately 55%, whereas XDR TB is barely 39%. New drugs and shorter drug regimens are actively sought to increase these success rates. This article covers TB drugs specifically targeting the mycobacterial cell wall currently used in clinics or in clinical development, focusing on their discovery, activity, toxicity, mode of action and resistance.

2. The Mycobacterial Cell Wall

The biosynthesis of the mycobacterial cell wall components has been extensively described recently [20–22], and only a summary of the most pertinent points for this article is presented here. The proteins implicated or targeted by TB drugs discussed below are underlined.

The three main components of the cell wall are the peptidoglycan (PG), the lipopolysaccharides (arabinogalactan, lipoarabinomannan, and lipomannan) and the outer membrane, which contains mycolic acids, various glycolipids and phthiocerol dimycocerosates (Figure 1).

The ***M. tuberculosis*** peptidoglycan is located outside of the mycobacterial inner membrane, conferring rigidity, integrity and shape to the cell [22]. The peptidoglycan is a polysaccharide composed of alternating ***N***-acetylglucosamine and muramic acid (either ***N***-acetylated or ***N***-glycolylated) residues linked by β (1→4) bonds [23–26]. Strands of polysaccharides are acylated on the muramic acid residues by the pentapeptide L-alanyl-D-isoglutaminyl-***meso***-diaminopimelyl-D-alanyl-D-alanine synthesized by the Mur ligases (MurC/D/E/F). The acylation reaction is performed by the D-Ala:D-Ala ligase DdlA. The pentapeptides are cross-linked to form the peptidoglycan. Two types of cross-linkages are observed in ***M. tuberculosis***: (i) the D,D-transpeptidase activity of the penicillin binding proteins PonA1 and PonA2 cross-links meso-diaminopimelic acid and D-alanine to form a 3→4 linkage; (ii) the

L,D-transpeptidases (LdtMt1 to 5) cross-link two meso-diaminopimelate residues to form a 3→3 linkage [22].

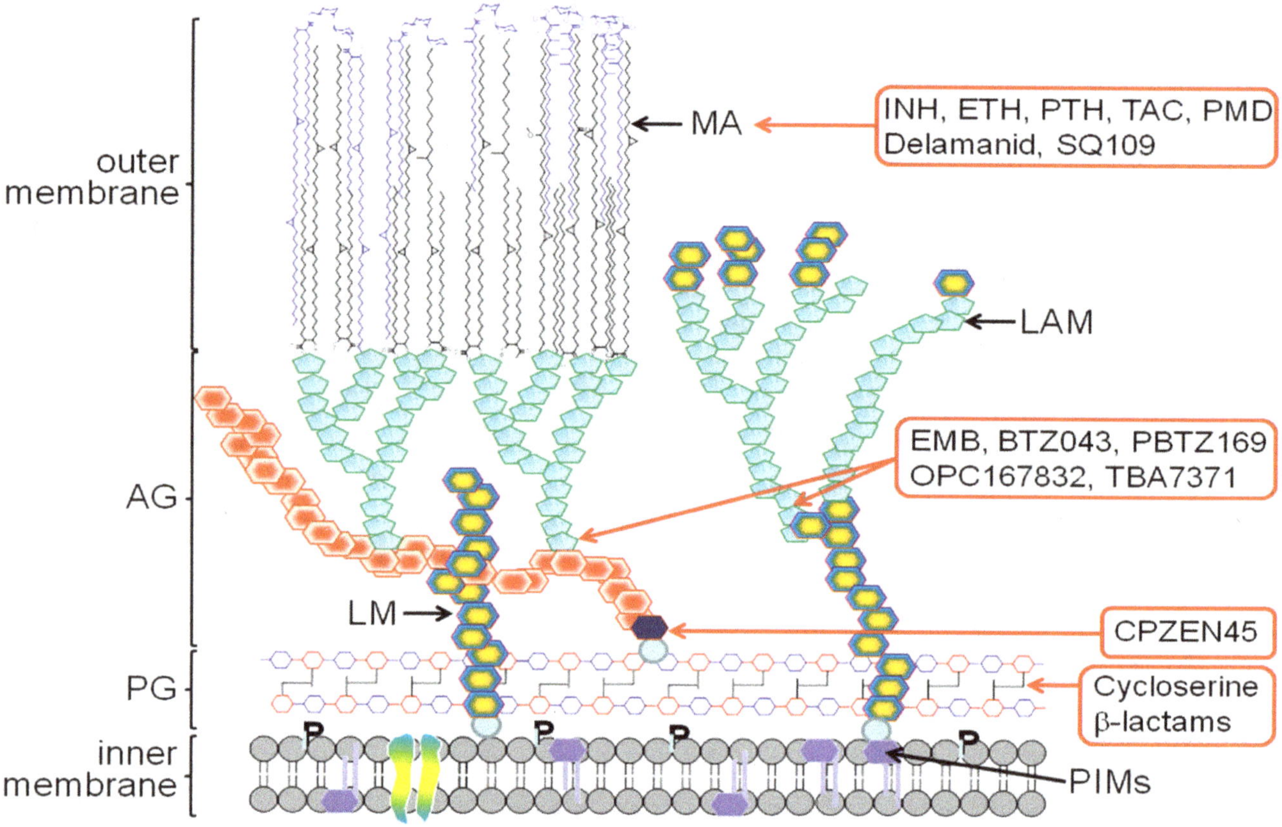

Figure 1. Illustration of the mycobacterial cell wall. The outermost layer of the cell wall, the capsule, is omitted. The cell wall components/sites inhibited by the tuberculosis (TB) drugs discussed herein are indicated. Abbreviations: AG, arabinogalactan; LAM, lipoarabinomannan; LM, lipomannan; MA, mycolic acids; PG, peptidoglycan; P, phospholipid; PIMs, phosphatidyl-*myo*-inositol mannosides; INH, isoniazid; ETH, ethionamide; PTH, prothionamide; TAC, thiacetazone; PMD, pretomanid; EMB, ethambutol.

The arabinogalactan is a branched polysaccharide composed of arabinose (Ara*f*) and galactose (Gal*f*) residues in the furanose configuration [27]. The first step in the arabinogalactan biosynthesis is the formation of the linker that anchors the arabinogalactan complex to the peptidoglycan via the *N*-glycolylated-muramic acid residues [28]. This linker is a decaprenyl-diphospho-*N*-acetylglucosamine-rhamnosyl molecule produced by the successive transfer of *N*-acetylglucosamine-1-phosphate to decaprenyl-phosphate by WecA followed by the transfer of L-rhamnose by WbbL. On this linker, 30 linear Gal*f* residues are added by the galactofuranosyl transferases GlfT1 and GlfT2. An Ara*f* unit is then transferred to the galactan chain using the arabinose donor decaprenylphosphoryl-D-arabinose (DPA). DPA is formed through several steps, starting with phospho-α-D-ribosyl-1-pyrophosphate (pRpp). UbiA adds a decaprenyl group to form decaprenol-1-monophosphate 5-phosphoribose (DPPR), which is dephosphorylated and epimerized by DprE1 and DprE2 to form DPA. The arabinofuranosyltransferase AftA catalyzes the transfer of the first unit of Ara*f* to the galactan chain. The arabinosyltransferases EmbA and EmbB catalyze the further addition of Ara*f* to form the arabinan. The final product, the arabinogalactan, is a linear galactan to which highly branched arabinans are attached. The arabinan anchors the mycolic acids forming the mycolyl-arabinogalactan-peptidoglycan (mAGP) complex.

Mycolic acids are the hallmark of the ***M. tuberculosis*** cell wall, an essential component regulating the permeability, acid-fast staining, viability and virulence of ***M. tuberculosis*** [29]. As stated above, mycolic acids are found attached to the arabinose part of the arabinogalactan complex but can also be found as a free form or bound to other saccharides to form trehalose mono/dimycolates (TMM/TDM) and glucose monomycolate. Mycolic acids are long-chain fatty acids composed of a meromycolate chain containing up to 62 carbons with various modifications (***cis/trans*** cyclopropane, keto, or methoxy groups) to which a saturated C_{26} alkyl chain is attached at the α position (Figure 2). The biosynthesis of mycolic acids starts with two fatty acid synthases (FAS): the eukaryotic-like type I (FAS-I) and the prokaryotic-like type II (FAS-II) (Figure 2). FAS-I is a multidomain polypeptide [30] that synthesizes the α-C_{26} alkyl chain and also provides a $C_{14/16}$ fatty acyl-CoA to be elongated into the meromycolate chain by the FAS-II system. This elongation reaction starts with the condensation of $C_{14/16}$ fatty acyl-CoA with malonyl-Acyl Carrier Protein (ACP) by the β-ketoacyl-ACP synthase III FabH. The resulting β-ketoacyl-ACP intermediate is delivered to FAS-II, which performs cycles of elongation using independent enzymes: the reductase MabA, the heterodimer dehydratases HadAB and HadBC, the enoyl-reductase InhA and the condensases KasA and KasB (Figure 2). The modifications (***cis/trans*** cyclopropane, keto, or methoxy groups) of the meromycolate chains are introduced either during the elongation by FAS-II or when the meromycolate chain is fully formed [31]. The meromycolate chain is activated by the fatty acid AMP synthase FadD32 to a meromycolyl-AMP, which is coupled to the carboxylated α-C_{26} fatty acyl-CoA (from FAS-I) by the polyketide synthase Pks13. Reduction of the resulting mycolic β-ketoester by the mycolyl reductase CmrA yields a mature mycolic acid. The biosynthesis of mycolic acids takes place in the cytoplasm. Transfer of the mycolic acids to the cell envelope occurs via the formation of a trehalose monomycolate (TMM) which is translocated by the efflux pump MmpL3 (Mycobacterial membrane protein Large). The mycolyltransferase Antigen 85 complex (***fbpA, fbpB, fbpC***) then condenses mycolic acids to the arabinogalactan releasing a molecule of trehalose.

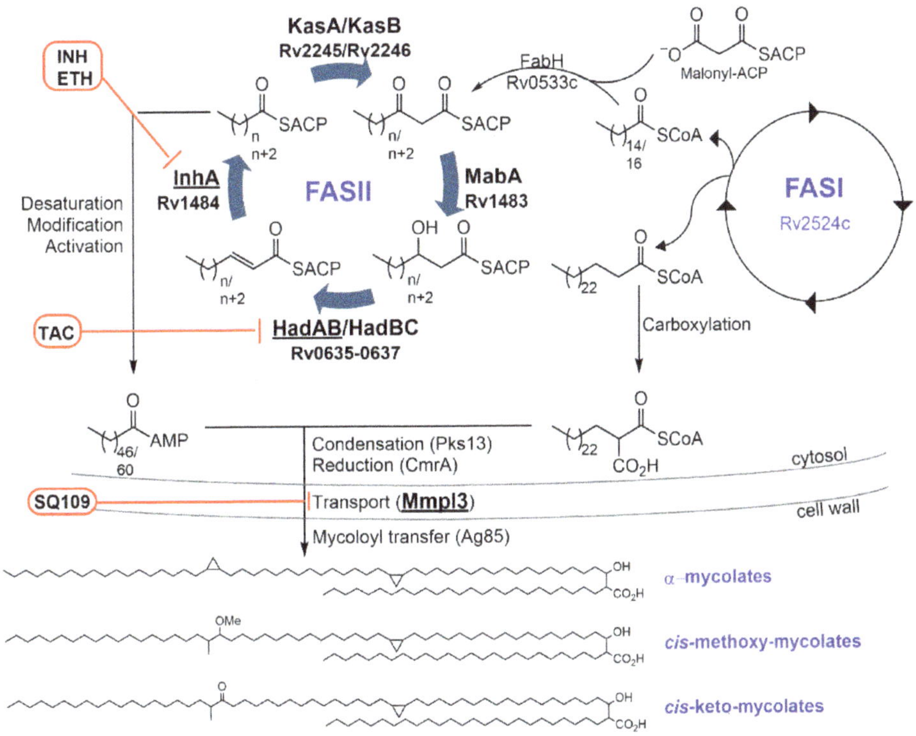

Figure 2. Schematic representation of the biosynthesis of mycolic acids. The three families of mycolic acids in *Mycobacterium tuberculosis* are the α-, methoxy- and keto-mycolic acids. Only the cis configuration of the cyclopropane group of the methoxy- and keto-mycolic acids is shown, but *M. tuberculosis* also produces the trans-methoxy- and trans-keto-mycolic acids. The known targets of the mycolic acid inhibitors in clinical use or in clinical trial are InhA for isoniazid (INH) and ethionamide (ETH); HadAB for thiacetazone (TAC); and Mmpl3 for SQ109.

Besides the mAGP complex, the mycobacterial cell wall also includes lipomannan (LM), lipoarabinomannan (LAM) and phosphatidyl-*myo*-inositol mannosides (PIMs). These lipids are anchored in the inner membrane and play an important role in ***M. tuberculosis*** growth, survival and virulence [32–34]. In the outer membrane, trehalose-containing glycolipids and phthiocerol dimycoserates are found interlaced with the mycolic acids. These lipids are crucial for their interactions with the host and its immune system [35].

Specific components of the cell wall are essential for ***M. tuberculosis*** survival in the host. It is, therefore, not surprising that two of the four first-line TB drugs target the cell wall. In the past 20 years, potent new TB drugs have been discovered that target the peptidoglycan, arabinogalactan, LAM, and mycolic acids or their transfer to the cell wall. This article focuses on the cell wall inhibitors included in the TB pharmacopeia since the 1950s/1960s (old TB drugs) and the new ones in clinical development.

3. Old TB Drugs

3.1. Isoniazid—Target: Mycolic Acids

Discovery. In 1949, Colin Hinshaw and Walsh McDermott went to Germany to investigate reports that TB patients were successfully treated with a new synthetic compound, Conteben [36]. Conteben, a thiosemicarbazone also known as thiacetazone and Tibione (see thiacetazone section below), had been discovered by Gerhard Domagk at Bayer in West Germany. Hinshaw and McDermott returned to the USA with a supply of Conteben. After testing of Conteben in US hospitals, they concluded that "a prompt and thorough series of experimental and clinical trials in the United States" was justified along with experimenting with other thiosemicarbazones [37]. Two US pharmaceutical companies, Hoffman-La Roche and E. R. Squibb & Sons, quickly developed a series of thiosemicarbazone analogs but none showed better activity than Conteben [38–40] until the benzene ring in Conteben was replaced with a pyridine ring leading to the simultaneous discovery of Rimifon at Hoffman-La Roche [39] and Nydrazid at Squibb [41]. In parallel, Domagk at Bayer developed the thiosemicarbazone analog Neoteben [42]. Rimifon, Nydrazid and Neoteben had antiTB activity that far exceeded streptomycin, PAS and any other analog synthesized so far and share the same chemical structure: 4-pyridinecarboxylic acid hydrazide. Hoffman-La Roche, Squibb and Bayer had simultaneously and independently discovered the most potent TB drug at the time: isoniazid (INH). Ironically, none of the pharmaceutical companies could patent their discovery, as INH had been synthesized 40 years earlier by two Polish graduate students Hans Meyer and Josef Mally [36]. The results with INH were so striking that chemotherapy became the leading route for TB treatment, and soon after the sanatoria closed. Almost 70 years later, INH remains the cornerstone of TB chemotherapy for the treatment of drug-susceptible and latent ***M. tuberculosis*** infections.

Activity and toxicity. INH is a first-line TB drug. INH is an oral, highly soluble in water (140 g/L), bactericidal drug with a minimum inhibitory concentration (MIC) ranging from 0.1 to 0.7 μm against ***M. tuberculosis***. In vitro, INH rapidly reduces the number of ***M. tuberculosis*** bacteria by 2- to 3-$\log_{10}$s during the first four days of treatment [43]. This bactericidal activity is only observed in exponentially growing ***M. tuberculosis*** cultures. INH has no activity in stationary or persistent ***M. tuberculosis***. In mice, a similar pattern is observed, where INH is bactericidal only on actively dividing ***M. tuberculosis*** [44]. INH is readily absorbed and reaches concentrations in tissues and organs above its MIC.

The main adverse effect of INH is hepatotoxicity. TB patients more likely to develop liver damage when taking INH are slow acetylators [45,46]. INH is acetylated into the inactive molecule AcINH by the human *N*-acetyltransferase-2 (NAT2), which is expressed mostly in the liver and gastrointestinal tract. Genetic polymorphisms in NAT2 renders this acetylation reaction either slow or fast, dividing TB patients between slow and fast acetylators. INH metabolism also involves an amidase metabolizing INH into an hydrazine (Hz), which is then acetylated by NAT2 to form a toxic acylhydrazine (AcHz) and a non-toxic diacylhydrazine (DiAcHz) [46]. Hz, AcHz and their metabolites generated by the liver microsomal cytochrome P450 enzymes have been linked to liver toxicity [47,48]. Fast acetylators have a lower risk of liver toxicity by producing more of the DiAcHz metabolite and less of the AcHz metabolite(s) [49].

Mode of action. INH enters ***M. tuberculosis*** cells by passive diffusion as a prodrug. A prodrug is the ideal drug where the compound has, if possible, no effect on eukaryotic cells, yet, once activated by a pathogen-specific enzyme, leads to the death of the pathogen [50]. Curiously, the TB pharmacopeia is composed of an array of prodrugs approved for clinical therapy as well as in the developmental phase [51]. INH is activated by the mycobacterial catalase peroxidase KatG (Rv1908c) [52] into what is most likely an isonicotinoyl radical that reacts with nicotinamide adenine dinucleotide (NAD^+) to form the INH-NAD adduct [53–56]. This adduct binds to and inhibits InhA [54,57–60], the NADH-dependent enoyl-ACP reductase [61,62] of the FAS-II system [63], leading to the inhibition of mycolic acid biosynthesis and mycobacterial cell death [60,64–66]. Although the mechanism of INH action seems rather straightforward, elucidation of the molecular details took almost fifty years [67].

Resistance. Shortly after the antimycobacterial activity of INH was published in 1952, the first report of INH-resistant clinical isolates appeared less than one year later [68]. In 1954, Gardner Middlebrook demonstrated that INH-resistant mutants isolated in vitro were catalase-negative [69]. It will then take another 40 years to discover the genetic basis of this phenotype and decipher the main mechanism of resistance to INH: mutation in ***katG,*** the gene encoding the INH activator. Zhang and colleagues showed that 1) complementation of an INH-resistant ***Mycobacterium smegmatis*** mutant with a single copy of ***katG*** restored INH susceptibility [52]; 2) two highly INH-resistant clinical isolates had ***katG*** deletion [52]; and 3) ***M. tuberculosis*** INH-resistant mutants regained INH susceptibility when transformed with ***katG*** [70]. Since then, more than 300 ***katG*** mutations covering 99% of the gene's length (***katG*** has 2223 base pairs (bp)) have been identified in INH-resistant laboratory and clinical strains [71]. The most frequent mutation in clinical isolates is the Ser315Thr. Actually, each of the three bases of the serine codon (AGC) can be mutated leading to Asn, Arg, Ile, Gly or Leu amino acid change. Mutations in KatG alter its catalase peroxidase and oxidase activities causing a defect in KatG's ability to activate INH [72–74]. Thus, most ***M. tuberculosis*** clinical strains carrying ***katG*** mutations are highly resistant to INH [75]. KatG enzymatic activities can also be disrupted by mutations in ***furA*** (***Rv1909c***), a gene encoding a ferric uptake regulation protein and a negative regulator of ***katG*** transcription. Isogenic strains carrying the mutations a-10c and g-7a in the intergenic region between ***katG*** and ***furA*** had reduced ***katG*** expression leading to a decrease in INH oxidase activity and a modest increase in INH resistance [76].

Resistance to a drug can occur through either target mutation (preventing the binding of the drug to its target) or target overexpression (titration of the drug). This is the case for the second most common mutations in INH-resistant clinical isolates: mutations in ***inhA*** and its promoter region. The c-15t mutation in the ***inhA*** promoter region increases ***inhA*** mRNA levels by 20-fold resulting in higher InhA protein levels and an 8-fold MIC increase in ***M. tuberculosis*** [60]. This mutation is found in about one third of the INH-resistant clinical isolates but more often in XDR TB cases than MDR or INH-monoresistant TB cases, suggesting that the c-15t mutation could be a marker for XDR TB [77]. In contrast to ***katG*** mutations, clinical strains with ***inhA*** mutations (either in the gene or in the promoter region) have a low INH resistance phenotype [75]. There are another 20 different mutations identified in the ***inhA*** promoter region [71]. Mutations in the target of INH ***inhA***, an essential gene, are rare, with only 17 identified so far [71]. The first ***inhA*** mutation (Ser94Ala) was isolated in vitro in ***M. smegmatis*** during a screening for mutants co-resistant to INH and ethionamide (ETH), a second-line TB drug [57]. This mutant led to the hypothesis that InhA was the primary target of both INH and ETH [57]. Introduction of the Ser94Ala mutation into wild-type ***M. tuberculosis*** H37Rv was shown to be sufficient to confer INH and ETH resistance [60] and to decrease the binding of the INH-NAD adduct to InhA [60,78]. These observations strongly supported the conclusion that INH and ETH target InhA. The Ser94Ala mutation has been found in INH-resistant ***M. tuberculosis*** clinical isolates carrying no mutations in ***katG*** [75,79–81].

Mutations in many other genes have been identified in INH-resistant laboratory and clinical strains such as ***kasA, mshA, ndh, nudC, ahpC,*** and ***nat*** (the ***M. tuberculosis*** *N*-acetyltransferase) to cite a few, but very often these mutations were present in clinical strains already carrying a ***katG*** or ***inhA*** mutation or were also found in INH-susceptible strains questioning their roles in INH resistance [71].

Area of investigation. For the past 70 years, INH has had an essential role in TB treatment and control. One of INH downsides is its lack of activity against dormant/persistent ***M. tuberculosis***. The reasons for this lack of activity in the dormant form of ***M. tuberculosis*** are still up for debate; however, it is known that KatG has limited activity in the dormant state [44]. With KatG being a major factor in INH resistance and a potential player in INH shortcoming in dormant ***M. tuberculosis***, new InhA inhibitors that would not require activation by KatG have been actively sought [82–89]. Compounds such as GlaxoSmithKline's thiadiazole GSK693 [90] or the diazaborine AN12855 [91,92] are promising leads with good oral bioavailability, low toxicity, activity against ***katG***-deficient ***M. tuberculosis*** and in vivo efficacy similar to INH.

3.2. *Ethambutol—Target: Arabinogalactan/LAM*

Discovery. Ethambutol ((+)-2,2′-(ethylenediimino)di-1-butanol, EMB) was discovered at the Lederle Laboratories division of the American Cyanamid Company in New York (USA) in 1961. During a random screening of synthetic compounds in mice, ***N,N′***-diisopropylethylenediamine was found to protect mice from an ***M. tuberculosis*** infection. Following an intensive campaign of structure–activity relationship (SAR), ethambutol, a di-hydroxylated derivative of ***N,N′***-diisopropylethylenediamine, was synthesized [93–95]. Its activity against ***M. tuberculosis*** in infected mice was four times more potent than streptomycin and protected mice infected with streptomycin- or isoniazid-resistant ***M. tuberculosis*** strains.

Activity and toxicity. EMB is water soluble (solubility 7.58 g/L) and easily taken up by ***M. tuberculosis*** [96]. EMB is bacteriostatic, with a MIC ranging from 5 to 34 μm against ***M. tuberculosis***. EMB is a first-line TB drug, given for the first two months of TB treatment alongside INH, RIF and PZA. EMB adverse effects include liver and ocular toxicity (decreased vision, color blindness) although these effects are reversible once EMB treatment is stopped [97].

Mode of action. The target of EMB has not been definitively determined. It was initially thought that EMB inhibited the synthesis of metabolites needed for ***M. tuberculosis*** replication [96] or hampered RNA synthesis [98]. A set of studies in ***M. smegmatis*** determined that EMB treatment resulted in the inhibition of mycolic acid transfer to the cell wall [99]; the cellular accumulation of TMM, TDM and free mycolic acids [100]; the inhibition of D-arabinose incorporation into the arabinogalactan complex and arabinomannan [101]; and the accumulation of DPA [102], the arabinose donor in the synthesis of arabinan [103]. While the synthesis of arabinan for the arabinogalactan complex was completely inhibited by EMB, EMB only partially inhibited the synthesis of the arabinan of LAM [104], leading to the conclusion that EMB inhibited different arabinosyl transferases responsible for the formation of arabinan in the cell wall [105].

Recently, EMB was postulated to target the glutamate racemase, MurI (Rv1338) [106]. MurI racemizes L-glutamate to D-glutamate, which is required for peptidoglycan biosynthesis. In an enzymatic assay, EMB partially inhibited the MurI racemisation reaction. Docking experiments suggested that EMB could bind to MurI and act as a competitive inhibitor of MurI substrate. Further experiments are required to confirm the role of MurI in ***M. tuberculosis*** inhibition by EMB.

Resistance. Characterization of EMB-resistant ***M. tuberculosis*** clinical isolates revealed a connection between EMB resistance and a cluster of genes (***embCAB, Rv3793–3795***) [107,108] encoding arabinosyltransferases involved in the biosynthesis of the mycobacterial cell wall arabinan [109]. Initially, the most common mutations found in EMB-resistant but not in EMB-susceptible clinical isolates were at position 306 of ***embB*** (M306I, M306V and M306L) [107]. When the ***embB*** mutations M306L, M306V and M306I were introduced into wild-type ***M. tuberculosis*** strains, the resulting strains were found to be EMB-resistant, suggesting that the ***embB*** mutations were a molecular marker for EMB resistance [110,111]. However, ***embB*** mutations were found in EMB-susceptible clinical isolates, leading to questioning the role of ***embB*** in EMB resistance [112–115]. Additionally, EMB-monoresistant clinical isolates did not harbor mutation in ***embB***, suggesting a different target for EMB [113]. EMB-susceptible strains carrying ***embB*** mutations were resistant to other antituberculosis drugs pointing to the ***emb*** locus as a marker for MDR or XDR ***M. tuberculosis*** strains [110,112,115].

Safi and colleagues have postulated that the high-level EMB resistance found in clinical isolates was a result of an accumulation of various mutations, each individually causing a low-level resistance to EMB but together provided a high degree of resistance [110]. The authors demonstrated that, in vitro, a stepwise introduction of specific mutations in ***embB, Rv3806c*** (***ubiA***) and ***embC*** in ***M. tuberculosis*** led to a strain 8-fold more resistant to EMB than wild-type ***M. tuberculosis***. ***ubiA*** encodes a DPPR synthase involved in DPA biosynthesis. Mutations in ***ubiA*** increase intracellular DPA levels, which might bind to Emb, leading to EMB resistance [116]. However, the role of ***ubiA*** in EMB resistance is questionable since mutations in ***ubiA*** are found in both EMB-susceptible and EMB-resistant ***M. tuberculosis*** clinical isolates [117].

Area of investigation. SAR on ethambutol was performed to improve EMB antimycobacterial activity while reducing its toxicity. The outcome was SQ109, a compound now in phase 2 clinical trial, and with a very different mechanism of action than EMB (see below).

3.3. Ethionamide/Prothionamide—Target: Mycolic Acids

Discovery. In 1954, Thomas Gardner and colleagues published the synthesis of an INH analog, where a thioamide group replaced the acyl hydrazide group in INH [118]. This thioisonicotinamide compound was active in a mouse model of ***M. tuberculosis*** infection but was found to be less potent than INH. This publication was noticed by a French team who found that the thioamide derivative was more active than streptomycin and more importantly, potent against INH-, streptomycin- and PAS-resistant ***M. tuberculosis*** strains. They synthesized a series of α-alkyl derivatives of the thioisonicotinamide and found that adding an ethyl or propyl group at the α position generated two compounds with activity in vitro and in mice greater than streptomycin but not as potent as INH [119]. They had synthesized ethionamide (ETH) and prothionamide (PTH).

Activity and toxicity. ETH is a bactericidal drug, with a MIC ranging from 6 to 15 μm against drug-susceptible ***M. tuberculosis***. ETH and PTH are poorly soluble in water (0.84 and 0.28 g/L, respectively). ETH and PTH are in the group C (other core second-line agents) of second-line TB drugs used interchangeably for the treatment of MDR and XDR TB cases. ETH and PTH are oral drugs with some severe adverse effects (hepatoxicity, gastrointestinal disorders, neurotoxicity) [120].

Mode of action. Winder and colleagues were the first to demonstrate that ETH inhibited mycolic acid biosynthesis [121]. They noticed that ETH affected ***Mycobacterium bovis*** BCG similarly to INH although they observed no cross resistance between INH and ETH leading to the conclusion that the mode of action of INH and ETH were not identical [121]. Actually, cross resistance between INH and ETH had been observed in TB patients a few years earlier. Several studies noted that TB patients treated with INH developed resistance to both INH and ETH although the patients had never received ETH [122–124]. This suggested that ETH and INH shared a common mechanism of action. Winder and colleagues had postulated that INH and ETH "might differ in the means by which they reach the sensitive site". That was prescient since INH and ETH were eventually revealed as prodrugs activated by different enzymes. While INH is activated by a catalase peroxidase, ETH is activated by the NADPH-specific flavin adenine dinucleotide-containing Baeyer–Villiger monooxygenase EthA (Rv3854c also called EtaA) [125,126]. In vitro, activation of ETH by EthA leads first to the formation of ethionamide S-oxide, which is further metabolized by EthA to form either 2-ethyl-4-amidopyridine [126] or (2-ethyl-pyridin-4-yl) methanol [125] via radical intermediate(s). Once activated, the mechanism of action of ETH is very similar to INH. The activated form of ETH reacts with NAD^+ to form an ETH*-NAD adduct [127]. The structures of this adduct as well as the PTH*-NAD adduct were determined by X-ray crystallography, revealing an ethyl-isonicotinoyl or a propyl-isonicotinoyl covalently attached to the nicotinamide portion of reduced NAD^+ and bound to InhA. Inhibition of InhA by these adducts results in mycolic acid biosynthesis inhibition.

Wang and colleagues postulated that the activated form of ETH was an iminoyl radical but expressed doubt that this activation reaction was caused by EthA alone and hypothesized that additional enzymes might be involved [127]. Another study also concluded that another mechanism of activation might exist for ETH when demonstrating that deletion of ***ethA*** and its regulator ***ethR*** (***Rv3855***) in ***M. tuberculosis*** caused only a modest increase (3-fold) in ETH resistance [128]. EthA has two close homologs: the monooxygenases Rv3083 (MymA) and Rv0565c [125]. Grant and colleagues determined that MymA was indeed an activator of ETH by showing that loss of function of MymA or overexpression of *mymA* conferred resistance or hypersusceptibility to ETH, respectively [129]. In this study, the authors also noted that transposon mutants in ***Rv0565c*** as well as in two other genes encoding Baeyer–Villiger monooxygenases (***Rv1393c*** and ***Rv3049c***) did not lead to ETH resistance. However, a recent study determined that overexpression or deletion of ***Rv0565c*** led to ETH hypersusceptibility or low resistance, respectively, in ***M. tuberculosis***, leading the authors to conclude that Rv0565c was an additional activator of ETH in ***M. tuberculosis*** [130]. In both studies on ***mymA*** and ***Rv0565c***, no biochemical evidence was provided to show that MymA or Rv0565c actually activates ETH and what would be the resulting activated molecule(s).

Resistance. Mutations in ETH-resistant laboratory and clinical ***M. tuberculosis*** strains are found in the activators of ETH (***ethA, mymA, Rv0565c***), the negative regulator of ***ethA*** (***ethR***) and ETH target (***inhA*** gene and promoter region) [129–131]. Mutations in the ***inhA*** promoter region are more frequent than mutations in the activator(s) of ETH [131]. Mutations in ***inhA*** or in its promoter region are found in up to 68% of ETH-resistant clinical isolates while mutations in ETH activator ***ethA*** are usually found in no more than 55% of ETH-resistant clinical isolates, and some of these ***ethA*** mutations can also be found in ETH-susceptible strains [131]. The mutations in ***ethA*** cover 91% of the gene (from 2 to 1341 bp; ***ethA*** has 1470 bp) [71]. Mutations in ***ethR*** have been identified in ETH-resistant clinical strains carrying the c-15t mutation in the ***inhA*** promoter region [131]. Recently, cyclic dimeric guanosine monophosphate, a bacterial second messenger, was shown to boost the binding of EthR to ***ethA*** promoter, causing a decrease in ***ethA*** transcription levels and ETH resistance [132].

Other genes have been implicated in ETH resistance. ***M. tuberculosis*** strains deleted for *mshA*, a gene encoding the glycosyltransferase involved in the biosynthesis of mycothiol, a major low-molecular-weight thiol, are eight times more resistant to ETH than their parental strains [133]. Mycothiol is thought to play a role in ETH resistance by increasing the rate of ETH activation by EthA [133]. In ***M. smegmatis*** and ***M. bovis*** BCG, mutants co-resistant to INH and ETH were isolated carrying mutations in ***ndh***, a gene encoding an NADH dehydrogenase whose function is to oxidize NADH into NAD^+. In this case, ***ndh*** mutants were shown to accumulate NADH. Excess NADH could act as a competitive inhibitor for the binding of the ETH-NAD to InhA, triggering ETH resistance [134].

Area of investigation. Regulation of ***ethR*** expression plays a role in ETH resistance and susceptibility. While overexpression of ***ethR*** was shown to cause ETH resistance, inhibition of ***ethR*** triggers higher levels of ***ethA*** expression and increases ETH susceptibility [135]. Baulard and colleagues have taken advantage of this point and generated EthR inhibitors to boost ETH activity. Screening of chemical libraries and SAR on potential EthR inhibitors led to a first series of EthR inhibitors, which by themselves had no activity on ***M. tuberculosis***, yet, when combined with ETH, significantly "boosted" ETH activity in vitro and in ***M. tuberculosis***-infected mice [136]. The most active of this first generation of boosters, the oxadiazole BDM41906, decreased the MIC for ETH to the nM range [137]; however, BDM41906 had no "boosting" activity in ***M. tuberculosis*** strains carrying ***ethA*** mutations [138]. The second generation of ETH booster, the spiroisoxazoline SMARt (Small Molecule Aborting Resistance)-420, does not inhibit EthR but instead triggers a different activation mechanism for ETH. This new activation system uses the oxidoreductase Rv0077c as the activator, which is negatively regulated by Rv0078. SMARt-420 binds to Rv0078, releasing the activity of Rv0077c. SMARt-420 increases the susceptibility of ***M. tuberculosis*** to ETH 40-fold. In addition, ETH-resistant ***M. tuberculosis*** strains carrying an ***ethA*** mutation regain ETH susceptibility when SMARt-420 is present, both in vitro and in mice [138]. SMARt-420 can, therefore, be used in the context of ETH resistance due to ***ethA*** mutations but not due to ***inhA*** mutations.

3.4. Cycloserine—Target: Peptidoglycan

Discovery. In contrast to INH, EMB and ETH, which are synthetic compounds, cycloserine is a natural product produced by *Streptomyces* with broad-spectrum activity. Cycloserine (D-4-amino-3-isoxazolidone, also called oxamycin or seromycin) was isolated from ***Streptomyces garyphalus*** **[139]**, ***Streptomyces lavendulae*** **[140]**, ***Streptomyces roseochromogenus*** [141] and ***Streptomyces orchidaceus*** [142] in the early 1950s.

Activity and toxicity. Cycloserine is an oral drug, highly soluble in water (877 g/L). Cycloserine is a bacteriostatic second-line TB drug, with a MIC ranging from 50 to 250 μm against drug-susceptible ***M. tuberculosis***. An analog of cycloserine, terizidone, a compound made of two molecules of cycloserine, is also used as a second-line TB drug to treat MDR TB. Cycloserine was shown to inhibit the growth of ***M. tuberculosis*** in vitro [143]. In vivo, cycloserine is rather inactive in a mouse or guinea pig model of ***M. tuberculosis*** infection [143–145] but effective in ***M. tuberculosis***-infected monkeys and humans [146–148]. The differences in cycloserine activity in animal models were correlated with levels of D-alanine in sera [149] and rate of cycloserine excretion [146]. In a cohort study in China, TB patients with MDR TB had a better outcome when cycloserine was added to the treatment but that was not the case for TB patients infected with pre-XDR or XDR ***M. tuberculosis*** strains [150]. As an inhibitor of peptidoglycan biosynthesis, cycloserine has the distinctive feature of having a unique mechanism of action thus preventing any cross resistance with other first-line and second-line TB drugs. Cycloserine is, therefore, a useful addition to second-line TB drugs, although its use might be limited by its severe toxicity. Serious adverse effects were observed during cycloserine treatment such as neuropathy and behavioral changes [151]. Cycloserine is, therefore, contraindicated in patients suffering from severe depression, suicidal tendencies, kidney failure, epilepsy or seizures.

Mode of action. The mechanism of action of cycloserine was primarily deciphered in ***Staphylococcus aureus***. Cycloserine is an analog of D-alanine and works as an antagonist of D-alanine [152]. Cycloserine inhibits the alanine racemase Alr (Rv3423c), which converts L-alanine to D-alanine, and the D-Ala:D-Ala ligase DdlA (Rv2981c) [153] preventing the integration of alanine into the pentapeptide core of the peptidoglycan. In ***M. tuberculosis***, DdlA is thought to be the primary target of cycloserine [154–156].

Resistance. D-cycloserine-resistant ***M. tuberculosis*** mutants were isolated as early as 1957 in TB patients treated with cycloserine [157]. Cycloserine resistance has been associated with mutations in the genes encoding the alanine transporter CycA (Rv1704c), the L-alanine dehydrogenase Ald (Rv2780) and the alanine racemase Alr. A Gly122Ser mutation in ***cycA*** is present in the naturally cycloserine-resistant ***M. bovis*** BCG vaccine strain [158]. Complementation of BCG with a cosmid containing ***M. tuberculosis cycA*** renders BCG more susceptible to cycloserine than the parental strain leading the authors to conclude that ***cycA*** may be a factor in cycloserine resistance in BCG [158]. Desjardins and colleagues demonstrated that deletion of ***ald*** increased the resistance to cycloserine 2-fold in ***M. tuberculosis***, while complementation of the ***ald*** mutant with a plasmid expressing ***M. tuberculosis ald*** only partially restored cycloserine susceptibility. Notably, complementation of BCG with the ***ald*** plasmid did not alter the strain resistance to cycloserine [159]. Mutations in ***alr*** (M319T, Y364D, R373L and c-8t in the promoter region) have been identified in XDR TB strains isolated from TB patients treated with cycloserine [160]. Further, the clinical isolate with the R373L mutation in ***alr*** also contained a deletion in ***ald***.

In an in vitro experiment, 18 cycloserine-resistant mutants were obtained by culturing ***M. tuberculosis*** H37Rv on plates containing increasing concentrations of cycloserine (from 0.2 to

3 mM) and characterized using whole-genome sequencing [161]. Mutants were only obtained on plates containing less than 0.8 mM of cycloserine. A mutation was identified in ***alr*** (D344N), but no mutations in ***ddlA, ald*** or ***cycA*** were found. Fifteen novel mutations were identified in genes involved in various pathways however no complementation or allelic exchange experiments were performed to confirm that these novel mutations were indeed involved in cycloserine resistance.

In a recent in vitro study [162], the authors showed that spontaneous cycloserine-resistant mutants emerged at a lower frequency (10^{-10}–10^{-11}) than rifampicin- (10^{-9}) or isoniazid-resistant (10^{-8}) mutants in ***M. tuberculosis***. The authors characterized 11 independent cycloserine-resistant ***M. tuberculosis*** mutants by whole-genome sequencing and found mutations in ***alr*** (gene (D322N) and promoter region) but again not in ***ddlA, ald*** or ***cycA***. None of these 11 cycloserine-resistant mutants showed any cross-resistance to other first-line and second-line TB drugs. The ***alr*** promoter mutation upregulated ***alr*** gene transcript, causing an increase in Alr protein level by up to 30-fold. The ***alr*** D322N mutation present in 8/11 mutants reduced the binding affinity for cycloserine by 240 fold while having limited effect on Alr enzymatic activity. Evangelopoulos and colleagues postulated that the ***alr*** mutations protected the enzymatic function of both cycloserine targets by decreasing the affinity of cycloserine to Alr and increasing the levels of D-alanine preventing the binding of cycloserine to DdlA. Their main conclusion was that DdlA was the "lethal target" for cycloserine.

3.5. Thiacetazone—Target: Mycolic Acids

Discovery. Gerhard Domagk was awarded the Nobel Prize in 1939 for the discovery of prontosil, a prodrug that releases ***p***-aminobenzenesulfonamide, the first sulfonamide drug active against ***Staphylococcus*** and ***Streptococcus*** infections, but not against ***M. tuberculosis*** infections [163]. While prontosil was quickly replaced by penicillin to fight antibacterial infections, Domagk and his team continued working on the synthesis of related compounds, the thiosemicarbazides, and discovered that one in particular, thiacetazone (TAC, also called Tibione, Tb I, Conteben), had impressive activity against ***M. tuberculosis*** in guinea pigs [164]. In the late 1940s, TAC was tested in Germany on patients with various forms of TB and found to have promising activity although severe adverse effects were recorded [37,165].

Activity and toxicity. TAC is an oral, inexpensive, effective and bacteriostatic drug, with a MIC ranging from 0.3 to 5 µm against drug-susceptible ***M. tuberculosis***. TAC is poorly soluble in water (0.09 g/L). TAC is part of the group D3 (add-on agents) of second-line TB drugs. TAC has been given in combination with INH in resource-poor countries [166,167]. Its utilization as a TB drug was mostly discontinued because of its high toxicity (skin disorder, gastrointestinal symptoms, conjunctivitis, vertigo, liver and kidney damage) especially in HIV-positive TB patients [168]. TAC is, therefore, not recommended in HIV-positive TB patients.

Mode of action. TAC is a prodrug that is activated by the monooxygenase EthA [127,169]. Once activated, TAC inhibits the dehydratase HadAB of the FAS-II system by forming a disulfide bound with a cysteine (Cys61) residue of HadA [170,171]. During the elongation of fatty acyl-ACPs by FAS-II, HadA binds the acyl-ACP while HadB performs the dehydratase reaction. When covalently bound to the Cys61 residue of HadA, TAC obstructs the acyl-ACP channel preventing the binding of the fatty acyl-ACP [172]. The covalent bond between TAC and HadA Cys61 blocks the activity of HadAB leading to inhibition of mycolic acid biosynthesis [173].

Resistance.The mode of action of TAC was discovered through analysis of TAC resistance. Since TAC treatment of ***M. tuberculosis***results in inhibition of mycolic acids, Belardinelli and Morbidoni overexpressed every gene involved in the FAS-II system. Only overexpression of the dehydratase operon ***hadABC***or its dimer ***hadBC***resulted in highly TAC-resistant ***M. tuberculosis***strains (MIC > 0.2 mm) [170]. Curiously, the level of TAC resistance was much lower when the dimer ***hadAB*** was overexpressed in ***M. tuberculosis*** (MIC 10 µm). This was puzzling since HadAB is the target of TAC. Moreover, sequencing of spontaneous ***M. tuberculosis*** TAC-resistant mutants revealed mutations in HadA (Cys61Ser, Cys61Gly) but also in HadC (Val85Phe, Thr123Ala, Lys157Arg, Ala151Val) [170,174].

Grzegorzewicz and colleagues set up to unmask the role of ***hadC*** in TAC resistance [175]. The authors found that mutations in ***hadC*** protected ***M. tuberculosis*** from TAC and compensated for HadAB inhibition by TAC. The authors proposed that ***hadC*** mutations prevented TAC from reaching the active site of HadAB [175].

TAC resistance is also mediated by mutations in ***mmaA4*** (***Rv0642c***), a gene encoding a methoxy mycolic acid synthase required for the synthesis of keto- and methoxy-mycolic acids [170,176]. The methyltransferases involved in the modifications of the meromycolic acids such as MmaA4 interact with the proteins of the FAS-II system including the dehydratase heterodimers HadAB and HadBC [31]. Mutations in ***mmaA4*** might, therefore, modify the conformation of HadAB preventing the binding of TAC to HadA and causing TAC resistance [175].

Area of investigation.In the late 1940s, the discovery of the antiTB activity of the thiosemicarbazide TAC propelled pharmaceutical companies into an extensive search for TAC analogs with antiTB properties. This led to the discovery of the most important antimycobacterial drug INH (see above). This family of compounds might still reveal interesting molecules with pharmaceutical properties. Recently, new TAC analogs were synthesized with promising activities against ***M. tuberculosis*** [174].

4. New Generation of Cell Wall Inhibitors

4.1. Target: Mycolic Acids

4.1.1. SQ109

Discovery. A collaboration between a pharmaceutical laboratory (Sequella) and an academic (Laboratory of Host Defenses NIAID/NIH) laboratory led to the synthesis and screening of a chemical library composed of 63,238 molecules based on the ethylenediamine core of EMB [177]. EMB was targeted for its good antimycobacterial activity in TB patients and lack of previous SAR studies. The goal was to create a more potent yet less toxic EMB analog. The screening selected 170 compounds that had an MIC of less than 6 mg/L against ***M. tuberculosis*** (discarding inactive or compounds that could not cross the cell wall) and had an inhibitory effect on the cell wall (determined by monitoring upregulation of the ***iniBAC*** operon promoter, a phenotype observed in cell wall inhibitors [178]). Based on the molecular structures of these 170 compounds, a new chemical library composed of 30,000 molecules was synthesized and retested against ***M. tuberculosis*** (in vitro and in macrophages). Eleven compounds passed those screens and were then assessed in mice [179]. The compound with the best antimycobacterial activity, pharmacological and toxicity data was SQ109.

Activity. SQ109 is a lipophilic, oral drug with poor water solubility (1.7 mg/L). SQ109 is bactericidal against drug-susceptible, MDR and XDR ***M. tuberculosis*** strains, with a MIC ranging from 0.4 to 3 μm. In vitro, SQ109 synergizes with the first-line TB drugs INH and RIF as well as with second-line TB drugs such as cycloserine, moxifloxacin, amikacin and bedaquiline (BDQ) [180]. In ***M. tuberculosis***-infected mice, treatment with SQ109 for 28 days resulted in a dose-dependent reduction in lung and spleen burdens [181]. SQ109 was not as effective as INH in eliminating ***M. tuberculosis*** with organ burdens between 1 and 2.5 $\log_{10}$ higher in the SQ109 treatment compared to INH treatment [181]. However, SQ109 peak concentration in the lung and spleen was higher than SQ109 MIC and 45-fold higher than in plasma [181].

Mode of action. Surprisingly, this double SAR based on EMB resulted in a drug, SQ109, with a different mode of action than EMB. EMB-resistant ***M. tuberculosis*** strains were fully susceptible to SQ109 [179]. Transcriptional response of SQ109-treated ***M. tuberculosis,*** while consistent with other cell wall inhibitors, did not match EMB's response [182]. Lipid analysis of SQ109-treated ***M. tuberculosis*** revealed an inhibition of mycolic acid attachment to the arabinogalactan, a depletion of TDM and an accumulation of TMM [183]. To decipher the mechanism behind this result, isolation of spontaneous SQ109-resistant mutants was attempted without success (the mutation rate for SQ109 is exceptionally low (10^{-11})) [183]. Instead, an analog of SQ109 was used to isolate spontaneous resistant mutants. These mutants were co-resistant to SQ109 and carried a mutation in the mycolic acid flippase encoded by ***mmpl3*** (***Rv0206c***), involved in the translocation of TMM across the plasma membrane [184]. Analyses carried out in ***M. smegmatis*** revealed that SQ109 binds to Mmpl3 at the proton transportation site inhibiting the proton motive force for substrate translocation [185].

Clinical trial. In a 14 day study where SQ109 was given alone or in combination with RIF, SQ109 was shown to be safe in TB patients, with only gastrointestinal issues being disclosed [186]. The SQ109 plasma concentration was lower than the MIC for the drug and, in contrast to the in vitro results, the combination of SQ109 and RIF led to a decrease in SQ109 availability [186]. In mice, SQ109 had been shown to be metabolized by the cytochrome P450 isoenzymes CYP_2D_6 and CYP_2C_{19} [181]. Since RIF induces the expression of CYP_2C enzymes in humans [187], RIF might lower the effective dose of SQ109. On the other hand, the presence of SQ109 had no effect on the plasma concentration of RIF. The result of this 14 day trial was that SQ109 alone had no bactericidal effect, and there was no synergy or additive effect with the combination RIF and SQ109 [186]. In a phase 2 trial (NCT01785186) performed in newly diagnosed pulmonary TB patients, treatment with SQ109 in combination with RIF/INH/PZA failed to improve culture conversion compared to RIF/INH/PZA [188]. A phase 2b clinical trial in Russia on MDR TB patients revealed that SQ109, combined with standard drug therapy, was safe, well tolerated and effective (80% of sputum negative patients after 24 weeks of treatment with SQ109 compared to 61% without SQ109) [189].

Area of investigation. With the success of SQ109 and the essentiality of ***mmpl3*** in ***M. tuberculosis***, novel inhibitors of Mmpl3 have been actively sought. Inhibition of Mmpl3 is not specific to the chemical structure of SQ109 and numerous chemical scaffolds are being identified as Mmpl3 inhibitors [185,190,191].

4.1.2. Pretomanid (PA-824)

Discovery. Another challenge in TB drug discovery is to discover new molecules that will eliminate dormant or persistent ***M. tuberculosis***, a subpopulation of bacteria that are genetically drug-susceptible but 'resistant' (or tolerant) to drug treatment. One of the most used methods to study persistent ***M. tuberculosis*** is the Wayne model where ***M. tuberculosis*** is subjected to gradual oxygen depletion to allow for a slow entry into anaerobiosis. To find potential inhibitors of dormant ***M. tuberculosis***, nitroimidazoles were tested, as they inhibit bacterial anaerobes. Metronidazole, an antibacterial and antiprotozoal drug with activity against Gram-positive and Gram-negative anaerobes [192] showed little, if any, activity against ***M. tuberculosis*** in mice [193]. However, a bicyclic nitroimidazole (CGI 17341) was reported to have potent in vitro and in vivo antimycobacterial activity. CGI 17341 showed no cross-resistance with other TB drugs but was highly mutagenic [194]. A series of more than 300 analogs was then synthesized to solve the CGI 17341 mutagenicity issue [195]. This led to the discovery of the nitroimidazole PA-824 now called pretomanid (PMD).

Activity. PMD is an oral drug, poorly soluble in water (0.012 g/L). PMD is active against replicating and non-replicating (anaerobic), drug-susceptible and drug-resistant (MIC ranging from 0.08 to 0.7 μm) ***M. tuberculosis*** strains. In a mouse model of ***M. tuberculosis*** infection, PMD given orally for 10 days performed as well as INH in lowering organ bacterial burdens. Increasing the concentration of PMD (from 25 mg/kg to 100 mg/kg) led to a significant reduction in organ burden compared to INH [195]. Similar results were obtained in ***M. tuberculosis***-infected guinea pigs treated with PMD. The toxic threshold in mice was 1 g/kg for a single dose of PMD and 0.5 g/kg for a daily dose given for 28 days [195]. In a drug combination experiment, the lung burden in mice infected with the drug-susceptible ***M. tuberculosis*** H37Rv strain was 2.5 $\log_{10}$ lower in mice receiving PMD/BDQ/PZA than in mice treated with standard regimen (INH/RIF/EMB/PZA) after one month of treatment. None of the mice treated for 2 months with PMD/BDQ/PZA relapsed (mice were kept for an additional three months at the end of the treatment to assess relapse). The addition of moxifloxacin (MXF) to this combination did not improve the outcome during the first month of treatment but did decrease the number of mice relapsing after 1.5 month treatment [196]. In a subsequent experiment,

M. tuberculosis-infected mice were treated with BDQ/MXF/PZA +/− PMD [197]. The addition of PMD to the BDQ/MXF/PZA treatment decreased the lung burden an extra 1 $\log_{10}$ after one month of treatment compared to BDQ/MXF/PZA alone. In both groups, mice were relapse free after two months of treatment [197]. In addition, treatment of ***M. tuberculosis***-infected mice with BDQ/linezolid (LZD) +/− PMD revealed that the addition of PMD had a significant impact on the lung burden. PMD in combination with BDQ/LZD resulted in a 7.2 $\log_{10}$ CFU ***M. tuberculosis*** killing in the lungs and relapse-free mice after two and three months of treatment, respectively. In contrast, the BDQ/LZD treatment resulted in a 5.2 log reduction in CFU in the lungs, but more than 90% of the mice relapsed even after 4 months of treatment [197].

Mode of action. Like many other TB drugs, PMD is a prodrug. PMD is activated by a deazaflavin (F420)-dependent nitroreductase (Ddn, Rv3547) to generate a des nitro metabolite releasing nitric oxide (NO) [198]. The presence of the des nitro metabolite and rate of NO release were linked specifically to the anaerobic killing activity of PMD. PMD treatment of ***M. tuberculosis*** also causes a decrease in ketomycolates production and an accumulation of hydroxymycolates leading to the hypothesis that PMD inhibits an enzyme or affects a cofactor responsible for the oxidation of hydroxymycolic acids to ketomycolic acids [195]. A transcriptional analysis of ***M. tuberculosis*** treated with PMD under replicating conditions revealed that PMD action had similarity with cell wall inhibitors as well as inhibitors of the respiratory chain [199]. This data confirmed the dual action of PMD as an inhibitor of a subfamily of mycolic acids as well as a NO generator leading to the inhibition of the respiratory chain under anaerobic conditions. This combination of a cell wall inhibitor and NO generator makes PMD a unique antimycobacterial drug, effective against active and dormant TB that can shorten the duration of chemotherapy.

Resistance. The main mechanism of resistance to PMD is through mutations in its activator Ddn. In vitro selection of spontaneous PMD-resistant mutants in ***M. tuberculosis*** led to the isolation of 183 mutants [200]. The mutation rate was relatively high ranging from 10^{-5} to 10^{-7}. Most of the mutations were in ***ddn*** (SNPs, base pair deletion or insertion, early stop codon). Mutations in ***fbiABC*** (***Rv3261, Rv3262, Rv1173***) encoding F420 biosynthesis proteins and ***fgd1*** (***Rv0407***) encoding a F420-dependent glucose-6-phosphate dehydrogenase were also identified, but no complementation experiments were performed to confirm the role of these mutations in PMD resistance.

Clinical trial. A phase 2a clinical trial (NCT01215851) evaluated the early bactericidal activity (EBA), safety and tolerability of PMD combined with BDQ, PZA and/or MXF in newly diagnosed drug-susceptible, smear-positive pulmonary TB patients [201]. These combinations were well tolerated and seemed safe. The combination PMD/PZA/MXF was more bactericidal than PMD/BDQ or PMD/PZA and as potent as the standard regimen (INH/RIF/EMB/PZA) [201]. In a phase 2b clinical trial (NCT02193776), the efficacy, safety and tolerability of the combination PMD/BDQ/PZA were assessed in newly diagnosed drug-susceptible, smear-positive pulmonary TB patients treated for 8 weeks [202]. TB patients converted more rapidly to sputum negativity with PMD/BDQ/PZA than the standard regimen. One arm of the study also looked at the combination PMD/BDQ/PZA/MXF for the treatment of newly diagnosed, MXF-sensitive, MDR, pulmonary TB patients. MDR TB patients converted to sputum negativity within 8 weeks of treatment with PMD/BDQ/PZA/MXF. A phase 2c trial (NCT03338621) is currently in progress to evaluate the efficacy, safety and tolerability of a 4 month PMD/BDQ/PZA/MXF treatment given to patients infected with drug-sensitive TB or a 6 month treatment given to drug-resistant TB patients. No results have been posted yet.

The Nix-TB trial (phase 3, NCT02333799) was set to test the efficacy, tolerability, safety and pharmacodymanics of the combination PMD/BDQ/LZD given for six months on 50 patients infected with XDR TB and 24 patients infected with treatment-intolerant or non-responsive MDR TB. 88% of XDR TB cases and 92% of MDR TB cases had favorable outcomes at the end of treatment (no clinical infection, culture negative 6 months post treatment). 23% of the patients had manageable adverse effects [203]. On August 14, 2019, the Food and Drug Administration (FDA) approved the use of PMD in combination with BDQ and LZD for the treatment of pulmonary TB only in the case of non-responsive MDR, XDR and treatment-intolerant ***M. tuberculosis*** infections. This new regimen is all oral, short (6 months), more efficacious (sputum conversion in less than 6 weeks) and uses fewer drugs (3) compared to the treatment for highly resistant TB, which entails daily injections for 6 months followed by daily treatment with five drugs for 12 to 18 months (https://www.fda.gov/media/128001/download).

4.1.3. Delamanid (OPC-67683)

Discovery. Upon the discovery of the activity of CGI 17341 against ***M. tuberculosis***, researchers at Otsuka Pharmaceutical Co., Japan, performed a SAR study on the compound to reduce its mutagenicity and increase its potency against ***M. tuberculosis*** [204]. The result was the nitroimidazole OPC-67683, now called delamanid.

Activity. Delamanid is an oral, non-mutagenic compound, poorly soluble in water (0.002 g/L). Delamanid is active in vitro (MIC 8–45 nM [205]) against drug-susceptible and MDR ***M. tuberculosis*** strains and highly efficacious in vivo [206]. Delamanid is also active against non-replicating ***M. tuberculosis*** [207]. Delamanid is only active against members of the MTB complex as well as some non-tuberculous mycobacteria and shows no activity against bacterial microflora [205]. In a mouse model of acute and chronic ***M. tuberculosis*** infections, delamanid performed better than PMD. After 3 weeks of treatment, in the acute model of infection, delamanid and PMD reduced the lung bacterial burden by 1 $\log_{10}$ and 0, respectively. In the chronic model of infection, delamanid and PMD reduced the lung bacterial burden by 3 and 2 $\log_{10}$, respectively [207]. Delamanid is included in the Group D2 (add-on agents) of second-line TB drugs to treat RIF-resistant and MDR TB patients.

Mode of action. Similar to PMD, delamanid is a prodrug activated by the deazaflavin-dependent nitroreductase Ddn to form a des nitro metabolite and release NO. Delamanid inhibits the biosynthesis of methoxy- and keto-mycolic acids but not of α-mycolic acids [206]. Deciphering the mechanism of action of delamanid by isolating spontaneous in vitro resistant mutants has led to the identification of mutations in genes involved only in delamanid activation (***ddn, fgd1, fbiABC***), not in its target [208]. Frequency of mutation was relatively high (10^{-5} to 10^{-6}). Complementation restored drug susceptibility except for one ***fbiB*** mutant that required complementation with a plasmid containing both ***fbiB*** and ***fbiA***. Two delamanid-resistant clinical isolates were also analyzed in that study and shown to have mutations in ***ddn*** (L107P and a 59–101 bp deletion). The target of delamanid is yet to be discovered, as no mutant in pathways independent to delamanid's mode of activation has been isolated. The question remains as to whether delamanid and PMD target mycolic acid biosynthesis or whether the inhibition of the biosynthesis of these specific mycolic acids observed during delamanid or PMD treatment of ***M. tuberculosis*** is only a consequence of the inhibition of these compounds' target(s).

Clinical trial. As of 2019, delamanid is one of three new TB drugs in phase 3 clinical development along with PMD and BDQ (www.newtbdrugs.org). In a clinical trial in MDR TB patients, delamanid was added for 2 months to an optimized background treatment regimen (OBR), resulting in 45% sputum culture conversion compared to 30% sputum culture conversion for the patients getting OBR and placebo [209]. In this study, the group of patients receiving higher doses of delamanid (200 mg, twice a day) had a higher incidence of palpitation and prolonged QT intervals than the groups that received a lower concentration (100 mg, twice a day) of delamanid or placebo. In a subsequent six-month delamanid trial, a lower mortality rate was observed in TB patients that received delamanid for 6 months rather than the previous 2 months trial, but no significant difference in successful treatment outcome was recorded between the 2 month and 6 month delamanid trial [210,211]. A phase 3 clinical trial on MDR TB patients tested the addition of delamanid for the first six months of the 24 month OBR regimen. There was no statistical difference in time to sputum culture conversion or rate of adverse events whether the patients received delamanid or not with their OBR treatment [212]. Overall, delamanid is a well-tolerated drug with good safety data. In 2014, delamanid was approved for the treatment of pulmonary MDR TB in adults in Europe, Japan and Korea.

Delamanid, PMD and SQ109 are the only drugs in advanced clinical development so far targeting mycolic acid biosynthesis or mycolic acid incorporation into the cell wall. Academic and pharmaceutical laboratories are developing new inhibitors of enzymes involved in mycolic acid biosynthesis. Inhibitors of KasA [213], InhA [83,90–92], Pks13 [214–217] and Mmpl3 [185,190,191,218,219] are being tested.

4.2. Target: Arabinogalactan/LAM

4.2.1. CPZEN-45

Discovery. Caprazamycin B, a liponucleoside isolated from ***Streptomyces,*** is a non-toxic antibiotic with good activity in vitro (MIC 3–11 μm) against drug-susceptible and MDR ***M. tuberculosis*** strains but insoluble in water [220]. To increase its hydrophilicity, SAR was performed and led to the nucleoside caprazene-45 (CPZEN-45) [221].

Activity. CPZEN-45 is a water-soluble drug (solubility ≈ 10 g/L) with an MIC of 2–5 μm and 10 μm against drug-susceptible and MDR ***M. tuberculosis,*** respectively. Unlike caprazamycin B, which is active against several Gram-positive bacteria, CPZEN-45 has no activity against ***S. aureus, Streptococcus pneumonia*** or ***Enterococcus faecalis*** [222]. CPZEN-45 is specific to slow-growing pathogens. In mice intravenously infected with the drug-susceptible ***M. tuberculosis*** H37Rv strain, a 30-day subcutaneous treatment with CPZEN-45 was as effective in reducing lung burden as INH and better than RIF alone [223]. Furthermore, the combination INH/RIF/CPZEN-45 resulted in at least a 1 $\log_{10}$ better killing of ***M. tuberculosis*** than the combination INH/RIF. In a subsequent experiment, mice were intravenously infected with an XDR ***M. tuberculosis*** strain and treated with CPZEN-45 at doses ranging from 6.3 to 200 mg/kg. After 30 days, the mice treated with the highest concentration of CPZEN-45 had a 1.5 $\log_{10}$ better reduction in CFUs in the lungs than the mice receiving the lowest concentration [223].

Mode of action. CPZEN-45 is an inhibitor of ***M. tuberculosis*** WecA (Rv1302) with an IC_{50} of 7 nM [222]. WecA is involved in the first step of the arabinogalactan biosynthesis forming the anchor point between peptidoglycan and arabinogalactan. Transcriptionally silencing ***wecA*** is bactericidal in ***M. tuberculosis*** in vitro and bacteriostatic ex vivo, validating WecA as candidate for drug development [224].

Clinical trial. CPZEN-45 is in the early stage of clinical development.

4.2.2. BTZ043

Discovery. A sulfur-based chemical library was tested for antibacterial and antifungal activities. A class of compounds, the nitrobenzothiazinones, was found to have specific activity against mycobacteria. The most promising hit BTZ038 was a racemic molecule and synthesis of its ***S*** enantiomer gave BTZ043 [225].

Activity. BTZ043 is lipophilic, bactericidal, and is active against drug-susceptible, MDR and XDR ***M. tuberculosis*** strains, with an MIC ranging from 2 to 70 nM. In contrast to the novel TB drugs targeting the mycolic acids, BTZ043 was less effective in non-replicating conditions, suggesting that BTZ043 would have to be used in combination with other drugs to be effective against TB [225]. BTZ043 was tested with first-, second-line and in-development TB drugs and showed no antagonistic effects. BTZ043 was additive with most of the drugs tested and synergistic with BDQ [226]. The compound is as effective in a mouse model of ***M. tuberculosis*** infection as INH. BTZ043 was well tolerated in rats, had low interaction with the CYP450 enzymes and showed no mutagenic or genotoxic properties [227].

Mode of action. BTZ043 is a prodrug activated by DprE1 (Rv3790). DprE1 reduces the nitro group in BTZ043, yielding a nitroso metabolite. This metabolite reacts with the thiol group of a cysteine (Cys387) residue in the substrate-binding site of DprE1 to form a covalent bond that irreversibly inhibits DprE1, classifying BTZ043 as a suicide inhibitor [228]. DprE1 catalyzes the first step in the epimerisation of decaprenylphosphoryl ribose (DPR) to decaprenylphosphoryl arabinose (DPA), the arabinose donor for the synthesis of arabinogalactan and LAM. Treatment of ***M. tuberculosis*** with BTZ043, therefore, results in inhibition of DPA formation and ultimately inhibition of both arabinogalactan and LAM [225].

Resistance. Mutation at the Cys387 position of ***dprE1*** is the main mechanism of resistance to BTZ043. Frequency of mutation is low ($<10^{-8}$); however, the resulting mutants ***dprE1*** Cys387Ser and Cys387Gly are highly resistant to BTZ043 (250-10,000-fold) [225].

Clinical trial. As of December 2019, BTZ043 is in Phase 1b/2a clinical trial to assess safety, tolerability, interaction with first-line TB drugs and early bactericidal activity in newly diagnosed patients infected with uncomplicated, smear-positive, drug-susceptible TB.

4.2.3. PBTZ169

Discovery. SAR on BTZ043 to improve its pharmacologic properties yielded PBTZ169 (now called macozinone), a piperazine derivative. Compared to BTZ043, PBTZ169 has the advantage of having no chiral center which facilitates its chemical synthesis.

Activity. PBTZ169 is a very potent bactericidal benzothiazinone with an MIC of 0.6 nM against ***M. tuberculosis***. PBTZ169 has better potency, pharmacodynamics and is 10 times less cytotoxic than BTZ043. PBTZ169 has poor solubility in water (0.9 g/L). PBTZ169 is synergistic with BDQ and clofazimine (CFZ) but not with other new TB drugs such as delamanid, linezolid, meropenem or sutezolid [229]. Interestingly, this synergistic phenotype was also observed in non-replicating conditions where PBTZ169 has no activity [230]. In a mouse model of chronic ***M. tuberculosis*** infection, the reduction in lung and spleen burden was similar between INH and PBTZ169 after 4 weeks of treatment [231]. Furthermore, in a mouse model of chronic ***M. tuberculosis*** infection, the lung burden was reduced by 2, 4 and 4.6 $\log_{10}$ after 28 days of treatment with PBTZ169, CFZ and the combination PBTZ169/CFZ, respectively [230]. In a similar experiment, the combination PBTZ169/BDQ/PZA was also shown to be more efficient in reducing lung and spleen burden of chronically ***M. tuberculosis***-infected mice than the standard INH/RIF/PZA treatment [231].

Mode of action. PBTZ169 mode of action is similar to BTZ043. PBTZ169 is a prodrug, activated by DprE1 to yield a nitroso metabolite that covalently binds to the Cys387 residue of DprE1.

Clinical trial. A phase I study (NCT03423030) in healthy male subjects receiving increasing doses of PBTZ169 showed that PBTZ169 was well tolerated and safe. No result has been posted for a phase 2a EBA study (NCT03334734) where PBTZ169 was given as a single dose to TB patients.

4.2.4. OPC167832

Activity. OPC167832 was developed by Otsuka pharmaceuticals. OPC167832 is a lipophilic, bactericidal compound, active against drug-susceptible, MDR and XDR ***M. tuberculosis*** strains, with a MIC ranging from 0.5 to 5 nM. OPC167832 is active in macrophage and in mouse model of ***M. tuberculosis*** infection at a dose of 1.25 mg/kg. OPC167832 is not antagonistic with other TB drugs. The combination of OPC167832 with delamanid and other TB drugs showed better efficacy than standard TB treatment in a mouse model of chronic drug-susceptible and MDR ***M. tuberculosis*** infections [232].

Mode of action. OPC167832 is a DprE1 inhibitor. OPC167832 does not contain a nitro group, and so it inhibits DprE1 via other interactions than a covalent bond with DprE1 Cys387 (see below).

Resistance. Spontaneous OPC167832-resistant mutants isolated at 16 × MIC occurred at a frequency of 2.6×10^{-9} to 1.5×10^{-7} in ***M. tuberculosis*** H37Rv. Mutations in ***dprE1*** and ***Rv0678*** encoding a transcriptional regulator of the efflux pumps MmpS5 and Mmpl5 [233] drive resistance to OPC167832.

Clinical trial. A phase 1/2 clinical trial (NCT03678688) is recruiting to test the safety, tolerability and pharmacokinetics of OPC167832 given at increasing concentrations to patients infected with uncomplicated, smear-positive, drug-susceptible TB (phase I). A phase II study will compare delamanid and OPC167832 vs. delamanid only or INH/RIF/EMB/PZA to demonstrate that this new regimen, which uses only oral drugs, is safer and can shorten TB treatment [232].

4.2.5. TBA-7371

Discovery. TBA-7371 was developed in collaboration between Astra Zeneca and the TB Global Alliance. TBA-7371 is a derivative of 1,4-azaindoles developed through scaffold morphing of an imidazopyridine compound with good MIC but low minimum bactericidal activity (MBC) against ***M. tuberculosis*** [234]. SAR on the hit azaindole compound led to TBA-7371.

Activity. TBA-7371 is bactericidal against ***M. tuberculosis***, with a MIC ranging from 0.78 to 3.12 μm against drug-susceptible and drug-resistant clinical isolates of ***M. tuberculosis*** [235]. Solubility of TBA-7371 is 170 μm. TBA-7371 does not exhibit toxicity in THP1 cell line up to concentration of 0.1 mM [235].

Mode of action. TBA-7371 inhibits DprE1 with an IC_{50} of 10–30 nm but, unlike BTZ043 and PBTZ169, TBA-7371 is a non-covalent inhibitor of DprE1 [234].

Resistance. Resistance to TBA-7371 was observed in strains overexpressing ***M. tuberculosis dprE1*** or carrying the mutation Y314H in ***dprE1***, but not in strains with a mutated Cys387 in ***dprE1*** [234].

Clinical trial. TBA-7371 is in phase I clinical trial (NCT03199339) for safety, tolerability and pharmacokinetic studies in healthy adults. No results have been posted.

DprE1 is a successful drug target. Since the discovery of BTZ043 and its target DprE1 [225], numerous groups have uncovered novel molecules that target DprE1. DprE1 inhibitors can be divided into two groups depending on whether or not they bind covalently to DprE1. The presence of the nitro group is a requirement for the covalent binding to the Cys387 amino acid of DprE1. Among the covalent inhibitors are benzothiazinethione [236], dinitrobenzamides [237], nitroquinoxalines [238] and nitroimidazoles [239]. Several non-covalent DprE1 inhibitors have been identified with various chemical structures: azaindoles [234], benzothiazoles [240], pyrazolopyridones [241], aminoquinolone piperidine amides [242], carboxyquinoxalines [243], pyrrole-benzothiazinones [244], pyridobenzimidazole [245], sulfonylpiperazin-benzothiazinones [246] and piperidinopyrimidines [247]. These compounds inhibit DprE1 through electrostatic or hydrophobic interactions with different sites of DprE1. Most of these compounds have low MICs (in the nM range), are active against MDR and XDR TB as well as in a mouse model of ***M. tuberculosis*** infection. Considering the promiscuity of the DprE1 target, better DprE1 inhibitors might still be discovered to improve TB treatment.

4.3. Target: Peptidoglycan

4.3.1. β-Lactams and Clavulanic Acid

Discovery. The first class of synthetic drugs that successfully treated bacterial infections were the sulfa drugs in the early 1930s [163]; however, by the early 1940s, penicillin had quickly eclipsed the sulfa drugs. Penicillin, a β-lactam compound, was active against Gram-positive and Gram-negative, yet penicillin, like the sulfa drugs, had no activity against ***M. tuberculosis***. For penicillin, the lack of activity was due to the presence in ***M. tuberculosis*** of a potent β-lactamase BlaC. The innate resistance of ***M. tuberculosis*** to β-lactams decreased when blaC was deleted from ***M. tuberculosis*** or when the β-lactamase irreversible inhibitor clavulanic acid [248] was used in combination with β-lactams [249]. Hugonnet and colleagues used this knowledge to validate the combination of meropenem, a carbapenem with poor affinity for BlaC, and clavulanic acid as an efficacious ***M. tuberculosis*** inhibitor [250].

Activity. The combination meropenem plus clavulanate is part of the group D3 (add-on agents) of second-line TB drugs. Meropenem is a potent inhibitor of drug-susceptible and XDR ***M. tuberculosis*** strains (MIC range from 0.6 μm to 3.3 μm) when combined with clavulanate [250]. Interestingly, this combination also inhibits non-replicating ***M. tuberculosis*** [250]. In a chronic model of ***M. tuberculosis*** infection in mice, meropenem had a modest activity in reducing lung burdens [251]. Surprisingly, the addition of clavulanate to the meropenem treatment did not increase meropenem activity in mice. In mice intravenously infected with ***M. tuberculosis***, the lung burden had increased by almost a 1 $\log_{10}$ after 4 weeks of treatment with meropenem and clavulanate showing no inhibitory activity of this combination in vivo [252]. However, studies in mice are problematic since the mice dehydropeptidase (DHP) rapidly cleaves the β-lactam ring.

Meropenem is administered via intravenous injection and new regimens are steering away from injectables. Therefore, Dhar and colleagues tested faropenem, an ***oral*** β-lactam, and demonstrated activity against ***M. tuberculosis*** (MIC 4.6 μm) without clavulanate addition (meropenem MIC is 8-fold higher without clavulanate) [253]. Faropenem is also more soluble in water than meropenem (solubility 14.7 g/L vs. 8 g/L for meropenem). Using the dehydropeptidase inhibitor, probenecid, Dhar and colleagues demonstrated that ***M. tuberculosis***-infected mice had a small but significant reduction in lung burden after 9 days of treatment with a combination faropenem/clavulanate/probenecid. In a study using DHP-I knockout mice [254], mice were infected intratracheally with ***M. tuberculosis*** H37Rv and treated for 8 consecutive days, 10 to 12 days post infection. Meropenem was given subcutaneously three times a day in combination with amoxicillin and clavulanate. Another group of mice received faropenem orally with amoxicillin and clavulanate. A control group was treated with moxifloxacin. Treatment also consisted of a dose of probenecid prior to drug administration. While the lung burden was 7.7 $\log_{10}$ CFU/mouse at the beginning of the treatment, the lung burdens at the end of the treatment were 7.8 and 7.5 $\log_{10}$ CFU/mouse for the meropenem and faropenem groups, respectively. Only the mice receiving moxifloxacin had a 2-$\log_{10}$ reduction in lung burden [254].

Experiments performed in other animal models (rabbits and monkeys) revealed that intravenous injections of meropenem with or without clavulanate and dehydropeptidase inhibitor led to serious adverse effects (diarrhea, weight loss and death) [251].

Mode of action. Meropenem binds to and inhibits the L,D-transpeptidase Ldt_{Mt1} (Rv0116c), which catalyzes the 3→3 cross-linkage in the peptidoglycan [255,256]. Faropenem is 14-fold more potent in inactivating Ldt_{Mt1} than meropenem, but this did not correlate with increasing killing against intracellular ***M. tuberculosis*** [253]. Dhar and colleagues demonstrated that the addition of faropenem to ***M. tuberculosis*** quickly arrested growth, which did not translate into an immediate lysis of the cells. This is opposite to the current understanding that β-lactams induce cell lysis by inhibiting peptidoglycan cross-linking while cells are still actively dividing. Dhar and colleagues concluded that the mechanism of ***M. tuberculosis*** killing by β-lactam should be revisited [253].

Clinical trial. A clinical study on MDR and XDR TB patients receiving meropenem/clavulanate (intravenous injections three times a day for an average of 85 days) in combination with an MDR/XDR drug regimen showed that the addition of meropenem/clavulanate did not improve: (1) sputum smear or culture conversion; (2) treatment outcome; or (3) treatment success [257]. A phase 2 clinical trial evaluated the early bactericidal activity, safety and tolerability of intravenously administered meropenem with amoxicillin and clavulanate versus orally-administered faropenem with amoxicillin and clavulanate (NCT02349841). Results have not been posted yet.

4.3.2. Sanfetrinem

Activity. Sanfetrinem is a tricyclic β-lactam developed by GlaxoSmithKline in the 1990s. Sanfetrinem has broad-spectrum activity against Gram-negative and Gram-positive bacteria. Sanfetrinem is also very stable to β-lactamases and to human renal dehydropeptidase (DHP) [258]. The MICs for sanfetrinem against ***M. tuberculosis*** H37Rv ranged from 1.25 to 5 μm with clavulanate (2.5 to 7.5 μm without clavulanate). In a checkerboard assay, the combination of sanfetrinem with RIF or amoxicillin was synergistic, but not with delamanid or ethambutol. Sanfetrinem cilexetil is an oral prodrug ester of sanfetrinem and has an MIC ranging from 5 to 20 μm with clavulanate (7.5 to 20 μm without clavulanate) against ***M. tuberculosis***. The compounds performed better against intracellular ***M. tuberculosis***. In THP1 monocytes, the MIC for sanfetrinem and sanfetrinem cilexetil ranged from 2.1 to 7.7 μm without clavulanate (6.1 to 8.8 μm with clavulanate) and 3.4 to 7.0 μm without clavulanate (4.6 to 5.3 μm with clavulanate), respectively. In a mouse model of acute ***M. tuberculosis*** infection, DHP-1 KO mice were infected intratracheally with ***M. tuberculosis*** H37Rv. Treatment started 9 days post infection, twice a day, for 5 days. Sanfetrinem was given subcutaneously, while sanfetrinem cilexetil and clavulanate were given orally. Growth arrest but not killing of ***M. tuberculosis*** was observed during this five-day treatment [259].

Clinical trial. A phase 2a clinical study is projected to start the first quarter of 2021 [260].

5. Conclusions

In 1882, when Robert Koch discovered the causative agent of TB, there was no valid treatment for the disease. In the past 70 years, with the introduction of multidrug chemotherapy, the cure rate for drug-susceptible ***M. tuberculosis*** infection has reached up to 95%. The treatment is effective but very long, with drugs that may not be well tolerated. New chemotherapy regimens are needed with drugs that are less toxic and more efficacious, so that a shorter treatment can be achieved. The pursuit of mycobacterial cell wall inhibitors has offered several hits with novel modes of action and remarkable potency that have reached clinical trials. Those pioneering compounds can lead the way to more valuable therapeutics. Numerous new compounds are being studied that either derive from the known hits or target other biosynthetic pathways of the cell wall [261,262]. In the past 20 years, ***M. tuberculosis*** has been unraveling many of its secrets: its niches in the host, its metabolism and its way of fighting drugs. New tools were developed to study ***M. tuberculosis*** and to search for new TB drugs more efficiently combining target and whole-cell screenings. We should be closer to a new TB regimen for a shorter treatment of drug-susceptible TB and a more successful treatment of MDR and XDR TB. The collaboration between academic and pharmaceutical laboratories and the involvement of funding foundations have opened the doors to the clinical testing of new drugs and new regimens [263].

In Selman Waksman's book "The Conquest of Tuberculosis" [264], a quote from Georges Canetti's speech at the 1961 Sixteenth International Conference on Tuberculosis, as reported by the chairman, stated: "We are not concerned with eradication in the absolutely literal sense of the word because this is something that many of us believe to be biologically impossible. What we are talking about, however, is tuberculosis 'eradication' in the sense of reducing the problem to the point where the disease is a scientific curiosity. This is a biologic possibility". With better diagnostic tools, a more efficient vaccine and sterilizing therapeutics, this might become a biologic reality.

A summary of the cell wall inhibitors discussed herein is presented in Table 1 with their chemical structures and targets.

Table 1. TB drugs targeting the mycobacterial cell wall.

Name	Structure	Cell Wall Component Inhibited	Prodrug/Activator	Target
Isoniazid	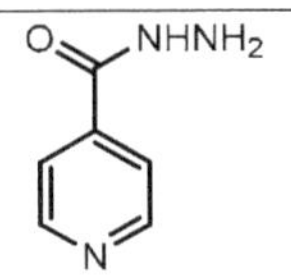	Mycolic acids	+ KatG	InhA
Ethionamide Prothionamide	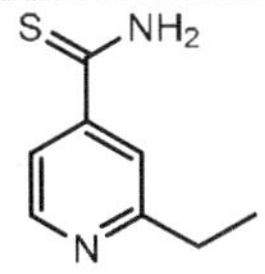 ETH 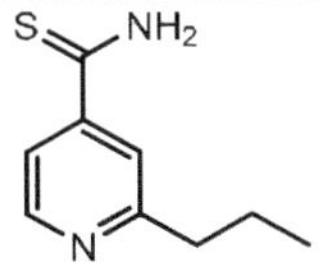 PTH	Mycolic acids	+ EthA, MymA, Rv0565c	InhA
Thiacetazone	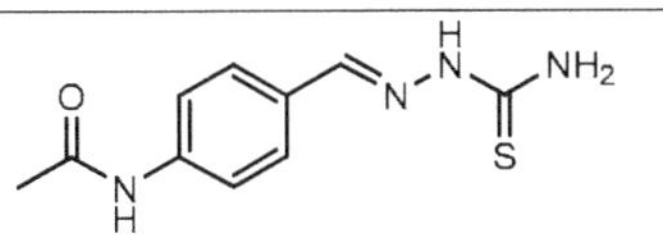	Mycolic acids	+ EthA	HadAB
Pretonamid	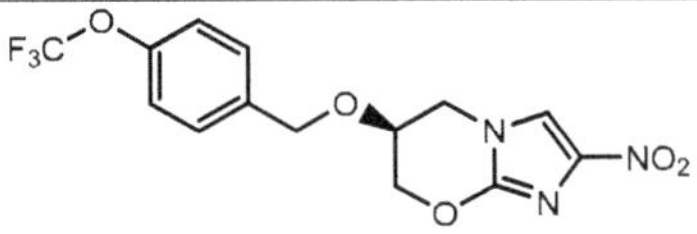	Keto-mycolic acids	+ Ddn	?

Table 1. *Cont.*

Name	Structure	Cell Wall Component Inhibited	Prodrug/Activator	Target
Delamanid	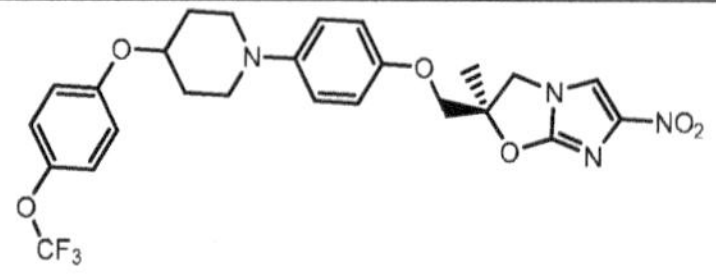	Methoxy- and keto-mycolic acids	+ Ddn	?
SQ109	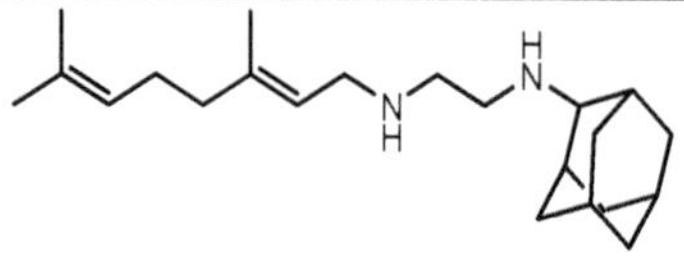	Mycolic acid transport	-	Mmpl3
CPZEN45	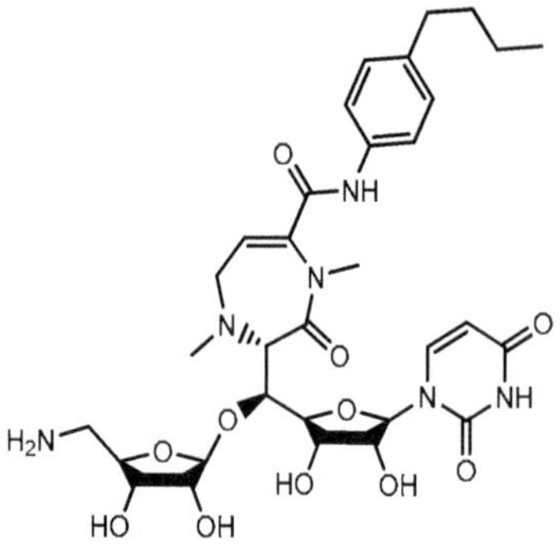	Arabinogalactan	-	WecA
Ethambutol	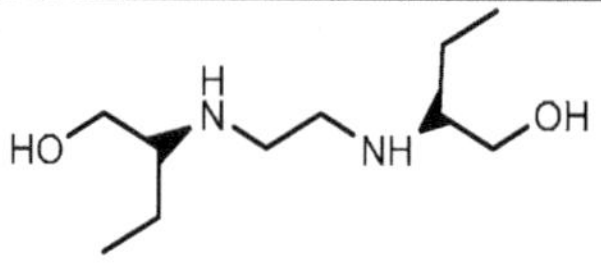	Arabinogalactan LAM	-	EmbCAB
BTZ043	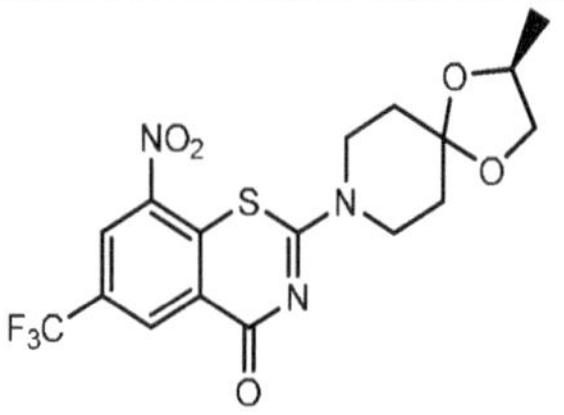	Arabinogalactan LAM	+ DprE1	DprE1
PBTZ169	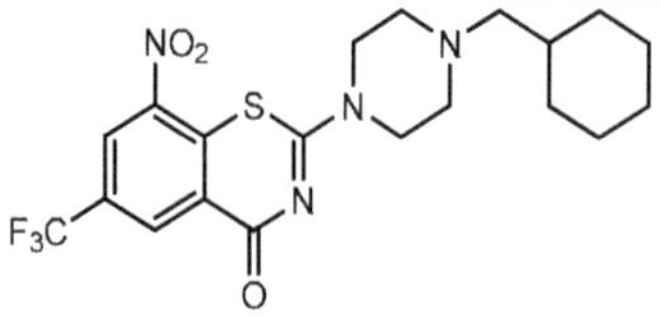	Arabinogalactan LAM	+ DprE1	DprE1
OPC167832	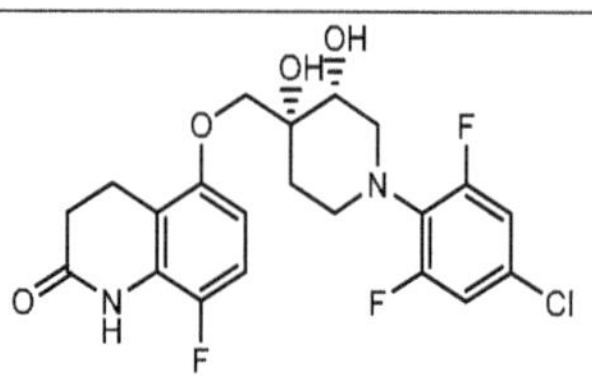	Arabinogalactan LAM	-	DprE1
TBA7371	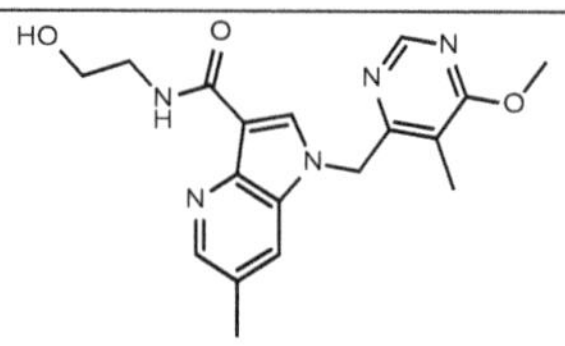	Arabinogalactan LAM	-	DprE1
Cycloserine	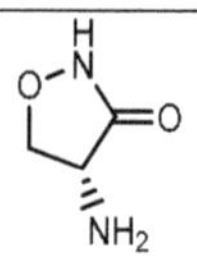	Peptidoglycan	-	DdlA

Table 1. *Cont.*

Name	Structure	Cell Wall Component Inhibited	Prodrug/Activator	Target
Meropenem/ clavulanate	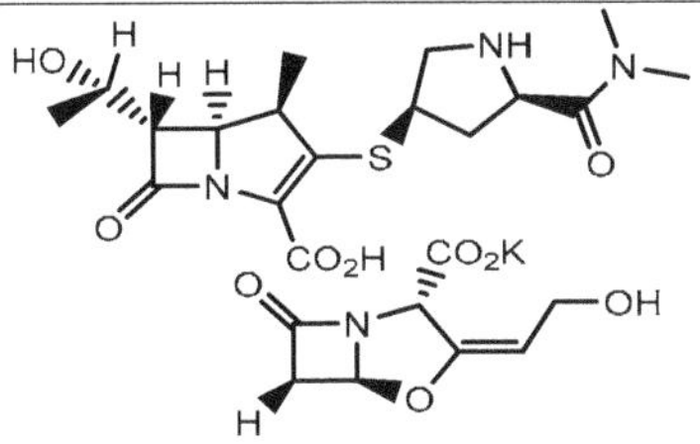	Peptidoglycan	-	LdtM1
sanfetrinem	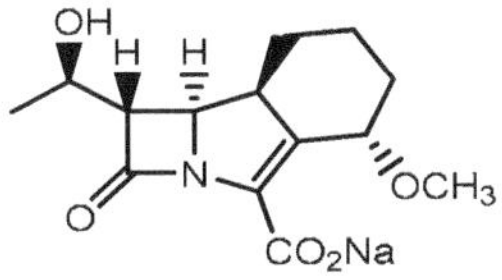	Peptidoglycan	-	

Acknowledgments: I thank Lawrence Leung, Claire Mulholland and Saranathan Rajagopalan for their critical reading, comments and feedback on this manuscript.

References

1. Daniel, T.M. The history of tuberculosis. *Respir. Med.* **2006**, *100*, 1862–1870. [CrossRef] [PubMed]
2. Keers, R.Y. Two forgotten pioneers. James Carson and George Bodington. *Thorax* **1980**, *35*, 483–489. [CrossRef] [PubMed]
3. Bodington, G. Reviews of Books. An essay on the treatment and cure of pulmunory consumption, on principles natural, ratinal and succesful. *Lancet* **1840**, *34*, 575–577.
4. George Bodington, M.D. Obituary. *Lancet* **1882**, *119*, 477.
5. McCarthy, O.R. The key to the sanatoria. *J. R. Soc. Med.* **2001**, *94*, 413–417. [CrossRef] [PubMed]
6. Latour, A. Review of Books. On the preservative and curative treatment of pulmunory consumption. *Lancet* **1840**, *34*, 616–619.
7. Cox, G.L. Sanatorium treatment contrasted with home treatment. After-histories of 4067 cases. *Br. J. Tuberc.* **1923**, *17*, 27–30.
8. Schatz, A.; Bugie, E.; Waksman, S.A. Streptomycin, a substance exhibiting antibiotic activity against gram-positive and gram-negative bacteria. *Proc. Exp. Biol. Med.* **1944**, *55*, 66–69. [CrossRef]
9. Schatz, A.; Waksman, S.A. Effect of streptomycin upon *Mycobacterium tuberculosis* and related organisms. *Proc. Soc. Exp. Biol. Med.* **1944**, *57*, 244–248. [CrossRef]
10. Pfuetze, K.H.; Pyle, M.M.; Hinshaw, H.C.; Feldman, W.H. The first clinical trial of streptomycin in human tuberculosis. *Am. Rev. Tuberc.* **1955**, *71*, 752–754. [CrossRef]
11. Waksman, S.A. Tenth anniversary of the discovery of streptomycin, the first chemotherapeutic agent found to be effective against tuberculosis in humans. *Am. Rev. Tuberc.* **1954**, *70*, 1–8. [CrossRef]
12. Hinshaw, H.C.; Pyle, M.M.; Feldman, W.H. Streptomycin in tuberculosis. *Am. J. Med.* **1947**, *2*, 429–435. [CrossRef]
13. Crofton, J.; Mitchison, D.A. Streptomycin resistance in pulmonary tuberculosis. *Br. Med. J.* **1948**, *2*, 1009–1015. [CrossRef] [PubMed]
14. Lehmann, J. *Para*-Aminosalicylic acid in the treatment of tuberculosis. *Lancet* **1946**, *247*, 15. [CrossRef]
15. Medical Research Council Investigation. Treatment of pulmonary tuberculosis with streptomycin and *para*-amino-salicylic acid. *Br. Med. J.* **1950**, *2*, 4688.
16. Crofton, J. Chemotherapy of pulmonary tuberculosis. *Br. Med. J.* **1959**, *1*, 1610–1614. [CrossRef]
17. Koul, A.; Arnoult, E.; Lounis, N.; Guillemont, J.; Andries, K. The challenge of new drug discovery for tuberculosis. *Nature* **2011**, *469*, 483–490. [CrossRef]
18. Payne, D.J.; Gwynn, M.N.; Holmes, D.J.; Pompliano, D.L. Drugs for bad bugs: Confronting the challenges of antibacterial discovery. *Nat. Rev. Drug Discov.* **2007**, *6*, 29–40. [CrossRef]
19. World Health Organization. Global Tuberculosis Report 2019. Available online: https://apps.who.int/iris/bitstream/handle/10665/329368/9789241565714-eng.pdf?ua=1 (accessed on 15 February 2020).

20. Abrahams, K.A.; Besra, G.S. Mycobacterial cell wall biosynthesis: A multifaceted antibiotic target. *Parasitology* **2018**, *145*, 116–133. [CrossRef]
21. Konyarikova, Z.; Savkova, K.; Kozmon, S.; Mikusova, K. Biosynthesis of Galactan in *Mycobacterium tuberculosis* as a Viable TB Drug Target? *Antibiotics* **2020**, *9*, 20. [CrossRef]
22. Maitra, A.; Munshi, T.; Healy, J.; Martin, L.T.; Vollmer, W.; Keep, N.H.; Bhakta, S. Cell wall peptidoglycan in *Mycobacterium tuberculosis*: An Achilles' heel for the TB-causing pathogen. *FEMS Microbiol. Rev.* **2019**, *43*, 548–575. [CrossRef] [PubMed]
23. Lederer, E.; Adam, A.; Ciorbaru, R.; Petit, J.F.; Wietzerbin, J. Cell walls of Mycobacteria and related organisms; chemistry and immunostimulant properties. *Mol. Cell. Biochem.* **1975**, *7*, 87–104. [CrossRef] [PubMed]
24. Mahapatra, S.; Crick, D.C.; Brennan, P.J. Comparison of the UDP-*N*-acetylmuramate:L-alanine ligase enzymes from *Mycobacterium tuberculosis* and *Mycobacterium leprae*. *J. Bacteriol.* **2000**, *182*, 6827–6830. [CrossRef] [PubMed]
25. Mahapatra, S.; Scherman, H.; Brennan, P.J.; Crick, D.C. *N*-Glycolylation of the nucleotide precursors of peptidoglycan biosynthesis of *Mycobacterium* spp. is altered by drug treatment. *J. Bacteriol.* **2005**, *187*, 2341–2347. [CrossRef] [PubMed]
26. Raymond, J.B.; Mahapatra, S.; Crick, D.C.; Pavelka, M.S., Jr. Identification of the *namH* gene, encoding the hydroxylase responsible for the *N*-glycolylation of the mycobacterial peptidoglycan. *J. Biol. Chem.* **2005**, *280*, 326–333. [CrossRef]
27. McNeil, M.; Wallner, S.J.; Hunter, S.W.; Brennan, P.J. Demonstration that the galactosyl and arabinosyl residues in the cell-wall arabinogalactan of *Mycobacterium leprae* and *Mycobacterium tuberculosis* are furanoid. *Carbohydr. Res.* **1987**, *166*, 299–308. [CrossRef]
28. McNeil, M.; Daffe, M.; Brennan, P.J. Evidence for the nature of the link between the arabinogalactan and peptidoglycan of mycobacterial cell walls. *J. Biol. Chem.* **1990**, *265*, 18200–18206.
29. Marrakchi, H.; Laneelle, M.A.; Daffe, M. Mycolic acids: Structures, biosynthesis, and beyond. *Chem. Biol.* **2014**, *21*, 67–85. [CrossRef]
30. Brindley, D.N.; Matsumura, S.; Bloch, K. *Mycobacterium phlei* Fatty Acid Synthetase—A Bacterial Multienzyme Complex. *Nature* **1969**, *224*, 666–669. [CrossRef]
31. Cantaloube, S.; Veyron-Churlet, R.; Haddache, N.; Daffe, M.; Zerbib, D. The *Mycobacterium tuberculosis* FAS-II dehydratases and methyltransferases define the specificity of the mycolic acid elongation complexes. *PLoS ONE* **2011**, *6*, e29564. [CrossRef]
32. Fukuda, T.; Matsumura, T.; Ato, M.; Hamasaki, M.; Nishiuchi, Y.; Murakami, Y.; Maeda, Y.; Yoshimori, T.; Matsumoto, S.; Kobayashi, K.; et al. Critical roles for lipomannan and lipoarabinomannan in cell wall integrity of mycobacteria and pathogenesis of tuberculosis. *MBio* **2013**, *4*, e00472-12. [CrossRef] [PubMed]
33. Nigou, J.; Gilleron, M.; Rojas, M.; Garcia, L.F.; Thurnher, M.; Puzo, G. Mycobacterial lipoarabinomannans: Modulators of dendritic cell function and the apoptotic response. *Microbes Infect.* **2002**, *4*, 945–953. [CrossRef]
34. Patterson, J.H.; Waller, R.F.; Jeevarajah, D.; Billman-Jacobe, H.; McConville, M.J. Mannose metabolism is required for mycobacterial growth. *Biochem. J.* **2003**, *372*, 77–86. [CrossRef] [PubMed]
35. Stanley, S.A.; Cox, J.S. Host-pathogen interactions during *Mycobacterium tuberculosis* infections. *Curr. Top. Microbiol. Immunol.* **2013**, *374*, 211–241. [CrossRef] [PubMed]
36. McDermott, W. The story of INH. *J. Infect. Dis.* **1969**, *119*, 678–683. [CrossRef]
37. Hinshaw, H.C.; Mc, D.W. Thiosemicarbazone therapy of tuberculosis in humans. *Am. Rev. Tuberc.* **1950**, *61*, 145–157.
38. Donovick, R.; Pansy, F.; Stryker, G.; Bernstein, J. The chemotherapy of experimental tuberculosis. I. The in vitro activity of thiosemicarbazides, thiosemicarbazones, and related compounds. *J. Bacteriol.* **1950**, *59*, 667–674. [CrossRef]
39. Fox, H.H. The chemical approach to the control of tuberculosis. *Science* **1952**, *116*, 129–134. [CrossRef]
40. Hamre, D.; Bernstein, J.; Donovick, R. The chemotherapy of experimental tuberculosis. II. Thiosemicarbazones and analogues in experimental tuberculosis in the mouse. *J. Bacteriol.* **1950**, *59*, 675–680. [CrossRef]
41. Bernstein, J.W.; Lott, A.; Steinberg, B.A.; Yale, H.L. Chemotherapy of experimental tuberculosis. *Am. Rev. Tuberc.* **1952**, *65*, 357–374.
42. Domagk, G.; Offe, H.A.; Siefken, W. [Therapy of experimental tuberculosis with neoteben]. *Med. Colon.* **1952**, *20*, 517–528. [PubMed]

43. Jain, P.; Weinrick, B.C.; Kalivoda, E.J.; Yang, H.; Munsamy, V.; Vilcheze, C.; Weisbrod, T.R.; Larsen, M.H.; O'Donnell, M.R.; Pym, A.; et al. Dual-Reporter Mycobacteriophages (Phi2DRMs) Reveal Preexisting *Mycobacterium tuberculosis* Persistent Cells in Human Sputum. *MBio* **2016**, *7*. [CrossRef] [PubMed]
44. Karakousis, P.C.; Williams, E.P.; Bishai, W.R. Altered expression of isoniazid-regulated genes in drug-treated dormant *Mycobacterium tuberculosis*. *J. Antimicrob. Chemother.* **2008**, *61*, 323–331. [CrossRef] [PubMed]
45. Ohno, M.; Yamaguchi, I.; Yamamoto, I.; Fukuda, T.; Yokota, S.; Maekura, R.; Ito, M.; Yamamoto, Y.; Ogura, T.; Maeda, K.; et al. Slow *N*-acetyltransferase 2 genotype affects the incidence of isoniazid and rifampicin-induced hepatotoxicity. *Int. J. Tuberc. Lung Dis.* **2000**, *4*, 256–261. [PubMed]
46. Wang, P.; Pradhan, K.; Zhong, X.B.; Ma, X. Isoniazid metabolism and hepatotoxicity. *Acta Pharm. Sin. B* **2016**, *6*, 384–392. [CrossRef]
47. Mitchell, J.R.; Zimmerman, H.J.; Ishak, K.G.; Thorgeirsson, U.P.; Timbrell, J.A.; Snodgrass, W.R.; Nelson, S.D. Isoniazid liver injury: Clinical spectrum, pathology, and probable pathogenesis. *Ann. Intern. Med.* **1976**, *84*, 181–192. [CrossRef]
48. Nelson, S.D.; Mitchell, J.R.; Timbrell, J.A.; Snodgrass, W.R.; Corcoran, G.B., 3rd. Isoniazid and iproniazid: Activation of metabolites to toxic intermediates in man and rat. *Science* **1976**, *193*, 901–903. [CrossRef]
49. Lauterburg, B.H.; Smith, C.V.; Todd, E.L.; Mitchell, J.R. Pharmacokinetics of the toxic hydrazino metabolites formed from isoniazid in humans. *J. Pharmacol. Exp. Ther.* **1985**, *235*, 566–570.
50. Gajdacs, M. The Concept of an Ideal Antibiotic: Implications for Drug Design. *Molecules* **2019**, *24*, 892. [CrossRef]
51. Laborde, J.; Deraeve, C.; Bernardes-Genisson, V. Update of Antitubercular Prodrugs from a Molecular Perspective: Mechanisms of Action, Bioactivation Pathways, and Associated Resistance. *ChemMedChem* **2017**, *12*, 1657–1676. [CrossRef]
52. Zhang, Y.; Heym, B.; Allen, B.; Young, D.; Cole, S. The catalase-peroxidase gene and isoniazid resistance of *Mycobacterium tuberculosis*. *Nature* **1992**, *358*, 591–593. [CrossRef] [PubMed]
53. Johnsson, K.; Schultz, P.G. Mechanistic Studies of the Oxidation of Isoniazid by the Catalase Peroxidase from *Mycobacterium tuberculosis*. *J. Am. Chem. Soc.* **1994**, *116*, 7425–7426. [CrossRef]
54. Lei, B.; Wei, C.J.; Tu, S.C. Action mechanism of antitubercular isoniazid. Activation by *Mycobacterium tuberculosis* KatG, isolation, and characterization of *inhA* inhibitor. *J. Biol. Chem.* **2000**, *275*, 2520–2526. [CrossRef] [PubMed]
55. Rozwarski, D.A.; Grant, G.A.; Barton, D.H.; Jacobs, W.R., Jr.; Sacchettini, J.C. Modification of the NADH of the isoniazid target (InhA) from *Mycobacterium tuberculosis*. *Science* **1998**, *279*, 98–102. [CrossRef]
56. Wilming, M.; Johnsson, K. Spontaneous Formation of the Bioactive Form of the Tuberculosis Drug Isoniazid. *Angew. Chem. Int. Ed. Engl.* **1999**, *38*, 2588–2590. [CrossRef]
57. Banerjee, A.; Dubnau, E.; Quemard, A.; Balasubramanian, V.; Um, K.S.; Wilson, T.; Collins, D.; de Lisle, G.; Jacobs, W.R., Jr. *inhA*, a gene encoding a target for isoniazid and ethionamide in *Mycobacterium tuberculosis*. *Science* **1994**, *263*, 227–230. [CrossRef]
58. Nguyen, M.; Quemard, A.; Broussy, S.; Bernadou, J.; Meunier, B. Mn(III) pyrophosphate as an efficient tool for studying the mode of action of isoniazid on the InhA protein of *Mycobacterium tuberculosis*. *Antimicrob. Agents Chemother.* **2002**, *46*, 2137–2144. [CrossRef]
59. Rawat, R.; Whitty, A.; Tonge, P.J. The isoniazid-NAD adduct is a slow, tight-binding inhibitor of InhA, the *Mycobacterium tuberculosis* enoyl reductase: Adduct affinity and drug resistance. *Proc. Natl. Acad. Sci. USA* **2003**, *100*, 13881–13886. [CrossRef]
60. Vilcheze, C.; Wang, F.; Arai, M.; Hazbon, M.H.; Colangeli, R.; Kremer, L.; Weisbrod, T.R.; Alland, D.; Sacchettini, J.C.; Jacobs, W.R., Jr. Transfer of a point mutation in *Mycobacterium tuberculosis inhA* resolves the target of isoniazid. *Nat. Med.* **2006**, *12*, 1027–1029. [CrossRef]
61. Dessen, A.; Quemard, A.; Blanchard, J.S.; Jacobs, W.R., Jr.; Sacchettini, J.C. Crystal structure and function of the isoniazid target of *Mycobacterium tuberculosis*. *Science* **1995**, *267*, 1638–1641. [CrossRef]
62. Quemard, A.; Sacchettini, J.C.; Dessen, A.; Vilcheze, C.; Bittman, R.; Jacobs, W.R., Jr.; Blanchard, J.S. Enzymatic characterization of the target for isoniazid in *Mycobacterium tuberculosis*. *Biochemistry* **1995**, *34*, 8235–8241. [CrossRef] [PubMed]
63. Marrakchi, H.; Laneelle, G.; Quemard, A. InhA, a target of the antituberculous drug isoniazid, is involved in a mycobacterial fatty acid elongation system, FAS-II. *Microbiology* **2000**, *146 Pt 2*, 289–296. [CrossRef]
64. Takayama, K.; Wang, L.; David, H.L. Effect of isoniazid on the in vivo mycolic acid synthesis, cell growth,

and viability of *Mycobacterium tuberculosis*. *Antimicrob. Agents Chemother.* **1972**, *2*, 29–35. [CrossRef]
65. Vilcheze, C.; Morbidoni, H.R.; Weisbrod, T.R.; Iwamoto, H.; Kuo, M.; Sacchettini, J.C.; Jacobs, W.R., Jr. Inactivation of the *inhA*-encoded fatty acid synthase II (FASII) enoyl-acyl carrier protein reductase induces accumulation of the FASI end products and cell lysis of *Mycobacterium smegmatis*. *J. Bacteriol.* **2000**, *182*, 4059–4067. [CrossRef]
66. Winder, F.G.; Collins, P.B. Inhibition by isoniazid of synthesis of mycolic acids in *Mycobacterium tuberculosis*. *J. Gen. Microbiol.* **1970**, *63*, 41–48. [CrossRef]
67. Vilcheze, C.; Jacobs, W.R., Jr. The mechanism of isoniazid killing: Clarity through the scope of genetics. *Annu. Rev. Microbiol.* **2007**, *61*, 35–50. [CrossRef] [PubMed]
68. Middlebrook, G.; Cohn, M.L. Some observations on the pathogenicity of isoniazid-resistant variants of tubercle bacilli. *Science* **1953**, *118*, 297–299. [CrossRef] [PubMed]
69. Middlebrook, G. Isoniazid resistance and catalase activity of tubercle bacilli. *Am. Rev. Tuberc.* **1954**, *69*, 471–472. [PubMed]
70. Zhang, Y.; Garbe, T.; Young, D. Transformation with *katG* restores isoniazid-sensitivity in *Mycobacterium tuberculosis* isolates resistant to a range of drug concentrations. *Mol. Microbiol.* **1993**, *8*, 521–524. [CrossRef]
71. Vilcheze, C.; Jacobs, W.R., Jr. Resistance to Isoniazid and Ethionamide in *Mycobacterium tuberculosis*: Genes, Mutations, and Causalities. *Microbiol. Spectr.* **2014**, *2*. [CrossRef]
72. Ando, H.; Kondo, Y.; Suetake, T.; Toyota, E.; Kato, S.; Mori, T.; Kirikae, T. Identification of *katG* mutations associated with high-level isoniazid resistance in *Mycobacterium tuberculosis*. *Antimicrob. Agents Chemother.* **2010**, *54*, 1793–1799. [CrossRef] [PubMed]
73. Sekiguchi, J.; Miyoshi-Akiyama, T.; Augustynowicz-Kopec, E.; Zwolska, Z.; Kirikae, F.; Toyota, E.; Kobayashi, I.; Morita, K.; Kudo, K.; Kato, S.; et al. Detection of multidrug resistance in *Mycobacterium tuberculosis*. *J. Clin. Microbiol.* **2007**, *45*, 179–192. [CrossRef] [PubMed]
74. Wei, C.J.; Lei, B.; Musser, J.M.; Tu, S.C. Isoniazid activation defects in recombinant *Mycobacterium tuberculosis* catalase-peroxidase (KatG) mutants evident in InhA inhibitor production. *Antimicrob. Agents Chemother.* **2003**, *47*, 670–675. [CrossRef]
75. Brossier, F.; Veziris, N.; Truffot-Pernot, C.; Jarlier, V.; Sougakoff, W. Performance of the genotype MTBDR line probe assay for detection of resistance to rifampin and isoniazid in strains of *Mycobacterium tuberculosis* with low- and high-level resistance. *J. Clin. Microbiol.* **2006**, *44*, 3659–3664. [CrossRef] [PubMed]
76. Ando, H.; Kitao, T.; Miyoshi-Akiyama, T.; Kato, S.; Mori, T.; Kirikae, T. Downregulation of *katG* expression is associated with isoniazid resistance in *Mycobacterium tuberculosis*. *Mol. Microbiol.* **2011**, *79*, 1615–1628. [CrossRef] [PubMed]
77. Muller, B.; Streicher, E.M.; Hoek, K.G.; Tait, M.; Trollip, A.; Bosman, M.E.; Coetzee, G.J.; Chabula-Nxiweni, E.M.; Hoosain, E.; Gey van Pittius, N.C.; et al. *inhA* promoter mutations: A gateway to extensively drug-resistant tuberculosis in South Africa? *Int. J. Tuberc. Lung Dis.* **2011**, *15*, 344–351. [PubMed]
78. Shaw, D.J.; Robb, K.; Vetter, B.V.; Tong, M.; Molle, V.; Hunt, N.T.; Hoskisson, P.A. Disruption of key NADH-binding pocket residues of the *Mycobacterium tuberculosis* InhA affects DD-CoA binding ability. *Sci. Rep.* **2017**, *7*, 4714. [CrossRef]
79. Machado, D.; Perdigao, J.; Ramos, J.; Couto, I.; Portugal, I.; Ritter, C.; Boettger, E.C.; Viveiros, M. High-level resistance to isoniazid and ethionamide in multidrug-resistant *Mycobacterium tuberculosis* of the Lisboa family is associated with *inhA* double mutations. *J Antimicrob. Chemother.* **2013**, *68*, 1728–1732. [CrossRef]
80. Morlock, G.P.; Metchock, B.; Sikes, D.; Crawford, J.T.; Cooksey, R.C. *ethA*, *inhA*, and *katG* loci of ethionamide-resistant clinical *Mycobacterium tuberculosis* isolates. *Antimicrob. Agents Chemother.* **2003**, *47*, 3799–3805. [CrossRef]
81. Nimmo, C.; Doyle, R.; Burgess, C.; Williams, R.; Gorton, R.; McHugh, T.D.; Brown, M.; Morris-Jones, S.; Booth, H.; Breuer, J. Rapid identification of a *Mycobacterium tuberculosis* full genetic drug resistance profile through whole genome sequencing directly from sputum. *Int. J. Infect. Dis.* **2017**, *62*, 44–46. [CrossRef]
82. Encinas, L.; O'Keefe, H.; Neu, M.; Remuinan, M.J.; Patel, A.M.; Guardia, A.; Davie, C.P.; Perez-Macias, N.; Yang, H.; Convery, M.A.; et al. Encoded library technology as a source of hits for the discovery and lead optimization of a potent and selective class of bactericidal direct inhibitors of *Mycobacterium tuberculosis* InhA. *J. Med. Chem.* **2014**, *57*, 1276–1288. [CrossRef] [PubMed]
83. Hartkoorn, R.C.; Sala, C.; Neres, J.; Pojer, F.; Magnet, S.; Mukherjee, R.; Uplekar, S.; Boy-Rottger, S.; Altmann, K.H.; Cole, S.T. Towards a new tuberculosis drug: Pyridomycin—Nature's isoniazid. *EMBO Mol.*

Med. **2012**, *4*, 1032–1042. [CrossRef] [PubMed]

84. Lu, X.Y.; You, Q.D.; Chen, Y.D. Recent progress in the identification and development of InhA direct inhibitors of *Mycobacterium tuberculosis*. *Mini Rev. Med. Chem.* **2010**, *10*, 181–192. [CrossRef] [PubMed]
85. Manjunatha, U.H.; SP, S.R.; Kondreddi, R.R.; Noble, C.G.; Camacho, L.R.; Tan, B.H.; Ng, S.H.; Ng, P.S.; Ma, N.L.; Lakshminarayana, S.B.; et al. Direct inhibitors of InhA are active against *Mycobacterium tuberculosis*. *Sci. Transl. Med.* **2015**, *7*, 269ra263. [CrossRef] [PubMed]
86. Pan, P.; Tonge, P.J. Targeting InhA, the FASII enoyl-ACP reductase: SAR studies on novel inhibitor scaffolds. *Curr. Top. Med. Chem.* **2012**, *12*, 672–693. [CrossRef] [PubMed]
87. Shirude, P.S.; Madhavapeddi, P.; Naik, M.; Murugan, K.; Shinde, V.; Nandishaiah, R.; Bhat, J.; Kumar, A.; Hameed, S.; Holdgate, G.; et al. Methyl-thiazoles: A novel mode of inhibition with the potential to develop novel inhibitors targeting InhA in *Mycobacterium tuberculosis*. *J. Med. Chem.* **2013**, *56*, 8533–8542. [CrossRef]
88. Sink, R.; Sosic, I.; Zivec, M.; Fernandez-Menendez, R.; Turk, S.; Pajk, S.; Alvarez-Gomez, D.; Lopez-Roman, E.M.; Gonzales-Cortez, C.; Rullas-Triconado, J.; et al. Design, synthesis, and evaluation of new thiadiazole-based direct inhibitors of enoyl acyl carrier protein reductase (InhA) for the treatment of tuberculosis. *J. Med. Chem.* **2015**, *58*, 613–624. [CrossRef]
89. Vilcheze, C.; Baughn, A.D.; Tufariello, J.; Leung, L.W.; Kuo, M.; Basler, C.F.; Alland, D.; Sacchettini, J.C.; Freundlich, J.S.; Jacobs, W.R., Jr. Novel inhibitors of InhA efficiently kill *Mycobacterium tuberculosis* under aerobic and anaerobic conditions. *Antimicrob. Agents Chemother.* **2011**, *55*, 3889–3898. [CrossRef]
90. Martinez-Hoyos, M.; Perez-Herran, E.; Gulten, G.; Encinas, L.; Alvarez-Gomez, D.; Alvarez, E.; Ferrer-Bazaga, S.; Garcia-Perez, A.; Ortega, F.; Angulo-Barturen, I.; et al. Antitubercular drugs for an old target: GSK693 as a promising InhA direct inhibitor. *EBioMedicine* **2016**, *8*, 291–301. [CrossRef]
91. Robertson, G.T.; Ektnitphong, V.A.; Scherman, M.S.; McNeil, M.B.; Dennison, D.; Korkegian, A.; Smith, A.J.; Halladay, J.; Carter, D.S.; Xia, Y.; et al. Efficacy and Improved Resistance Potential of a Cofactor-Independent InhA Inhibitor of *Mycobacterium tuberculosis* in the C3HeB/FeJ Mouse Model. *Antimicrob. Agents Chemother.* **2019**, *63*. [CrossRef]
92. Xia, Y.; Zhou, Y.; Carter, D.S.; McNeil, M.B.; Choi, W.; Halladay, J.; Berry, P.W.; Mao, W.; Hernandez, V.; O'Malley, T.; et al. Discovery of a cofactor-independent inhibitor of *Mycobacterium tuberculosis* InhA. *Life Sci. Alliance* **2018**, *1*, e201800025. [CrossRef] [PubMed]
93. Shepherd, R.G.; Wilkinson, R.G. Antituberculous Agents. Ii. *N,N'*-Diisopropylethylenediamine and Analogs. *J. Med. Chem.* **1962**, *91*, 823–835. [CrossRef] [PubMed]
94. Thomas, J.P.; Baughn, C.O.; Wilkinson, R.G.; Shepherd, R.G. A new synthetic compound with antituberculous activity in mice: Ethambutol (dextro-2,2'-(ethylenediimino)-di-l-butanol). *Am. Rev. Respir. Dis.* **1961**, *83*, 891–893. [CrossRef] [PubMed]
95. Wilkinson, R.G.; Shepherd, R.G.; Thomas, J.P.; Baughn, C.O. Stereospecificity in a new type of synthetic antituberculous agent. *J. Am. Chem. Soc.* **1961**, *83*, 2212. [CrossRef]
96. Kuck, N.A.; Peets, E.A.; Forbes, M. Mode of action of ethambutol on *Mycobacterium tuberculosis*, strain H37R V. *Am. Rev. Respir. Dis.* **1963**, *87*, 905–906. [CrossRef]
97. Koul, P.A. Ocular toxicity with ethambutol therapy: Timely recaution. *Lung India* **2015**, *32*, 1–3. [CrossRef]
98. Forbes, M.; Kuck, N.A.; Peets, E.A. Effect of Ethambutol on Nucleic Acid Metabolism in *Mycobacterium Smegmatis* and Its Reversal by Polyamines and Divalent Cations. *J. Bacteriol.* **1965**, *89*, 1299–1305. [CrossRef]
99. Takayama, K.; Armstrong, E.L.; Kunugi, K.A.; Kilburn, J.O. Inhibition by ethambutol of mycolic acid transfer into the cell wall of *Mycobacterium smegmatis*. *Antimicrob. Agents Chemother.* **1979**, *16*, 240–242. [CrossRef]
100. Kilburn, J.O.; Takayama, K. Effects of ethambutol on accumulation and secretion of trehalose mycolates and free mycolic acid in *Mycobacterium smegmatis*. *Antimicrob. Agents Chemother.* **1981**, *20*, 401–404. [CrossRef]
101. Takayama, K.; Kilburn, J.O. Inhibition of synthesis of arabinogalactan by ethambutol in *Mycobacterium smegmatis*. *Antimicrob. Agents Chemother.* **1989**, *33*, 1493–1499. [CrossRef]
102. Wolucka, B.A.; McNeil, M.R.; de Hoffmann, E.; Chojnacki, T.; Brennan, P.J. Recognition of the lipid intermediate for arabinogalactan/arabinomannan biosynthesis and its relation to the mode of action of ethambutol on mycobacteria. *J. Biol. Chem.* **1994**, *269*, 23328–23335. [PubMed]
103. Mikusova, K.; Huang, H.; Yagi, T.; Holsters, M.; Vereecke, D.; D'Haeze, W.; Scherman, M.S.; Brennan, P.J.; McNeil, M.R.; Crick, D.C. Decaprenylphosphoryl arabinofuranose, the donor of the D-arabinofuranosyl residues of mycobacterial arabinan, is formed via a two-step epimerization of decaprenylphosphoryl ribose.

J. Bacteriol. **2005**, *187*, 8020–8025. [CrossRef] [PubMed]

104. Deng, L.; Mikusova, K.; Robuck, K.G.; Scherman, M.; Brennan, P.J.; McNeil, M.R. Recognition of multiple effects of ethambutol on metabolism of mycobacterial cell envelope. *Antimicrob. Agents Chemother.* **1995**, *39*, 694–701. [CrossRef] [PubMed]
105. Mikusova, K.; Slayden, R.A.; Besra, G.S.; Brennan, P.J. Biogenesis of the mycobacterial cell wall and the site of action of ethambutol. *Antimicrob. Agents Chemother.* **1995**, *39*, 2484–2489. [CrossRef]
106. Pawar, A.; Jha, P.; Konwar, C.; Chaudhry, U.; Chopra, M.; Saluja, D. Ethambutol targets the glutamate racemase of *Mycobacterium tuberculosis*-an enzyme involved in peptidoglycan biosynthesis. *Appl. Microbiol. Biotechnol.* **2019**, *103*, 843–851. [CrossRef]
107. Sreevatsan, S.; Stockbauer, K.E.; Pan, X.; Kreiswirth, B.N.; Moghazeh, S.L.; Jacobs, W.R., Jr.; Telenti, A.; Musser, J.M. Ethambutol resistance in *Mycobacterium tuberculosis*: Critical role of *embB* mutations. *Antimicrob. Agents Chemother.* **1997**, *41*, 1677–1681. [CrossRef] [PubMed]
108. Telenti, A.; Philipp, W.J.; Sreevatsan, S.; Bernasconi, C.; Stockbauer, K.E.; Wieles, B.; Musser, J.M.; Jacobs, W.R., Jr. The *emb* operon, a gene cluster of *Mycobacterium tuberculosis* involved in resistance to ethambutol. *Nat. Med.* **1997**, *3*, 567–570. [CrossRef]
109. Belanger, A.E.; Besra, G.S.; Ford, M.E.; Mikusova, K.; Belisle, J.T.; Brennan, P.J.; Inamine, J.M. The *embAB* genes of *Mycobacterium avium* encode an arabinosyl transferase involved in cell wall arabinan biosynthesis that is the target for the antimycobacterial drug ethambutol. *Proc. Natl. Acad. Sci. USA* **1996**, *93*, 11919–11924. [CrossRef]
110. Safi, H.; Sayers, B.; Hazbon, M.H.; Alland, D. Transfer of *embB* codon 306 mutations into clinical *Mycobacterium tuberculosis* strains alters susceptibility to ethambutol, isoniazid, and rifampin. *Antimicrob. Agents Chemother.* **2008**, *52*, 2027–2034. [CrossRef]
111. Starks, A.M.; Gumusboga, A.; Plikaytis, B.B.; Shinnick, T.M.; Posey, J.E. Mutations at *embB* codon 306 are an important molecular indicator of ethambutol resistance in *Mycobacterium tuberculosis*. *Antimicrob. Agents Chemother.* **2009**, *53*, 1061–1066. [CrossRef]
112. Hazbon, M.H.; Bobadilla del Valle, M.; Guerrero, M.I.; Varma-Basil, M.; Filliol, I.; Cavatore, M.; Colangeli, R.; Safi, H.; Billman-Jacobe, H.; Lavender, C.; et al. Role of *embB* codon 306 mutations in *Mycobacterium tuberculosis* revisited: A novel association with broad drug resistance and IS6110 clustering rather than ethambutol resistance. *Antimicrob. Agents Chemother.* **2005**, *49*, 3794–3802. [CrossRef] [PubMed]
113. Lee, A.S.; Othman, S.N.; Ho, Y.M.; Wong, S.Y. Novel mutations within the *embB* gene in ethambutol-susceptible clinical isolates of *Mycobacterium tuberculosis*. *Antimicrob. Agents Chemother.* **2004**, *48*, 4447–4449. [CrossRef] [PubMed]
114. Mokrousov, I.; Otten, T.; Vyshnevskiy, B.; Narvskaya, O. Detection of *embB306* mutations in ethambutol-susceptible clinical isolates of *Mycobacterium tuberculosis* from Northwestern Russia: Implications for genotypic resistance testing. *J. Clin. Microbiol.* **2002**, *40*, 3810–3813. [CrossRef] [PubMed]
115. Shen, X.; Shen, G.M.; Wu, J.; Gui, X.H.; Li, X.; Mei, J.; DeRiemer, K.; Gao, Q. Association between *embB* codon 306 mutations and drug resistance in *Mycobacterium tuberculosis*. *Antimicrob. Agents Chemother.* **2007**, *51*, 2618–2620. [CrossRef]
116. Safi, H.; Lingaraju, S.; Amin, A.; Kim, S.; Jones, M.; Holmes, M.; McNeil, M.; Peterson, S.N.; Chatterjee, D.; Fleischmann, R.; et al. Evolution of high-level ethambutol-resistant tuberculosis through interacting mutations in decaprenylphosphoryl-beta-D-arabinose biosynthetic and utilization pathway genes. *Nat. Genet.* **2013**, *45*, 1190–1197. [CrossRef]
117. Tulyaprawat, O.; Chaiprasert, A.; Chongtrakool, P.; Suwannakarn, K.; Ngamskulrungroj, P. Association of *ubiA* mutations and high-level of ethambutol resistance among *Mycobacterium tuberculosis* Thai clinical isolates. *Tuberculosis* **2019**, *114*, 42–46. [CrossRef]
118. Gardner, T.S.; Wenis, E.; Lee, J.H. The synthesis of compounds for the chemotherapy of tuberculosis. IV. The amide function. *J. Org. Chem.* **1954**, *19*, 753–757. [CrossRef]
119. Grumbach, F.; Rist, N.; Libermann, D.; Moyeux, M.; Cals, S.; Clavel, S. Experimental antituberculous activity of certain isonicotinic thioamides substituted on the nucleus. *C. R. Hebd. Seances Acad. Sci.* **1956**, *242*, 2187–2189.
120. Scardigli, A.; Caminero, J.A.; Sotgiu, G.; Centis, R.; D'Ambrosio, L.; Migliori, G.B. Efficacy and tolerability of ethionamide versus prothionamide: A systematic review. *Eur. Respir. J.* **2016**, *48*, 946–952. [CrossRef]
121. Winder, F.G.; Collins, P.B.; Whelan, D. Effects of ethionamide and isoxyl on mycolic acid synthesis in *Mycobacterium tuberculosis* BCG. *J. Gen. Microbiol.* **1971**, *66*, 379–380. [CrossRef]

122. Hok, T.T. A comparative study of the susceptibility to ethionamide, thiosemicarbazone, and isoniazid of tubercle bacilli from patients never treated with ethionamide or thiosemicarbazone. *Am. Rev. Respir. Dis.* **1964**, *90*, 468–469. [PubMed]
123. Lefford, M.J. The ethionamide sensitivity of British pre-treatment strains of *Mycobacterium tuberculosis*. *Tubercle* **1966**, *47*, 198–206. [CrossRef]
124. Stewart, S.M.; Hall, E.; Riddell, R.W.; Somner, A.R. Bacteriological aspects of the use of ethionamide, pyrazinamide and cycloserine in the treatment of chronic pulmonary tuberculosis. *Tubercle* **1962**, *43*, 417–431. [CrossRef]
125. DeBarber, A.E.; Mdluli, K.; Bosman, M.; Bekker, L.G.; Barry, C.E., 3rd. Ethionamide activation and sensitivity in multidrug-resistant *Mycobacterium tuberculosis*. *Proc. Natl. Acad. Sci. USA* **2000**, *97*, 9677–9682. [CrossRef]
126. Vannelli, T.A.; Dykman, A.; Ortiz de Montellano, P.R. The antituberculosis drug ethionamide is activated by a flavoprotein monooxygenase. *J. Biol. Chem.* **2002**, *277*, 12824–12829. [CrossRef]
127. Wang, F.; Langley, R.; Gulten, G.; Dover, L.G.; Besra, G.S.; Jacobs, W.R., Jr.; Sacchettini, J.C. Mechanism of thioamide drug action against tuberculosis and leprosy. *J. Exp. Med.* **2007**, *204*, 73–78. [CrossRef]
128. Ang, M.L.T.; Zainul Rahim, S.Z.; de Sessions, P.F.; Lin, W.; Koh, V.; Pethe, K.; Hibberd, M.L.; Alonso, S. EthA/R-Independent Killing of *Mycobacterium tuberculosis* by Ethionamide. *Front. Microbiol.* **2017**, *8*, 710. [CrossRef]
129. Grant, S.S.; Wellington, S.; Kawate, T.; Desjardins, C.A.; Silvis, M.R.; Wivagg, C.; Thompson, M.; Gordon, K.; Kazyanskaya, E.; Nietupski, R.; et al. Baeyer-Villiger Monooxygenases EthA and MymA Are Required for Activation of Replicating and Non-replicating *Mycobacterium tuberculosis* Inhibitors. *Cell Chem. Biol.* **2016**, *23*, 666–677. [CrossRef]
130. Hicks, N.D.; Carey, A.F.; Yang, J.; Zhao, Y.; Fortune, S.M. Bacterial Genome-Wide Association Identifies Novel Factors That Contribute to Ethionamide and Prothionamide Susceptibility in *Mycobacterium tuberculosis*. *MBio* **2019**, *10*. [CrossRef]
131. Brossier, F.; Veziris, N.; Truffot-Pernot, C.; Jarlier, V.; Sougakoff, W. Molecular investigation of resistance to the antituberculous drug ethionamide in multidrug-resistant clinical isolates of *Mycobacterium tuberculosis*. *Antimicrob. Agents Chemother.* **2011**, *55*, 355–360. [CrossRef]
132. Zhang, H.N.; Xu, Z.W.; Jiang, H.W.; Wu, F.L.; He, X.; Liu, Y.; Guo, S.J.; Li, Y.; Bi, L.J.; Deng, J.Y.; et al. Cyclic di-GMP regulates *Mycobacterium tuberculosis* resistance to ethionamide. *Sci. Rep.* **2017**, *7*, 5860. [CrossRef] [PubMed]
133. Vilcheze, C.; Av-Gay, Y.; Attarian, R.; Liu, Z.; Hazbon, M.H.; Colangeli, R.; Chen, B.; Liu, W.; Alland, D.; Sacchettini, J.C.; et al. Mycothiol biosynthesis is essential for ethionamide susceptibility in *Mycobacterium tuberculosis*. *Mol. Microbiol.* **2008**, *69*, 1316–1329. [CrossRef] [PubMed]
134. Vilcheze, C.; Weisbrod, T.R.; Chen, B.; Kremer, L.; Hazbon, M.H.; Wang, F.; Alland, D.; Sacchettini, J.C.; Jacobs, W.R., Jr. Altered NADH/NAD^+ ratio mediates coresistance to isoniazid and ethionamide in mycobacteria. *Antimicrob. Agents Chemother.* **2005**, *49*, 708–720. [CrossRef] [PubMed]
135. Baulard, A.R.; Betts, J.C.; Engohang-Ndong, J.; Quan, S.; McAdam, R.A.; Brennan, P.J.; Locht, C.; Besra, G.S. Activation of the pro-drug ethionamide is regulated in mycobacteria. *J. Biol. Chem.* **2000**, *275*, 28326–28331. [CrossRef] [PubMed]
136. Willand, N.; Dirie, B.; Carette, X.; Bifani, P.; Singhal, A.; Desroses, M.; Leroux, F.; Willery, E.; Mathys, V.; Deprez-Poulain, R.; et al. Synthetic EthR inhibitors boost antituberculous activity of ethionamide. *Nat. Med.* **2009**, *15*, 537–544. [CrossRef]
137. Flipo, M.; Desroses, M.; Lecat-Guillet, N.; Villemagne, B.; Blondiaux, N.; Leroux, F.; Piveteau, C.; Mathys, V.; Flament, M.P.; Siepmann, J.; et al. Ethionamide boosters. 2. Combining bioisosteric replacement and structure-based drug design to solve pharmacokinetic issues in a series of potent 1,2,4-oxadiazole EthR inhibitors. *J. Med. Chem.* **2012**, *55*, 68–83. [CrossRef]
138. Blondiaux, N.; Moune, M.; Desroses, M.; Frita, R.; Flipo, M.; Mathys, V.; Soetaert, K.; Kiass, M.; Delorme, V.; Djaout, K.; et al. Reversion of antibiotic resistance in *Mycobacterium tuberculosis* by spiroisoxazoline SMARt-420. *Science* **2017**, *355*, 1206–1211. [CrossRef]
139. Harris, D.A.; Ruger, M.; Reagan, M.A.; Wolf, F.J.; Peck, R.L.; Wallick, H.; Woodruff, H.B. Discovery, development, and antimicrobial properties of D-4-amino-3-isoxazolidone (oxamycin), a new antibiotic produced by *Streptomyces garyphalus* n. sp. *Antibiot. Chemother.* **1955**, *5*, 183–190.
140. Shull, G.M.; Sardinas, J.L. PA-94, an antibiotic identical with D-4-amino-3-isoxazolidinone (cycloserine,

oxamycin). *Antibiot. Chemother.* **1955**, *5*, 398–399.
141. Kurosawa, H. The isolation of an antibiotic produced by a strain of streptomyces K-300. *Yokohama Med. Bull.* **1952**, *3*, 386–399.
142. Harned, R.L.; Hidy, P.H.; La Baw, E.K. Cycloserine. I. A preliminary report. *Antibiot. Chemother.* **1955**, *5*, 204–205.
143. Steenken, W., Jr.; Wolinsky, E. Cycloserine: Antituberculous activity in vitro and in the experimental animal. *Am. Rev. Tuberc.* **1956**, *73*, 539–546. [CrossRef] [PubMed]
144. Cuckler, A.C.; Frost, B.M.; Mc, C.L.; Solotorovsky, M. The antimicrobial evaluation of oxamycin (D-4-amino-3-isoxazolidone), a new broad-spectrum antibiotic. *Antibiot. Chemother.* **1955**, *5*, 191–197.
145. Patnode, R.A.; Hudgins, P.C.; Cummings, M.M. Effect of cycloserine on experimental tuberculosis in guinea pigs. *Am. Rev. Tuberc.* **1955**, *72*, 117–118. [CrossRef]
146. Conzelman, G.M., Jr.; Jones, R.K. On the physiologic disposition of cycloserine in experimental animals. *Am. Rev. Tuberc.* **1956**, *74*, 802–806. [CrossRef]
147. Epstein, I.G.; Nair, K.G.; Boyd, L.J. Cycloserine, a new antibiotic, in the treatment of human pulmonary tuberculosis: A preliminary report. *Antibiot. Med. Clin. Ther.* **1955**, *1*, 80–93.
148. Lester, W., Jr.; Salomon, A.; Reimann, A.F.; Shulruff, E.; Berg, G.S. Cycloserine therapy in tuberculosis in humans. *Am. Rev. Tuberc.* **1956**, *74*, 121–127. [CrossRef]
149. Hoeprich, P.D. Alanine: Cycloserine Antagonism. Vi. Demonstration of D-Alanine in the Serum of Guinea Pigs and Mice. *J. Biol. Chem.* **1965**, *240*, 1654–1660.
150. Li, Y.; Wang, F.; Wu, L.; Zhu, M.; He, G.; Chen, X.; Sun, F.; Liu, Q.; Wang, X.; Zhang, W. Cycloserine for treatment of multidrug-resistant tuberculosis: A retrospective cohort study in China. *Infect. Drug Resist.* **2019**, *12*, 721–731. [CrossRef]
151. Walker, W.C.; Murdoch, J.M. Cycloserine in the treatment of pulmonary tuberculosis; a report on toxicity. *Tubercle* **1957**, *38*, 297–302. [CrossRef]
152. Bondi, A.; Kornblum, J.; Forte, C. Inhibition of antibacterial activity of cycloserine by alpha-alanine. *Proc. Soc. Exp. Biol. Med.* **1957**, *96*, 270–272. [CrossRef] [PubMed]
153. Strominger, J.L.; Ito, E.; Threnn, R.H. Competitive inhibition of enzymatic reactions by oxamycin. *J. Am. Chem. Soc.* **1960**, *82*, 998–999. [CrossRef]
154. Halouska, S.; Fenton, R.J.; Zinniel, D.K.; Marshall, D.D.; Barletta, R.G.; Powers, R. Metabolomics analysis identifies d-Alanine-d-Alanine ligase as the primary lethal target of d-Cycloserine in mycobacteria. *J. Proteome Res.* **2014**, *13*, 1065–1076. [CrossRef] [PubMed]
155. Prosser, G.A.; de Carvalho, L.P. Reinterpreting the mechanism of inhibition of *Mycobacterium tuberculosis* D-alanine:D-alanine ligase by D-cycloserine. *Biochemistry* **2013**, *52*, 7145–7149. [CrossRef]
156. Prosser, G.A.; de Carvalho, L.P. Kinetic mechanism and inhibition of *Mycobacterium tuberculosis* D-alanine:D-alanine ligase by the antibiotic D-cycloserine. *FEBS J.* **2013**, *280*, 1150–1166. [CrossRef]
157. Viallier, J.; Cayre, R.M.; Biot, N. Sensitivity and resistance of *Mycobacterium tuberculosis* to cycloserine; study of 115 strains isolated from human pathological materials. *Ann. Inst. Pasteur (Paris)* **1957**, *93*, 127–131.
158. Chen, J.M.; Uplekar, S.; Gordon, S.V.; Cole, S.T. A point mutation in *cycA* partially contributes to the D-cycloserine resistance trait of *Mycobacterium bovis* BCG vaccine strains. *PLoS ONE* **2012**, *7*, e43467. [CrossRef]
159. Desjardins, C.A.; Cohen, K.A.; Munsamy, V.; Abeel, T.; Maharaj, K.; Walker, B.J.; Shea, T.P.; Almeida, D.V.; Manson, A.L.; Salazar, A.; et al. Genomic and functional analyses of *Mycobacterium tuberculosis* strains implicate *ald* in D-cycloserine resistance. *Nat. Genet.* **2016**, *48*, 544–551. [CrossRef]
160. Nakatani, Y.; Opel-Reading, H.K.; Merker, M.; Machado, D.; Andres, S.; Kumar, S.S.; Moradigaravand, D.; Coll, F.; Perdigao, J.; Portugal, I.; et al. Role of Alanine Racemase Mutations in *Mycobacterium tuberculosis* d-Cycloserine Resistance. *Antimicrob. Agents Chemother.* **2017**, *61*. [CrossRef]
161. Chen, J.; Zhang, S.; Cui, P.; Shi, W.; Zhang, W.; Zhang, Y. Identification of novel mutations associated with cycloserine resistance in *Mycobacterium tuberculosis*. *J. Antimicrob. Chemother.* **2017**, *72*, 3272–3276. [CrossRef]
162. Evangelopoulos, D.; Prosser, G.A.; Rodgers, A.; Dagg, B.M.; Khatri, B.; Ho, M.M.; Gutierrez, M.G.; Cortes, T.; de Carvalho, L.P.S. Comparative fitness analysis of D-cycloserine resistant mutants reveals both fitness-neutral and high-fitness cost genotypes. *Nat. Commun.* **2019**, *10*, 4177. [CrossRef] [PubMed]
163. Hager, T. *The Demon under the Microscope. From Battlefield Hospitals to Nazi Labs, One Doctor's Heroic Search for the World's First Miracle Drug*, 1st ed.; Three River Press: New York, NY, USA, 2006; p. 340.

164. Domagk, G. Investigations on the antituberculous activity of the thiosemicarbazones in vitro and in vivo. *Am. Rev. Tuberc.* **1950**, *61*, 8–19. [PubMed]
165. Mertens, A.; Bunge, R. The present status of the chemotherapy of tuberculosis with conteben a substance of the thiosemicarbazone series; a review. *Am. Rev. Tuberc.* **1950**, *61*, 20–38. [CrossRef] [PubMed]
166. Cavanagh, P.; McPherson, K. The thiacetazone sensitivity of *Mycobacterium tuberculosis*. *J. Med. Microbiol.* **1969**, *2*, 237–242. [CrossRef]
167. Rieder, H.L.; Enarson, D.A. Rebuttal: Time to call a halt to emotions in the assessment of thioacetazone. *Tuber. Lung Dis.* **1996**, *77*, 109–111. [CrossRef]
168. Falzon, D.; Hill, G.; Pal, S.N.; Suwankesawong, W.; Jaramillo, E. Pharmacovigilance and tuberculosis: Applying the lessons of thioacetazone. *Bull. World Health Organ.* **2014**, *92*, 918–919. [CrossRef]
169. Dover, L.G.; Alahari, A.; Gratraud, P.; Gomes, J.M.; Bhowruth, V.; Reynolds, R.C.; Besra, G.S.; Kremer, L. EthA, a common activator of thiocarbamide-containing drugs acting on different mycobacterial targets. *Antimicrob. Agents Chemother.* **2007**, *51*, 1055–1063. [CrossRef]
170. Belardinelli, J.M.; Morbidoni, H.R. Mutations in the essential FAS II beta-hydroxyacyl ACP dehydratase complex confer resistance to thiacetazone in *Mycobacterium tuberculosis* and *Mycobacterium kansasii*. *Mol. Microbiol.* **2012**, *86*, 568–579. [CrossRef]
171. Grzegorzewicz, A.E.; Kordulakova, J.; Jones, V.; Born, S.E.; Belardinelli, J.M.; Vaquie, A.; Gundi, V.A.; Madacki, J.; Slama, N.; Laval, F.; et al. A common mechanism of inhibition of the *Mycobacterium tuberculosis* mycolic acid biosynthetic pathway by isoxyl and thiacetazone. *J. Biol. Chem.* **2012**, *287*, 38434–38441. [CrossRef]
172. Dong, Y.; Qiu, X.; Shaw, N.; Xu, Y.; Sun, Y.; Li, X.; Li, J.; Rao, Z. Molecular basis for the inhibition of beta-hydroxyacyl-ACP dehydratase HadAB complex from *Mycobacterium tuberculosis* by flavonoid inhibitors. *Protein Cell* **2015**, *6*, 504–517. [CrossRef]
173. Grzegorzewicz, A.E.; Eynard, N.; Quemard, A.; North, E.J.; Margolis, A.; Lindenberger, J.J.; Jones, V.; Kordulakova, J.; Brennan, P.J.; Lee, R.E.; et al. Covalent modification of the *Mycobacterium tuberculosis* FAS-II dehydratase by Isoxyl and Thiacetazone. *ACS Infect. Dis.* **2015**, *1*, 91–97. [CrossRef] [PubMed]
174. Coxon, G.D.; Craig, D.; Corrales, R.M.; Vialla, E.; Gannoun-Zaki, L.; Kremer, L. Synthesis, antitubercular activity and mechanism of resistance of highly effective thiacetazone analogues. *PLoS ONE* **2013**, *8*, e53162. [CrossRef] [PubMed]
175. Grzegorzewicz, A.E.; Gee, C.; Das, S.; Liu, J.; Belardinelli, J.M.; Jones, V.; McNeil, M.R.; Lee, R.E.; Jackson, M. Mechanisms of Resistance Associated with the Inhibition of the Dehydration Step of Type II Fatty Acid Synthase in *Mycobacterium tuberculosis*. *ACS Infect. Dis.* **2019**. [CrossRef]
176. Alahari, A.; Alibaud, L.; Trivelli, X.; Gupta, R.; Lamichhane, G.; Reynolds, R.C.; Bishai, W.R.; Guerardel, Y.; Kremer, L. Mycolic acid methyltransferase, MmaA4, is necessary for thiacetazone susceptibility in *Mycobacterium tuberculosis*. *Mol. Microbiol.* **2009**, *71*, 1263–1277. [CrossRef] [PubMed]
177. Sacksteder, K.A.; Protopopova, M.; Barry, C.E., 3rd; Andries, K.; Nacy, C.A. Discovery and development of SQ109: A new antitubercular drug with a novel mechanism of action. *Future Microbiol.* **2012**, *7*, 823–837. [CrossRef] [PubMed]
178. Alland, D.; Steyn, A.J.; Weisbrod, T.; Aldrich, K.; Jacobs, W.R., Jr. Characterization of the *Mycobacterium tuberculosis iniBAC* promoter, a promoter that responds to cell wall biosynthesis inhibition. *J. Bacteriol.* **2000**, *182*, 1802–1811. [CrossRef] [PubMed]
179. Protopopova, M.; Hanrahan, C.; Nikonenko, B.; Samala, R.; Chen, P.; Gearhart, J.; Einck, L.; Nacy, C.A. Identification of a new antitubercular drug candidate, SQ109, from a combinatorial library of 1,2-ethylenediamines. *J. Antimicrob. Chemother.* **2005**, *56*, 968–974. [CrossRef]
180. Chen, P.; Gearhart, J.; Protopopova, M.; Einck, L.; Nacy, C.A. Synergistic interactions of SQ109, a new ethylene diamine, with front-line antitubercular drugs in vitro. *J. Antimicrob. Chemother.* **2006**, *58*, 332–337. [CrossRef]
181. Jia, L.; Tomaszewski, J.E.; Hanrahan, C.; Coward, L.; Noker, P.; Gorman, G.; Nikonenko, B.; Protopopova, M. Pharmacodynamics and pharmacokinetics of SQ109, a new diamine-based antitubercular drug. *Br. J. Pharmacol.* **2005**, *144*, 80–87. [CrossRef]
182. Boshoff, H.I.; Myers, T.G.; Copp, B.R.; McNeil, M.R.; Wilson, M.A.; Barry, C.E., 3rd. The transcriptional responses of *Mycobacterium tuberculosis* to inhibitors of metabolism: Novel insights into drug mechanisms of action. *J. Biol. Chem.* **2004**, *279*, 40174–40184. [CrossRef]
183. Tahlan, K.; Wilson, R.; Kastrinsky, D.B.; Arora, K.; Nair, V.; Fischer, E.; Barnes, S.W.; Walker, J.R.; Alland, D.;

Barry, C.E., 3rd; et al. SQ109 targets MmpL3, a membrane transporter of trehalose monomycolate involved in mycolic acid donation to the cell wall core of *Mycobacterium tuberculosis*. *Antimicrob. Agents Chemother.* **2012**, *56*, 1797–1809. [CrossRef] [PubMed]
184. Grzegorzewicz, A.E.; Pham, H.; Gundi, V.A.; Scherman, M.S.; North, E.J.; Hess, T.; Jones, V.; Gruppo, V.; Born, S.E.; Kordulakova, J.; et al. Inhibition of mycolic acid transport across the *Mycobacterium tuberculosis* plasma membrane. *Nat. Chem. Biol.* **2012**, *8*, 334–341. [CrossRef] [PubMed]
185. Zhang, B.; Li, J.; Yang, X.; Wu, L.; Zhang, J.; Yang, Y.; Zhao, Y.; Zhang, L.; Cheng, X.; Liu, Z.; et al. Crystal Structures of Membrane Transporter MmpL3, an Anti-TB Drug Target. *Cell* **2019**, *176*, 636–648.e13. [CrossRef] [PubMed]
186. Heinrich, N.; Dawson, R.; du Bois, J.; Narunsky, K.; Horwith, G.; Phipps, A.J.; Nacy, C.A.; Aarnoutse, R.E.; Boeree, M.J.; Gillespie, S.H.; et al. Early phase evaluation of SQ109 alone and in combination with rifampicin in pulmonary TB patients. *J. Antimicrob. Chemother.* **2015**, *70*, 1558–1566. [CrossRef]
187. Niemi, M.; Backman, J.T.; Fromm, M.F.; Neuvonen, P.J.; Kivisto, K.T. Pharmacokinetic interactions with rifampicin: Clinical relevance. *Clin. Pharmacokinet.* **2003**, *42*, 819–850. [CrossRef]
188. Boeree, M.J.; Heinrich, N.; Aarnoutse, R.; Diacon, A.H.; Dawson, R.; Rehal, S.; Kibiki, G.S.; Churchyard, G.; Sanne, I.; Ntinginya, N.E.; et al. High-dose rifampicin, moxifloxacin, and SQ109 for treating tuberculosis: A multi-arm, multi-stage randomised controlled trial. *Lancet Infect. Dis.* **2017**, *17*, 39–49. [CrossRef]
189. Tiberi, S.; du Plessis, N.; Walzl, G.; Vjecha, M.J.; Rao, M.; Ntoumi, F.; Mfinanga, S.; Kapata, N.; Mwaba, P.; McHugh, T.D.; et al. Tuberculosis: Progress and advances in development of new drugs, treatment regimens, and host-directed therapies. *Lancet Infect. Dis.* **2018**, *18*, e183–e198. [CrossRef]
190. Poce, G.; Consalvi, S.; Biava, M. MmpL3 Inhibitors: Diverse Chemical Scaffolds Inhibit the Same Target. *Mini Rev. Med. Chem.* **2016**, *16*, 1274–1283. [CrossRef]
191. Williams, J.T.; Haiderer, E.R.; Coulson, G.B.; Conner, K.N.; Ellsworth, E.; Chen, C.; Alvarez-Cabrera, N.; Li, W.; Jackson, M.; Dick, T.; et al. Identification of New MmpL3 Inhibitors by Untargeted and Targeted Mutant Screens Defines MmpL3 Domains with Differential Resistance. *Antimicrob. Agents Chemother.* **2019**, *63*. [CrossRef]
192. Samuelson, J. Why metronidazole is active against both bacteria and parasites. *Antimicrob. Agents Chemother.* **1999**, *43*, 1533–1541. [CrossRef]
193. Brooks, J.V.; Furney, S.K.; Orme, I.M. Metronidazole therapy in mice infected with tuberculosis. *Antimicrob. Agents Chemother.* **1999**, *43*, 1285–1288. [CrossRef] [PubMed]
194. Ashtekar, D.R.; Costa-Perira, R.; Nagrajan, K.; Vishvanathan, N.; Bhatt, A.D.; Rittel, W. In vitro and in vivo activities of the nitroimidazole CGI 17341 against *Mycobacterium tuberculosis*. *Antimicrob. Agents Chemother.* **1993**, *37*, 183–186. [CrossRef] [PubMed]
195. Stover, C.K.; Warrener, P.; VanDevanter, D.R.; Sherman, D.R.; Arain, T.M.; Langhorne, M.H.; Anderson, S.W.; Towell, J.A.; Yuan, Y.; McMurray, D.N.; et al. A small-molecule nitroimidazopyran drug candidate for the treatment of tuberculosis. *Nature* **2000**, *405*, 962–966. [CrossRef] [PubMed]
196. Li, S.Y.; Tasneen, R.; Tyagi, S.; Soni, H.; Converse, P.J.; Mdluli, K.; Nuermberger, E.L. Bactericidal and Sterilizing Activity of a Novel Regimen with Bedaquiline, Pretomanid, Moxifloxacin, and Pyrazinamide in a Murine Model of Tuberculosis. *Antimicrob. Agents Chemother.* **2017**, *61*. [CrossRef] [PubMed]
197. Xu, J.; Li, S.Y.; Almeida, D.V.; Tasneen, R.; Barnes-Boyle, K.; Converse, P.J.; Upton, A.M.; Mdluli, K.; Fotouhi, N.; Nuermberger, E.L. Contribution of Pretomanid to Novel Regimens Containing Bedaquiline with either Linezolid or Moxifloxacin and Pyrazinamide in Murine Models of Tuberculosis. *Antimicrob. Agents Chemother.* **2019**, *63*. [CrossRef] [PubMed]
198. Singh, R.; Manjunatha, U.; Boshoff, H.I.; Ha, Y.H.; Niyomrattanakit, P.; Ledwidge, R.; Dowd, C.S.; Lee, I.Y.; Kim, P.; Zhang, L.; et al. PA-824 kills nonreplicating *Mycobacterium tuberculosis* by intracellular NO release. *Science* **2008**, *322*, 1392–1395. [CrossRef]
199. Manjunatha, U.; Boshoff, H.I.; Barry, C.E. The mechanism of action of PA-824: Novel insights from transcriptional profiling. *Commun. Integr. Biol.* **2009**, *2*, 215–218. [CrossRef]
200. Haver, H.L.; Chua, A.; Ghode, P.; Lakshminarayana, S.B.; Singhal, A.; Mathema, B.; Wintjens, R.; Bifani, P. Mutations in genes for the F420 biosynthetic pathway and a nitroreductase enzyme are the primary resistance determinants in spontaneous in vitro-selected PA-824-resistant mutants of *Mycobacterium tuberculosis*. *Antimicrob. Agents Chemother.* **2015**, *59*, 5316–5323. [CrossRef]
201. Diacon, A.H.; Dawson, R.; von Groote-Bidlingmaier, F.; Symons, G.; Venter, A.; Donald, P.R.; van Niekerk, C.;

Everitt, D.; Winter, H.; Becker, P.; et al. 14-day bactericidal activity of PA-824, bedaquiline, pyrazinamide, and moxifloxacin combinations: A randomised trial. *Lancet* **2012**, *380*, 986–993. [CrossRef]
202. Tweed, C.D.; Dawson, R.; Burger, D.A.; Conradie, A.; Crook, A.M.; Mendel, C.M.; Conradie, F.; Diacon, A.H.; Ntinginya, N.E.; Everitt, D.E.; et al. Bedaquiline, moxifloxacin, pretomanid, and pyrazinamide during the first 8 weeks of treatment of patients with drug-susceptible or drug-resistant pulmonary tuberculosis: A multicentre, open-label, partially randomised, phase 2b trial. *Lancet Respir. Med.* **2019**, *7*, 1048–1058. [CrossRef]
203. Conradie, F.; Diacon, A.; Everitt, D.; Mendel, C.M.; Crook, A.M.; Howell, P.; Comins, K.; Spigelman, M. Sustained High Rate of Successful Treatment Outcomes: Interim Results of 75 Patients in the Nix-TB Clinical Study of Pretomanid, Bedaquiline and Linezolid. Available online: https://www.dropbox.com/s/gu8l27grq38psul/Nix%20TB%20interim%20results%20-%2010-25-18.pdf?dl=0 (accessed on 30 January 2020).
204. Sasaki, H.; Haraguchi, Y.; Itotani, M.; Kuroda, H.; Hashizume, H.; Tomishige, T.; Kawasaki, M.; Matsumoto, M.; Komatsu, M.; Tsubouchi, H. Synthesis and antituberculosis activity of a novel series of optically active 6-nitro-2,3-dihydroimidazo[2,1-b]oxazoles. *J. Med. Chem.* **2006**, *49*, 7854–7860. [CrossRef] [PubMed]
205. Liu, Y.; Matsumoto, M.; Ishida, H.; Ohguro, K.; Yoshitake, M.; Gupta, R.; Geiter, L.; Hafkin, J. Delamanid: From discovery to its use for pulmonary multidrug-resistant tuberculosis (MDR-TB). *Tuberculosis* **2018**, *111*, 20–30. [CrossRef]
206. Matsumoto, M.; Hashizume, H.; Tomishige, T.; Kawasaki, M.; Tsubouchi, H.; Sasaki, H.; Shimokawa, Y.; Komatsu, M. OPC-67683, a nitro-dihydro-imidazooxazole derivative with promising action against tuberculosis in vitro and in mice. *PLoS Med.* **2006**, *3*, e466. [CrossRef] [PubMed]
207. Upton, A.M.; Cho, S.; Yang, T.J.; Kim, Y.; Wang, Y.; Lu, Y.; Wang, B.; Xu, J.; Mdluli, K.; Ma, Z.; et al. In vitro and in vivo activities of the nitroimidazole TBA-354 against *Mycobacterium tuberculosis*. *Antimicrob. Agents Chemother.* **2015**, *59*, 136–144. [CrossRef] [PubMed]
208. Fujiwara, M.; Kawasaki, M.; Hariguchi, N.; Liu, Y.; Matsumoto, M. Mechanisms of resistance to delamanid, a drug for *Mycobacterium tuberculosis*. *Tuberculosis* **2018**, *108*, 186–194. [CrossRef] [PubMed]
209. Gler, M.T.; Skripconoka, V.; Sanchez-Garavito, E.; Xiao, H.; Cabrera-Rivero, J.L.; Vargas-Vasquez, D.E.; Gao, M.; Awad, M.; Park, S.K.; Shim, T.S.; et al. Delamanid for multidrug-resistant pulmonary tuberculosis. *N. Engl. J. Med.* **2012**, *366*, 2151–2160. [CrossRef]
210. Gupta, R.; Geiter, L.J.; Wells, C.D.; Gao, M.; Cirule, A.; Xiao, H. Delamanid for Extensively Drug-Resistant Tuberculosis. *N. Engl. J. Med.* **2015**, *373*, 291–292. [CrossRef]
211. Wells, C.D.; Gupta, R.; Hittel, N.; Geiter, L.J. Long-term mortality assessment of multidrug-resistant tuberculosis patients treated with delamanid. *Eur. Respir. J.* **2015**, *45*, 1498–1501. [CrossRef]
212. Von Groote-Bidlingmaier, F.; Patientia, R.; Sanchez, E.; Balanag, V., Jr.; Ticona, E.; Segura, P.; Cadena, E.; Yu, C.; Cirule, A.; Lizarbe, V.; et al. Efficacy and safety of delamanid in combination with an optimised background regimen for treatment of multidrug-resistant tuberculosis: A multicentre, randomised, double-blind, placebo-controlled, parallel group phase 3 trial. *Lancet Respir. Med.* **2019**, *7*, 249–259. [CrossRef]
213. Kumar, P.; Capodagli, G.C.; Awasthi, D.; Shrestha, R.; Maharaja, K.; Sukheja, P.; Li, S.G.; Inoyama, D.; Zimmerman, M.; Ho Liang, H.P.; et al. Synergistic Lethality of a Binary Inhibitor of *Mycobacterium tuberculosis* KasA. *MBio* **2018**, *9*. [CrossRef]
214. Aggarwal, A.; Parai, M.K.; Shetty, N.; Wallis, D.; Woolhiser, L.; Hastings, C.; Dutta, N.K.; Galaviz, S.; Dhakal, R.C.; Shrestha, R.; et al. Development of a Novel Lead that Targets *M. tuberculosis* Polyketide Synthase 13. *Cell* **2017**, *170*, 249–259.e25. [CrossRef] [PubMed]
215. Dal Molin, M.; Selchow, P.; Schafle, D.; Tschumi, A.; Ryckmans, T.; Laage-Witt, S.; Sander, P. Identification of novel scaffolds targeting *Mycobacterium tuberculosis*. *J. Mol. Med.* **2019**, *97*, 1601–1613. [CrossRef]
216. Wilson, R.; Kumar, P.; Parashar, V.; Vilcheze, C.; Veyron-Churlet, R.; Freundlich, J.S.; Barnes, S.W.; Walker, J.R.; Szymonifka, M.J.; Marchiano, E.; et al. Antituberculosis thiophenes define a requirement for Pks13 in mycolic acid biosynthesis. *Nat. Chem. Biol.* **2013**, *9*, 499–506. [CrossRef] [PubMed]
217. Zhang, W.; Lun, S.; Wang, S.H.; Jiang, X.W.; Yang, F.; Tang, J.; Manson, A.L.; Earl, A.M.; Gunosewoyo, H.; Bishai, W.R.; et al. Identification of Novel Coumestan Derivatives as Polyketide Synthase 13 Inhibitors against *Mycobacterium tuberculosis*. *J. Med. Chem.* **2018**, *61*, 791–803. [CrossRef] [PubMed]
218. Li, W.; Sanchez-Hidalgo, A.; Jones, V.; de Moura, V.C.; North, E.J.; Jackson, M. Synergistic Interactions of MmpL3 Inhibitors with Antitubercular Compounds In Vitro. *Antimicrob. Agents Chemother.* **2017**, *61*. [CrossRef] [PubMed]

219. Poce, G.; Bates, R.H.; Alfonso, S.; Cocozza, M.; Porretta, G.C.; Ballell, L.; Rullas, J.; Ortega, F.; De Logu, A.; Agus, E.; et al. Improved BM212 MmpL3 inhibitor analogue shows efficacy in acute murine model of tuberculosis infection. *PLoS ONE* **2013**, *8*, e56980. [CrossRef] [PubMed]
220. Igarashi, M.; Nakagawa, N.; Doi, N.; Hattori, S.; Naganawa, H.; Hamada, M. Caprazamycin B, a novel anti-tuberculosis antibiotic, from *Streptomyces* sp. *J. Antibiot.* **2003**, *56*, 580–583. [CrossRef]
221. Takahashi, Y.; Igarashi, M.; Miyake, T.; Soutome, H.; Ishikawa, K.; Komatsuki, Y.; Koyama, Y.; Nakagawa, N.; Hattori, S.; Inoue, K.; et al. Novel semisynthetic antibiotics from caprazamycins A-G: Caprazene derivatives and their antibacterial activity. *J. Antibiot.* **2013**, *66*, 171–178. [CrossRef]
222. Ishizaki, Y.; Hayashi, C.; Inoue, K.; Igarashi, M.; Takahashi, Y.; Pujari, V.; Crick, D.C.; Brennan, P.J.; Nomoto, A. Inhibition of the first step in synthesis of the mycobacterial cell wall core, catalyzed by the GlcNAc-1-phosphate transferase WecA, by the novel caprazamycin derivative CPZEN-45. *J. Biol. Chem.* **2013**, *288*, 30309–30319. [CrossRef]
223. Takahashi, Y.; Igarashi, M.; Okada, M. Anti-XDR-TB, Anti-MDR-TB Drug, and Combination Anti-Tuberculoses Drug. U.S. Patent 9040502 B2, 26 May 2015.
224. Huszar, S.; Singh, V.; Polcicova, A.; Barath, P.; Barrio, M.B.; Lagrange, S.; Leblanc, V.; Nacy, C.A.; Mizrahi, V.; Mikusova, K. *N*-Acetylglucosamine-1-Phosphate Transferase, WecA, as a Validated Drug Target in *Mycobacterium tuberculosis*. *Antimicrob. Agents Chemother.* **2017**, *61*. [CrossRef]
225. Makarov, V.; Manina, G.; Mikusova, K.; Mollmann, U.; Ryabova, O.; Saint-Joanis, B.; Dhar, N.; Pasca, M.R.; Buroni, S.; Lucarelli, A.P.; et al. Benzothiazinones kill *Mycobacterium tuberculosis* by blocking arabinan synthesis. *Science* **2009**, *324*, 801–804. [CrossRef]
226. Lechartier, B.; Hartkoorn, R.C.; Cole, S.T. In vitro combination studies of benzothiazinone lead compound BTZ043 against *Mycobacterium tuberculosis*. *Antimicrob. Agents Chemother.* **2012**, *56*, 5790–5793. [CrossRef]
227. New TB Drugs. BTZ-043. Available online: https://www.newtbdrugs.org/pipeline/compound/btz-043 (accessed on 15 February 2020).
228. Trefzer, C.; Skovierova, H.; Buroni, S.; Bobovska, A.; Nenci, S.; Molteni, E.; Pojer, F.; Pasca, M.R.; Makarov, V.; Cole, S.T.; et al. Benzothiazinones are suicide inhibitors of mycobacterial decaprenylphosphoryl-beta-D-ribofuranose 2′-oxidase DprE1. *J. Am. Chem. Soc.* **2012**, *134*, 912–915. [CrossRef] [PubMed]
229. Lupien, A.; Vocat, A.; Foo, C.S.; Blattes, E.; Gillon, J.Y.; Makarov, V.; Cole, S.T. Optimized Background Regimen for Treatment of Active Tuberculosis with the Next-Generation Benzothiazinone Macozinone (PBTZ169). *Antimicrob. Agents Chemother.* **2018**, *62*. [CrossRef] [PubMed]
230. Lechartier, B.; Cole, S.T. Mode of Action of Clofazimine and Combination Therapy with Benzothiazinones against *Mycobacterium tuberculosis*. *Antimicrob. Agents Chemother.* **2015**, *59*, 4457–4463. [CrossRef] [PubMed]
231. Makarov, V.; Lechartier, B.; Zhang, M.; Neres, J.; van der Sar, A.M.; Raadsen, S.A.; Hartkoorn, R.C.; Ryabova, O.B.; Vocat, A.; Decosterd, L.A.; et al. Towards a new combination therapy for tuberculosis with next generation benzothiazinones. *EMBO Mol. Med.* **2014**, *6*, 372–383. [CrossRef] [PubMed]
232. Workshop "Critical Path to TB Drug Regimens". Available online: http://www.cptrinitiative.org/wp-content/uploads/2017/05/Jeffrey_Hafkin_CPTR2017_JH.pdf (accessed on 26 January 2020).
233. Hartkoorn, R.C.; Uplekar, S.; Cole, S.T. Cross-Resistance between Clofazimine and Bedaquiline through Upregulation of MmpL5 in *Mycobacterium tuberculosis*. *Antimicrob. Agents Chemother.* **2014**, *58*, 2979–2981. [CrossRef]
234. Shirude, P.S.; Shandil, R.; Sadler, C.; Naik, M.; Hosagrahara, V.; Hameed, S.; Shinde, V.; Bathula, C.; Humnabadkar, V.; Kumar, N.; et al. Azaindoles: Noncovalent DprE1 inhibitors from scaffold morphing efforts, kill *Mycobacterium tuberculosis* and are efficacious in vivo. *J. Med. Chem.* **2013**, *56*, 9701–9708. [CrossRef]
235. Chatterji, M.; Shandil, R.; Manjunatha, M.R.; Solapure, S.; Ramachandran, V.; Kumar, N.; Saralaya, R.; Panduga, V.; Reddy, J.; Prabhakar, K.R.; et al. 1,4-azaindole, a potential drug candidate for treatment of tuberculosis. *Antimicrob. Agents Chemother.* **2014**, *58*, 5325–5331. [CrossRef] [PubMed]
236. Gao, C.; Peng, C.; Shi, Y.; You, X.; Ran, K.; Xiong, L.; Ye, T.H.; Zhang, L.; Wang, N.; Zhu, Y.; et al. Benzothiazinethione is a potent preclinical candidate for the treatment of drug-resistant tuberculosis. *Sci. Rep.* **2016**, *6*, 29717. [CrossRef] [PubMed]
237. Christophe, T.; Jackson, M.; Jeon, H.K.; Fenistein, D.; Contreras-Dominguez, M.; Kim, J.; Genovesio, A.; Carralot, J.P.; Ewann, F.; Kim, E.H.; et al. High content screening identifies decaprenyl-phosphoribose 2′ epimerase as a target for intracellular antimycobacterial inhibitors. *PLoS Pathog.* **2009**, *5*, e1000645. [CrossRef]

[PubMed]

238. Magnet, S.; Hartkoorn, R.C.; Szekely, R.; Pato, J.; Triccas, J.A.; Schneider, P.; Szantai-Kis, C.; Orfi, L.; Chambon, M.; Banfi, D.; et al. Leads for antitubercular compounds from kinase inhibitor library screens. *Tuberculosis* **2010**, *90*, 354–360. [CrossRef] [PubMed]
239. Stanley, S.A.; Grant, S.S.; Kawate, T.; Iwase, N.; Shimizu, M.; Wivagg, C.; Silvis, M.; Kazyanskaya, E.; Aquadro, J.; Golas, A.; et al. Identification of novel inhibitors of *M. tuberculosis* growth using whole cell based high-throughput screening. *ACS Chem. Biol.* **2012**, *7*, 1377–1384. [CrossRef] [PubMed]
240. Wang, F.; Sambandan, D.; Halder, R.; Wang, J.; Batt, S.M.; Weinrick, B.; Ahmad, I.; Yang, P.; Zhang, Y.; Kim, J.; et al. Identification of a small molecule with activity against drug-resistant and persistent tuberculosis. *Proc. Natl. Acad. Sci. USA* **2013**, *110*, E2510–E2517. [CrossRef] [PubMed]
241. Panda, M.; Ramachandran, S.; Ramachandran, V.; Shirude, P.S.; Humnabadkar, V.; Nagalapur, K.; Sharma, S.; Kaur, P.; Guptha, S.; Narayan, A.; et al. Discovery of pyrazolopyridones as a novel class of noncovalent DprE1 inhibitor with potent anti-mycobacterial activity. *J. Med. Chem.* **2014**, *57*, 4761–4771. [CrossRef] [PubMed]
242. Naik, M.; Humnabadkar, V.; Tantry, S.J.; Panda, M.; Narayan, A.; Guptha, S.; Panduga, V.; Manjrekar, P.; Jena, L.K.; Koushik, K.; et al. 4-aminoquinolone piperidine amides: Noncovalent inhibitors of DprE1 with long residence time and potent antimycobacterial activity. *J. Med. Chem.* **2014**, *57*, 5419–5434. [CrossRef]
243. Neres, J.; Hartkoorn, R.C.; Chiarelli, L.R.; Gadupudi, R.; Pasca, M.R.; Mori, G.; Venturelli, A.; Savina, S.; Makarov, V.; Kolly, G.S.; et al. 2-Carboxyquinoxalines kill *Mycobacterium tuberculosis* through noncovalent inhibition of DprE1. *ACS Chem. Biol.* **2015**, *10*, 705–714. [CrossRef]
244. Makarov, V.; Neres, J.; Hartkoorn, R.C.; Ryabova, O.B.; Kazakova, E.; Sarkan, M.; Huszar, S.; Piton, J.; Kolly, G.S.; Vocat, A.; et al. The 8-Pyrrole-Benzothiazinones Are Noncovalent Inhibitors of DprE1 from *Mycobacterium tuberculosis*. *Antimicrob. Agents Chemother.* **2015**, *59*, 4446–4452. [CrossRef]
245. Warrier, T.; Kapilashrami, K.; Argyrou, A.; Ioerger, T.R.; Little, D.; Murphy, K.C.; Nandakumar, M.; Park, S.; Gold, B.; Mi, J.; et al. *N*-methylation of a bactericidal compound as a resistance mechanism in *Mycobacterium tuberculosis*. *Proc. Natl. Acad. Sci. USA* **2016**, *113*, E4523–E4530. [CrossRef]
246. Piton, J.; Vocat, A.; Lupien, A.; Foo, C.S.; Riabova, O.; Makarov, V.; Cole, S.T. Structure-Based Drug Design and Characterization of Sulfonyl-Piperazine Benzothiazinone Inhibitors of DprE1 from *Mycobacterium tuberculosis*. *Antimicrob. Agents Chemother.* **2018**, *62*. [CrossRef]
247. Borthwick, J.A.; Alemparte, C.; Wall, I.; Whitehurst, B.C.; Argyrou, A.; Burley, G.; de Dios-Anton, P.; Guijarro, L.; Monteiro, M.C.; Ortega, F.; et al. *Mycobacterium tuberculosis* Decaprenylphosphoryl-beta-d-ribose Oxidase Inhibitors: Expeditious Reconstruction of Suboptimal Hits into a Series with Potent in Vivo Activity. *J. Med. Chem.* **2020**. [CrossRef] [PubMed]
248. Hugonnet, J.E.; Blanchard, J.S. Irreversible inhibition of the *Mycobacterium tuberculosis* beta-lactamase by clavulanate. *Biochemistry* **2007**, *46*, 11998–12004. [CrossRef] [PubMed]
249. Flores, A.R.; Parsons, L.M.; Pavelka, M.S. Genetic analysis of the beta-lactamases of *Mycobacterium tuberculosis* and *Mycobacterium smegmatis* and susceptibility to beta-lactam antibiotics. *Microbiology* **2005**, *151*, 521–532. [CrossRef] [PubMed]
250. Hugonnet, J.E.; Tremblay, L.W.; Boshoff, H.I.; Barry, C.E., 3rd; Blanchard, J.S. Meropenem-clavulanate is effective against extensively drug-resistant *Mycobacterium tuberculosis*. *Science* **2009**, *323*, 1215–1218. [CrossRef]
251. England, K.; Boshoff, H.I.; Arora, K.; Weiner, D.; Dayao, E.; Schimel, D.; Via, L.E.; Barry, C.E., 3rd. Meropenem-clavulanic acid shows activity against *Mycobacterium tuberculosis* in vivo. *Antimicrob. Agents Chemother.* **2012**, *56*, 3384–3387. [CrossRef]
252. Veziris, N.; Truffot, C.; Mainardi, J.L.; Jarlier, V. Activity of carbapenems combined with clavulanate against murine tuberculosis. *Antimicrob. Agents Chemother.* **2011**, *55*, 2597–2600. [CrossRef]
253. Dhar, N.; Dubee, V.; Ballell, L.; Cuinet, G.; Hugonnet, J.E.; Signorino-Gelo, F.; Barros, D.; Arthur, M.; McKinney, J.D. Rapid cytolysis of *Mycobacterium tuberculosis* by faropenem, an orally bioavailable beta-lactam antibiotic. *Antimicrob. Agents Chemother.* **2014**, *59*, 1308–1319. [CrossRef]
254. Rullas, J.; Dhar, N.; McKinney, J.D.; Garcia-Perez, A.; Lelievre, J.; Diacon, A.H.; Hugonnet, J.E.; Arthur, M.; Angulo-Barturen, I.; Barros-Aguirre, D.; et al. Combinations of beta-Lactam Antibiotics Currently in Clinical Trials Are Efficacious in a DHP-I-Deficient Mouse Model of Tuberculosis Infection. *Antimicrob. Agents Chemother.* **2015**, *59*, 4997–4999. [CrossRef]

255. Dubee, V.; Triboulet, S.; Mainardi, J.L.; Etheve-Quelquejeu, M.; Gutmann, L.; Marie, A.; Dubost, L.; Hugonnet, J.E.; Arthur, M. Inactivation of *Mycobacterium tuberculosis* L,D-transpeptidase Ldt_{Mt1} by carbapenems and cephalosporins. *Antimicrob. Agents Chemother.* **2012**, *56*, 4189–4195. [CrossRef]
256. Lavollay, M.; Arthur, M.; Fourgeaud, M.; Dubost, L.; Marie, A.; Veziris, N.; Blanot, D.; Gutmann, L.; Mainardi, J.L. The peptidoglycan of stationary-phase *Mycobacterium tuberculosis* predominantly contains cross-links generated by L,D-transpeptidation. *J. Bacteriol.* **2008**, *190*, 4360–4366. [CrossRef]
257. Tiberi, S.; Payen, M.C.; Sotgiu, G.; D'Ambrosio, L.; Alarcon Guizado, V.; Alffenaar, J.W.; Abdo Arbex, M.; Caminero, J.A.; Centis, R.; De Lorenzo, S.; et al. Effectiveness and safety of meropenem/clavulanate-containing regimens in the treatment of MDR- and XDR-TB. *Eur. Respir. J.* **2016**, *47*, 1235–1243. [CrossRef] [PubMed]
258. Di Modugno, E.; Erbetti, I.; Ferrari, L.; Galassi, G.; Hammond, S.M.; Xerri, L. In vitro activity of the tribactam GV104326 against gram-positive, gram-negative, and anaerobic bacteria. *Antimicrob. Agents Chemother.* **1994**, *38*, 2362–2368. [CrossRef] [PubMed]
259. Barros Aguirre, D.; Bates, R.H.; Gonzalez Del Rio, R.; Mendoza Losana, A.; Ramón García, S. Sanfetrinem or a Salt or Ester Thereof for Use in Treating Mycobacterial Infection. Patent No. WO/2018/206466, 15 November 2018.
260. New TB Drugs. Sanfetrinem. Available online: https://www.newtbdrugs.org/pipeline/compound/sanfetrinem (accessed on 31 January 2020).
261. Campanico, A.; Moreira, R.; Lopes, F. Drug discovery in tuberculosis. New drug targets and antimycobacterial agents. *Eur. J. Med. Chem.* **2018**, *150*, 525–545. [CrossRef] [PubMed]
262. Libardo, M.; Boshoff, H.I.; Barry, C.E., 3rd. The present state of the tuberculosis drug development pipeline. *Curr. Opin. Pharmacol.* **2018**, *42*, 81–94. [CrossRef] [PubMed]
263. Tiberi, S.; Munoz-Torrico, M.; Duarte, R.; Dalcolmo, M.; D'Ambrosio, L.; Migliori, G.B. New drugs and perspectives for new anti-tuberculosis regimens. *Pulmonology* **2018**, *24*, 86–98. [CrossRef]
264. Waksman, S.A. *The Conquest of Tuberculosis*; University of California Press: Berkeley, CA, USA, 1964; p. 211.

5

Structure-Based Drug Design for Tuberculosis: Challenges Still Ahead

Eduardo M. Bruch, Stéphanie Petrella and Marco Bellinzoni *

Unité de Microbiologie Structurale, Institut Pasteur, CNRS, Université de Paris, F-75015 Paris, France; eduardo.bruch@pasteur.fr (E.M.B.); stephanie.petrella@pasteur.fr (S.P.)

* Correspondence: marco.bellinzoni@pasteur.fr

Abstract: Structure-based and computer-aided drug design approaches are commonly considered to have been successful in the fields of cancer and antiviral drug discovery but not as much for antibacterial drug development. The search for novel anti-tuberculosis agents is indeed an emblematic example of this trend. Although huge efforts, by consortiums and groups worldwide, dramatically increased the structural coverage of the *Mycobacterium tuberculosis* proteome, the vast majority of candidate drugs included in clinical trials during the last decade were issued from phenotypic screenings on whole mycobacterial cells. We developed here three selected case studies, i.e., the serine/threonine (Ser/Thr) kinases—protein kinase (Pkn) B and PknG, considered as very promising targets for a long time, and the DNA gyrase of *M. tuberculosis*, a well-known, pharmacologically validated target. We illustrated some of the challenges that rational, target-based drug discovery programs in tuberculosis (TB) still have to face, and, finally, discussed the perspectives opened by the recent, methodological developments in structural biology and integrative techniques.

Keywords: tuberculosis; structure-based drug design; target-based drug design; PknB; PknG; DNA gyrase; antibiotic

---

1. Introduction

Although the drug discovery process has historically relied on high-throughput screening (HTS) to identify hits to be developed into drug candidates, either on a given target (in most cases, an essential enzyme) or through whole-cell screenings, it still remains an experimentally laborious, expensive, and time-consuming process. Unlike traditional drug discovery, however, drug design is not necessarily based on the screening of large libraries, which is intrinsically a trial and error process, but builds on the available knowledge for a given biological target. A particular, well-known case of drug design is called structure-based drug design (SBDD), which uses the three-dimensional structural knowledge of the target to find or optimize molecules that can bind to the target with high affinity and selectivity. The potential of using structural information for discovering candidate drugs was apparent from the early days of structural biology [1], but it took several years to achieve the first successful examples, i.e., human immunodeficiency virus (HIV) protease inhibitors [2] and carbonic anhydrase inhibitors for the treatment of glaucoma [3].

A three-dimensional model of the target is, therefore, a prerequisite for SBDD. The structure can be obtained experimentally in different ways, in most cases by X-ray crystallography, although nuclear magnetic resonance (NMR) and, more recently, cryo-electron microscopy (cryo-EM) have also attracted attention [4], especially following the spectacular increase in the resolution capabilities of single-particle cryo-EM, which is commonly referred to as the resolution revolution [5,6]. For targets whose experimental structure is elusive, in silico structure prediction is also routinely performed and can be achieved, whenever suitable models are available, through homology modeling from a closely related homologous protein [7].

The identification of potential drug binding sites can be obvious when ligand-bound target structures are available. However, the capability to detect binding sites for substrates or modulators becomes highly relevant not only for targets for which no ligand-bound three-dimensional structure is available, but also to detect allosteric sites or protein–protein interaction surfaces that might be specifically targeted [8], and for these, dedicated libraries are now available [9]. Considering that binding site identification is not always straightforward, tools have been developed to infer "druggable" pockets from the identification of concave regions—that could accommodate drug-size molecules—by screening for appropriate binding properties, such as volume, hydrophobicity, hydrogen bonding, energy potential, solvent accessibility, and desolvation energy [10].

The search for potential ligands on a given target can then follow two different approaches, commonly referred to as ligand-based drug design (LBDD) or target-based drug design (TBDD). LBDD does not require, a priori, direct structural knowledge of the target, but relies on the identification of hits, usually congeneric compounds, with an established biological effect; hit-to-lead optimization can then proceed through the definition of appropriate chemical descriptors of the series, quantitative structure-activity relationship analysis (QSAR), and pharmacophore modeling [11], all followed by experimental validation. QSAR-based virtual screening approaches, alone or in combination with HTS screenings, can also be used to enlarge the panel of bioactive compounds against the target or pathway of interest, increasing the overall hit rate [12]. TBDD, in contrast, uses the physical-chemical constrains from the target three-dimensional structure, and possibly a well-defined binding pocket, to perform virtual screening of libraries, either of natural or synthetic compounds, usually applying appropriate filters like compliance to Lipinski's rules or QSAR models, or to design molecules de novo in a step-wise manner. A particular case of de novo molecule design is fragment-based drug design (FBDD), in which low-affinity target binding molecules are identified from appropriate libraries, using a variety of biophysical approaches, and then merged or linked together using the available three-dimensional information to achieve larger binders with improved properties [13,14].

It is common knowledge in the field that although SBDD approaches have proven to be successful for non-transmissible diseases and viral diseases, they have proven to be much less effective in the antibiotic discovery field [15,16]. Unfortunately, tuberculosis represents no exception to this trend [17], despite the considerable progress achieved during the last twenty years in the understanding of the pathogen molecular physiology, starting from the seminal publication of the *M. tuberculosis* genome sequence in 1998 [18], the extensive structural genomics campaigns during the following years [19–21], the advances in understanding host-pathogen interactions and the development of the disease [22,23], and notwithstanding the development of genetic and biochemical tools to allow the in vivo and in vitro validation of targets [24,25].

The purpose of this review was not to provide an exhaustive overview of the capabilities now offered by in silico approaches for antibiotic development against *M. tuberculosis*, already reviewed elsewhere [26,27], nor to make a survey of the current state of structural knowledge of the pathogen proteome and the experimental structures relevant for drug discovery, for which we point the reader to very recent, extensive work [28]. Rather, we focused here on three emblematic case studies of *M. tuberculosis* targets that attracted most efforts for anti-tuberculosis compound development by HTS campaigns, computer-aided, and structure-driven compound identification: the serine/threonine (Ser/Thr) kinases—protein kinase (Pkn)B and PknG—two amongst the most known, supposedly promising new targets offered by the post-genomic era, and the DNA gyrase, the 'old' but the well-proven target of fluoroquinolones.

2. Protein Ser/Thr Kinases as Drug Targets

Protein phosphorylation is a well-known, widespread mechanism for signal transduction and regulation of several biological functions. Protein kinases have long been known as major drug targets [29], especially for the treatment of cancer, where the deregulation of signaling mechanisms is a hallmark of the disease [30]. Protein kinases are not only pharmaceutical targets in cancer chemotherapy but also for the treatment of parasitic infections, ranging from the ones caused by Trypanosomatids or *Leishmania* [31] to malaria [32]. Since the sequence of *M. tuberculosis* H37Rv genome was first reported in 1998 [18], the pathogen has been known to possess eleven genes coding for Hanks-type Ser/Thr kinases [33], named from *pknA* to *pknL* (but no *pknC*), providing one of the first challenges to the paradigm of prokaryotic cell signaling as being entirely driven by two-component systems. One gene coding for a transmembrane Ser/Thr phosphatase, *pstP*, was also identified as lying on the same cluster as *pknA* and *pknB*, forming a putative operon [34], in addition to two genes (*ptpA* and *ptpB*) coding for Tyr phosphatases [35]. Nine out of eleven Ser/Thr kinases (all but PknG and PknK) were predicted to be integral membrane proteins, all sharing the same topology with an N-terminal catalytic domain in which the archetypal Hanks motifs could be identified [33], a single transmembrane segment and a very variable extracellular, C-terminal domain, hypothesized to be acting as a signal sensing domain. The role of such C-terminal domains is, in most cases, still puzzling, although, in some kinases like PknB, it has been suggested to be involved in the kinase activation process, possibly by controlling the kinase oligomerization state as a function of the external signal [36]. Work from Tom Alber's group in Berkeley indeed demonstrated the role of the 'back-to-back' dimerization to promote an active kinase conformation, not only for PknB [37,38] but also for PknD [39], notwithstanding the observation that mutations in the dimerization interface do not abolish kinase activity, as reported by separate groups [37,40]. PknB was also the first *M. tuberculosis* kinase for which the crystal structure of the catalytic domain was described in 2003 [41,42]. Indeed, this first crystal structure confirmed the overall conservation of the bi-lobed protein kinase fold and the initial assumptions about the presence of the known structural features of eukaryotic protein kinases, as predicted by the detection of the Hanks motifs [42], thus underlining the common origin of eukaryotic and prokaryotic kinases. Following these first milestones and the genetic proof of the in vitro essentiality of *pknB* coming both from transposon mutagenesis [43] and targeted studies [44,45], PknB then attracted the attention of tuberculosis (TB) research community as an ideal target for structure-based drug design. The community's interest rise when considering the increasing evidence, over the years, of its role in the control of peptidoglycan synthesis and cell division (recently reviewed in [46]). The first description of the potential use of PknB inhibitors as anti-mycobacterial agents reported the compound H-7 (1-(5-isoquinolinesulfonyl)-2-methylpiperazine; Table 1), well before any bacterial protein kinase structure was available [47]. Once the PknB catalytic domain structure was solved, virtual screening carried out on a library of about 40,000 compounds for hits into the PknB adenosine triphosphate-binding (ATP-binding) pocket was performed. The screening led to identifying mitoxantrone, a chemotherapeutic agent known for its DNA intercalating properties, as a sub-micromolar PknB inhibitor [48], similar to staurosporine, K-252-a, and K-252-b (Table 1), who were identified as hits after testing a few commercially available eukaryotic kinase inhibitors [44]. The crystal structure of the PknB-mitoxantrone complex was the first showing the kinase catalytic domain in complex with a non-ATP analog, kinase inhibitor. Two crucial, hydrogen bonding interactions were evidenced between the mitoxantrone hydroxyl groups and main chain atoms from the PknB hinge region that connects the two kinase lobes, i.e., the carbonyl oxygen of Glu93 and the amino group of Val95 [48], opening the way to compound optimization (Figure 1A,B). Several other PknB inhibitors were proposed in the course of the following years, starting from hits developed either from known kinase inhibitors like staurosporine analogs [37], 2-aminopurine and its derivatives, including organometallic compounds [49]), or from hits obtained from HTS on public or proprietary libraries using GarA as the substrate [50–53], or phytocompounds [54] (Table 1). Most of the published work deals with compounds inhibiting the kinase in the micro and sub-micromolar range but with limited activity on mycobacteria. The exception to this trend is IMB-YH-8 (Table 1), a compound that, despite showing an IC_{50} (half maximal inhibitory concentration) on PknB in the 20 μM range, shows good selectivity for mycobacterial PknB and PknA and a MIC (minimal inhibitory concentration) in the sub-micromolar range [53]. Compounds highly active on both PknB and PknA have also been reported recently by others in the form of substituted quinazolines, and, for a compound derived from this series (a pyrimidine analog), the crystal structures of the respective complexes with both kinases have been described [55] (Figure 1, Table 1). Both structures underline the common binding mode in the ATP pocket and the crucial interaction with the hinge region (Figure 1B). Despite the inhibition constant for both kinases falls in the nanomolar range, these dual-targeting inhibitors display promising but yet limited antibacterial effect with MIC on *M. tuberculosis* in the lower micromolar range [55]. A different PknB inhibitor for which a crystal structure in complex with the target is available is GSK690693 (Figure 1C, Table 1), also identified through a virtual screening approach on known kinase inhibitors [56]. This compound, member of the imidazopyridine aminofurazans class, also displays conserved features in its binding mode to the PknB hinge region (Figure 1B), and sub-micromolar affinity to the kinase, but no significant antimycobacterial activity on *Mycobacterium smegmatis* or *Mycobacterium bovis* BCG (bacillus Calmette-Guerin). However, the MIC is significantly lowered if the compound is associated with a sub-MIC50 concentration of meropenem, suggesting a synergistic action between PknB inhibitors and β-lactams [56].

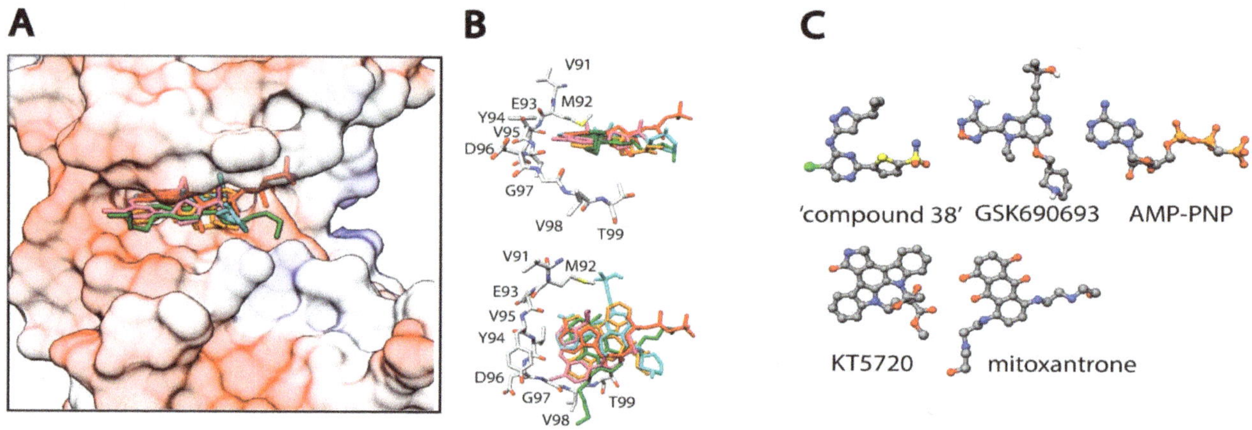

Figure 1. Experimental structures of protein kinase B (PknB)-inhibitor complexes. (**A**) Electrostatic surface from the X-ray structure of PknB in complex with AMP-PCP (β,γ-methyleneadenosine 5′-triphosphate) in red (pdb: 1O6Y), superimposed with the coordinates of four other PknB complexes with, respectively, mitoxantrone in green (pdb: 2FUM), KT5720 in orange (pdb: 3F69), GSK690693 in cyan (pdb: 5U94), and 'compound 38' in pink (pdb: 6B2P). This compound has been reported as active on both PknA and PknB [55]. (**B**) Side and top view of the superimposed ligands with the hinge region from the pdb entry 6B2P. Kinase residues are indicated. (**C**) Ball-and-stick representation of the ligands kept in the same relative binding orientation as in (**B**) and colored by element.

Table 1. *M. tuberculosis* PknB inhibitors.

Family	Name	Structure	IC_{50} (μM)	Reference
Isoquinolines	H-7	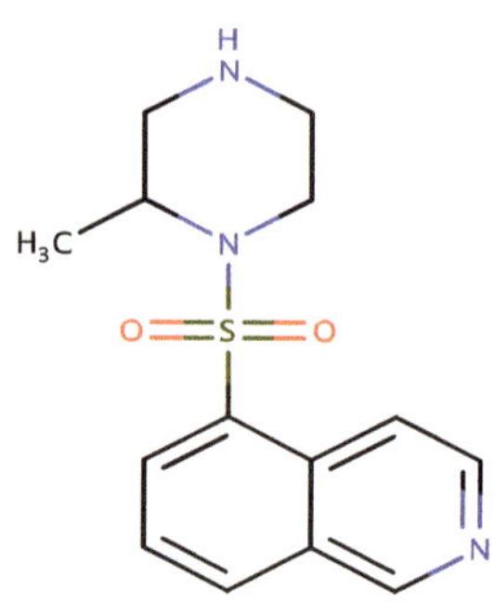	ND	[47]

Table 1. *Cont.*

Family	Name	Structure	IC_{50} (μM)	Reference
Staurosporine analogues	Staurosporine	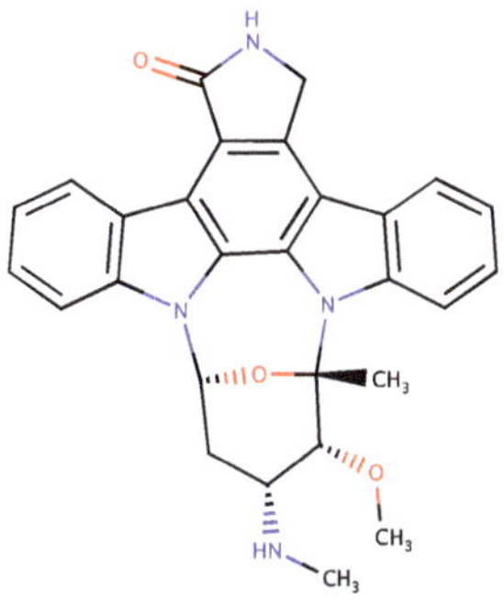	0.6	[44]
	K-252-a	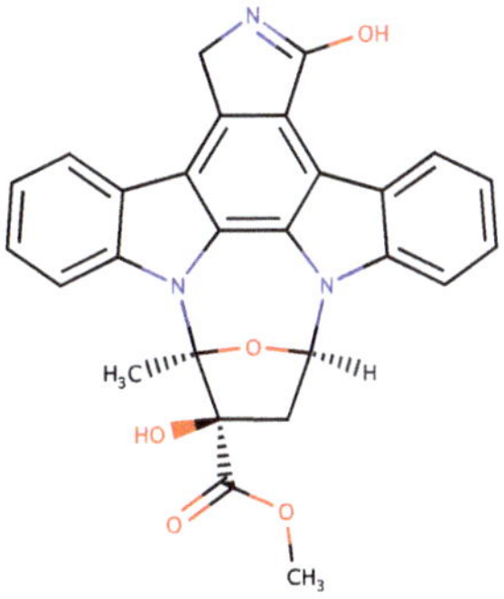	0.096	
	K-252-b	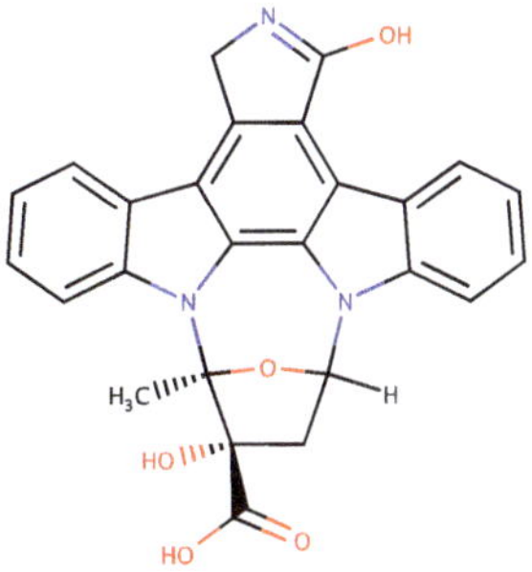	0.106	
	KT5720	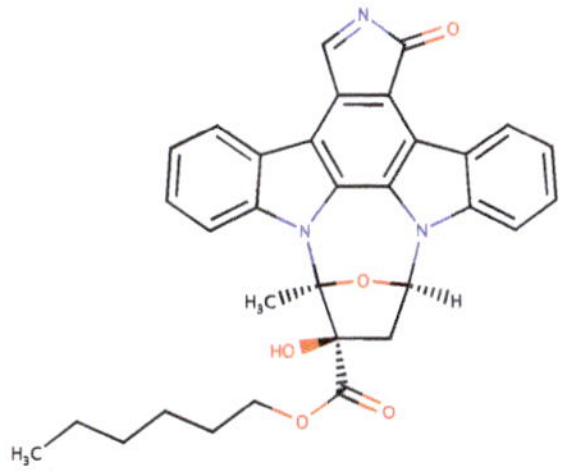	~1 [a]	[37]
Anthracenediones	Mitoxantrone	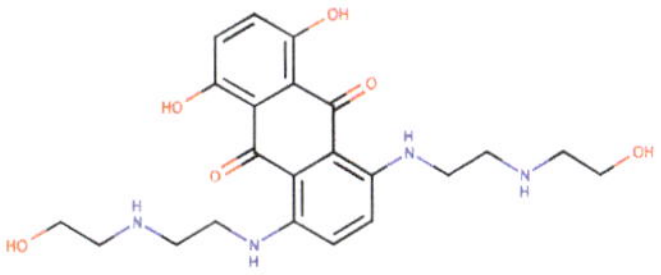	0.8	[48]
Aminopurines	2-A9P	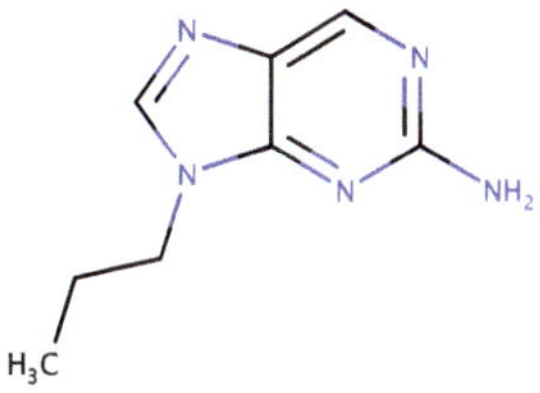	1300	[49]

Table 1. *Cont.*

Family	Name	Structure	IC_{50} (μM)	Reference
Quinazolines	Disubstituted series	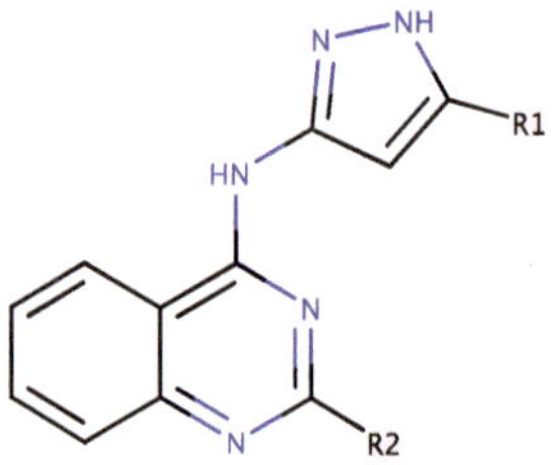	≤ 1.1	[51]
Pyrimidines	Disubstituted (-R1 also as -NHR1)	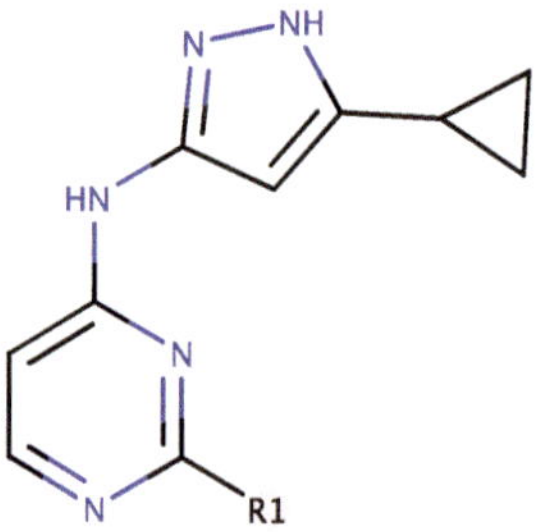	≤ 0.4	[51]
	'Compound 38'	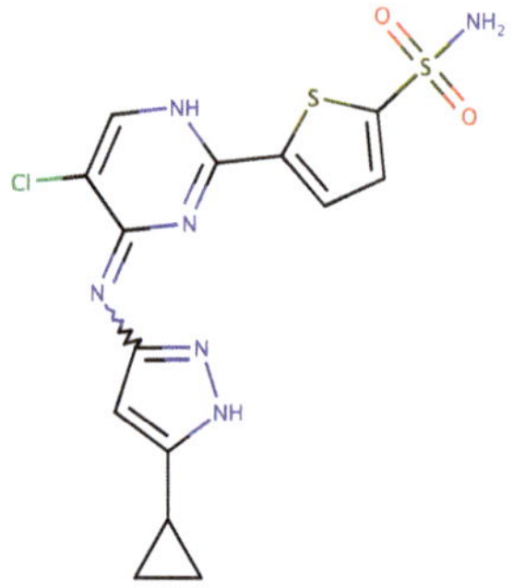	Ki ~ 1 nM	[55]
Phytocompounds	Demethylcalabaxanthone	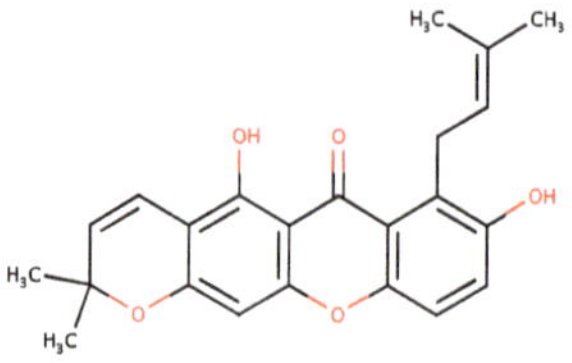	ND	[54]
4-oxo-crotonic acid derivatives	IMB-YH-8	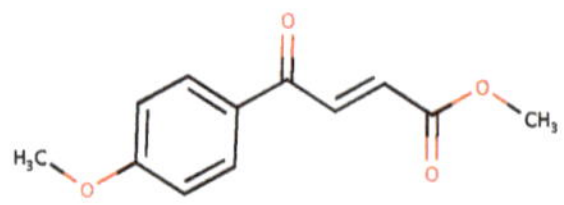	20.2	[53]
Imidazopyridine aminofurazans	GSK690693	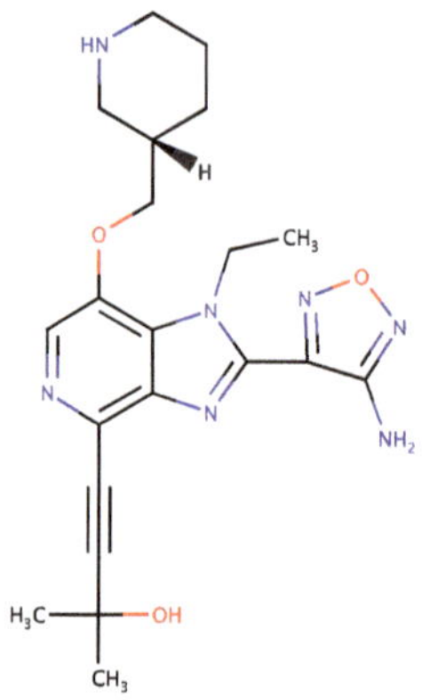	0.34	[56]

ND: not determined. [a] measured on a PknB mutant (M145L, M155V) [37].

On the other hand, another *M. tuberculosis* kinase that attracted as much attention for its potential druggability is PknG, a soluble Ser/Thr kinase that was described, by Jean Pieters and coworkers, as a virulence factor secreted into the human macrophage, where it would inhibit the phagosome-lysosome fusion [57]. Most notably, in the same work, the authors showed that chemical inhibition of PknG by the compound AX20017 (a tetrahydrobenzothiophene identified by HTS and found to inhibit PknG with IC_{50} in the sub-micromolar range; Table 2) led to the accumulation of *M. tuberculosis* inside lysosomes [57]. Noteworthy, the 2.4 Å resolution crystal structure of an N-terminal truncated form of PknG in complex with AX20017, published later [58], shows a great similarity between the AX20017 binding to PknG and the binding of ATP and mitoxantrone to PknB. Not only the compound occupies the adenine binding pocket but also makes similar interactions with the main chain atoms of residues Glu233 and Val235 (Figure 1). It was only a few years later that further structural work allowed to elucidate the binding mode of ATP to PknG and suggested a regulatory role of the rubredoxin-like domain by a reversible occlusion of the active site entrance [59]. These initial findings paved the way to further structure-based lead optimization and undoubtedly generated excitement for the potential chemical targeting of this kinase, which would allow preventing the arrest of phagosome maturation, directing *M. tuberculosis* to lysosomes.

Attempts to develop more potent compounds starting from AX20017 yielded sub-micromolar inhibitors, some of which had no activity in macrophage assays [50], and no other structure of a PknG-inhibitor complex has so far been reported. It is, however, worth noting that, more than ten years later, the role of PknG in arresting the phagosome maturation is still elusive. Although progress has been made in identifying the SecA2 system as responsible for the export of PknG outside *M. tuberculosis* [60,61], and interference by PknG on the host Rab7l1 signaling pathway has been reported [62], it is largely accepted that several mechanisms, and not a single virulence factor, contribute to the *M. tuberculosis* capability to escape the phagocytic route and survive into macrophages [22,63]. Moreover, an increasing amount of evidence has since validated PknG as a key signaling element in the control of central metabolism, as first shown in *Corynebacterium glutamicum* [64,65], then in mycobacteria [66,67], where genetic and metabolomic evidence point to a role of PknG in regulating the 2-oxoglutarate node according to nutrient availability [68]. Alternative roles of PknG in biofilm formation, adaptation to oxidative stress [69], and hypoxia [70] have also been proposed. Therefore, the observed effects of the lack of PknG on the phagosome-lysosome fusion, and the decreased viability of a *pknG*-deprived *M. tuberculosis* mutant, both in vitro and in the mouse model [71], may not necessarily indicate a direct interference of the kinase on the host signaling pathways but could be ascribed to metabolic alterations caused by the depletion of PknG [68,72].

During the last years, further search for PknG inhibitors has allowed identifying sclerotiorin, an azaphilone derivative isolated from *Penicillium* sp. ZJ27 (Table 2), a known inhibitor of other unrelated enzymes like lipoxygenase, that, despite showing an IC_{50} on PknG around 76 μM and no inhibition on *M. tuberculosis* growth in vitro, displays capability to partially reduce the growth of *Mycobacterium bovis* BCG inside macrophages, and to enhance the effect of rifampicin [73]. On the other hand, the recently described PknG inhibitor NU-6027 (2,6-diamino-4-cyclohexylmethoxy-5-nitrosopyrimidine; Table 2) was identified from phenotypic screening as having an MIC99 value of 1.56 μMon*M. bovis* BCG and shown to partially inhibit PknG and PknD autophosphorylation in vitro [74]. Another series of four compounds, all inhibiting PknG in the micromolar range, was also recently reported after the screening of an 80-compound, commercially available kinase inhibitor library (Table 2); three of them were found to promote the transfer of mycobacteria to lysosomes, and two to inhibit *M. bovis* BCG growth in macrophages [75]. None of the reported compounds, however, issued from a structure-based screening approach.

Table 2. *M. tuberculosis* PknG inhibitors.

Family	Name	Structure	IC_{50} (μM)	Reference
Tetrahydrobenzothiophenes	AX20017	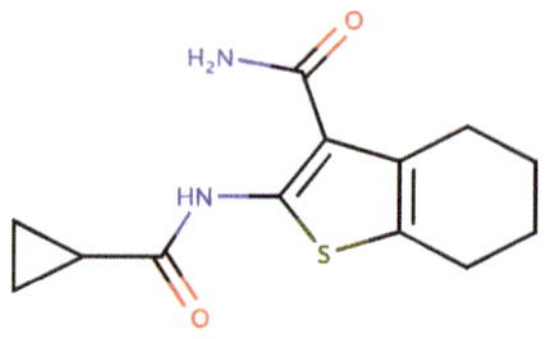	0.39 5.5	[57] [75]
Azaphilones	Sclerotiorin	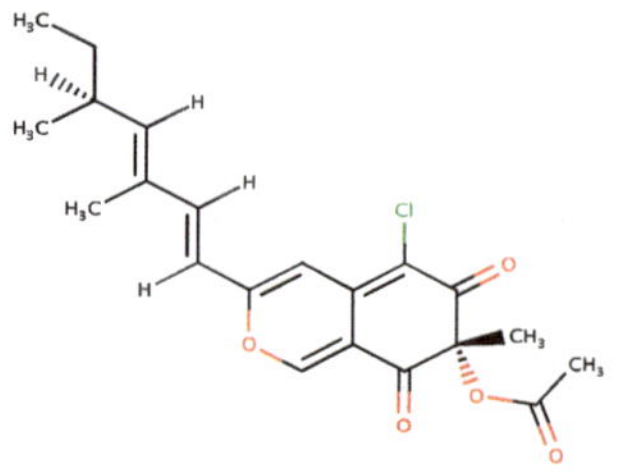	76	[73]
Pyrimidines	NU-6027	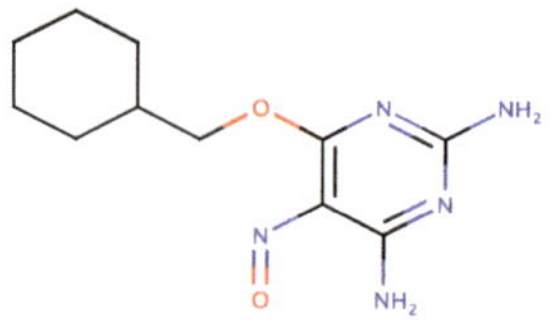	ND	[74]
	CYC116	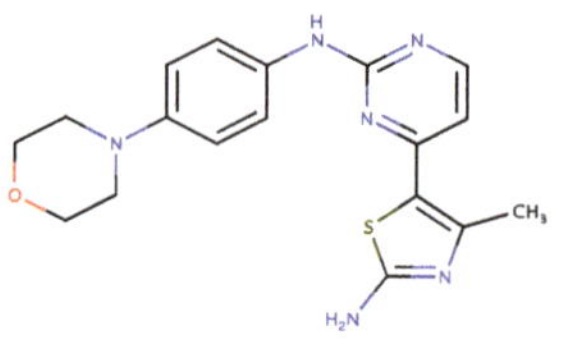	35.1	[75]
Thiophenes	AZD7762	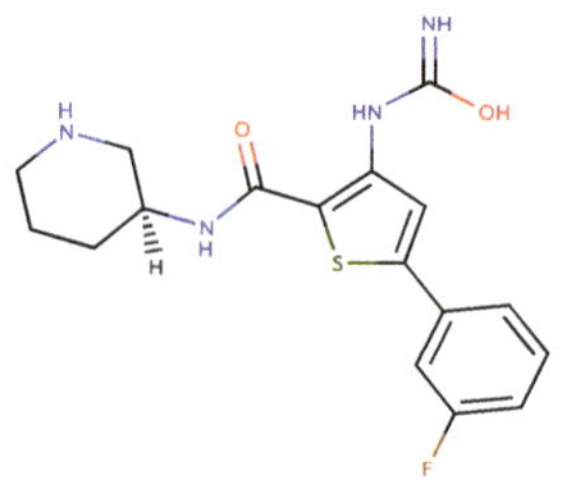	30.3	[75]
Methoxybenzenes	R406 (benzenesulfonate) and its free base R406f (also known as Tamatinib)	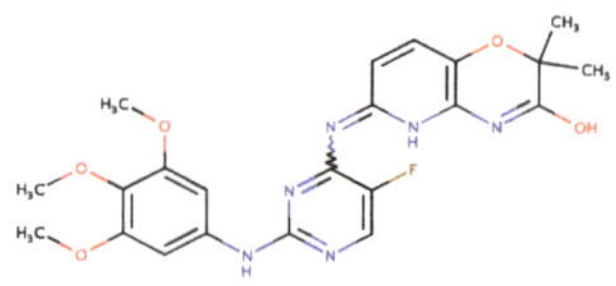	8.0 (R406) 16.1 (R406f)	[75]

ND: not determined.

3. DNA Gyrase: A Validated Drug Target

Topoisomerases are enzymes that participate in the overwinding or underwinding of DNA. They are commonly split into two classes, depending on the number of DNA strands cut during a single catalysis cycle: class I topoisomerases, which include eukaryotic topoisomerase I, prokaryotic topoisomerase IIIa, or reverse gyrase among others, and class II topoisomerases, whose members include (but are not restricted to) topoisomerase IV and DNA gyrase [76]. In *M. tuberculosis*, DNA gyrase is a heterotetrameric nanomachine, consisting of two GyrB and two GyrA subunits, and is essential for DNA replication, transcription, and repair in living cells [77].

M. tuberculosis is an exception in the prokaryotic world because of the presence of only one type I and one type II topoisomerase, whereas most other eubacteria have two enzymes of each type. In the canonical situation, DNA gyrase and topoisomerase IV, both type IIA topoisomerases, have distinct specific activities: DNA gyrase removes positive supercoils that accumulate ahead of replication forks [78], whereas topoisomerase IV decatenates replication intermediates [79]. Thus, in *M. tuberculosis*, DNA gyrase being the unique topoisomerase IIA, it must be able to carry out both activities in vivo [80]. Furthermore, with no other topoisomerase IIA in *M. tuberculosis*, the DNA gyrase is the unique target of antibiotics from the fluoroquinolones (FQ) family (quinolones with higher cellular penetration efficiency), which bind and stabilize the DNA–DNA gyrase complex. Stabilization of this ternary complex leads to the cytotoxic accumulation of double-strand cleaved DNA fragments within the cell, inducing bacterial death [81]. Crystallographic structures of the isolated domain and the cleavage core, either in its *apo* form or co-crystallized with several FQ, brought crucial information to elucidate the mode of binding of these drugs [82–87]. The ratio FQ/DNA–DNA gyrase in the ternary complex is two FQ molecules per complex, with one molecule binding in each cleavage site, wedging between the two ends of the cleaved DNA strands on both halves of the complex, in a drug-binding pocket whose walls are formed by DNA base stacking (Figure 2A) [82]. The emergence of strains with multidrug resistance (MDR) phenotype, or extensively-drug resistance (XDR) phenotype in which drug resistance includes this family of antibiotics, has made improving the activity of this family of drugs by using structural data to be of utmost importance. The main goals of these studies are to increase specific drug/enzyme interactions, but also to find new molecules that inhibit this validated target without cross-resistance with FQ [88].

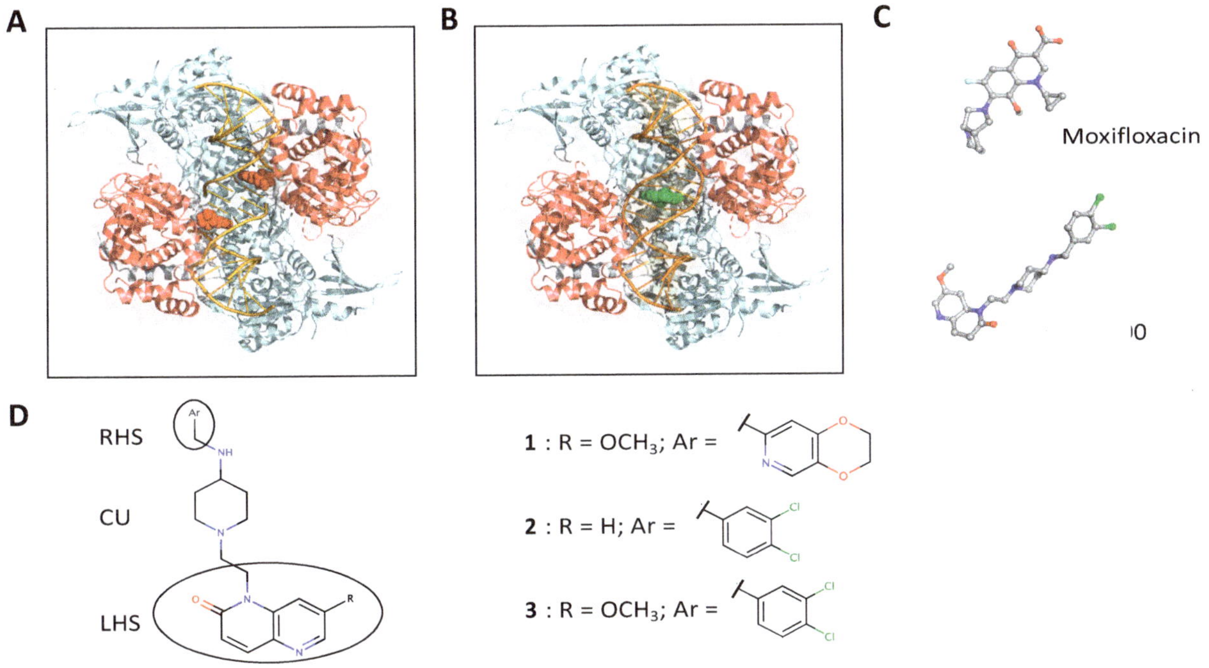

Figure 2. Inhibitors of DNA gyrase. (**A**) Top view of the X-ray structure of *M. tuberculosis* gyrase cleavage core in complex with DNA and moxifloxacin. Protein is shown in cartoon representation with transparent surfaces, with GyrB in blue and GyrA in pink. DNA is shown in orange, with moxifloxacin as red spheres (pdb: 5BS8). (**B**) Top view of the model of a complex of GSK000 (green spheres) with *M. tuberculosis* gyrase cleavage core and uncleaved DNA (in orange), based on the crystal structure of GSK299423 with *Staphylococcus aureus* gyrase (pdb: 2XCR). The same representation, as in panel A, was used for the protein. (**C**) Ball-and-stick representation of the ligands colored by element. (**D**) Generic chemical structure of the novel bacterial topoisomerase inhibitor (NBTI) series of compounds. Analog 1 is a classical NBTI, whereas analogs 2 and 3 combine the three favorable features for *M. tuberculosis* DNA gyrase inhibitor (MGI).

A significant amount of effort has thus been invested in discovering new *M. tuberculosis* gyrase inhibitors, mostly centered on the ATP- and DNA-binding sites, and particularly using in silico methods based on the emerging gyrase structural information, as extensively reviewed by Nagaraja and coworkers [89]. Although the ATP binding sites have been less successfully exploited as antibacterial targets, with the exception of the natural products, such as coumarins [90,91], it is worth noting that a candidate drug emerged from these studies. SPR720 (Table 3) is an orally bioavailable prodrug of SPR719, an aminobenzimidazole inhibitor of both gyrase and topoisomerase IV. Indeed, this novel class of antimicrobials targets the ATPase subunits of gyrase and topoisomerase IV, and it was optimized using SSBD and structure-activity relationship (SAR) studies of potency against both Gram-positive and some Gram-negative bacterial species [92,93]. Crystal structures of novobiocin (Table 3) bound to *Escherichia coli* GyrB subunit served as a starting point for ligand optimization [94], while further optimization of the metabolic profile led to the identification of SPR720 (formerly VXc-486) [95], whose suitability to be a drug candidate for the treatment of tuberculosis and non-tuberculosis mycobacterial infections was thoroughly evaluated [96,97]. The compound completed Phase I clinical trials in 2019 (study ID NCT03796910, sponsored by Spero Therapeutics, LLC), aimed at evaluating the safety, tolerability, and pharmacokinetics (PK) profile in healthy volunteers. Moreover, an in vivo combination of SPR720 with rifampicin and pyrazinamide (two first-line drugs used in TB treatment) showed comparable efficacy to the combination of three drugs, including moxifloxacin, rifampicin, and pyrazinamide [98].

Work on the DNA-binding site has also been productive, as GlaxoSmithKline (GSK) created a new class of type IIA topoisomerase inhibitors, called novel bacterial topoisomerase inhibitors (NBTIs) (Table 3) [99]. The crystallographic structures of the DNA-bound *Staphylococcus aureus* DNA gyrase with either NBTI or FQ, all obtained at high resolution, revealed that the binding sites for each drug are different [100]. Indeed, the NBTI 'bridges' the DNA and a transient non-catalytic pocket on the two-fold axis at the GyrA dimer interface, remaining close to the active sites and FQs binding sites (Figure 2B). As NBTIs display relatively poor activity against the *M. tuberculosis* DNA gyrase, the antitubercular profiles of 3000 compounds, representative of the chemical diversity of this family, were evaluated by high-throughput phenotypic screenings in vitro and in vivo [101]. MIC determination on *M. tuberculosis* H37Rv showed a high hit rate (68% of compounds with MIC values lower than 10 μM), with the most potent derivatives matching or even improving the MIC values for currently used TB drugs, including last-generation FQs. Overall, 29% of the compounds had MICs of < 1 μM, and 18% had MICs of < 0.1 μM. By using structural data provided by the work of Bax et al., the general structures of these TB-active compounds were divided into three different regions, each of them interacting with one of the three topologically important target-gyrase interacting regions [100]. While a left-hand side (LHS) is responsible for key contacts with the gyrase DNA substrate, a right-hand side (RHS) is embedded into the enzyme, potentially contributing to the protein target selectivity (Figure 2D). Last, a central linker unit (CU) establishes key interactions with the gyrase and offers the opportunity to modulate key physicochemical properties (Figure 2D). These SAR observations helped to schematize synthesis and to rationalize how to balance antimycobacterial potency with oral exposure, safety, and synthetic complexity, leading to the identification of the 7-substituted-1,5-naphthyridin-2-one core as a privileged LHS binder, the N-ethyl-4-aminopiperidines as a linker, and monocyclic aromatic rings with different substitution patterns as the best RHS binding option, in contrast to NBTIs bearing bicyclic rings as the RHS (Figure 2D, analogs 2 and 3) [101]. This work led to the identification of a subclass of naphthytidone/aminopiperidine-containing compounds that displayed activity against *M. tuberculosis*, both in vitro and in the mouse model, known as '*M. tuberculosis* DNA gyrase inhibitors' (MGIs) due to structural and activity differences with respect to NBTIs [101]. More recently, the mechanism of action of two such compounds, i.e., GSK000 and GSK325 (Figure 2C; Table 3), was assessed on the *M. tuberculosis* gyrase, showing that MGIs greatly enhanced DNA cleavage mediated by the bacterial enzyme, but they induced only single-stranded DNA breaks [102]. Their mechanism of action involves stabilizing covalent gyrase-cleaved DNA complexes and appears to suppress the ability of the enzyme to induce double-stranded breaks. Furthermore, these compounds maintained activity against mutant versions of DNA gyrase, bearing the three most commonly observed FQs resistance mutations, but displayed no activity against human topoisomerase IIα [102], suggesting good potential as candidate drugs, especially in the presence of FQ resistance. Modeling studies were carried out by the authors using the crystal structure of the *M. tuberculosis* gyrase cleavage core and the NBTI crystal structure complex of *S. aureus* gyrase [100] (Figure 2B). Most importantly, these studies allowed to confirm that FQs and MGIs do not share the same binding site and bind in a mutually exclusive manner (Figure 2), considerably reducing the risk of developing cross-resistance phenotypes.

Table 3. *M. tuberculosis* DNA gyrase inhibitors.

Family	Name	Structure	IC_{50} (μM)	Reference
Fluoroquinolones	Moxifloxacin	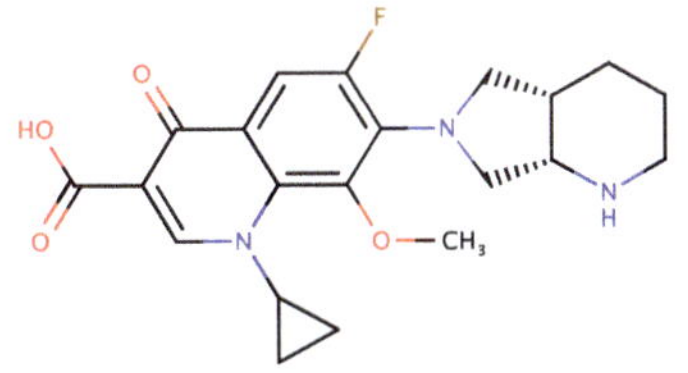	1 2.5	[102] [101]
SPR	SPR720 (VXc-100, VXc-486)	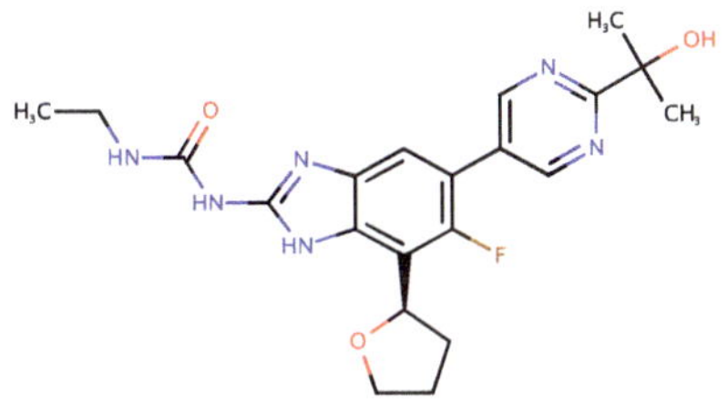	ND	[92,93]
Coumarins	Novobiocin	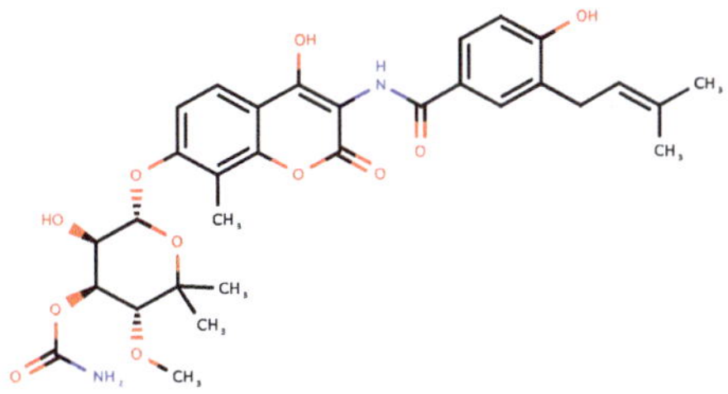	0.5	[80]
NBTI	GSK000	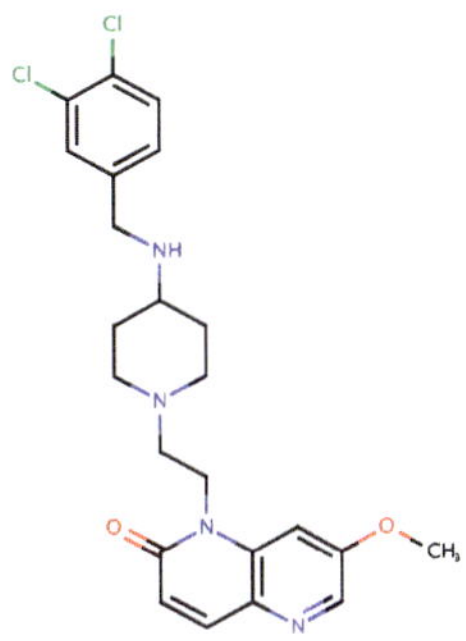	0.5 5.4	[102] [101]
	GSK325	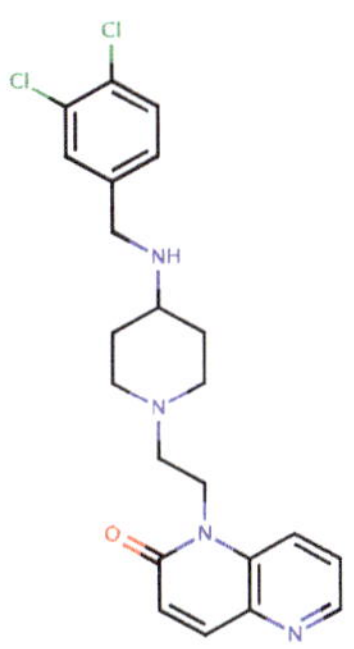	10.98	[101]

ND: not determined.

4. General Remarks

Several challenges need to be overcome for therapeutic molecules to be active against *M. tuberculosis*. Due to its metabolic adaptability and its known capabilities to occupy different niches inside the human host, from free aerobic bacteria to granulomas, an ideal molecule should be able to act against bacteria in very different, environmentally adapted states. The unique structure and composition of the *M. tuberculosis* cell wall are also well known to act as a barrier for potentially active compounds. To be active against latent and active infections, an ideal drug candidate should thus be able to reach bacteria in all the tubercular lesions and niches inside the human host [103], permeate the mycobacterial cell wall or be actively internalized, and deliver the desired bioactivity in bacteria under different metabolic states. To overcome these limitations and reduce the risk of further resistance development, TB drugs are delivered in combinations, starting from the standard DOTS (directly observed therapy short-course). Drug combinations, however, have to take in due account the bioavailability and pharmacokinetic properties of the single components and their associations, as extensively treated in this same journal issue [104].

In the course of the last ten years, it has become increasingly clear that some of the criteria commonly used to classify a given *M. tuberculosis* biological process, in many cases, an enzymatic step in a pathway, as a 'good' target for drug development, needed to be revised. This is particularly true for in vitro genetic essentiality. Even targets confirmed to be essential by the construction of specific conditional mutants do not necessarily show a good 'druggability', even when highly potent hits become available. The case of PknB is an emblematic example: despite the gene was early shown to be essential for *M. tuberculosis* growth, first by transposon mutagenesis [43], then through attempts to generate a knock-out mutant [44], yet several research groups, including ours, had to face the problem of the lack of correlation between hit potency in vitro and efficacy in vivo [50–52]. Similar issues were also reported for other *M. tuberculosis* kinase inhibitors, in addition to the cross-reactivity sometimes reported towards eukaryotic kinases, and the cytotoxicity shown by some compounds on human cell lines [105]. In addition, although the availability of crystal structures of both PknB and PknG in complex with hits issued from medium-throughput screens (mitoxantrone and AX20017, respectively) has looked as a promising 'proof-of-concept' [48,58], further structure-based work on these kinases has, so far, failed to produce suitable drug candidates. Many reasons might be evoked to explain the lack of *M. tuberculosis* kinase inhibitors that display significant antibacterial activity, ranging from the poor capacity to penetrate the mycobacterial cell and reach their target to the kinase redundancy in *M. tuberculosis* and their, relatively poor, substrate specificity [46], which prompted groups to seek for multiple kinase inhibition [105]. Yet, the main causes should perhaps be looked for in our, still limited, knowledge of mycobacterial molecular physiology and the regulatory networks in *M. tuberculosis*, in which Ser/Thr kinases are actors of a complex interplay [46,106]. Indeed, the activation mechanisms of both PknB and PknG are still a matter of speculation, and changes to *pknB* expression, either as depletion or overexpression, have been reported to alter the bacterial growth significantly [34]. Given the known *M. tuberculosis* metabolic plasticity, whose complexity has only recently started to be elucidated, thanks to the development of genetic and 'omics' tools [107], and the adaptability of the pathogen in the course of infection, it is now largely accepted that genetic essentiality of a putative target in laboratory conditions is not necessarily an indication of chemical vulnerability [15], and even more in clinical conditions. For these reasons, phenotypic screens have increasingly been employed in TB drug development to the detriment of target and structure-based methods, including for lead optimization [15], and the vast majority of candidate TB drugs that have been able to enter clinical trials in the last years were issued from this kind of screens [17,108].

Nevertheless, structure-based and computer-aided drug design maintain a clear potential for the future development of new anti-tubercular drug candidates. For instance, a recent, very promising success of structure-based and fragment-based approaches in TB drug discovery is the development of the so-called ethionamide boosters directed against the EthR repressor, one of which has been shown to be active both in vitro and in vivo [109]. In addition, the recent developments in X-ray crystallography [110], cryo-EM [4], and integrative structural biology methods [111] will all contribute to increasing the number of tools available to tackle the challenges that lay ahead. These opportunities are well exemplified by the case of mycobacterial DNA gyrase that, considering our capacity to obtain high-resolution structures of an almost full-length form of the *M. tuberculosis* enzyme [112], and the recent, high-resolution cryo-EM structure of *E. coli* gyrase in complex with NBTI [113], let us believe that SBDD will deliver a key contribution to developing new compounds against this 'old' but validated target. High-resolution snapshots of the complete mycobacterial gyrase machinery, especially if in complex with representative members of each known family of inhibitors, might revolutionize our knowledge of this key target and substantially increase chances of improving our therapeutic bullets. For instance, combining crystallographic and cryo-EM data could allow to perform structure-guided drug design to target these flexible complexes and identify new conformations of mycobacterial gyrase that could not, otherwise, be obtained by conventional structural methods. More generally, the integration of biophysical and structural biology data, with the notable contribution of high-resolution EM, will allow the drug discovery pipelines to work on a higher complexity level that was previously not achievable, now looking at targets in their larger biological context (e.g., complexes or cellular compartments). It is, therefore, foreseeable that, despite the technical challenges, target-based and structure-based approaches will have increasing relevance in future drug discovery and will give significant contributions in the search for new tuberculosis drugs.

Author Contributions: All authors contributed to conceptualization, the preparation of the draft, and the review of this work. All authors have read and agreed to the published version of the manuscript.

Acknowledgments: We are grateful to all our past and present colleagues from the Structural Microbiology Unit, as well as collaborators from the former MM4TB Consortium, for so many fruitful exchanges and insightful discussions.

References

1. Perutz, M.F. Fundamental research in molecular biology: Relevance to medicine. *Nature* **1976**, *262*, 449–453. [CrossRef] [PubMed]
2. Wlodawer, A. Rational approach to AIDS drug design through structural biology. *Annu. Rev. Med.* **2002**, *53*, 595–614. [CrossRef] [PubMed]
3. Greer, J.; Erickson, J.W.; Baldwin, J.J.; Varney, M.D. Application of the three-dimensional structures of protein target molecules in structure-based drug design. *J. Med. Chem.* **1994**, *37*, 1035–1054. [CrossRef] [PubMed]
4. Renaud, J.-P.; Chari, A.; Ciferri, C.; Liu, W.-T.; Rémigy, H.-W.; Stark, H.; Wiesmann, C. Cryo-EM in drug discovery: Achievements, limitations and prospects. *Nat. Rev. Drug. Discov.* **2018**, *17*, 471–492. [CrossRef] [PubMed]
5. Kuehlbrandt, W. The Resolution Revolution. *Science* **2014**, *343*, 1443–1444. [CrossRef]
6. Mitra, A.K. Visualization of biological macromolecules at near-atomic resolution: Cryo-electron microscopy comes of age. *Acta Crystallogr. F Struct. Biol. Commun.* **2019**, *75*, 3–11. [CrossRef]
7. Muhammed, M.T.; Aki-Yalcin, E. Homology modeling in drug discovery: Overview, current applications, and future perspectives. *Chem. Biol. Drug. Des.* **2019**, *93*, 12–20. [CrossRef]
8. Kuenemann, M.A.; Sperandio, O.; Labbé, C.M.; Lagorce, D.; Miteva, M.A.; Villoutreix, B.O. In silico design of low molecular weight protein-protein interaction inhibitors: Overall concept and recent advances. *Prog. Biophys. Mol. Biol.* **2015**, *119*, 20–32. [CrossRef]
9. Bosc, N.; Muller, C.; Hoffer, L.; Lagorce, D.; Bourg, S.; Derviaux, C.; Gourdel, M.-E.; Rain, J.-C.; Miller, T.W.; Villoutreix, B.O.; et al. Fr-PPIChem: An academic compound library dedicated to protein–protein interactions. *ACS Chem. Biol.* **2020**. [CrossRef]
10. Yuan, Y.; Pei, J.; Lai, L. Binding site detection and druggability prediction of protein targets for structure-based drug design. *Curr. Pharm. Des.* **2013**, *19*, 2326–2333. [CrossRef]

11. Acharya, C.; Coop, A.; Polli, J.E.; Mackerell, A.D. Recent advances in ligand-based drug design: Relevance and utility of the conformationally sampled pharmacophore approach. *Curr. Comput. Aided. Drug. Des.* **2011**, *7*, 10–22. [CrossRef] [PubMed]
12. Neves, B.J.; Braga, R.C.; Melo-Filho, C.C.; Moreira-Filho, J.T.; Muratov, E.N.; Andrade, C.H. QSAR-based virtual screening: Advances and applications in drug discovery. *Front. Pharmacol.* **2018**, *9*, 1275. [CrossRef] [PubMed]
13. Davis, B.J.; Hubbard, R.E. Fragment-Based Ligand Discovery. In *Structural Biology in Drug Discovery Methods, Techniques, and Practices*; Renaud, J.-P., Ed.; Wiley: Hoboken, NJ, USA, 2020; Volume 10, pp. 79–98.
14. Mendes, V.; Blundell, T.L. Targeting tuberculosis using structure-guided fragment-based drug design. *Drug Discov. Today* **2017**, *22*, 546–554. [CrossRef] [PubMed]
15. Kana, B.D.; Karakousis, P.C.; Parish, T.; Dick, T. Future target-based drug discovery for tuberculosis? *Tuberculosis* **2014**, *94*, 551–556. [CrossRef] [PubMed]
16. Payne, D.J.; Gwynn, M.N.; Holmes, D.J.; Pompliano, D.L. Drugs for bad bugs: Confronting the challenges of antibacterial discovery. *Nat. Rev. Drug Discov.* **2007**, *6*, 29–40. [CrossRef] [PubMed]
17. Koul, A.; Arnoult, E.; Lounis, N.; Guillemont, J.; Andries, K. The challenge of new drug discovery for tuberculosis. *Nature* **2011**, *469*, 483–490. [CrossRef]
18. Cole, S.T.; Brosch, R.; Parkhill, J.; Garnier, T.; Churcher, C.; Harris, D.; Gordon, S.V.; Eiglmeier, K.; Gas, S.; Barry, C.E.; et al. Deciphering the biology of *Mycobacterium tuberculosis* from the complete genome sequence. *Nature* **1998**, *393*, 537–544. [CrossRef]
19. Holton, S.J.; Weiss, M.S.; Tucker, P.A.; Wilmanns, M. Structure-based approaches to drug discovery against tuberculosis. *Curr. Protein Pept. Sci.* **2007**, *8*, 365–375. [CrossRef]
20. Terwilliger, T.C.; Park, M.S.; Waldo, G.S.; Berendzen, J.; Hung, L.W.; Kim, C.Y.; Smith, C.V.; Sacchettini, J.C.; Bellinzoni, M.; Bossi, R.; et al. The TB structural genomics consortium: A resource for *Mycobacterium tuberculosis* biology. *Tuberculosis* **2003**, *83*, 223–249. [CrossRef]
21. Ehebauer, M.T.; Wilmanns, M. The progress made in determining the *Mycobacterium tuberculosis* structural proteome. *Proteomics* **2011**, *11*, 3128–3133. [CrossRef]
22. Huang, L.; Nazarova, E.V.; Russell, D.G. *Mycobacterium tuberculosis*: Bacterial Fitness within the Host Macrophage. *Microbiol. Spectr.* **2019**, *7*, PMC6459685. [CrossRef] [PubMed]
23. Sia, J.K.; Rengarajan, J. Immunology of *Mycobacterium tuberculosis* Infections. *Microbiol. Spectr.* **2019**, *7*, PMC6636855. [CrossRef] [PubMed]
24. Woong Park, S.; Klotzsche, M.; Wilson, D.J.; Boshoff, H.I.; Eoh, H.; Manjunatha, U.; Blumenthal, A.; Rhee, K.; Barry, C.E.; Aldrich, C.C.; et al. Evaluating the sensitivity of *Mycobacterium tuberculosis* to biotin deprivation using regulated gene expression. *PLoS Pathog.* **2011**, *7*, e1002264. [CrossRef]
25. Wei, J.-R.; Krishnamoorthy, V.; Murphy, K.; Kim, J.-H.; Schnappinger, D.; Alber, T.; Sassetti, C.M.; Rhee, K.Y.; Rubin, E.J. Depletion of antibiotic targets has widely varying effects on growth. *Proc. Natl. Acad. Sci. USA* **2011**, *108*, 4176–4181. [CrossRef]
26. Aleksandrov, A.; Myllykallio, H. Advances and challenges in drug design against tuberculosis: Application of in silico approaches. *Expert Opin. Drug Discov.*. **2019**, *14*, 35–46. [CrossRef] [PubMed]
27. Waman, V.P.; Vedithi, S.C.; Thomas, S.E.; Bannerman, B.P.; Munir, A.; Skwark, M.J.; Malhotra, S.; Blundell, T.L. Mycobacterial genomics and structural bioinformatics: Opportunities and challenges in drug discovery. *Emerg. Microbes Infect.* **2019**, *8*, 109–118. [CrossRef]
28. Pedelacq, J.D.; Nguyen, M.C.; Terwilliger, T.C.; Mourey, L. A Comprehensive Review on *Mycobacterium tuberculosis* Targets and Drug Development from a Structural Perspective. In *Structural Biology in Drug Discovery Methods, Techniques, and Practices*; Renaud, J.-P., Ed.; Wiley: Hoboken, NJ, USA, 2020; Volume 3, pp. 545–566.
29. Cohen, P. Protein kinases–the major drug targets of the twenty-first century? *Nat. Rev. Drug Discov.* **2002**, *1*, 309–315. [CrossRef]
30. Knapp, S. New opportunities for kinase drug repurposing and target discovery. *Br. J. Cancer* **2018**, *118*, 936–937. [CrossRef]
31. Schoijet, A.C.; Sternlieb, T.; Alonso, G.D. Signal Transduction Pathways as Therapeutic Target for Chagas Disease. *Curr. Med. Chem.* **2019**, *26*, 6572–6589. [CrossRef]

32. Lima, M.N.N.; Cassiano, G.C.; Tomaz, K.C.P.; Silva, A.C.; Sousa, B.K.P.; Ferreira, L.T.; Tavella, T.A.; Calit, J.; Bargieri, D.Y.; Neves, B.J.; et al. Integrative Multi-Kinase Approach for the Identification of Potent Antiplasmodial Hits. *Front. Chem.* **2019**, *7*, 773. [CrossRef]
33. Av-Gay, Y.; Everett, M. The eukaryotic-like Ser/Thr protein kinases of *Mycobacterium tuberculosis*. *Trends Microbiol.* **2000**, *8*, 238–244. [CrossRef]
34. Kang, C.-M.; Abbott, D.W.; Park, S.T.; Dascher, C.C.; Cantley, L.C.; Husson, R.N. The *Mycobacterium tuberculosis* serine/threonine kinases PknA and PknB: Substrate identification and regulation of cell shape. *Genes Dev.* **2005**, *19*, 1692–1704. [CrossRef] [PubMed]
35. Wehenkel, A.; Bellinzoni, M.; Graña, M.; Duran, R.; Villarino, A.; Fernandez, P.; Andre-Leroux, G.; England, P.; Takiff, H.; Cerveñansky, C.; et al. Mycobacterial Ser/Thr protein kinases and phosphatases: Physiological roles and therapeutic potential. *Biochim. Biophys. Acta Proteins Proteom.* **2008**, *1784*, 193–202. [CrossRef] [PubMed]
36. Alber, T. Signaling mechanisms of the *Mycobacterium tuberculosis* receptor Ser/Thr protein kinases. *Curr. Opin. Struct. Biol.* **2009**, *19*, 650–657. [CrossRef]
37. Mieczkowski, C.; Iavarone, A.T.; Alber, T. Auto-activation mechanism of the *Mycobacterium tuberculosis* PknB receptor Ser/Thr kinase. *EMBO J.* **2008**, *27*, 3186–3197. [CrossRef]
38. Lombana, T.N.; Echols, N.; Good, M.C.; Thomsen, N.D.; Ng, H.-L.; Greenstein, A.E.; Falick, A.M.; King, D.S.; Alber, T. Allosteric activation mechanism of the *Mycobacterium tuberculosis* receptor Ser/Thr protein kinase, PknB. *Structure* **2010**, *18*, 1667–1677. [CrossRef]
39. Greenstein, A.E.; Echols, N.; Lombana, T.N.; King, D.S.; Alber, T. Allosteric activation by dimerization of the PknD receptor Ser/Thr protein kinase from *Mycobacterium tuberculosis*. *J. Biol. Chem.* **2007**, *282*, 11427–11435. [CrossRef]
40. Wagner, T.; Andre-Leroux, G.; Hindie, V.; Barilone, N.; Lisa, M.-N.; Hoos, S.; Raynal, B.; Vulliez-Le Normand, B.; O'Hare, H.M.; Bellinzoni, M.; et al. Structural insights into the functional versatility of an FHA domain protein in mycobacterial signaling. *Sci. Signal.* **2019**, *12*, eaav9504. [CrossRef]
41. Young, T.A.; Delagoutte, B.; Endrizzi, J.A.; Falick, A.M.; Alber, T. Structure of *Mycobacterium tuberculosis* PknB supports a universal activation mechanism for Ser/Thr protein kinases. *Nat. Struct. Biol.* **2003**, *10*, 168–174. [CrossRef]
42. Ortiz-Lombardía, M.; Pompeo, F.; Boitel, B.; Alzari, P.M. Crystal structure of the catalytic domain of the PknB serine/threonine kinase from *Mycobacterium tuberculosis*. *J. Biol. Chem.* **2003**, *278*, 13094–13100. [CrossRef]
43. Sassetti, C.M.; Boyd, D.H. Genes required for mycobacterial growth defined by high density mutagenesis. *Mol. Microbiol.* **2003**, *48*, 77–84. [CrossRef] [PubMed]
44. Fernandez, P.; Saint-Joanis, B.; Barilone, N.; Jackson, M.; Gicquel, B.; Cole, S.T.; Alzari, P.M. The Ser/Thr protein kinase PknB is essential for sustaining mycobacterial growth. *J. Bacteriol.* **2006**, *188*, 7778–7784. [CrossRef] [PubMed]
45. Chawla, Y.; Upadhyay, S.; Khan, S.; Nagarajan, S.N.; Forti, F.; Nandicoori, V.K. Protein kinase B (PknB) of *Mycobacterium tuberculosis* is essential for growth of the pathogen in vitro as well as for survival within the host. *J. Biol. Chem.* **2014**, *289*, 13875. [CrossRef] [PubMed]
46. Bellinzoni, M.; Wehenkel, A.M.; Duran, R.; Alzari, P.M. Novel mechanistic insights into physiological signaling pathways mediated by mycobacterial Ser/Thr protein kinases. *Genes Immun.* **2019**, *20*, 383–393. [CrossRef] [PubMed]
47. Drews, S.J.; Hung, F.; Av-Gay, Y. A protein kinase inhibitor as an antimycobacterial agent. *FEMS Microbiol. Lett.* **2001**, *205*, 369–374. [CrossRef] [PubMed]
48. Wehenkel, A.; Fernandez, P.; Bellinzoni, M.; Catherinot, V.; Barilone, N.; Labesse, G.; Jackson, M.; Alzari, P.M. The structure of PknB in complex with mitoxantrone, an ATP-competitive inhibitor, suggests a mode of protein kinase regulation in mycobacteria. *FEBS Lett.* **2006**, *580*, 3018–3022. [CrossRef]
49. Bais, V.S.; Mohapatra, B.; Ahamad, N.; Boggaram, S.; Verma, S.; Prakash, B. Investigating the inhibitory potential of 2-Aminopurine metal complexes against serine/threonine protein kinases from *Mycobacterium tuberculosis*. *Tuberculosis* **2018**, *108*, 47–55. [CrossRef]
50. Székely, R.; Waczek, F.; Szabadkai, I.; Németh, G.; Hegymegi-Barakonyi, B.; Eros, D.; Szokol, B.; Pato, J.; Hafenbradl, D.; Satchell, J.; et al. A novel drug discovery concept for tuberculosis: Inhibition of bacterial and host cell signalling. *Immunol. Lett.* **2008**, *116*, 225–231. [CrossRef]

51. Chapman, T.M.; Bouloc, N.; Buxton, R.S.; Chugh, J.; Lougheed, K.E.A.; Osborne, S.A.; Saxty, B.; Smerdon, S.J.; Taylor, D.L.; Whalley, D. Substituted aminopyrimidine protein kinase B (PknB) inhibitors show activity against *Mycobacterium tuberculosis*. *Bioorg. Med. Chem. Lett.* **2012**, *22*, 3349–3353. [CrossRef]
52. Lougheed, K.E.A.; Osborne, S.A.; Saxty, B.; Whalley, D.; Chapman, T.; Bouloc, N.; Chugh, J.; Nott, T.J.; Patel, D.; Spivey, V.L.; et al. Effective inhibitors of the essential kinase PknB and their potential as anti-mycobacterial agents. *Tuberculosis* **2011**, *91*, 277–286. [CrossRef]
53. Xu, J.; Wang, J.-X.; Zhou, J.-M.; Xu, C.-L.; Huang, B.; Xing, Y.; Wang, B.; Luo, R.; Wang, Y.-C.; You, X.-F.; et al. A novel protein kinase inhibitor IMB-YH-8 with anti-tuberculosis activity. *Sci. Rep.* **2017**, *7*, 5093–5110. [CrossRef] [PubMed]
54. Appunni, S.; Rajisha, P.M.; Rubens, M.; Chandana, S.; Singh, H.N.; Swarup, V. Targeting PknB, an eukaryotic-like serine/threonine protein kinase of *Mycobacterium tuberculosis* with phytomolecules. *Comput. Biol. Chem.* **2017**, *67*, 200–204. [CrossRef] [PubMed]
55. Wang, T.; Bemis, G.; Hanzelka, B.; Zuccola, H.; Wynn, M.; Moody, C.S.; Green, J.; Locher, C.; Liu, A.; Gao, H.; et al. Mtb PKNA/PKNB Dual Inhibition Provides Selectivity Advantages for Inhibitor Design To Minimize Host Kinase Interactions. *ACS Med. Chem. Lett.* **2017**, *8*, 1224–1229. [CrossRef] [PubMed]
56. Wlodarchak, N.; Teachout, N.; Beczkiewicz, J.; Procknow, R.; Schaenzer, A.J.; Satyshur, K.; Pavelka, M.; Zuercher, W.; Drewry, D.; Sauer, J.-D.; et al. In Silico Screen and Structural Analysis Identifies Bacterial Kinase Inhibitors which Act with β-Lactams To Inhibit Mycobacterial Growth. *Mol. Pharm.* **2018**, *15*, 5410–5426. [CrossRef] [PubMed]
57. Walburger, A.; Koul, A.; Ferrari, G.; Nguyen, L.; Prescianotto-Baschong, C.; Huygen, K.; Klebl, B.; Thompson, C.; Bacher, G.; Pieters, J. Protein kinase G from pathogenic mycobacteria promotes survival within macrophages. *Science* **2004**, *304*, 1800–1804. [CrossRef] [PubMed]
58. Scherr, N.; Honnappa, S.; Kunz, G.; Mueller, P.; Jayachandran, R.; Winkler, F.; Pieters, J.; Steinmetz, M.O. Structural basis for the specific inhibition of protein kinase G, a virulence factor of *Mycobacterium tuberculosis*. *Proc. Natl. Acad. Sci. USA* **2007**, *104*, 12151–12156. [CrossRef]
59. Lisa, M.-N.; Gil, M.; Andre-Leroux, G.; Barilone, N.; Duran, R.; Biondi, R.M.; Alzari, P.M. Molecular Basis of the Activity and the Regulation of the Eukaryotic-like S/T Protein Kinase PknG from Mycobacterium tuberculosis. *Structure* **2015**, *23*, 1039–1048. [CrossRef]
60. van der Woude, A.D.; Stoop, E.J.M.; Stiess, M.; Wang, S.; Ummels, R.; van Stempvoort, G.; Piersma, S.R.; Cascioferro, A.; Jiménez, C.R.; Houben, E.N.G.; et al. Analysis of SecA2-dependent substrates in *Mycobacterium marinum* identifies protein kinase G (PknG) as a virulence effector. *Cell Microbiol.* **2014**, *16*, 280–295. [CrossRef]
61. Zulauf, K.E.; Sullivan, J.T.; Braunstein, M. The SecA2 pathway of *Mycobacterium tuberculosis* exports effectors that work in concert to arrest phagosome and autophagosome maturation. *PLoS Pathog.* **2018**, *14*, e1007011. [CrossRef]
62. Pradhan, G.; Shrivastva, R.; Mukhopadhyay, S. Mycobacterial PknG targets the Rab7l1 signaling pathway to inhibit phagosome-lysosome fusion. *J. Immunol.* **2018**, *201*, 1421–1433. [CrossRef]
63. Bussi, C.; Gutierrez, M.G. *Mycobacterium tuberculosis* infection of host cells in space and time. *FEMS Microbiol. Rev.* **2019**, *43*, 341–361. [CrossRef] [PubMed]
64. Schultz, C.; Niebisch, A.; Gebel, L.; Bott, M. Glutamate production by *Corynebacterium glutamicum*: Dependence on the oxoglutarate dehydrogenase inhibitor protein OdhI and protein kinase PknG. *Appl. Microbiol. Biotechnol.* **2007**, *76*, 691–700. [CrossRef] [PubMed]
65. Niebisch, A.; Kabus, A.; Schultz, C.; Weil, B.; Bott, M. Corynebacterial protein kinase G controls 2-oxoglutarate dehydrogenase activity via the phosphorylation status of the OdhI protein. *J. Biol. Chem.* **2006**, *281*, 12300–12307. [CrossRef] [PubMed]
66. Ventura, M.; Rieck, B.; Boldrin, F.; Degiacomi, G.; Bellinzoni, M.; Barilone, N.; Alzaidi, F.; Alzari, P.M.; Manganelli, R.; O'Hare, H.M. GarA is an essential regulator of metabolism in *Mycobacterium tuberculosis*. *Mol. Microbiol.* **2013**, *90*, 356–366.
67. O'Hare, H.M.; Duran, R.; Cerveñansky, C.; Bellinzoni, M.; Wehenkel, A.M.; Pritsch, O.; Obal, G.; Baumgartner, J.; Vialaret, J.; Johnsson, K.; et al. Regulation of glutamate metabolism by protein kinases in mycobacteria. *Mol. Microbiol.* **2008**, *70*, 1408–1423. [CrossRef]
68. Rieck, B.; Degiacomi, G.; Zimmermann, M.; Cascioferro, A.; Boldrin, F.; Lazar-Adler, N.R.; Bottrill, A.R.; Le Chevalier, F.; Frigui, W.; Bellinzoni, M.; et al. PknG senses amino acid availability to control metabolism and virulence of Mycobacterium tuberculosis. *PLoS Pathog.* **2017**, *13*, e1006399. [CrossRef]

69. Wolff, K.A.; de la Peña, A.H.; Nguyen, H.T.; Pham, T.H.; Amzel, L.M.; Gabelli, S.B.; Nguyen, L. A redox regulatory system critical for mycobacterial survival in macrophages and biofilm development. *PLoS Pathog.* **2015**, *11*, e1004839. [CrossRef]
70. Khan, M.Z.; Bhaskar, A.; Upadhyay, S.; Kumari, P.; Rajmani, R.S.; Jain, P.; Singh, A.; Kumar, D.; Bhavesh, N.S.; Nandicoori, V.K. Protein kinase G confers survival advantage to *Mycobacterium tuberculosis* during latency-like conditions. *J. Biol. Chem.* **2017**, *292*, 16093–16108. [CrossRef]
71. Cowley, S.; Ko, M.; Pick, N.; Chow, R.; Downing, K.J.; Gordhan, B.G.; Betts, J.C.; Mizrahi, V.; Smith, D.A.; Stokes, R.W.; et al. The *Mycobacterium tuberculosis* protein serine/threonine kinase PknG is linked to cellular glutamate/glutamine levels and is important for growth in vivo. *Mol. Microbiol.* **2004**, *52*, 1691–1702. [CrossRef]
72. Chao, J.; Wong, D.; Zheng, X.; Poirier, V.; Bach, H.; Hmama, Z.; Av-Gay, Y. Protein kinase and phosphatase signaling in *Mycobacterium tuberculosis* physiology and pathogenesis. *Biochim. Biophys. Acta Proteins Proteom.* **2010**, *1804*, 620–627. [CrossRef]
73. Chen, D.; Ma, S.; He, L.; Yuan, P.; She, Z.; Lu, Y. Sclerotiorin inhibits protein kinase G from *Mycobacterium tuberculosis* and impairs mycobacterial growth in macrophages. *Tuberculosis* **2017**, *103*, 37–43. [CrossRef] [PubMed]
74. Kidwai, S.; Bouzeyen, R.; Chakraborti, S.; Khare, N.; Das, S.; Priya Gosain, T.; Behura, A.; Meena, C.L.; Dhiman, R.; Essafi, M.; et al. NU-6027 Inhibits Growth of *Mycobacterium tuberculosis* by Targeting Protein Kinase D and Protein Kinase G. *Antimicrob. Agents Chemother.* **2019**, *63*, 39. [CrossRef] [PubMed]
75. Kanehiro, Y.; Tomioka, H.; Pieters, J.; Tatano, Y.; Kim, H.; Iizasa, H.; Yoshiyama, H. Identification of Novel Mycobacterial Inhibitors Against Mycobacterial Protein Kinase G. *Front. Microbiol.* **2018**, *9*, 1517. [CrossRef] [PubMed]
76. Schoeffler, A.J.; Berger, J.M. DNA topoisomerases: Harnessing and constraining energy to govern chromosome topology. *Quart. Rev. Biophys.* **2008**, *41*, 41–101. [CrossRef] [PubMed]
77. Gellert, M.; Mizuuchi, K.; O'Dea, M.H.; Nash, H.A. DNA gyrase: An enzyme that introduces superhelical turns into DNA. *Proc. Natl. Acad. Sci. USA* **1976**, *73*, 3872–3876. [CrossRef]
78. Sissi, C.; Palumbo, M. In front of and behind the replication fork: Bacterial type IIA topoisomerases. *Cell. Mol. Life Sci.* **2010**, *67*, 2001–2024. [CrossRef]
79. Peng, H.; Marians, K.J. Decatenation activity of topoisomerase IV during oriC and pBR322 DNA replication in vitro. *Proc. Natl. Acad. Sci. USA* **1993**, *90*, 8571–8575. [CrossRef]
80. Aubry, A.; Fisher, L.M.; Jarlier, V.; Cambau, E. First functional characterization of a singly expressed bacterial type II topoisomerase: The enzyme from *Mycobacterium tuberculosis*. *Biochem. Biophys. Res. Commun.* **2006**, *348*, 158–165. [CrossRef]
81. Hooper, D.C.; Jacoby, G.A. Topoisomerase Inhibitors: Fluoroquinolone Mechanisms of Action and Resistance. *Cold Spring Harb. Perspect. Med.* **2016**, *6*, a025320. [CrossRef]
82. Blower, T.R.; Williamson, B.H.; Kerns, R.J.; Berger, J.M. Crystal structure and stability of gyrase–fluoroquinolone cleaved complexes from *Mycobacterium tuberculosis*. *Proc. Natl. Acad. Sci. USA* **2016**, *113*, 1706–1713. [CrossRef]
83. Fu, G.; Wu, J.; Liu, W.; Zhu, D.; Hu, Y.; Deng, J.; Zhang, X.-E.; Bi, L.; Wang, D.-C. Crystal structure of DNA gyrase B′ domain sheds lights on the mechanism for T-segment navigation. *Nucleic Acids Res.* **2009**, *37*, 5908–5916. [CrossRef] [PubMed]
84. Tretter, E.M.; Schoeffler, A.J.; Weisfield, S.R.; Berger, J.M. Crystal structure of the DNA gyrase GyrA N-terminal domain from *Mycobacterium tuberculosis*. *Proteins* **2010**, *78*, 492–495. [CrossRef] [PubMed]
85. Agrawal, A.; Roue, M.; Spitzfaden, C.; Petrella, S.; Aubry, A.; Hann, M.; Bax, B.; Mayer, C. *Mycobacterium tuberculosis* DNA gyrase ATPase domain structures suggest a dissociative mechanism that explains how ATP hydrolysis is coupled to domain motion. *Biochem. J.* **2013**, *456*, 263–273. [CrossRef] [PubMed]
86. Bouige, A.; Darmon, A.; Piton, J.; Roue, M.; Petrella, S.; Capton, E.; Forterre, P.; Aubry, A.; Mayer, C. *Mycobacterium tuberculosis* DNA gyrase possesses two functional GyrA-boxes. *Biochem. J.* **2013**, *455*, 285–294. [CrossRef] [PubMed]
87. Piton, J.; Petrella, S.; Delarue, M.; Andre-Leroux, G.; Jarlier, V.; Aubry, A.; Mayer, C. Structural Insights into the Quinolone Resistance Mechanism of *Mycobacterium tuberculosis* DNA Gyrase. *PLoS ONE* **2010**, *5*, e12245. [CrossRef]

88. World Health Organization. Global Tuberculosis Report 2019. Available online: https://www.who.int/tb/publications/global_report/en/ (accessed on 19 June 2020).
89. Nagaraja, V.; Godbole, A.A.; Henderson, S.R.; Maxwell, A. DNA topoisomerase I and DNA gyrase as targets for TB therapy. *Drug Discov. Today* **2017**, *22*, 510–518. [CrossRef]
90. Vanden Broeck, A.; McEwen, A.G.; Chebaro, Y.; Potier, N.; Lamour, V. Structural Basis for DNA Gyrase Interaction with Coumermycin A1. *J. Med. Chem.* **2019**, *62*, 4225–4231. [CrossRef]
91. Mizuuchi, K.; O'Dea, M.H.; Gellert, M. DNA gyrase: Subunit structure and ATPase activity of the purified enzyme. *Proc. Natl. Acad. Sci. USA* **1978**, *75*, 5960–5963. [CrossRef]
92. Grossman, T.H.; Bartels, D.J.; Mullin, S.; Gross, C.H.; Parsons, J.D.; Liao, Y.; Grillot, A.-L.; Stamos, D.; Olson, E.R.; Charifson, P.S.; et al. Dual targeting of GyrB and ParE by a novel aminobenzimidazole class of antibacterial compounds. *Antimicrob. Agents Chemother.* **2007**, *51*, 657–666. [CrossRef]
93. Charifson, P.S.; Grillot, A.-L.; Grossman, T.H.; Parsons, J.D.; Badia, M.; Bellon, S.; Deininger, D.D.; Drumm, J.E.; Gross, C.H.; LeTiran, A.; et al. Novel dual-targeting benzimidazole urea inhibitors of DNA gyrase and topoisomerase IV possessing potent antibacterial activity: Intelligent design and evolution through the judicious use of structure-guided design and structure-activity relationships. *J. Med. Chem.* **2008**, *51*, 5243–5263. [CrossRef]
94. Holdgate, G.A.; Tunnicliffe, A.; Ward, W.H.; Weston, S.A.; Rosenbrock, G.; Barth, P.T.; Taylor, I.W.; Pauptit, R.A.; Timms, D. The entropic penalty of ordered water accounts for weaker binding of the antibiotic novobiocin to a resistant mutant of DNA gyrase: A thermodynamic and crystallographic study. *Biochemistry* **1997**, *36*, 9663–9673. [CrossRef] [PubMed]
95. Grillot, A.-L.; Le Tiran, A.; Shannon, D.; Krueger, E.; Liao, Y.; O'Dowd, H.; Tang, Q.; Ronkin, S.; Wang, T.; Waal, N.; et al. Second-generation antibacterial benzimidazole ureas: Discovery of a preclinical candidate with reduced metabolic liability. *J. Med. Chem.* **2014**, *57*, 8792–8816. [CrossRef] [PubMed]
96. Brown-Elliott, B.A.; Rubio, A.; Wallace, R.J., Jr. In Vitro Susceptibility Testing of a Novel Benzimidazole, SPR719, against Nontuberculous Mycobacteria. *Antimicrob. Agents Chemother.* **2018**, *62*, 545. [CrossRef] [PubMed]
97. Locher, C.P.; Jones, S.M.; Hanzelka, B.L.; Perola, E.; Shoen, C.M.; Cynamon, M.H.; Ngwane, A.H.; Wiid, I.J.; van Helden, P.D.; Betoudji, F.; et al. A Novel Inhibitor of Gyrase B Is a Potent Drug Candidate for Treatment of Tuberculosis and Nontuberculosis Mycobacterial Infections. *Antimicrob. Agents Chemother.* **2015**, *59*, 1455–1465. [CrossRef]
98. Shoen, C.M.; DeStefano, M.; Pucci, M.; Cynamon, M.H. Evaluating the Sterilizing Activity of SPR720 in Combination Therapy against Mycobacterium tuberculosis Infection in Mice. In Proceedings of the Conference of ASM Microbes 2019, San Francisco, CA, USA, 20–24 June 2019.
99. Coates, W.J.; Gwynn, M.N.; Hatton, I.K.; Masters, P.J.; Pearson, N.D.; Rahman, S.S.; Slocombe, B.; Warrack, J.D.; SmithKline Beecham Ltd. Quinoline Derivatives as Antibacterials. European Patent EP1051413, 4 June 2003.
100. Bax, B.D.; Chan, P.F.; Eggleston, D.S.; Fosberry, A.; Gentry, D.R.; Gorrec, F.; Giordano, I.; Hann, M.M.; Hennessy, A.; Hibbs, M.; et al. Type IIA topoisomerase inhibition by a new class of antibacterial agents. *Nature* **2010**, *466*, 935–940. [CrossRef]
101. Blanco, D.; Perez-Herran, E.; Cacho, M.; Ballell, L.; Castro, J.; González del Río, R.; Lavandera, J.L.; Remuiñán, M.J.; Richards, C.; Rullas, J.; et al. Mycobacterium tuberculosis Gyrase Inhibitors as a New Class of Antitubercular Drugs. *Antimicrob. Agents Chemother.* **2015**, *59*, 1868–1875. [CrossRef]
102. Gibson, E.G.; Blower, T.R.; Cacho, M.; Bax, B.; Berger, J.M.; Osheroff, N. Mechanism of Action of *Mycobacterium tuberculosis* Gyrase Inhibitors: A Novel Class of Gyrase Poisons. *ACS Infect. Dis.* **2018**, *4*, 1211–1222. [CrossRef]
103. Tanner, L.; Denti, P.; Wiesner, L.; Warner, D.F. Drug permeation and metabolism in *Mycobacterium tuberculosis*: Prioritising local exposure as essential criterion in new TB drug development. *IUBMB Life* **2018**, *70*, 926–937. [CrossRef]
104. Van Wijk, R.C.; Ayoun Alsoud, R.; Lennernäs, H.; Simonsson, U.S.H. Model-Informed Drug Discovery and Development Strategy for the Rapid Development of Anti-Tuberculosis Drug Combinations. *Appl. Sci.* **2020**, *10*, 2376. [CrossRef]
105. Mori, M.; Sammartino, J.C.; Costantino, L.; Gelain, A.; Meneghetti, F.; Villa, S.; Chiarelli, L.R. An Overview on the Potential Antimycobacterial Agents Targeting Serine/Threonine Protein Kinases from Mycobacterium tuberculosis. *Curr. Top. Med. Chem.* **2019**, *19*, 646–661. [CrossRef]

106. Prisic, S.; Husson, R.N. *Mycobacterium tuberculosis* Serine/Threonine Protein Kinases. *Microbiol. Spectr.* **2014**, 2. [CrossRef] [PubMed]
107. Ehrt, S.; Schnappinger, D.; Rhee, K.Y. Metabolic principles of persistence and pathogenicity in *Mycobacterium tuberculosis*. *Nat. Rev. Microbiol.* **2018**, *16*, 496–507. [CrossRef] [PubMed]
108. Sala, C.; Hartkoorn, R.C. Tuberculosis drugs: New candidates and how to find more. *Future Microbiol.* **2011**, *6*, 617–633. [CrossRef] [PubMed]
109. Villemagne, B.; Machelart, A.; Tran, N.C.; Flipo, M.; Moune, M.; Leroux, F.; Piveteau, C.; Wohlkönig, A.; Wintjens, R.; Li, X.; et al. Fragment-Based Optimized EthR Inhibitors with in Vivo Ethionamide Boosting Activity. *ACS Infect. Dis.* **2020**, *6*, 366–378. [CrossRef]
110. Maveyraud, L.; Mourey, L. Protein X-ray Crystallography and Drug Discovery. *Molecules* **2020**, *25*, 1030. [CrossRef]
111. Rout, M.P.; Sali, A. Principles for Integrative Structural Biology Studies. *Cell* **2019**, *177*, 1384–1403. [CrossRef]
112. Petrella, S.; Capton, E.; Raynal, B.; Giffard, C.; Thureau, A.; Bonneté, F.; Alzari, P.M.; Aubry, A.; Mayer, C. Overall Structures of *Mycobacterium tuberculosis* DNA Gyrase Reveal the Role of a *Corynebacteriales* GyrB-Specific Insert in ATPase Activity. *Structure* **2019**, *27*, 579–589.e5. [CrossRef]
113. Vanden Broeck, A.; Lotz, C.; Ortiz, J.; Lamour, V. Cryo-EM structure of the complete *E. coli* DNA gyrase nucleoprotein complex. *Nat. Commun.* **2019**, *10*, 4935. [CrossRef]

6

Two Decades of TB Drug Discovery Efforts—What Have we Learned?

Balachandra Bandodkar [1], Radha Krishan Shandil [2], Jagadeesh Bhat [3] and Tanjore S. Balganesh [3,*]

1 Pharmaron Beijing Co., Ltd., 6, Taihe Road, BDA, Beijing 100176, China; balachandra.bandodkar@pharmaron.com

2 Foundation for Neglected Disease Research [FNDR], Plot 20A, KIADB Industrial Area, Doddaballapur, Bengaluru 561203, India; rk.shandil@fndr.in

3 Gangagen Biotechnologies P Ltd., #12, 5th Cross, Raghavendra Layout, Tumkur Road, Yeshwantpur, Bengaluru 560022, India; bjagadeesh@gangagen.com

* Correspondence: balganesh@gangagen.com

Abstract: After several years of limited success, an effective regimen for the treatment of both drug-sensitive and multiple-drug-resistant tuberculosis is in place. However, this success is still incomplete, as we need several more novel combinations to treat extensively drug-resistant tuberculosis, as well newer emerging resistance. Additionally, the goal of a shortened therapy continues to evade us. A systematic analysis of the tuberculosis drug discovery approaches employed over the last two decades shows that the lead identification path has been largely influenced by the improved understanding of the biology of the pathogen *Mycobacterium tuberculosis*. Interestingly, the drug discovery efforts can be grouped into a few defined approaches that predominated over a period of time. This review delineates the key drivers during each of these periods. While doing so, the author's experiences at AstraZeneca R&D, Bangalore, India, on the discovery of new antimycobacterial candidate drugs are used to exemplify the concept. Finally, the review also discusses the value of validated targets, promiscuous targets, the current anti-TB pipeline, the gaps in it, and the possible way forward.

Keywords: tuberculosis; *Mycobacterium tuberculosis*; drug discovery; drug development; target-based screening; phenotypic screening; antituberculosis agents; antimycobacterial; anti-TB drug pipeline; privileged targets; promiscuous targets; lead generation

---

Chemotherapy for the treatment of tuberculosis has evolved over a period of several decades, starting from the 1950s. The discovery of drugs with superior effectiveness that are part of the current regimen has been facilitated through the success of several novel approaches and technologies. While the medical need has at times hastened newer approaches to be adopted, the main driver for the improvement has been the increased understanding of the biology of the pathogen, as well as its interaction with the human host. In this review, we try to discuss the discovery of new drugs in groups, with the groups sharing a common key driver that precipitated the changes of the treatment regimen. As 'newer aspects of the biology' of the pathogen became known, they provided opportunities to build novel drug discovery approaches. The paper also uses as examples the approaches, the results, and the learning gathered as a part of the antituberculosis (anti-TB) program at Astra Zeneca, R and D, Bangalore, India (AZI).

Several of the drugs that have been discovered are based on the learning that followed the introduction of each of the new compounds into the drug regimen. The data have several pointers; while each of the successful drugs was discovered building on the then state of the knowledge, the newer drugs themselves also helped in the further understanding of the pathogen biology. This is even reflected in the current set of drugs that are in late-stage development or have been recently introduced into the anti-TB regimen.

The anti-TB drugs currently in use, and those in the late stages of clinical development, can be broadly pooled into the following groups:

1. Serendipitous drug discovery—early chemotherapy;
2. Modification of drug scaffolds;
3. Revisiting targets that have clinically validated drugs against them (referred to as established targets);
4. Target-based screening;
5. Phenotypic screening.

1. Serendipitous Drug Discovery: Early Chemotherapy

The first successful chemotherapy and cure of an infectious disease is indeed the discovery and design of the 'first line' therapy for the treatment of tuberculosis—the design and development of which was completed in the 1960s. Even today, this regimen is the therapy of choice for treating drug-sensitive tuberculosis (DSTB). The drugs in the first-line treatment for DSTB, isoniazid, rifampicin, pyrazinamide, and ethambutol became anti-TB drugs based on their activity on *Mycobacterium tuberculosis* (MTB) cells in vitro, followed by testing in animal models and their rapid introduction into humans [1]. This progression was driven by the medical need, as no chemotherapy existed before these drugs were discovered.

It is interesting to note that two biological observations and a hypothesis on potential 'chemical structures' that may interfere with the observed biological process were the first starting points of anti-TB drug discovery. Aspirin was shown to be a potent stimulator of the TB bacilli's 'oxygen consumption'; analogs of aspirin were then postulated to be inhibitors of this process. This led to the synthesis of a number of aspirin-like structures, of which para-aminosalicylic acid (PAS) became a successful anti-TB drug [1–3]. The second observation was that niacin helped in the recovery of guinea pigs infected with MTB, as well as the observation that niacin helped in faster recovery of TB patients, raising the possibility that niacin was acting as a 'vitamin' [4,5]. Chemical synthesis focused on making derivatives of niacin led to the design of three anti-TB drugs, namely isoniazid (Inh), pyrazinamide (Pza) and ethionamide (Eth) [6]. Two of these are even today the most potent drugs for the treatment of TB. This early period of chemotherapy also included extensive search for natural products with antibacterial activity; Rifamycin and Streptomycin were natural products that showed potent activity against MTB cells and were also introduced into the treatment of TB.

In 1979, Mitchison observed that 10 to 12 drugs were available for the treatment of tuberculosis, which could be classified in terms of their effectiveness [7]. The choice of combinations was dictated by animal toxicity of the individual drugs and in human trials, which assessed time taken to the sputum negative state, cure as reflected by relapse rates, the emergence of resistant strains, and compliance. Once an effective combination had been proven, it became to be referred to as the 'Short Course Chemotherapy' and was adopted systematically all over the world [8]. This was the first successful conquering of an infectious disease. In about 20 years, TB patients went from complete helplessness to an effective cure achieved with drug treatment.

The key learning from this pioneering era was as follows:

1. In vitro MIC (Minimum Inhibitory Concentration) was insufficient to predict efficacy in humans. Requirement for a combination therapy of drugs.
2. The best regimen required six months of treatment to achieve cure.
3. Each of the drugs in the combination had a unique role to play in leading to the cure.

The cure was defined as the lack of relapse.

The last two points remain, to date, the biggest challenge in finding and developing novel combinations. The era of 1950 to 1980 had 10 drugs, of which the most efficacious combination of four drugs was identified through rapid testing in humans. In spite of more than two decades of sustained research into the biology of MTB, the traits of a new drug that could contribute to both the 'cure' and the shortening of therapy are still unknown.

2. Modification of Drug Scaffolds: Analogs of Known Drugs or the Literature Compounds

The initiation points for this approach were natural product scaffolds or scaffolds known to have activity against MTB cells in vitro but did not possess drug-like properties. Efforts to address this were mainly medicinal-chemistry driven, focused on understanding structure–activity relationship (SAR) on potency and animal toxicity. The advances in chemistry in terms of novel reactions and the use of combinatorial chemistry resulted in rapid diversification of key scaffolds to yield potent analogs. Some of the examples of scaffolds were the nitroimidazoles and several newer rifampicins, isoniazid, and ethambutol analogs [9–12].

2.1. Nitroimidazole as a Starting Point

Among the diverse scaffolds tested in this approach, the 'nitroimidazole' starting point has been the most successful. The antibiotic 5-nitroimidazole was used for treating bacterial infections of the gut and was also shown to be active on anaerobic bacteria [13]. Metronidazole, a drug still in use for the treatment of amoebic infections, was one of the first successful derivatives of 5-nitroimidazole. CGI-17341, a bicyclic imidazofuran, was one of the derivatives and was found to be a potent anti-Tb molecule [14]. Continued chemistry on this molecule led to several analogs, among which PA-824 (Pretomanid) [15], OPC-67683 (Delamanid) [16] have recently been registered as anti-TB drugs and are constituents of the current Multi drug resistant (MDR) regimen [15,16]. This progression is shown in Figure 1.

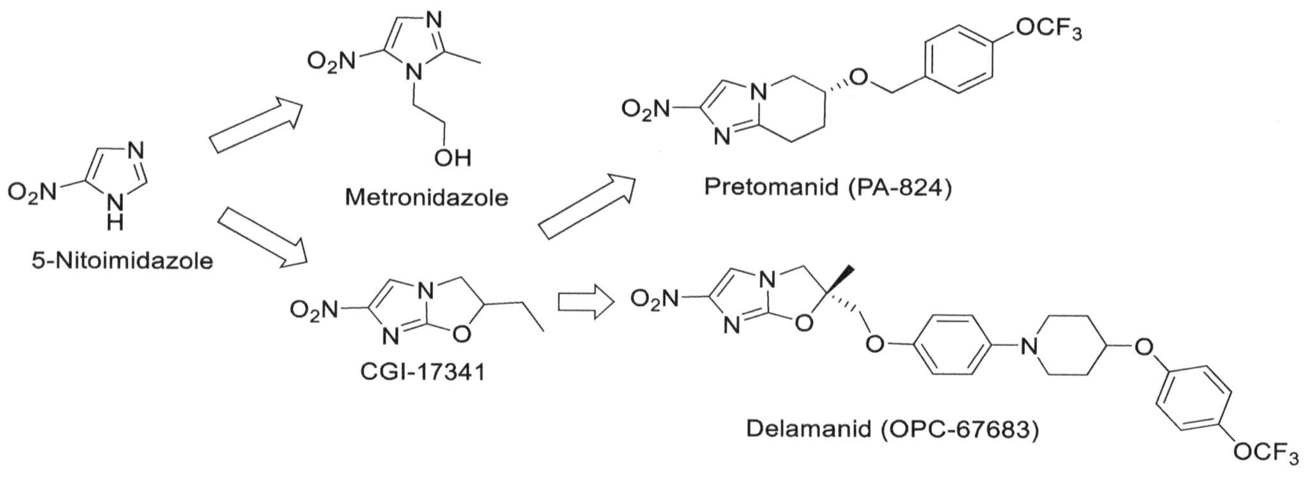

Figure 1. The progression of 5-Nitoimidazole derivatives.

2.2. Rifampicin Analogs

Rifampicin was obtained through the chemical modification of the natural product rifamycin [17]. Derivatives of rifampicin, like rifabutin, were synthesized and found to have favorable properties in terms of compatibility with anti-HIV drugs but could not overcome the cross-resistance with rifampicin [18].

2.3. Ethambutol Derivatives

Increased throughput in chemistry also contributed to finding new leads. A combinatorial library created around ethambutol led to the discovery of a clinical candidate SQ-109 [19,20]. SQ-109 was found to be active even on ethambutol-resistant strains of MTB. SQ109 has been shown to target the Mycobacterial Membrane Protein Large 3 (Mmpl3) [21]. It is interesting to note that ethambutol does not inhibit Mmpl3.

2.4. Isoniazid Analogs

Among the many Inh analogs synthesized, Sudoterb (LL 3858) was successfully progressed to Phase 1 [22,23]. Inh, because of its simplicity of structure, remains an attractive starting point for analog-based discovery.

The approach involving modifications of existing drug scaffolds has two important aims: firstly, to discover novel analogs that are active on MTB strains resistant to the parent drug, and secondly, to design 'drug-friendly' molecules. This approach has yielded two, drugs and a third is in development: Pretomanid (Pre), Delamanid (Del), and SQ-109, respectively.

The key learning from these examples is that sustained effort can lead to useful drugs, even though the starting scaffolds have issues.

3. Revisiting Established Targets: Revisiting Targets Proven as Druggable by Using Broad-Spectrum Compounds

TB was declared a global emergency by WHO in 1996 [24]. The emergence of drug-resistant TB and the complete lack of drugs capable of treating patients with MDR TB led the drug development community to investigate alternate approaches to rapidly induct novel drugs into the regimen. This prompted investigations into the feasibility of introducing the existing broad-spectrum antibacterial drugs into the TB treatment regimen. Several antibacterial classes that have been shown to be active on MTB in vitro were investigated in clinical trials.

This approach, which is now classified as 'repurposing', has successfully delivered new options for TB treatment. The key classes that have added to the anti-TB portfolio are the following:

3.1. Protein-Synthesis Inhibitors

Streptomycin, a protein-synthesis inhibitor and a well-established anti-TB drug, has been shown to be effective in treating MTB patients, but its use is limited because of it not being an oral drug and the toxicities associated with it for prolonged use [25]. Several novel protein-synthesis inhibitors that have been approved as antibacterials were also tested for their antimycobacterial activity. The oxazolidinone [26] class of compounds, despite its limitations of myelotoxicity, hold a significant position in the treatment of MDR and Extensively drug-resistant tuberculosis (XDR)TB in the current anti-TB treatment regimen. Linezolid [27,28] is currently a part of the drug regimen for the treatment of MDR TB, XDR and non-responding TB (NRTB), while newer oxazolidinones like Posizolid [29–31] and Sutezolid [32,33] have been tested in advanced clinical trials. Newer oxazolidinones like the Delpazolid [34] and Contezolid [35] are also in clinical trials.

3.2. Beta Lactams as Antimycobacterials

Several broad-spectrum antibacterials like meropenem, a beta-lactam, have also been shown to have activity against MTB in in vitro models, as well as in studies measuring Early Bactericidal Activity (EBA) in humans [36].

The key 'unknowns' in the development of broad-spectrum antibiotics as anti-TB treatment are twofold:

- Priming of resistance against the antibiotic among normal gut bacteria due to the long-term treatment required for TB. This priming could lead to the selection of resistant mutants and subsequently spread of resistance to other pathogens in the gut.
- Effect of the antibiotic on 'latent MTB bacteria': Latent bacteria could also be primed, leading to probability of a drug-resistant infection on reactivation.

Despite these concerns, even after several years of the use of rifampicin for the treatment of Drug sensitive (DS) TB and moxifloxacin for the treatment of MDR TB, the extent of 'priming' caused is not clear, and some of the fears could well be unfounded. This could also be a reflection of the use of these drugs only in combinations or our inability to monitor the impact systematically.

The key learning from this approach of including broad-spectrum antibiotics into the combination regimen to treat MTB patients has been as follows:

- Drugs with several new targets, like the ones discussed above, can be introduced into novel combinations, thus enabling the treatment of drug resistant (DR) MTB patients.
- The effectiveness of drugs like moxifloxacin or linezolid establish the vulnerability of the target, thus promoting the search for new compounds that can inhibit the same target. This approach of revisiting 'established/vulnerable targets' continues to be explored by using several newer assets, like new libraries, which are novel screening formats, including those enabled by the availability of the molecular structures. Two novel compounds that have entered clinical development, GSK070 shown in Figure 2a [37] and SPR20 shown in Figure 2b [38], are examples of this approach. GSK 3036656 (GSK-070) belongs to the oxaborole class of compounds and has been shown to be a Leucine tRNA synthase inhibitor. The compound is currently in Phase 2 clinical trials [37]. SPR 720 is a GyrB ATPase inhibitor that belongs to the benzimidazole class. The molecule is also in Phase 2 clinical trials [38,39]. A very recent report shows that SPR 720 obtained an orphan disease status from FDA to treat non-tuberculosis mycobacteria (NTM) [40].

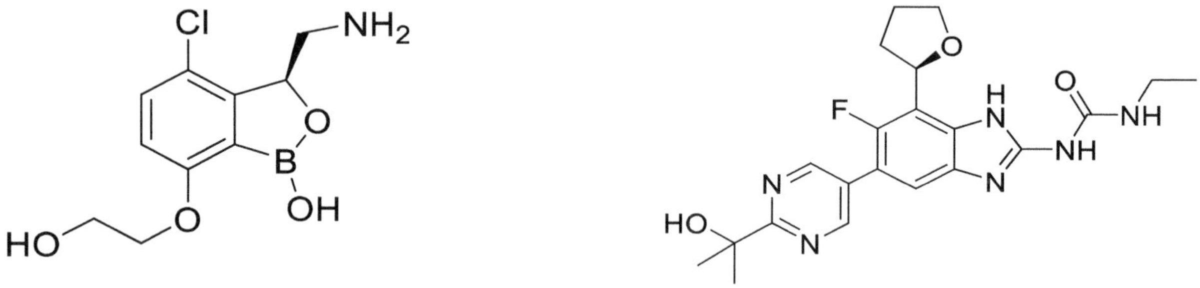

GSK 3036656 (GSK 070)

(a)

SPR720 (VXc-100, VXc-486)

(b)

Figure 2. Two novel compounds that have entered clinical development (**a**) GSK070 and (**b**) SPR20.

3.3. Gyrase Inhibitors

The fluoroquinolone class (Moxifloxacin, Levofloxacin, Ofloxacin, and Gatifloxacin) of compounds are potent inhibitors of the DNA gyrase enzyme and are proven antibacterials. Several of these were shown to be active on the MTB bacilli in vitro. Researchers at the National Tuberculosis Institute, India, tested the usefulness of ofloxacin as a part of the anti-TB regimen and showed it to be effective in the clinical trial [41]. Multiple members of this class of compounds have undergone clinical trials as part of an anti-TB regimen; moxifloxacin [42] is now a part of the standard regimen to treat drug-resistant TB infections. Section 3.4 covers the target-based TB drug discovery efforts at AstraZeneca, with major emphasis on gyrase inhibitors.

3.4. The AstraZeneca India (AZI) Effort

Gyrase as a target: One of the favorite targets for anti-TB drug discovery is the 'gyrase enzyme'. This is because of the multiple steps involved in the mechanistic of the 'negative supercoiling' enzyme reaction, several steps of which have been shown to be inhibitable [43]. Additionally, the availability of the several crystal structures of the enzyme has also helped in developing diverse screening approaches, as well as in building SAR of the identified inhibitors.

AZI employed multiple 'hit' generation approaches like high-throughput screening (HTS) of the AZ library, fragment library screening, targeted library screening, and pharmacophore-based screening, as well as virtual screening, in the quest for robust novel inhibitors. Shirude and Hameed [44] reviewed the features of the diverse set of inhibitors identified by the different groups. Several novel chemical entities were identified and are being investigated further (Table 1).

Table 1. Gyrase inhibitors identified at AstraZeneca (AZ).

Approach	Target	Inhibitor Series	Mechanism of Inhibition	Reference
Following known series	GyrB	Pyrrolamides	ATPase inhibitor	[45]
Pharmacophore based library	GyrB	Thiazolopyridine ureas	ATPase inhibitor	[46]
Pharmacophore based library, scaffold morphing	GyrB	Thiazolopyridone ureas	ATPase inhibitor	[47]
High throughput screening	GyrB	Aminopyrazinamides	ATPase, MTB gyrase specific. Novel binding mode.	[48]
Focused library screening	GyrB	Aminopiperidine	Non-ATP site binders, different from fluoroquinolones	[49]
Scaffold hopping	GyrB	Benzimidazoles	Non-ATP site binders, different from FQs	[50]

The key learning from these extensive efforts on 'revisiting gyrase as an established target' are as follows:

- A variety of novel chemical structures could be identified as potent starting points (Table 1).
- Several of these enzyme inhibitors showed an IC_{50}-MIC correlation.
- The inhibitors worked through different mechanisms; hence, they have a potential to avoid cross-resistance.
- These inhibitors were shown to have a higher potency against the MTB enzyme target, as compared to other bacterial gyrases, that translated into selectivity in their antimicrobial activity.

4. Target-Based Screening

The target-based lead identification approach was given a major impetus because of the following developments:

- The availability of the MTB genome sequence in 1998 [51] promised a new era both for studying the 'biology' of the pathogen and investigating novel pathways suitable for drug development. Several publications appeared, proving the essentiality of biochemical targets based on gene knockout studies in vitro, as well as investigations on the survival of the gene knockouts of MTB in the mouse model, confirming the essentiality of a variety of metabolic targets in vivo [52].
- Chris Lipinski et al. published the 'Lipinski rule of 5' for oral drugs [53]. The poor physiochemical properties of lead compounds vis a vis the 'Lipinski rule of 5' was shown to be the leading reason for the failure of potent compounds in the clinical trials, which was the direct result of poor pharmacokinetics. This led to the understanding of the concept of 'lead-like compounds' [54]. These rules served as guidelines for the selection/prioritization of 'hits' with a higher probability of being converted to drugs with favorable pharmacokinetics.

- This period also saw an enhanced efficiency in solving crystal structures; the macromolecular structures of several mycobacterial enzymes were solved and became key tools for the rationale design of novel inhibitors. A consortium of structural genomics groups was formed for facilitating the determination and analysis of structures of proteins from MTB [55].
- In addition to these facilitators of drug development, several public–private partnership consortia were also formed, which propelled interactions between the pharmaceutical industry and academic laboratories to engage in the TB drug discovery process. Examples include 'The Action TB program' (1996); the 'Global Alliance for TB' (GATB), which was launched in 2000; and the EU FW6/7 program entitled 'New Medicines for Tuberculosis' (NM4TB), which was launched in 2005, followed by the 'More Medicines for Tuberculosis' (MM4TB) program. Several pharmaceutical companies turned to target-based screening to find novel 'lead compounds' with a potential to inhibit the growth of MTB cells [56].
- Examples of efforts at AZI toward finding potent inhibitors by using target-based screening are summarized in Table 2. Though there are several publications on these efforts, it is interesting to view them in the context of the learning and the impact. A few of these programs were also in collaboration between AZI and partners of the NM4TB and MM4TB, the EU FW6, and seven programs, as well as with the Global Alliance for TB.

Table 2. Target-based efforts at AstraZeneca.

Approach	Target	Pathway	Inhibitor Class	Status Reached	Remarks	Reference
Known inhibitors	Acetolactate synthase	Branched chain amino acid biosynthesis	Triazolopyrimidine	IC_{50}~30 nM MIC0.5 μg/mL	Possible auxotrophy	[57,58]
Virtual screening	MtSK	Aromatic amino acid biosynthesis	Pyrazolones	IC_{50}~0. 6μM MIC 0.5 μg/mL	Possible promiscuity	[59,60]
Targeted Library	Pkn B	Cell division	Bis anilinopyrimidines (BAP)	IC_{50}~40 pM MIC 8 μg/mL	Possible redundancy	[61]
HTS	PanK	Coenzyme A (CoA) biosynthesis pathway	Triazoles (ATP competitive)	Nanomolar IC_{50}, not translating into microbial inhibition.	Possible Target vulnerability	[62–64]
HTS	PanK	Coenzyme A (CoA) biosynthesis pathway	Quinolones (ATP competitive)	Nanomolar IC_{50}, not translating into microbial inhibition.	Possible Target vulnerability	[62–64]
HTS	PanK	Coenzyme A (CoA) biosynthesis pathway	Biarylacetic acids (ATP non-competitive)	Nanomolar IC_{50}, not translating into microbial inhibition.	Possible Target vulnerability	[62–64]
HTS	TMK	DNA synthesis	3-Cyanopyridone	Nanomolar IC_{50}, not translating into microbial inhibition.	Possible redundancy	[65]
Fragment screening	TMK	DNA synthesis	1,6-Naphthyridinone	Nanomolar IC_{50}, not translating into microbial inhibition.	Possible redundancy	[65]
HTS	NdH2	Energy Metabolism	Quinolyl pyrimidines	Ndh2 IC_{50}: 96 nM MIC: <0.5 μg/mL	In progress	[66]

The key learning derived from these extensive studies are as follows:

a. The patterns obtained throw important light on both the characteristics of the target and the characteristics of the inhibitor.
b. The question of target vulnerability: Gene knockout studies for PanK demonstrated the essentiality of the gene product. However, elegant studies with the PanK target showed that modulation of enzyme levels (inferred based on regulating gene expression) altered the sensitivity of the MTB cell to inhibitors of the enzyme [62]. This change in vulnerability of the target was the reason attributed to the failure to obtaining bactericidal effects with the potent inhibitors.

c. Type of inhibition: Most of the inhibitors described in Table 2 were 'competitive' in nature, competing with the ATP site for binding. High-throughput screening mostly identifies 'competitive inhibitors' because of the design of the assay. The inhibition brought about by this type of inhibition is influenced by the 'substrate concentration', resulting in the modulation of target vulnerability [65].
d. Promiscuous targets: These types of targets are discussed later, in the lead generation approaches.
e. Established target: As described under Section 3.4, several inhibitors that have progressed to anti-TB drugs establish the 'vulnerability' of a target; ATP synthase (ATPS) is one such target. Bedaquiline, a non-competitive inhibitor of ATPS, is a front-line treatment for MDR TB [67,68].

5. Phenotypic Screening

This is a biology-driven effort where compound libraries are screened for antimycobacterial activity against mycobacterial cells in culture, and the 'hits' are progressed based on the potency both in vitro and in vivo [69]. This cell-based approach has been successful from the early days of TB discovery, and most of the frontline drugs were progressed based on the structure–activity relationship that was evaluated directly on the whole cells. Current-day phenotypic-screening approaches include the ability to identify inhibitors that are active against MTB cells growing in a variety of microenvironments that represent the replicating, the non-replicating, or bacilli in different physiological states [70]. Genetic probes have also facilitated the unravelling of the biological targets of the inhibitors.

Some of the examples of phenotypic-screening-derived compounds that have become drugs, or those in late clinical development, are discussed here.

a. **Bedaquiline:** Approved in 2012 for the treatment of MDR TB, Bedaquiline (TMC-207, R207910, shown in Figure 3) has the reputation of being the first FDA approved TB drug in more than four decades. It was discovered by Johnson & Johnson by screening more than 70,000 compounds against *Mycobacterium. smegmatis* (M.sm). The compound was first described in 2004, at the Interscience Conference on Antimicrobial Agents and Chemotherapy (ICAAC). The target of TMC-207 was later conclusively proven to be the MTB ATP synthase [68]. Subsequently, in 2012, Bedaquiline became an essential part of the MDR regimen [71,72]. Several combinations of Bedaquiline are also being investigated for their potential to reduce the duration of therapy [73]. Discovery of Bedaquiline and the target link has made MTB ATP synthase an attractive validated target.

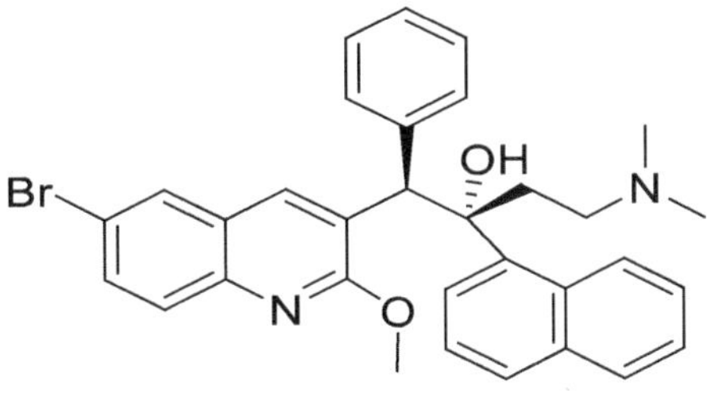

Bedaquiline (TMC-207, R207910)

Figure 3. Structure of Bedaquiline (TMC-207, R207910).

b. **Benzothiazinone (BTZ) and Macozinone (PBTZ):** BTZ was discovered at the Russian academy of science and developed with NM4TB, and it is presently being clinically evaluated under the Innovative Medicines for Tuberculosis (iM4TB). The target for BTZ has been shown as decaprenylphosphoryl-β-D-ribose-2′-oxidase (DprE1) by genetic and biochemical studies [74,75]. Based on SAR explorations, a piperazine derivative, PBTZ-169 (Macozinone), which has superior pharmacokinetics (PK), as compared to that of BTZ [76], was discovered and is currently in Phase 2 clinical trials, in addition to BTZ 043. Structures of BTZ and PBTZ are shown in Figure 4.

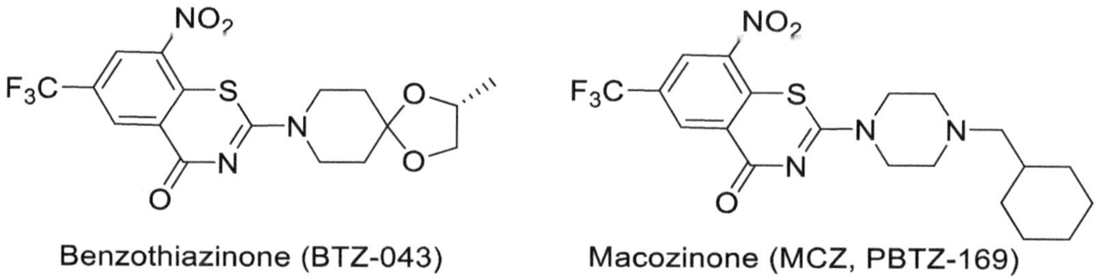

Figure 4. Structures of BTZ and PBTZ.

c. **Azaindoles:** These compounds emerged from a literature search for compounds similar to Q-203 [77,78]. The compound had an MIC but was not bactericidal. Scaffold morphing efforts on this compound at AZ Bangalore in a collaboration with TB alliance led to the identification of TBA 7371 [79–81], a potent DprE1 inhibitor with non-covalent binding. TBA 7371, jointly owned by Global Alliance for TB and the Foundation for Neglected Disease Research (FNDR), was developed by GATB through Phase 1 safety trials in humans. Recently, GATB has licensed TBA 7371 to Gates Medical Research Institute (GMRI); the news was disclosed in Union World conference of lung health at Hyderabad, India, in November 2019. GMRI is currently testing TBA7371 in Phase 2A clinical trials in TB patients [82]. The progression is depicted in Figure 5.

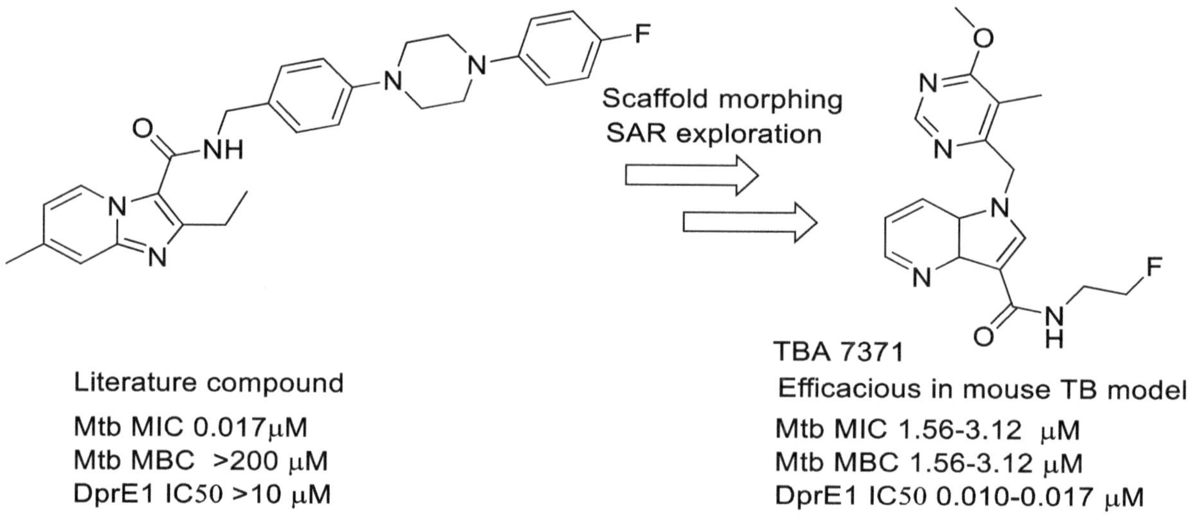

Figure 5. Evolution of TBA7371 which is in Phase 2A clinical trials in TB patients.

d. **Q203:** Telacebec (Q203) is a compound that was discovered by the researchers at Institute Pasteur, Korea, and is structurally very similar to the one discussed above [77,78]. This compound inhibits the cytochrome bc1 complex of MTB that is critical for the electron transport chain. The compound is in Phase 2 clinical trials [83]. Structure of Telacebec is shown in Figure 6.

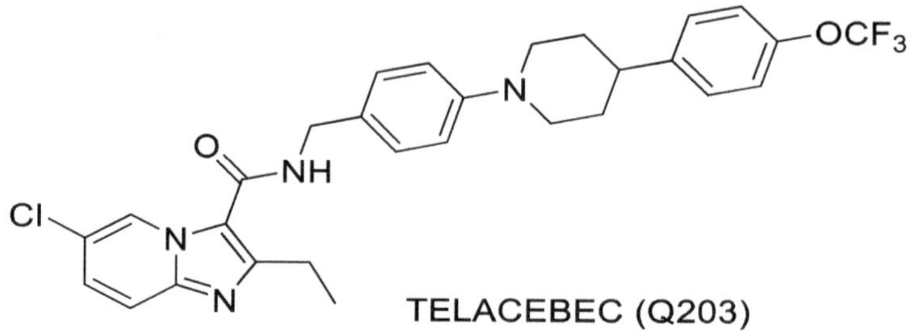

Figure 6. Structure of Telacebec.

e. **OPC-167832:** First discussed in 2016 at the 47th Union World Conference on Lung Health in Liverpool, UK, this is a carbostyril derivative that inhibits DPRE1. The structure shown in Figure 7 represents a balance of hydrophobic and hydrophilic residues. The compound is currently in Phase 2 clinical trials [84]. Structure of OPC-167832 is shown in Figure 7.

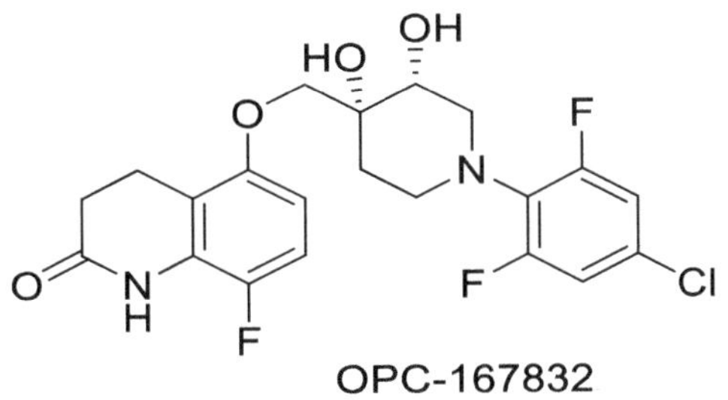

OPC-167832

Figure 7. Structure of OPC-167832.

Phenotypic-Screening Efforts at AstraZeneca India

The continued success of phenotypic screening as a viable alternative to discover novel inhibitors of MTB was based on its ability to circumvent the failure to convert enzyme inhibition into antibacterial activity. The advent of 'rapid sequencing technology' provided an impetus to this approach because of the ability to rapidly sequence the genome to elucidate mechanism of action. This led AZ India to focus on phenotypic screening for lead generation. A diversity library of 100,000 compounds was assembled and used for screening directly against both *M. smegmatis* or *Mycobacterium bovis* BCG cells as surrogates for MTB. Several novel scaffolds and their cognate targets were identified, confirming the validity of this approach; a short list of the results obtained is shown in Table 3. Many of the novel scaffolds identified were found to target DprE1 or the ATP synthase in target enzyme assays.

Table 3. Phenotypic screening-based efforts at AstraZeneca India (AZI).

Screening Mode	Target	Compound	Comments	Reference
HTS	DprE1	Benzothiazole	Promiscuous target	[85,86]
HTS	DprE1	4-Aminoquinoline piperidine amides	Promiscuous target	[87]
HTS	DprE1	Pyrazolopryridones	Promiscuous target	[88]
HTS	DprE1	Azaindoles	Promiscuous target	[79,80]
Scaffold hopping	DprE1	Benzimidazole	Promiscuous target	[81]
HTS	ATPS	Squaramide	Established/Validated Target	[89]
HTS	ATPS	Imidazopyridine	Established/Validated Target	[89]
Scaffold morphing	ATPS	Diaminoquinazoline	Established/Validated Target	[90]

6. The Anti-TB Pipeline—The Learning and the Gaps

6.1. The 'Evolution' of the Anti-TB Drug Pipeline

The anti-TB drug portfolio went from a 'no treatment' option to a successful therapy in ~20 years. The main properties of drugs in the regimen that was labeled 'Short Course Chemotherapy' were potency against the microbe, the ability to prevent relapse, and compatibility in terms of safety. The next phase, ~1980s, was the search for a compound that could shorten the course of the treatment. In the absence of 'physiologically' relevant in vitro and in vivo models to progress compounds for this property, it was indeed a 'black box' experimentation. However, with the spread of MDR TB, this focus turned to finding compounds 'active on MDR TB' and compatibility with the 'patient comorbidities', like HIV infection [91]. The concept of introducing 'broad-spectrum antibiotics' for the treatment of TB was a direct consequence of this shift; even the original trial that included 'ofloxacin' into the regimen was for reducing the duration of therapy [25]. Studies in animal models with a combination containing moxifloxacin showed that the combination had a potential to reduce the duration of therapy [92], and this was one of the end points in the trials with moxifloxacin in humans. However, the final results showed that, while the drug was effective, the combination did not reduce the duration of therapy, although it was efficacious on MDR, as well as on DS TB patients. The drug was introduced into the regimen to treat MDR TB [93].

The need for efficacious drugs for treating MDR TB became the 'new end point' for a drug. Both Bedaquiline and Delamanid fulfilled this criterion and are now parts of the new regimen [67,94].

There has been a concerted effort to understand the 'persister' population that is hypothesized to be difficult to eradicate and hence the need for prolonged duration of therapy [95,96]. The non-replicating persister (NRP) state has been the subject of intense investigations and several models representing this state have been developed. Both Bedaquiline and Delamanid are active against MTB bacilli growing under such conditions [16,67]. Further trials to investigate if this property of the new drugs will contribute to the reduction in therapy duration needs to be performed. In parallel, the portfolio is sure to see 'adjunct therapy' compounds that modulate the host response [92–95]. Repurposed candidate drugs offer faster development options and are also expected to enrich the TB portfolio [97–103]. These could also be weapons against the 'persister' population.

6.2. Lead Generation Approaches

The evolution of the anti-TB drug regimen, including the current portfolio, has followed a traceable pattern of periods. These periods are recognizable by the 'classes' of compounds that were introduced into the regimen. The different lead generation approaches and their accelerators are shown in Figure 8. Accelerators are defined as new knowledge or global exigencies. Each of these accelerators influenced lead generation methodology, to follow a certain approach during a certain period.

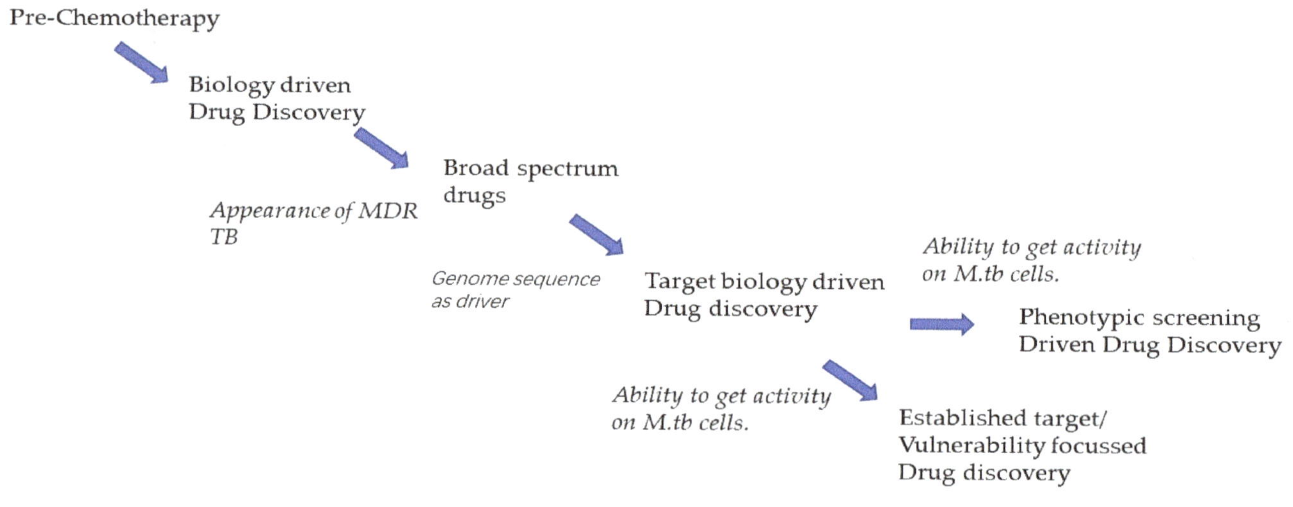

Figure 8. Evolution of lead generation approaches.

What is the current trend of preclinical 'hit' molecules being identified by using phenotypic screening? Mdluli et al. [104] have discussed this trend which indicates that the majority of these 'hits' act on the targets, namely DprE1, Mmpl3, and Cytochrome bcc complex. This has led to the coining of the term 'promiscuous targets'. The AstraZeneca 'hit' compound list also shows the same trend (Table 3). Why are these targets prone to get hit in phenotypic screens? The ultimate consequence of the so called 'promiscuity' on drug discovery will be fully answered by the clinical trial outcome of the compounds TBA737, BTZ043, PBTZ-169, OPC 167832 (DprE1 and Mmpl3), and Q203 (bcc1 complex) hitting such targets [105].

Another interesting trend is the increased number of compounds in later stages of development that are inhibitors of 'established targets'. This again adds to the concept of 'privileged targets' of MTB (privileged because the inhibition of these targets converts to an antimicrobial effect on MTB). Perhaps the so-called 'promiscuous targets' can also be classified as 'privileged targets'.

6.3. Has the Pipeline Evolved Based on the Significant Increase in the Knowledge of the 'Biology' of MTB?

In 1996, Mitchison in his Garrod lecture postulated the presence of different populations of MTB in the lungs of the TB patient [106]. Mitchison postulated the presence of the rapidly multiplying and the slow-growing populations of MTB, as well as the intracellular and extracellular niches of the organism. The last two decades have uncovered several shifts in the physiological state of the pathogen that are responses to both the immune mechanism of the host or the 'niche' in which the pathogen is proliferating [107]. The newer drugs like Bedaquiline, Pretomanid, and Delamanid have been shown to be active against MTB cells in the NRP state in vitro, as well as against the MTB bacilli multiplying within the macrophage [108,109]. However, these drugs were initially identified as inhibitors of the rapidly multiplying pathogen under in vitro culture conditions. It is generally accepted that the MTB population in the human host is a heterogeneous collection of the multiple 'physiological states' [69] that could indeed be a dynamic interchanging state. This raises two questions:

1. What is the value of having novel drugs that are active predominantly on one of the physiological states like the hypoxic or the intracellular state? Metronidazole is a known antiparasitic drug that is also active on MTB growing under oxygen-limiting conditions [110]. The addition of metronidazole to a cocktail of drugs for the treatment of MDR TB did not show clinical benefit [111]. On the other hand, several inhibitors of the intracellular survival of the pathogen in the macrophage have been identified, have been shown to be active in animal models of infection [34,67,77,83,112], and are undergoing clinical evaluation. These inhibitors potentially will facilitate the 'killing' of the pathogen within the macrophage, which in turn may reflect in 'faster' cure.
2. How do we develop molecules with activity against only specific subpopulations? The accepted path through the regulatory system is by showing superiority of the new combination over the existing standard of care (SOC) combination—a steep bar to cross. Until the beginning of this decade, very few efficacious drugs were available for the treatment of MDR TB patients. This provided the opportunity for newer efficacious drugs to show non-inferiority against the poorly active regimen, a bar, which was reasonable to go across. However, the current combination regimen for MDR TB treatment is efficacious, and newer compounds will have to demonstrate a clear advantage over the current regimen. Identification of novel biomarkers that can be evaluated during Phase 2a (Early Bactericidal Activity trials) could help in positioning these compounds that are active on specific populations to the best advantage.

Undoubtedly, there is a rapid expansion in the knowledge of the pathogen biology and its interaction with the host. Additionally, several novel inhibitors for pathways of the host that influence the survival of the bacilli have been identified. However, translational research must be supported to evaluate the potential of these compounds to become anti-TB drugs.

6.4. Combination Therapy: Finding Novel Combinations

What constitutes an 'ideal' combination? Faster time for sputum conversion, faster cure, tolerability, lower rates of drug resistance, lower relapse rates, combination suitable for treating pulmonary and extrapulmonary TB, and other properties, like compatible with comorbidities, etc. The concept of searching for novel combinations is recent; it was first advocated by the GATB [113] by studying a variety of combinations in humans using EBA. The two recently approved drugs, Bedaquiline and Delamanid, were progressed as add-ons to a cocktail of second-line drugs. Pretomanid, in combination with Bedaquiline and linezolid, has been approved for the treatment of XDR TB patients for whom there is very limited choice [73].

Another question is, can compounds active on the same target be compatible in the same combination? It is possible if the two inhibitors bind to different sites of the same targets, like in the examples of BTZ, PBTZ, and TBA7371. If the resistant mutants for the individual compounds do not confer cross-resistance, can such an approach bring additional advantage to the treatment? This can be relevant in the context of the so-called 'promiscuous targets' in TB and the diverse chemical inhibitors of these targets reported in recent years, e.g., benzothiazinones, azaindoles, and Q 203.

7. Going Forward

It is interesting to view the current anti-TB portfolio as a glass 'half full'. Novel efficacious compounds are in the late stages of clinical development [114–116]. This will offer the opportunity of designing new combinations. Several novel molecules are in the late discovery phase that will diversify the repertoire of potential anti-TB molecules. The challenge is to find simpler paths through the regulatory system that can demonstrate advantages with the molecule, as well as ensure safety. This will need concerted discussion with multiple stakeholders, which is already happening [117,118].

The secret to 'shortening therapy' needs to be unraveled, whether this will continue to be a hit-and-miss experimentation or further knowledge of the biology of the pathogen and will allow rational experimentation is not clear. Can adjunct therapy with immuno-modulators help, or will compounds acting on subpopulations that represent the 'difficult to treat' cells facilitate faster cure? Such questions need to be evaluated. This requires an urgent need to find novel translational approaches compatible with the regulatory framework to achieve this shift that, in turn, can create a paradigm shift in our modus operandi of how we treat this affliction.

8. Conclusions

Finding new drugs for the treatment of tuberculosis has been and continues to be a challenge despite the increased efforts over the last two decades. Lead generation approaches for MTB drug discovery have undergone several changes, mostly driven by an increased understanding of the biology of the pathogen, as well as the rapidly expanding knowledge on the biology of the interaction of the pathogen with the human host. This review chronicles the advances in a systematic study, starting from 'serendipitous discovery to phenotypic screening'. The technological advance mirrors the increased understanding of the biology of the pathogen. Interestingly, much of this increased understanding is also a consequence of the introduction of newer drugs for the treatment of tuberculosis.

Author Contributions: The authors contributed to the review in the following manner: Original idea of writing review (T.S.B., B.B. and R.K.S.), Conceptualization and frame work of the article (T.S.B., R.K.S., B.B. and J.B.), Data analysis (B.B., R.K.S. and J.B.) writing of review (T.S.B., B.B. and R.K.S.), data curation and editing (B.B., R.K.S. and J.B.) and writing of the article (T.S.B., B.B., R.K.S. and J.B.). All authors have read and agreed to the published version of the manuscript.

References

1. TB Facts.org, Information about Tuberculosis. Available online: https://tbfacts.org/history-of-tb-drugs/ (accessed on 13 April 2020).
2. Lehmann, J. Para-aminosalicylic acid in the treatment of Tuberculosis. *Lancet* **1946**, *247*, 15–16. [CrossRef]
3. Lehmann, J. Twenty years afterwards, Historical notes on the Discovery of the Antituberculosis Effect of Para-Aminosalicylic Acid (PAS) and the First Clinical Trials. *Am. Rev. Respir. Dis.* **1964**, *90*, 953–956.
4. Lehmann, E. Nicotinic acid in therapy of pulmonary tuberculosis; preliminary therapeutic report. *Dtsch. Med. Wochenschr.* **1952**, *77*, 1480–1481. [CrossRef]

5. Murray, F.M. Nicotinamide: An Oral Antimicrobial Agent with Activity against Both Mycobacterium tuberculosis and Human Immunodeficiency Virus. *Clin. Infect. Dis.* **2003**, *36*, 453–460. [CrossRef]
6. Thayer, J.D.; Seligman, R.B. The anti-tuberculous activity of some derivatives of p-aminosalicylic acid, nicotinic acid, and isonicotinic acid. *Antibiot. Chemother. (Northfield)* **1955**, *5*, 129–131.
7. Mitchison, D.A. Treatment of tuberculosis. The Mitchell lecture 1979. *J. R. Coll. Physicians Lond.* **1980**, *14*, 91.
8. Aquinas, M. Short-course therapy for tuberculosis. *Drugs* **1982**, *24*, 118–132. [CrossRef]
9. Mohammad, A. Rifampin and Their Analogs: A Development of Antitubercular Drugs. *World J. Org. Chem.* **2013**, *1*, 14–19.
10. Ramani, A.V.; Monika, A.; Indira, V.L.; Karyavardhi, G.; Venkatesh, J.; Jeankumar, V.U.; Manjashetty, T.H.; Yogeeswari, P.; Sriram, D. Synthesis of highly potent novel anti-tubercular isoniazid analogues with preliminary pharmacokinetic evaluation. *Bioorg. Med. Chem. Lett.* **2012**, *22*, 2764–2767. [CrossRef]
11. Yamamoto, S.; Toida, I.; Watanabe, N.; Ura, T. In vitro Antimycobacterial Activities of Pyrazinamide Analogs. *Antimicrob. Agents Chemother.* **1995**, *39*, 2088–2091. [CrossRef]
12. Häusler, H.; Kawakami, R.P.; Mlaker, E.; Severn, W.B.; Stütz, A.E. Ethambutol Analogues as Potential Antimycobacterial Agents. *Bioorg. Med. Chem. Lett.* **2001**, *11*, 1679–1681. [CrossRef]
13. Goldman, P. The development of 5-nitroimidazole for the treatment and prophylaxis of anaerobic bacterial infections. *J. Antimicrob. Chemother.* **1982**, *10*, 23–33. [CrossRef]
14. Ashtekar, D.R.; Costa-Perira, R.; Nagrajan, K.; Vishvanathan, N.; Bhatt, A.D.; Rittel, W. In vitro and in vivo activities of the nitroimidazole CGI 17341 against Mycobacterium tuberculosis. *Antimicrob. Agents Chemother.* **1993**, *37*, 183–186. [CrossRef]
15. Stover, C.K.; Warrener, P.; Van Devanter, D.R.; Sherman, D.R.; Arain, T.M.; Langhorne, M.H.; Anderson, S.W.; Towell, J.A.; Yuan, Y.; McMurray, D.N.; et al. A small-molecule nitroimidazopyran drug candidate for the treatment of tuberculosis. *Nature* **2000**, *405*, 962–966. [CrossRef]
16. Liu, Y.; Matsumoto, M.; Ishida, H.; Ohguro, K.; Yoshitake, M.; Gupta, R.; Geiter, L.; Hafkin, J. Delamanid: From discovery to its use for pulmonary multidrug-resistant tuberculosis (MDR-TB). *Tuberculosis* **2018**, *111*, 20–30. [CrossRef]
17. Sensi, P. History of the development of rifampin. *Rev. Infect. Dis.* **1983**, *5*, S402–S466. [CrossRef]
18. Janin, Y.L. Antituberculosis drugs: Ten years of research. *Bioorg. Med. Chem.* **2007**, *15*, 2479–2513. [CrossRef]
19. Bogatcheva, E.; Hanrahan, C.F.; Nikonenko, B.; Samala, R.; Chen, P.; Gearhart, J.; Barbosa, F.; Einck, L.; Nacy, A.C.A.; Protopopova, M. Identification of new diamine scaffolds with activity against Mycobacterium tuberculosis. *J. Med. Chem.* **2006**, *49*, 3045–3048. [CrossRef]
20. Yendapally, R.; Lee, R.E. Design, synthesis, and evaluation of novel ethambutol analogues. *Bioorg. Med. Chem. Lett.* **2008**, *18*, 1607–1611. [CrossRef]
21. Kapil, T.; Regina, W.; David, B.K.; Kriti, A.; Vinod, N.; Elizabeth, F.; Barnes, S.W.; John, R.W.; David, A.; Clifton, E.B., III; et al. SQ109 targets MmpL3, a membrane transporter of trehalose monomycolate involved in mycolic acid donation to the cell wall core of Mycobacterium tuberculosis. *Antimicrob. Agents Chemother.* **2012**, *56*, 1797–1809.
22. Sinha, N.; Jain, S.; Tilekar, A.; Upadhayaya, R.S.; Kishore, N.; Jana, G.H.; Arora, S.K. Synthesis of isonicotinic acid N′-arylidene-N-2-oxo-2-(4-aryl-piperazin-1-yl) ethyl-hydrazides as antituberculosis agents. *Bioorg. Med. Chem. Lett.* **2005**, *15*, 1573–1576. [CrossRef]
23. Sinha, R.K.; Arora, S.K.; Sinha, N.; Modak, V.M. In vivo activity of LL4858 against Mycobacterium tuberculosis. In Proceedings of the 44th Annual Interscience Conference on Antimicrobial Agents and Chemotherapy (ICAAC-2004), Washington, DC, USA, 30 October–2 November 2004.
24. World Health Organization. *Tuberculosis—A Global Emergency Case Notification Update: February 1996*; WHO Reference Number: WHO/TB/96.197; WHO: Geneva, Switzerland, 1996.
25. Hinshaw, H.; Pyle, M.M.; Feldman, W.H. Streptomycin in tuberculosis. *Am. J. Med.* **1947**, *2*, 429–435. [CrossRef]
26. Schecter, G.F.; Scott, C.; True, L.; Raftery, A.; Flood, J.; Mase, S. Linezolid in the Treatment of Multidrug-Resistant Tuberculosis. *Clin. Infect. Dis.* **2010**, *50*, 49–55. [CrossRef]
27. Maartens, G.; Benson, C.A. Linezolid for Treating Tuberculosis: A Delicate Balancing Act. *BioMedicine* **2015**, *2*, 1568–1569. [CrossRef]
28. Lee, M.; Song, T.; Kim, Y.; Jeong, I.; Cho, S.N.; Barry, C.E., III. Linezolid for XDR-TB—Final Study Outcomes. *N. Engl. J. Med.* **2015**, *373*, 290–291. [CrossRef]

29. Balasubramanian, V.; Solapure, S.; Shandil, R.; Gaonkar, S.; Mahesh, K.N.; Reddy, J.; Deshpande, A.; Bharath, S.; Kumar, N.; Wright, L.; et al. Pharmacokinetic and pharmacodynamic evaluation of AZD5847 in a mouse model of tuberculosis. *Antimicrob. Agents Chemother.* **2014**, *58*, 4185–4190. [CrossRef]
30. Balasubramanian, V.; Solapure, S.; Iyer, H.; Ghosh, A.; Sharma, S.; Kaur, P.; Deepthi, R.; Subbulakshmi, V.; Ramya, V.; Ramachandran, V.; et al. Bactericidal activity and mechanism of action of AZD5847, a novel oxazolidinone for treatment of tuberculosis. *Antimicrob. Agents Chemother.* **2013**, *58*, 495–502. [CrossRef]
31. Werngren, J.; Wijkander, M.; Perskvist, N.; Balasubramanian, V.; Sambandamurthy, V.K.; Rodrigues, C.; Hoffner, S. In vitro activity of AZD5847 against geographically diverse clinical isolates of Mycobacterium tuberculosis. *Antimicrob. Agents Chemother.* **2014**, *58*, 4222–4223. [CrossRef]
32. Williams, K.N.; Brickner, S.J.; Stover, C.K.; Zhu, T.; Ogden, A.; Tasneen, R.; Tyagi, S.; Grosset, J.H.; Nuermberger, E.L. Addition of PNU-100480 to First-Line Drugs Shortens the Time Needed to Cure Murine Tuberculosis. *Am. J. Respir. Crit. Care Med.* **2009**, *180*, 371–376. [CrossRef]
33. Lanoix, J.P.; Nuermberger, E. Sutezolid: Oxazolidinone antibacterial treatment of tuberculosis. *Drugs Future* **2013**, *38*, 387–394. [CrossRef]
34. Choi, Y.; Lee, S.W.; Kim, A.; Jang, K.; Nam, H.; Cho, Y.L.; Yu, K.-S.; Chung, J.-Y. Safety, tolerability and pharmacokinetics of 21 day multiple oral administration of a new oxazolidinone antibiotic, LCB01-0371, in healthy male subjects. *Antimicrob. Chemother.* **2018**, *73*, 183–190. [CrossRef]
35. Shoen, C.; DeStefano, M.; Hafkin, B.; Cynamon, M. In vitro and in vivo activity of contezolid (MRX-I) against M. tuberculosis. *Antimicrob. Agents Chemother.* **2018**, *62*, e00493-18. [CrossRef]
36. ClinicalTrails.gov. Phase 2 Trial to Evaluate the Early Bactericidal Activity, Safety and Tolerability of Meropenem Plus Amoxycillin/CA and Faropenem Plus Amoxycillin/CA in Adult Patients with Newly Diagnosed Pulmonary Tuberculosis. Available online: https://clinicaltrials.gov/ct2/show/NCT02349841 (accessed on 15 March 2020).
37. Palencia, A.; Li, X.; Bu, W.; Choi, W.; Ding, C.Z.; Easom, E.E.; Feng, L.; Hernandez, V.; Houston, P.; Liu, L.; et al. Discovery of Novel Oral Protein Synthesis Inhibitors of Mycobacterium tuberculosis That Target Leucyl-tRNA Synthetase. *Antimicrob. Agents Chemother.* **2016**, *60*, 6271–6280. [CrossRef]
38. Shoen, C.; DeStefano, M.; Pucci, M.; Cynamon, M. Evaluating the Sterilizing Activity of SPR720 in Combination Therapy against Mycobacterium Tuberculosis Infection in Mice, ASM Microbe 2019. Session P439 Poster AAR-749. Available online: https://www.newtbdrugs.org/pipeline/compound/spr720 (accessed on 19 March 2020).
39. Shoen, C.; Pucci, M.; DeStefano, M.; Cynamon, M. Efficacy of SPR720 and SPR750 Gyrase Inhibitors in a Mouse Mycobacterium tuberculosis Infection Model, ASM Microbe 2017. Session 336. Poster 43. Available online: https://www.abstractsonline.com/pp8/#!/4358/presentation/6167 (accessed on 25 March 2020).
40. Spero Therapeutics Receives FDA Orphan Drug Designation for SPR720 for the Treatment of on tuberculous Mycobacterial (NTM) Infection. Available online: https://www.globenewswire.com/news-release/2020/03/11/1998722 (accessed on 6 April 2020).
41. Narayanan, P. Shortening short course chemotherapy: A randomised clinical trial for treatment of smear positive pulmonary tuberculosis with regimens using ofloxacin in the intensive phase. *Indian J. Tuberc.* **2002**, *49*, 27–38.
42. Stephen, H.G. The role of moxifloxacin in tuberculosis therapy. *Eur. Respir. Rev.* **2016**, *25*, 19–28.
43. Nagaraja, V.; Godbole, A.A.; Henderson, S.R.; Maxwell, A. DNA topoisomerase I and DNA gyrase as targets for TB therapy. *Drug Discov. Today* **2017**, *22*, 510–518. [CrossRef]
44. Shirude, P.S.; Hameed, S. Nonfluoroquinolone-Based Inhibitors of Mycobacterial Type II Topoisomerase as Potential Therapeutic Agents for TB. *Annu. Rep. Med. Chem.* **2012**, *47*, 319–330.
45. Solapure, S.; Mukherjee, K.; Nandi, V.; Waterson, D.; Shandil, R.; Balganesh, M.; Sambandamurthy, V.K.; Raichurkar, A.K.; Deshpande, A.; Ghosh, A.; et al. Optimization of Pyrrolamides as Mycobacterial GyrB ATPase Inhibitors: Structure-Activity Relationship and In Vivo Efficacy in a Mouse Model of Tuberculosis. *Antimicrob. Agents Chemother.* **2014**, *58*, 61–70.
46. Kale, M.G.; Raichurkar, A.; Waterson, D.; McKinney, D.; Manjunatha, M.R.; Kranthi, U.; Koushik, K.; Jena, L.K.; Shinde, V.; Rudrapatna, S.; et al. Thiazolopyridine Ureas as Novel Antitubercular Agents Acting through Inhibition of DNA Gyrase B. *J. Med. Chem.* **2013**, *56*, 8834–8848.

47. Kale, R.R.; Kale, M.G.; Waterson, D.; Raichurkar, A.; Hameed, S.P.; Manjunatha, M.R.; Reddy, B.K.; Malolanarasimhan, K.; Shinde, V.; Koushik, K.; et al. Thiazolopyridoneureas as DNA gyrase B inhibitors: Optimization of antitubercular activity and efficacy. *Bioorg. Med. Chem. Lett.* **2014**, *24*, 870–879. [CrossRef]
48. Shirude, P.S.; Madhavapeddi, P.; Tucker, J.A.; Murugan, K.; Patil, V.; Basavarajappa, H.D.; Raichurkar, A.V.; Humnabadkar, V.; Hussein, S.; Sharma, S.; et al. Aminopyrazinamides: Novel and Specific GyrB Inhibitors that Kill Replicating and Nonreplicating Mycobacterium tuberculosis. *ACS Chem. Biol.* **2013**, *8*, 519–523. [CrossRef]
49. Hameed, P.S.; Patil, V.; Solapure, S.; Sharma, U.; Madhavapeddi, P.; Raichurkar, A.; Chinnapattu, M.; Manjrekar, P.; Shanbhag, G.; Puttur, J.; et al. Novel N-Linked Aminopiperidine-Based Gyrase Inhibitors with Improved hERG and in Vivo Efficacy against Mycobacterium tuberculosis. *J. Med. Chem.* **2014**, *57*, 4889–4905.
50. Hameed, P.S.; Raichurkar, A.; Madhavapeddi, P.; Menasinakai, S.; Sharma, S.; Kaur, P.; Nandishaiah, R.; Panduga, V.; Reddy, J.; Sambandamurthy, V.K.; et al. Benzimidazoles: Novel Mycobacterial Gyrase Inhibitors from Scaffold Morphing. *ACS Med. Chem. Lett.* **2014**, *5*, 820–825. [CrossRef]
51. Cole, S.T.; Brosch, R.; Parkhill, J.; Garnier, T.; Churcher, C.; Harris, D.; Gordon, S.; Eiglmeier, K.; Gas, S.; Barry, C.E.; et al. Deciphering the biology of Mycobacterium tuberculosis from the complete genome sequence. *Nature* **1998**, *393*, 537–544. [CrossRef]
52. Vashisht, R.; Bhat, A.G.; Kushwaha, S.; Bhardwaj, A.; OSDD Consortium; Brahmachari, S.K. Systems level mapping of metabolic complexity in Mycobacterium tuberculosis to identify high-value drug target. *J. Transl. Med.* **2014**, *12*, 263. [CrossRef]
53. Lipinski, C.A.; Lombardo, F.; Dominy, B.W.; Feeney, P.J. Experimental and computational approaches to estimate solubility and permeability in drug discovery and development settings. *Adv. Drug Deliv. Rev.* **1997**, *23*, 3–25. [CrossRef]
54. Teague, S.J.; Davis, A.M.; Leeson, P.D.; Oprea, T. The Design of Lead like Combinatorial Libraries. *Angew. Chem. Int. Ed. Eng.* **1999**, *28*, 3743–3748. [CrossRef]
55. Terwilliger, T.C.; Park, M.; Waldo, G.; Berendzen, J.; Hung, L.-W.; Kim, C.-Y.; Smith, C.; Sacchettini, J.; Bellinzoni, M.; Bossi, R.; et al. The TB structural genomics consortium: A resource for Mycobacterium tuberculosis biology. *Tuberculosis* **2003**, *83*, 223–249. [CrossRef]
56. Yuan, T.; Sampson, N.S. Hit Generation in TB Drug Discovery: From Genome to Granuloma. *Chem. Rev.* **2018**, *118*, 1887–1916. [CrossRef]
57. Patil, V.; Kale, M.; Raichurkar, A.; Bhaskar, B.; Prahlad, D.; Balganesh, M.; Nandan, S.; Shahul Hameed, P. Design and synthesis of triazolopyrimidineacylsulfonamides as novel anti-mycobacterial leads acting through inhibition of acetohydroxyacid synthase. *Bioorg. Med. Chem. Lett.* **2014**, *24*, 2222–2225. [CrossRef]
58. Balganesh, M.; Nandan, S. Combination Chemotherapy for Tuberculosis by Synergistic Action of Rifampicin as the RNA Polymerase Inhibitors with Acetolactate Synthase Inhibitors. PCT International Application WO 2007132189 A1 20071122, 22 November 2007.
59. Bandodkar, B.S.; Naik, M.; Ghorpade, S.; Kale, M.; Shanbhag, G.; Patil, V.; Solapure, S.; Balganesh, M.; Shandil, R.K.; Balasubramanian, B.; et al. Lead Generation via Virtual Screening: Discovery of Pyrazolones as Potent Antimycobacterial Leads through structure based virtual screening of shikimate kinase. In Proceedings of the ICAAC 2009, San Francisco, CA, USA, 12–15 September 2009.
60. Bandodkar, B.S.; Schmitt, S. Pyrazolone Derivatives for the Treatment of Tuberculosis. PCT International Application No. WO/2007/020426 A1, 22 February 2007.
61. Bandodkar, B.S. Oral presentation, "A decade of learning". In Proceedings of the CSIR-NM4TB Symposium, Bangalore, India, 14 December 2009.
62. Venkatraman, J.; Bhat, J.; Solapure, S.M.; Sandesh, J.; Sarkar, D.; Aishwarya, S.; Mukherjee, K.; Datta, S.; Malolanarasimhan, K.; Bandodkar, B.; et al. Screening, Identification, and Characterization of Mechanistically Diverse Inhibitors of the Mycobacterium Tuberculosis Enzyme, Pantothenate Kinase (CoaA). *J. Biomol. Screen.* **2012**, *17*, 293. [CrossRef] [PubMed]
63. Reddy, B.K.K.; Landge, S.; Ravishankar, S.; Patil, V.; Shinde, V.; Tantry, S.; Kale, M.; Raichurkar, A.; Menasinakai, S.; Mudugal, N.V.; et al. Assessment of Mycobacterium tuberculosis Pantothenate Kinase Vulnerability through Target Knockdown and Mechanistically Diverse Inhibitors. *Antimicrob. Agents Chemother.* **2014**, *8*, 3312–3326. [CrossRef]

64. Björkelid, C.; Bergfors, T.; Raichurkar, A.K.V.; Mukherjee, K.; Malolanarasimhan, K.; Bandodkar, B.; Jones, T.A. Structural and Biochemical Characterization of Compounds Inhibiting Mycobacterium tuberculosis Pantothenate Kinase. *J. Biol. Chem.* **2013**, *288*, 18260–18270. [CrossRef]
65. Naik, M.; Raichurkar, A.; Bandodkar, B.S.; Varun, B.V.; Bhat, S.; Kalkhambkar, R.; Murugan, K.; Menon, R.; Bhat, J.; Paul, B.; et al. Structure Guided Lead Generation for M. tuberculosis Thymidylate Kinase (Mtb TMK): Discovery of 3-Cyanopyridone and 1,6-Naphthyridin-2-one as Potent Inhibitors. *J. Med. Chem.* **2015**, *58*, 755–766.
66. Shirude, P.S.; Paul, B.; Choudhury, N.R.; Kedari, C.; Bandodkar, B.; Ugarkar, B.G. Quinolinyl Pyrimidines: Potent Inhibitors of NDH-2 as a Novel Class of Anti-TB Agents. *ACS Med. Chem. Lett.* **2012**, *3*, 736–740. [CrossRef]
67. Andries, K. A diarylquinoline drug active on the ATP Synthase of Mycobacterium tuberculosis. *Science* **2006**, *307*, 223–227. [CrossRef]
68. Koul, A.; Dendouga, N.; Vergauwen, K.; Molenberghs, B.; Vranckx, L.; Willebrords, R.; Ristic, Z.; Lill, H.; Dorange, I.; Guillemont, J.; et al. Diarylquinolines target subunit c of mycobacterial ATP synthase. *Nat. Chem. Biol.* **2007**, *3*, 323–324. [CrossRef]
69. Grzelak, E.M.; Choules, M.P.; Gao, W.; Cai, G.; Wan, B.; Wang, Y.; McAlpine, J.B.; Cheng, J.; Jin, Y.; Lee, H.; et al. Strategies in anti-Mycobacterium tuberculosis drug discovery based on phenotypic screening. *J. Antibiot.* **2019**, *72*, 719–728. [CrossRef]
70. Manjunatha, U.H.; Smith, P.W. Perspective: Challenges and opportunities in TB drug discovery from phenotypic screening. *Bioorg. Med. Chem.* **2015**, *23*, 5087–5097. [CrossRef]
71. Matteelli, A.; Carvalho, A.C.; E Dooley, K.; Kritski, A. TMC207: The first compound of a new class of potent anti-tuberculosis drugs. *Future Microbiol.* **2010**, *5*, 849–858. [CrossRef]
72. Deoghare, S. Bedaquiline: A new drug approved for treatment of multidrug-resistant tuberculosis. *Indian J. Pharmacol.* **2013**, *45*, 536–537. [CrossRef] [PubMed]
73. Conradie, F.; Diacon, A.H.; Ngubane, N.; Howell, P.; Everitt, D.; Crook, A.M.; Mendel, C.M.; Egizi, E.; Moreira, J.; Timm, J.; et al. Bedaquiline, pretomanid and linezolid for treatment of extensively drug resistant, intolerant or non-responsive multidrug resistant pulmonary tuberculosis. *N. Engl. J. Med.* **2020**, *382*, 893–902. [CrossRef] [PubMed]
74. Makarov, V.; Manina, G.; Mikusova, K.; Möllmann, U.; Ryabova, O.; Saint-Joanis, B.; Dhar, N.; Pasca, M.R.; Buroni, S.; Lucarelli, A.P.; et al. Benzothiazinones Kill Mycobacterium tuberculosis by Blocking Arabinan Synthesis. *Science* **2009**, *324*, 801–804. [CrossRef] [PubMed]
75. Trefzer, C.; Rengifo-Gonzalez, M.; Hinner, M.J.; Schneider, P.; Makarov, V.; Cole, S.T.; Johnsson, K. Benzothiazinones: Prodrugs That Covalently Modify the Decaprenylphosphoryl-D-ribose 2′-epimerase DprE1 of Mycobacterium tuberculosis. *J. Am. Chem. Soc.* **2010**, *132*, 13663–13665. [CrossRef] [PubMed]
76. Makarov, V.; Lechartier, B.; Zhang, M.; Neres, J.; Sar, A.M.; A Raadsen, S.; Hartkoorn, R.C.; Ryabova, O.B.; Vocat, A.; Decosterd, L.A.; et al. Towards a new combination therapy for tuberculosis with next generation benzothiazinones. *EMBO Mol. Med.* **2014**, *6*, 372–383. [CrossRef] [PubMed]
77. No, Z.; Kim, J.; Brodin, P.B.; Seo, M.J.; Kim, Y.M.; Cechetto, J.; Jeon, H.; Genovesio, A.; Lee, S.; Kang, S.; et al. Anti-Infective Compounds. PCT Publication No. WO 2011/113606 A1, 22 September 2011.
78. No, Z.; Kim, J.; Brodin, P.; Seo, M.J.; Park, E.; Cechetto, J.; Jeon, H.; Genovesio, A.; Lee, S.; Kang, S.; et al. Anti-Infective pyrido (1,2-a) pyrimidines. PCT Publication No. WO 2011/085990 A1, 21 July 2011.
79. Shirude, P.S.; Shandil, R.; Sadler, C.; Naik, M.; Hosagrahara, V.; Hameed, S.; Shinde, V.; Bathula, C.; Humnabadkar, V.; Kumar, N.; et al. Azaindoles: Noncovalent DprE1 Inhibitors from Scaffold Morphing Efforts, Kill Mycobacterium tuberculosis and Are Efficacious In Vivo. *J. Med. Chem.* **2013**, *56*, 9701–9708. [PubMed]
80. Chatterji, M.; Shandil, R.; Manjunatha, M.R.; Solapure, S.; Ramachandran, V.; Kumar, N.; Saralaya, R.; Panduga, V.; Reddy, J.; Kr, P.; et al. 1, 4-Azaindole, a Potential Drug Candidate for Treatment of Tuberculosis. *Antimicrob. Agents Chemother.* **2014**, *58*, 5325–5331. [CrossRef] [PubMed]
81. Manjunatha, M.R.; Shandil, R.K.; Panda, M.; Sadler, C.; Ambady, A.; Panduga, V.; Kumar, N.; Mahadevaswamy, J.; Sreenivasaiah, M.; Narayan, A.; et al. Scaffold Morphing to Identify Novel DprE1 Inhibitors with Antimycobacterial Activity. *ACS Med. Chem. Lett.* **2019**, *10*, 1480–1485.
82. Early Bactericidal Activity of TBA-7371 in Pulmonary Tuberculosis, Identifier: NCT04176250. Available online: https://clinicaltrials.gov (accessed on 2 April 2020).

83. Pethe, K.; Bifani, P.J.; Jang, J.; Kang, S.; Park, S.; Ahn, S.; Jiricek, J.; Jung, J.; Jeon, H.K.; Cechetto, J.; et al. Discovery of Q203, a potent clinical candidate for the treatment of tuberculosis. *Nat. Med.* **2013**, *19*, 1157–1160. [CrossRef]
84. Otsuka Awarded Grant to Advance Development of Novel Anti-Tuberculosis Compound OPC-167832 with Delamanid. Available online: https://www.businesswire.com/news/home/20180129005073/en/ (accessed on 11 April 2020).
85. Landge, S.; Mullick, A.B.; Nagalapur, K.; Neres, J.; Subbulakshmi, V.; Murugan, K.; Ghosh, A.; Sadler, C.; Fellows, M.D.; Humnabadkar, V.; et al. Discovery of benzothiazoles as antimycobacterial agents: Synthesis, structure–activity relationships and binding studies with Mycobacterium tuberculosis decaprenylphosphoryl-b-D-ribose 20-oxidase. *Bioorg. Med. Chem.* **2015**, *23*, 7694–7710. [CrossRef]
86. Landge, S.; Ramachandran, V.; Kumar, A.; Neres, J.; Murugan, K.; Sadler, C.; Fellows, M.D.; Humnabadkar, V.; Vachaspati, P.; Raichurkar, A.; et al. Nitroarenes as Antitubercular Agents: Stereoelectronic Modulation to Mitigate Mutagenicity. *Chemmedchem* **2016**, *11*, 331–339. [CrossRef] [PubMed]
87. Naik, M.; Humnabadkar, V.; Tantry, S.J.; Panda, M.; Narayan, A.; Guptha, S.; Panduga, V.; Manjrekar, P.; Jena, L.K.; Koushik, K.; et al. 4-Aminoquinolone Piperidine Amides: Noncovalent Inhibitors of DprE1 with Long Residence Time and Potent Antimycobacterial Activity. *J. Med. Chem.* **2014**, *57*, 5419–5434.
88. Panda, M.; Ramachandran, S.; Ramachandran, V.; Shirude, P.S.; Humnabadkar, V.; Nagalapur, K.; Sharma, S.; Kaur, P.; Guptha, S.; Narayan, A.; et al. Discovery of Pyrazolopyridones as a Novel Class of Noncovalent DprE1 Inhibitor with Potent Anti-Mycobacterial Activity. *J. Med. Chem.* **2014**, *57*, 4761–4771. [PubMed]
89. Tantry, S.J.; Markad, S.D.; Shinde, V.; Bhat, J.; Balakrishnan, G.; Gupta, A.K.; Ambady, A.; Raichurkar, A.; Kedari, C.; Sharma, S.; et al. Discovery of Imidazo[1,2-a]pyridine Ethers and Squaramides as Selective and Potent Inhibitors of Mycobacterial Adenosine Triphosphate (ATP) Synthesis. *J. Med. Chem.* **2017**, *60*, 1379–1399. [PubMed]
90. Tantry, S.J.; Shinde, V.; Balakrishnan, G.; Markad, S.D.; Gupta, A.K.; Bhat, J.; Narayan, A.; Raichurkar, A.; Jena, L.K.; Sharma, S.; et al. Scaffold morphing leading to evolution of 2,4-diaminoquinolines and aminopyrazolopyrimidines as inhibitors of the ATP synthesis pathway. *MedChemComm* **2016**, *7*, 1022–1032. [CrossRef]
91. Gandhi, N.R.; Nunn, P.; Dheda, K.; Schaaf, H.S.; Zignol, M.; Van Soolingen, D.; Jensen, P.; Bayona, J. Multidrug-resistant and extensively drug-resistant tuberculosis: A threat to global control of tuberculosis. *Lancet* **2010**, *375*, 1830–1843. [CrossRef]
92. Nuermberger, E.; Yoshimatsu, T.; Tyagi, S.; O'Brien, R.J.; Vernon, A.N.; Chaisson, R.E.; Bishai, W.R.; Grosset, J. 2004. Moxifloxacin-containing Regimen Greatly Reduces Time to Culture Conversion in Murine Tuberculosis. *Am. J. Respir. Crit. Care Med.* **2003**, *169*, 421–426. [CrossRef]
93. Gillespie, S.H.; Crook, A.M.; McHugh, T.D.; Mendel, C.M.; Meredith, S.K.; Murray, S.R.; Pappas, F.; Phillips, P.P.; Nunn, A.J. Four-Month Moxifloxacin-Based Regimens for Drug-Sensitive Tuberculosis. *N. Eng. J. Med.* **2014**, *351*, 1577–1587. [CrossRef]
94. Mabhula, A.; Singh, V. Drug-resistance in Mycobacterium tuberculosis: Where we stand. *MedChemComm* **2019**, *10*, 1342–1360. [CrossRef]
95. Muñoz-Elías, E.J.; Timm, J.; Botha, T.; Chan, W.T.; Gomez, J.E.; McKinney, J.D. Replication Dynamics of *Mycobacterium tuberculosis* in Chronically Infected Mice. *Infect. Immun.* **2005**, *73*, 546–551. [CrossRef]
96. Mitchison, D.A. Role of individual drugs in the chemotherapy of tuberculosis. *Int. J. Tuberc. Lung Dis.* **2004**, *4*, 796–806.
97. Rayasam, G.V.; Balganesh, T.S. Exploring the potential of adjunct therapy in tuberculosis. *Trends Pharmacol. Sci.* **2015**, *36*, 506–513. [CrossRef] [PubMed]
98. Zumla, A.; Chakaya, J.; Hoelscher, M.; Ntoumi, F.; Rustomjee, R.; Vilaplana, C.; Yeboah-Manu, D.; Rasolofo, V.; Munderi, P.; Singh, N.; et al. Towards host-directed therapies for tuberculosis. *Nat. Rev. Drug Discov.* **2015**, *14*, 511–512. [CrossRef] [PubMed]
99. Zumla, A.; Rao, M.; Wallis, R.S.; Kaufmann, S.H.; Rustomjee, R.; Mwaba, P.; Vilaplana, C.; Yeboah-Manu, D.; Chakaya, J.; Ippolito, G.; et al. Host-directed therapies for infectious diseases: Current status, recent progress and future prospects. *Lancet Infect. Dis.* **2016**, *16*, e47–e63. [CrossRef]
100. Kumar, D.; Nath, L.; Kamal, A.; Varshney, A.; Jain, A.; Singh, S.; Rao, K.V.; Singh, S. Genome-wide analysis of the host intracellular network that regulates survival of Mycobacterium tuberculosis. *Cell* **2010**, *140*, 731–743. [CrossRef]

101. Singhal, A.; Jie, L.; Kumar, P.; Hong, G.S.; Leow, M.K.-S.; Paleja, B.; Tsenova, L.; Kurepina, N.; Chen, J.; Zolezzi, F.; et al. Metformin as adjunct antituberculosis therapy. *Sci. Transl. Med.* **2014**, *263*, 263ra159. [CrossRef]
102. Mishra, R.; Kohli, S.; Malhotra, N.; Bandyopadhyay, P.; Mehta, M.; Munshi, M.; Adiga, V.; Ahuja, V.K.; Shandil, R.K.; Rajmani, R.S.; et al. Targeting redox heterogeneity to counteract drug tolerance in replicating Mycobacterium tuberculosis. *Sci. Transl. Med.* **2019**, *11*, eaaw6635. [CrossRef]
103. Padmapriyadarsini, C.; Bhavani, P.K.; Natrajan, M.; Ponnuraja, C.; Kumar, H.; Gomathy, S.N.; Guleria, R.; Jawahar, S.M.; Singh, M.; Balganesh, T.; et al. Evaluation of metformin in combination with rifampicin containing antituberculosis therapy in patients with new, smear-positive pulmonary tuberculosis (METRIF): Study protocol for a randomised clinical trial. *BMJ Open* **2019**, *9*, e024363. [CrossRef]
104. Mdluli, K.; Kaneko, T.; Upton, A. The Tuberculosis Drug Discovery andDevelopment Pipeline and Emerging Drug Targets. *Cold Spring Harb. Perspect. Med.* **2015**, *5*, a021154. [CrossRef]
105. Roy, K.K.; Wani, M.A. Emerging opportunities of exploiting electron transport chain pathway for drug resistant tuberculosis drug discovery. *Expert Opin. Drug Discov.* **2020**, *15*, 231–241. [CrossRef]
106. Mitchison, D.A. The action of antituberculosis drugs in short-course chemotherapy. *Tubercle* **1985**, *66*, 219–225. [CrossRef]
107. Jindani, A.; Doré, C.J.; Mitchison, D.A. The bactericidal and sterilising activities of antituberculosis drugs during the first 14 days. *Am. J. Respir. Crit. Care Med.* **2003**, *167*, 1348–1354. [CrossRef]
108. Hernandez-Pando, R. Persistence of DNA from Mycobacterium tuberculosis in superficially normal lung tissue during latent infection. *Lancet* **2004**, *356*, 2133–2137. [CrossRef]
109. Mitchison, D.A. The search for new sterilizing anti-tuberculosis drugs. *Front. Biosci.* **2004**, *9*, 1059–1072. [CrossRef] [PubMed]
110. Waynel, L.G.; Hilda, A. Metronidazole is bactericidal to dormant cells of Mycobacterium tuberculosis. *Antimicrob. Agents Chemother.* **1994**, *38*, 2054–2058. [CrossRef] [PubMed]
111. Carroll, M.W. Efficacy and safety of metronidazole for pulmonary multidrug resistant tuberculosis. *Antimicrob. Agents Chemother.* **2013**, *57*, 3903–3909. [CrossRef]
112. Tyagi, S.; Nuermberger, E.; Yoshimatsu, T.; Williams, K.; Rosenthal, I.; Lounis, N.; Bishai, W.; Grosset, J. Bactericidal activity of the nitroimidazopyranPA-824 in a murine model of tuberculosis. *Antimicrob. Agents Chemother.* **2005**, *49*, 2289–2293. [CrossRef]
113. Dooley, K.E.; Hanna, D.; Mave, V.; Eisenach, K.; Savic, R.M. Advancing the development of new tuberculosis treatment regimens: The essential role of translational and clinical pharmacology and microbiology. *PLoS Med.* **2019**, *16*, e1002842. [CrossRef]
114. Nimmo, C.; Naidoo, K.; O'Donnell, M.; Bolhuis, M.S.; Van Der Werf, T.S.; Akkerman, O.W.; Conradie, F.; Everitt, D.; Crook, A.M. Treatment of Highly Drug-Resistant Pulmonary Tuberculosis. *N. Engl. J. Med.* **2020**, *382*, 893–902.
115. Diacon, A.H.; Dawson, R.; Von Groote-Bidlingmaier, F.; Symons, G.; Venter, A.; Donald, P.R.; Van Niekerk, C.; Everitt, D.; Winter, H.; Becker, P.; et al. 14-Day bactericidal activity of PA-824, bedaquiline, pyrazinamide, and moxifloxacin combinations: A randomised trial. *Lancet* **2012**, *380*, 986–993. [CrossRef]
116. McHugh, T.D.; Honeyborne, I.; Lipman, M.; Zumla, A. Revolutionary new regimens for multidrug resistant tuberculosis. *Lancet* **2018**, *19*, 233–234. [CrossRef]
117. Working Group on New TB Drugs. Available online: https://www.newtbdrugs.org/ (accessed on 13 April 2020).
118. TB Facts.org, New-Tb-Drugs. Available online: https://tbfacts.org/new-tb-drugs/ (accessed on 13 April 2020).

7

Host-Directed Therapies and Anti-Virulence Compounds to Address Anti-Microbial Resistant Tuberculosis Infection

Raphael Gries [1,2], Claudia Sala [3] and Jan Rybniker [1,2,4,*]

1 Department I of Internal Medicine, Division of Infectious Diseases, University of Cologne, 50931 Cologne, Germany; raphael.gries@uk-koeln.de
2 Center for Molecular Medicine Cologne, University of Cologne, 50931 Cologne, Germany
3 Fondazione Toscana Life Sciences, 53100 Siena, Italy; c.sala@toscanalifesciences.org
4 German Center for Infection Research (DZIF), Partner Site Bonn-Cologne, 50931 Cologne, Germany
* Correspondence: jan.rybniker@uk-koeln.de.

Abstract: Despite global efforts to contain tuberculosis (TB), the disease remains a leading cause of morbidity and mortality worldwide, further exacerbated by the increased resistance to antibiotics displayed by the tubercle bacillus *Mycobacterium tuberculosis*. In order to treat drug-resistant TB, alternative or complementary approaches to standard anti-TB regimens are being explored. An area of active research is represented by host-directed therapies which aim to modulate the host immune response by mitigating inflammation and by promoting the antimicrobial activity of immune cells. Additionally, compounds that reduce the virulence of *M. tuberculosis*, for instance by targeting the major virulence factor ESX-1, are being given increased attention by the TB research community. This review article summarizes the current state of the art in the development of these emerging therapies against TB.

Keywords: tuberculosis; *Mycobacterium tuberculosis*; host-directed therapy; anti-virulence compounds

1. Introduction

Mycobacterium tuberculosis, the etiological agent of human tuberculosis (TB), is thought to latently infect approximately one fourth of the world's population and is responsible for over one million deaths every year [1], thus representing the leading cause of mortality by an infectious disease worldwide. Immunodeficiency caused by HIV [2] and co-morbidities like diabetes [3] constitute additional risk factors for the development of active TB disease.

The current anti-TB therapy consists of a combination of four antibiotics (rifampicin, isoniazid, pyrazinamide and ethambutol) that must be administered for at least 6 months in case of drug-sensitive pulmonary TB infection [4]. However, *M. tuberculosis* displays increased resistance to first-line drugs, which has resulted in multidrug-resistant (MDR) and extensively drug-resistant (XDR) TB cases [5]. Second-line treatment regimens are therefore employed but require longer duration to be effective and are associated with severe side effects that frequently decrease patient compliance [6].

To address the increasing need for new and potent therapeutic options against TB, alternative approaches are being explored. These include host-directed therapy (HDT) and anti-virulence compounds. Within the first choice, a number of molecules that reduce inflammation, modulate autophagy and potentiate the immune response are currently in preclinical and in clinical trials. On the other hand, drugs that affect *M. tuberculosis* ability to infect and kill host cells represent a promising complement to standard antibiotic treatment.

Here we review the current state of research in the areas of HDT and anti-virulence drugs as complementary approaches to TB therapy.

2. Host Directed Therapy

2.1. Promoting Phagosome Maturation and Enhancing Autophagy

Autophagy is a natural process which protects cells against unfolded proteins and potentially dangerous aggregates, viral and bacterial infections. By means of autophagy, macrophages deliver toxic macromolecules, organelles and phagocytosed pathogens to lysosomes for degradation [7]. Modulating autophagy in order to promote bacterial killing represents one example of HDT against TB infection. This statement is supported by studies conducted by Gutierrez and co-workers who reported that stimulation of autophagy in macrophages promotes phago-lysosome maturation and impacts mycobacterial survival [8]. More recent investigations revealed increased susceptibility to TB in mice defective in autophagy pathways [9] and a positive interplay between autophagy and interferon-gamma (IFN-γ) in TB patients [10].

2.1.1. mTOR Inhibition

The best described autophagy inducer is rapamycin (sirolimus), used in patients who underwent organ transplantation [11]. Rapamycin, a macrolide produced by *Streptomyces hygroscopicus* and originally discovered on Easter Island (Rapa Nui for the inhabitants, hence the name given to the compound), inhibits TOR, the Target Of Rapamycin [12]. The mammalian Target of Rapamycin mTOR is a negative regulator of autophagy [13]. Its clinical use in infectious diseases is restricted due to its broadly immunosuppressive effects. In addition, rapamycin is metabolized by CYP3A4 [14], a hepatic enzyme induced by the first-line TB drug rifampicin, thus hampering its exploitation as HDT in TB patients. However, other molecules capable of inducing autophagy have been discovered and are now under development. Among these, vadimezan [15], Tat-beclin 1 fusion peptide [16], the calcium-channel blocker verapamil [17] and the rapamycin analogue everolimus [18]. In particular, verapamil was shown to be efficacious when combined with rifampicin and with the recently approved medication bedaquiline in mouse models of infection, where it increased the bioavailability of the antibiotic [19–21]. On the other hand, everolimus, an anti-cancer agent, may be repurposed as an anti-TB HDT therapeutic capable of inhibiting mTOR although, as with rapamycin, immunosuppression [22] and toxicity [23] may represent issues in the clinical development as an anti-TB drug.

2.1.2. Metformin

One of the most promising drugs that promotes autophagy is currently used for treatment of type 2 diabetes: metformin [24]. This compound is characterized by a good safety profile, activates 5′-adenosine monophosphate-activated protein kinase (AMPK), induces production of mitochondrial reactive oxygen species (mROS), which are deleterious to *M. tuberculosis* and was found to reduce the severity of TB disease in humans [25]. Despite these promising data, combination therapies which involved metformin in mice had contradictory results. While in one case metformin enhanced the activity of isoniazid and ethionamide [25], in another one it did not improve the efficacy of the combined first-line drugs [26]. Recent retrospective studies reported a protective effect for metformin against reactivation of latent TB in diabetic patients [27–29]. Phase II clinical trials have been initiated (Table 1).

Activity of the major virulence factor ESX-1 can be blocked by compounds BBH7 and BTP15. While BBH7 hinders the secretion mechanism by inducing zinc stress, BTP15 was shown to act by downregulating expression of the *espA-espC-espD* operon upon interaction with MprB. The secreted proteins MptpB, SapM and Zmp1, which prevent phagosomal maturation, can be directly targeted extracellularly by their respective inhibitors. The dedicated secretion systems for these three proteins are not described yet. Gene expression of PhoP-dependent virulence genes can be controlled by PhoP inhibitors which prevent binding of PhoP to specific promoter regions, thus affecting transcription.

2.1.3. Imatinib and Other Tyrosine Kinase Inhibitors

A key feature of *M. tuberculosis* is represented by its ability to inhibit phago-lysosome fusion, and thus potentially limit the efficacy of the autophagy process, thanks to the presence of specific virulence factors like lipoarabinomannan in the cell wall [30], the ESX-1 secretion system [31,32] and other key components such as the Eis protein which modulates autophagy and inflammation and suppresses host innate immune responses [33]. This inhibitory effect can be overcome by tyrosine kinase inhibitors, such as imatinib and the second-generation inhibitors nilotinib and dasatinib, which target the BCR-ABL fusion protein and are used for treating chronic myeloid leukemia [34]. Different studies explored the effect of imatinib on *M. tuberculosis*-infected macrophages and revealed that it increases acidification of lysosomes thereby halting bacterial multiplication [35]. Moreover, imatinib was shown to reduce the number of granulomatous lesions in mice and to act synergistically with first-line anti-TB drug rifampicin [36].

2.1.4. Statins

Statins, i.e., agents that lower cholesterol through inhibition of the biosynthetic pathway, also impact autophagy [37]. Given the relevance of cholesterol in *M. tuberculosis* persistence [38], statins have received considerable attention. Indeed, in addition to their cholesterol-lowering effect, statins decrease lipid body biogenesis and limit *M. tuberculosis* survival [39]. Additionally, it was discovered that atorvarstatin potentiates the effect of rifampin in *M. leprae* infection of the mouse footpad [40]. These substances are currently investigated in clinical trials (Table 1).

2.2. Vitamin D and the Induction of Anti-Microbial Peptides

Anti-microbial peptides like cathelicidins are components of the innate immune system whose synthesis is induced by mycobacterial ligands through binding to Toll-like receptors (TLRs), especially TLR2 and TLR9 [41]. Cathelicidin LL37 represents a major example of this class of molecules, is expressed by neutrophils and macrophages and participates in anti-TB defense through pore-forming capability in the bacterial membranes [42,43].

It has been shown that vitamin D promotes synthesis and release of LL37 [44], which in turn helps in autophagy [45,46]. Moreover, vitamin D enhances the ability of monocytes to respond to interferon gamma (IFN-γ) [47]. Various clinical trials which included vitamin D in addition to the standard regimen have been performed, sometimes with variable results [48–50]. It seems evident that key issues for successful use of vitamin D in TB therapy are proper dosing and possibly also genetic background and comorbidities of the patient. A recently published study by Aibana and co-workers suggested that vitamin D deficiency is associated with increased probability of developing TB in HIV-positive people [51]. However, further investigations are needed to clarify whether vitamin D supplementation might play a significant role in reducing the risk of TB.

Another vitamin whose antitubercular effects have been evaluated is vitamin A, which limits *M. tuberculosis* replication in macrophages by promoting acidification [52,53]. However, while studies in rats showed a beneficial impact of vitamin A supplementation [54], the same was not observed in humans [55,56].

Regulation of anti-microbial peptide expression is also controlled by histone deacetylase inhibitors (for instance 4-phenylbutyrate) through epigenetic mechanisms [57,58]. In the context of *M. tuberculosis* infection of human macrophages, it was demonstrated that phenylbutyrate, alone or in combination with vitamin D3, was able to counteract the suppressive effect of the bacilli on LL-37 expression, thus promoting autophagy [59].

In addition to cathelicidins, another group of anti-microbial peptides plays an important role in anti-TB mechanisms. These are defensins. Defensins are arginine-rich, cationic peptides resistant to proteolysis. They are usually stored in the granules and in the lysosomes of innate immune cells, such as neutrophils, and are released upon pathogen invasion [60]. *M. tuberculosis* stimulates production of beta defensin-2 (HBD-2), which reduces bacterial multiplication and has a chemotactic effect [61] Despite these features, exploitation of HBD-2 in HDT against TB is far from clinical use, due to high costs and poor stability in vivo [62]. Clinical trials where these compounds are being investigated are listed in Table 1.

2.3. *IFN-γ and IL-2 as Adjunct Therapy*

Production of anti-microbial peptides and other antimicrobial activities exerted by macrophages are stimulated by a panel of cytokines that include TNF (Tumor Necrosis Factor), IFN-γ and interleukin 1 (IL-1). While IFN-γ plays its major role in promoting autophagy and phagosome maturation, TNF increases IFN-γ responsiveness and IL-1 counteracts the detrimental effects of Type I IFN in TB [63]. HDT against TB infection includes IFN-γ and modulators of TNF, which will be discussed later in this review. Concerning IFN-γ, it was demonstrated that its administration to TB patients via the aerosol route is well-tolerated and reduces time to sputum conversion while improving lung repair after the disease [64–66]. However, the role of IFN-γ in controlling TB is still under debate, as reported in a study by Sakai and co-workers, who showed that contribution of CD4-T cell derived IFN-γ is limited and, even worse, sometimes detrimental [67]. Another clinical study, where IL-2 was added during the first month of anti-TB treatment resulted in no benefit [68], thus questioning the relevance of adding cytokines to the existing therapy. Possible side effects and treatment costs should also be considered when exploring the administration of cytokines to TB patients.

2.4. *Inhibition of M. tuberculosis Induced Inflammation and Host Cell Death*

2.4.1. The Role of Corticosteroids in TB Treatment

It sounds counterintuitive to address the problem of active TB with anti-inflammatory drugs. However, for some clinical manifestations of the diseases, reduction of inflammation by using adjunctive corticosteroids has already become a well-established and lifesaving treatment approach. Addition of dexamethasone or prednisolone, two potent corticosteroids, to the antibiotic regimen for treatment of TB meningitis improves survival and is considered as a valid therapeutic approach for TB affecting the central nervous system (CNS) [69], although care should be taken since individual responses to steroid treatment might differ. Several studies have tried to improve the outcome of pulmonary TB by lowering the inflammatory response using high doses of corticosteroids in combination with antibiotics. While it was found that this therapy leads to faster resolution of symptoms and lesions in radiographic examinations and a more rapid discharge from hospitals, a statistically significant survival benefit could not be shown (Table 1) [70–72]. In addition, high dose corticosteroids may result in serious side effects such as diabetes and psychiatric symptoms. Today, corticosteroids remain the treatment of choice in specific clinical situations such as CNS TB or hyperinflammatory syndromes e.g., the immune reconstitution inflammatory syndrome (IRIS) in HIV/TB co-infected patients. Investigations at the molecular level proved that dysregulation of inflammasome signaling and of secretion of various cytokines, including IL-1γ, was associated with TB-IRIS in patients infected by HIV [73,74], thus supporting the inclusion of corticosteroids in the treatment of TB patients at risk of developing IRIS [75]. Despite these evidences, a broader application of the drugs in TB treatment is currently not justified. However, clinical studies as well as ex vivo and in vivo experiments performed with these substances indicate that a more specific or tailored modification of the TB inflammatory response may provide a suitable approach to improve patient outcomes. Understanding the exact mechanism of action of corticosteroids in TB may help overcome this hurdle. Corticosteroids are broadly immunosuppressive drugs with multiple modulatory effects on leukocytes once bound to the main target, the corticosteroid receptor. Downstream effects include repression of pro-inflammatory transcriptional regulators like NF-κB as well as impaired release of cytokines such as TNFα and IL-1 [76]. In addition, corticosteroids such as dexamethasone seem to have an *M. tuberculosis* specific inhibitory effect on necrotic host cell death in vitro [77]. This effect seems to depend on inhibition of p38 MAP kinase which impairs mitochondrial membrane stability upon infection with *M. tuberculosis*. p38 MAP kinase is activated during *M. tuberculosis* infection in vitro and in vivo and represents a possible host directed target with several clinically tested small molecule inhibitors available for repurposing.

2.4.2. Non-Steroidal Anti-Inflammatory Drugs (NSAID) and Leukotriene Inhibitors

A series of mouse studies have shown beneficial effects of non-steroidal anti-inflammatory drugs (NSAIDS) such as aspirin, diclofenac and ibuprofen when used alone or in combination with common antibiotics in *M. tuberculosis*-infected mice. The main mechanism of action seems to be inhibition of prostaglandin synthesis via inhibition of cyclooxygenase 1 and 2. Prostaglandins are known drivers of tissue damaging inflammation. It is important to note that diclofenac was shown to possess growth inhibitory effects on the bacterium itself in addition to its anti-inflammatory properties. The substances have been extensively discussed elsewhere [78]. NSAID Clinical trials initiated recently are listed in Table 1. Another category of anti-inflammatory drugs is represented by leukotriene receptor antagonists, such as zafirlukast, which was reported to have anti-mycobacterial activity in vitro and cause alterations in the transcription profile in *M. tuberculosis* [79]. The potential of these drugs in HDT against TB deserves deeper investigation given the role for leukotriene A(4) hydrolase (LTA4H) demonstrated by Tobin and colleagues in animal models of infection [80,81].

2.4.3. Necrosis

Necrotic host cell death is a highly dynamic research field increasingly linked to the release of pro-inflammatory cytokines. A better understanding of the mechanisms of *M. tuberculosis* induced cell death may provide additional starting points for HDTs. Most studies have been focusing on cell death in macrophages, however, necrosis of other cell types such as neutrophils seems to play a pivotal and additive role in *M. tuberculosis* pathogenicity. *M. tuberculosis* released by necrotic neutrophils displays improved survival and growth once phagocytosed by adjacent macrophages [82]. Neutrophil necrotic cell death is driven by reactive oxygen species (ROS) which can be abrogated by ROS inhibitors. In addition, ROS and nitric oxide (NO) have been found to show antimicrobial activity and to modulate neutrophil recruitment to the granuloma [83]. While ROS seems to increase cytokine production and to inhibit inflammasome activation, NO shows a regulatory effect on macrophages with increased expression of hypoxia-inducible factor 1 alpha (HIF-1α) and repression of nuclear factor kappa-light-chain-enhancer of activated B cells (NF-κB) [84,85]. A recent study highlights a role for ferroptotic cell death in TB. Ferroptosis is a type of regulated necrosis induced by accumulation of free iron and toxic lipid peroxides which seems to be mediated by decreased levels of glutathione peroxidase-4 (Gpx4) upon *M. tuberculosis* infection in vitro. Intraperitoneal treatment of *M. tuberculosis* infected mice with ferrostatin, a ferroptosis inhibitor resulted in reduced lung pathology and decreased bacterial load [86]. In addition to ferroptosis, efferocytosis (the physiological process of removing apoptotic cells by macrophages) is an anti-bacterial mechanism that seems to play a relevant role in TB as well [87]. Indeed, efferocytosis of apoptotic neutrophils was shown to improve control of *M. tuberculosis* in an in vitro model of HIV-*M. tuberculosis* macrophage co-infection [88,89].

2.4.4. TNF and TNF-Mediated Signaling

Further downstream of intracellular mediators or regulators of cell death, inflammation and cytokine release, there are more direct targets amenable to therapeutic interventions. These include the cytokines themselves. Biologicals targeting TNFα such as infliximab and adalimumab (monoclonal antibodies) or etanercept (TNF receptor fusion protein) may be used to limit exacerbated pathology and improve antibiotic activity. These substances are restricted for use in combination with antibiotics (adjuvant treatment) since TNFα is essential for protective immunity and granuloma integrity. Monotherapy with infliximab and other anti-TNF antibodies led to reactivation of latent TB [90]. However, when combined with anti-TB drugs, TNF neutralization enhanced *M. tuberculosis* clearance and reduced lung pathology [91]. A clinical study performed with adjuvant etanercept in patients with pulmonary TB and HIV showed a trend towards improved outcome when the TNF blocker was added to the antibiotic regimen [92].

TNF signaling is also the main target of other HDT candidates such as thalidomide, phosphodiesterase inhibitors or Janus kinase (JAK) inhibitors. Thalidomide has potent anti-inflammatory properties which led to successful application of the drug in cases where anti-TB or HIV treatment triggered hyperinflammatory syndromes such as paradoxical reactions or immune reconstitution syndrome (IRIS). A general application for adjuvant treatment approaches may be hampered due to side effects as seen in a study performed with children suffering from TB meningitis [93]. Phosphodiesterase (PDE) inhibitors seem to be more promising for broad application in TB patients. PDEs degrade cyclic AMP (cAMP), a second messenger negatively regulating TNF levels. Decreased levels of cAMP stimulate TNFα secretion, thus making PDE inhibitors interesting HDT targets. Among the five PDE subtypes, targeting PDE4 seems to be the most promising option in TB with adjuvant use of inhibitors leading to improved outcome in several animal models [94,95]. A phase II clinical trial with the PDE4 inhibitor CC-11050 is ongoing (Table 1).

2.4.5. Targeting Matrix Metalloproteinases for Improved Tissue Repair

Imbalanced inflammation eventually results in host tissue destruction, cavitation and dissemination of bacteria. A main driver of these end-stage events are matrix metalloproteinases (MMP) [96]. Once released from activated or necrotic cells, these zinc dependent proteases cleave the extracellular matrix, mostly collagen, and inhibition with small molecules should restrict tissue damage and exacerbation of the disease. Several in vitro and ex vivo studies identified elevated MMP levels in *M. tuberculosis* infected cells or tissue indicating that these enzymes are engaged [96]. In particular, Andrade and colleagues [97] evaluated the interplay between the levels of MMP and heme oxygenase-1 (HO) and discovered that the abundance of these two markers in plasma correlates with different inflammatory profiles and clinical presentations of TB. To date, the only FDA approved MMP inhibitor is doxycycline, an antibiotic with a dual mechanism of action targeting primarily MMP1 and MMP9. The drug suppressed MMP1 and 9 activities in *M. tuberculosis* infected primary human macrophages [98].

In the same study, doxycycline treatment of *M. tuberculosis*-infected guinea pigs led to reduction of the lung bacterial load compared to untreated animals. However, it is important to note that the substance shows a significant growth inhibitory effect on *M. tuberculosis* in broth (MIC 2.5 μg/mL) making it difficult to differentiate between selective host directed and antibacterial effects in these experiments. Experiments with more selective MMP inhibitors such as marimastat (BB-2516), a collagen peptidomimetic broad spectrum MMP inhibitor, showed adjuvant activity in *M. tuberculosis*-infected mice when combined with isoniazid or rifampicin [99]. In contrast to doxycycline, monotherapy with marimastat had no effect on lung bacterial burden [99].

Table 1. Candidate compounds for host-directed therapy (HDT) against tuberculosis (TB).

HDT Effect	Compound	Target or Mode of Action	Notes	Clinical Trials (ClinicalTrials.gov)	References
Promote phagosome maturation and enhance autophagy	Rapamycin (sirolimus)	Inhibition of mTOR	Metabolized by CYP3A4	–	[11–14]
	Everolimus	Inhibition of mTOR, rapamycin analogue	Anti-cancer agent	NCT02968927	[18,22,23]
	Metformin	Activates AMPK	Used to treat diabetes	Phase 2 studies planned CTRI/2018/01/011176	[25]
	Imatinib	Inhibition of BCR-ABL tyrosine kinase	Used to treat leukaemia	NCT03891901	[35,36]
	Statins	Inhibition of cholesterol biosynthetic pathway	Cholesterol is relevant in *M. tuberculosis* persistence	NCT03882177 NCT03456102 NCT04147286	[37,40]
Induce anti-microbial peptides	Vitamin D	Promotes synthesis of cathelicidin LL37	Variable results in clinical trials	NCT00918086 NCT01722396 NCT01130311 NCT01244204 NCT00677339 NCT01698476 NCT01137370 (all completed)	[44,47–50]
	Vitamin A	Promotes acidification of phagosome	Inconsistent results in rats and humans	NCT00057434 (completed)	[52–56]
	4-phenylbutyrate	Inhibition of histone deacetylase	Promotes autophagy	NCT01580007 NCT01698476 (all completed)	[57–59]
	Beta defensin 2 (HBD-2)	Reduces *M. tuberculosis* multiplication	High costs and poor stability	–	[60–62]

Table 1. *Cont.*

HDT Effect	Compound	Target or Mode of Action	Notes	Clinical Trials (ClinicalTrials.gov)	References
Adjunct cytokine therapy	Interferon gamma (IFN-γ)	Promotes autophagy and phagosome maturation	Reduces time to sputum conversion	NCT00201123 NCT00001407 (all completed)	[63–66]
	Interleukin 2 (IL-2)	Enhances cell-mediated response to infection	Contrasting results in clinical trials	NCT03069534	[63,68]
Reduce inflammation/Inhibit necrotic cell death	Corticosteroids	Multiple anti-inflammatory effects	Standard of care for CNS TB. Other forms of TB may require high doses for beneficial effects leading to unwanted side effects	Multiple clinical trials. See meta-analysis in Critchley et al. 2013 and 2014	[69–72]
	P38 MAPK inhibitors	Protect cells from mitochondria-induced necrosis			[77]
	Ferrostatin	Decrease of glutathione peroxidase-4 (Gpx4) levels	Mouse study showing beneficial effect		[86]
	Infliximab, adalimumab, etanercept	Inhibition of TNFα	Restricted for use in combination with antibiotics		[90–92]
	CC-11050	Phosphodiesterase (PDE) inhibition		NCT02968927	[94,95]
	Doxycycline, marimastat (BB-2516)	Inhibition of matrix metalloproteinases	Doxycycline shows growth inhibition of *M. tuberculosis*, effects probably not purely host directed	NCT02774993	[99]
	NSAID: aspirin, ibuprofen, diclofenac, etoricoxib, indomethacin	Cyclooxygenase 1 and/or 2 inhibition		NCT02781909 NCT02602509 NCT02503839	[78]

3. Targeting Bacterial Virulence

3.1. The ESX-1 Secretion System

Lately, the interest in finding novel lead compounds, which prevent infection and dissemination by inhibiting bacterial virulence factors, has increased. These anti-virulence molecules target one or more proteins in the virulence machinery with one prominent example being the ESX-1 secretion system as ESX-1 deletion mutants show strongly attenuated phenotypes in vitro and in vivo [100]. ESX-1 is a type VII secretion system essential for host cell infection, bacterial spread and macrophage escape but not for bacterial growth in axenic cultures [101]. In a whole-cell-based phenotypic screening assay selecting for compounds that abrogate ESX-1 dependent host cell death, the two ESX-1 inhibitors BTP15 and BBH7 have been found and characterized [102]. BTP15 inhibits the histidine kinase MprB that regulates ESX-1 via the *espA-espC-espD* operon. BBH7 on the other hand disturbs metal-ion homeostasis leading to zinc stress and thus hindering secretion of ESX-1 substrates such as EsxA and EsxB (Figure 1). These inhibitors can also be used to abrogate ESX-1 dependent activation of the cytosolic DNA sensor cyclic GMP-AMP synthase (cGAS), a main driver of type I interferon (IFN) secretion, thus nicely linking anti-virulence drugs to modulation of the inflammatory response [103].

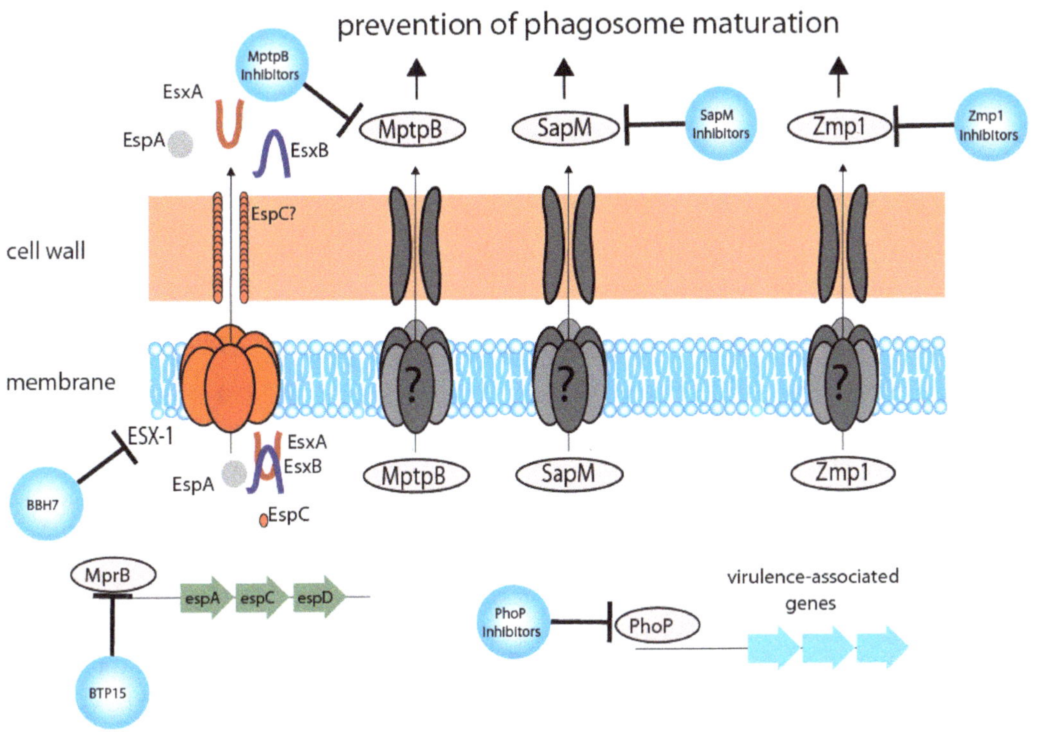

Figure 1. Schematic overview of antivirulence targets in *M. tuberculosis*.

3.2. PhoPR Inhibitors

The PhoPR two-component system plays a central role in regulating the expression of several proteins relevant for virulence of *M. tuberculosis* as mutants deficient in the effector response regulator PhoP show attenuated growth in infected THP-1 cells and in mice [104]. A microarray-based transcriptional profiling study of *M. tuberculosis* strain H37Rv revealed 110 genes that have been differently expressed in PhoP-deficient mutants [105]. This attenuated strain harbors a single nucleotide polymorphism (S219L) in the DNA-binding domain of PhoP resulting in a reduced DNA-binding capacity [105]. Further studies revealed that PhoP is involved in regulating ESX-1 and in biosynthesis of cell wall components such as sulfolipids, polyacyltrehaloses and diacyltrehaloses [106–108]. Two different approaches identified inhibitors of the PhoPR regulon.

3.2.1. Ethoxzolamide

Using a pH-inducible fluorescence reporter system Johnson et al. phenotypically screened for inhibitors of the PhoPR regulon (Figure 1). This screening discovered the carbonic anhydrase inhibitor ethoxzolamide, which inhibits PhoPR while not reducing mycobacterial growth in vitro. Chromatin immunoprecipitation followed by deep sequencing (ChIP-seq) of compound-exposed *M. tuberculosis* cultivated in medium at pH 5.7 showed downregulation of several PhoPR regulated genes involved in lipid synthesis, carbon metabolism and virulence. In addition, the presence of ethoxzolamide did not modulate the expression levels of PhoP itself indicating that the substance acts as a direct inhibitor of the core PhoPR regulon [109].

3.2.2. Inhibitors of the PhoP-DNA Complex

Three active compounds (NCGC00093547, NCGC00244580 and NCGC00161636) that directly bind to PhoP and therefore inhibit PhoP-DNA interactions were found in a screening assay based on Foster resonance energy transfer (FRET). For this screening a DNA-Protein complex of Cy3-labeled DNA and Cy5-labeled PhoP protein was exposed to compounds of interest. Inhibitors of this DNA-Protein complex led to dissociation and consequently to a reduced FRET signal [110]. Direct binding of inhibitors to PhoP was confirmed by thermal shift assays in which target-bound inhibitors stabilize the protein and increase the melting temperature, which can be quantified using the fluorescence signal of fluorophore-protein complexes. Compounds NCGC00093547 and NCGC00161636 increased PhoP melting temperature by 14 °C and 18 °C with an IC_{50} of 15.6 and 15.5 μM, respectively. Data on in vivo or ex vivo activity of these compounds is not available yet.

3.3. Phagosomal Regulation/Hindering Intracellular Survival

3.3.1. MptpB Inhibitors

The *M. tuberculosis* protein-tyrosine-phosphatase B (MptpB) is another putative target for anti-virulence compounds (Figure 1). This kinase is secreted into the cytoplasm of host macrophages allowing for inhibition outside the thick and difficult to overcome mycobacterial cell wall [111]. The function of MptpB is not fully described yet, but the protein has been reported to be necessary for bacterial survival in guinea pigs [112]. So far, it was shown that MptpB dephosphorylates host phosphotyrosine substrates, phosphoserine/threonine substrates and phosphoinositides, with the latter being essential for host macrophage maturation [113].

Several isoxazole-based molecules were created to block the primary and secondary phosphate-binding pockets of MptpB followed by phenotypic testing for activity. In these ex vivo assays, the compounds led to a reduction of mycobacterial burden in macrophages (J774 and THP-1) and in a guinea pig model, without affecting extracellular growth in broth. Additionally, attenuated growth of MDR strains of *M. tuberculosis* in the presence of compound 13 was shown in macrophages. In addition, this inhibitor caused increased sensitivity of a BCG strain to rifampicin and isoniazid in an ex vivo macrophage infection experiment [114]. A similar effect has not been published for *M. tuberculosis* yet.

3.3.2. SapM Inhibitors

Another virulence factor that affects phagocytosis and phagosome formation is the secreted acid phosphatase M (SapM) (Figure 1). SapM shows activity as a monoester alkaline phosphatase and targets two phosphoinositides ($PI(4,5)P_2$ and PI3P) important for phagosome maturation [115]. In inhibition studies, it was shown that 2-phospho-L-ascorbic acid interferes with SapM activity without attenuating extracellular bacterial growth. At 4 mM, this drug could reduce intracellular growth of *M. tuberculosis* by 39% [116].

3.3.3. Zmp1 Inhibitors

Although its role is not fully understood yet, Zmp1 is involved in mycobacterial pathogenicity as it inhibits the inflammasome and therefore prevents phagosome maturation (Figure 1) [117]. Zinc peptidases like Zmp1 are often inhibited by molecules with specific zinc binding groups (ZBG) like 8-hydroxyquinolines. 8-hydroxyquinolines are already in use as metal-interacting structures in pharmacological applications [118]. Based on this, Vickers et al. synthesized compounds consisting of an 8-hydroxyquinoline ring and a hydroxamate moiety and isosteric analogues of these. One 8-hydroxyquinoline-2-hydroxamate derivative showed a reduction in colony forming units (CFU) in infected J774 mouse macrophages while no extracellular, anti-mycobacterial activity was observed. Treatment of infected human monocyte-derived macrophages with this substance led to a decrease in bacterial burden in a dose-dependent matter. In in-vitro inhibition assays the compound inhibited Zmp1 with an IC_{50} of 0.011 μM [119].

3.4. Stress Associated Approaches

DosRST Signaling

M. tuberculosis exploits its two-component system DosRST to establish a dormant state of nonreplicating persistence (NRP) [120]. As *dosRST* mutants show attenuated growth in animal models, including nonhuman primates and guinea pigs, DosRST might be a potential target to reduce mycobacterial virulence [121]. When investigating compounds for their effect on the DosRST system, Zheng et al. identified two candidates (HC104A and HC106A) which interact with distinct members of the two-component system and decrease production of hypoxia-induced triacylglycerol by around 50% during NRP [122]. In a hypoxic shift-down model using a DosR-dependent fluorescent strain CDC1551(*hspX'*::GFP) HC106A was found to affect *M. tuberculosis* survival during NRP. HC104A on the other hand did not attenuate growth in this setting. The in vivo relevance for these interesting findings still needs to be established in a suitable animal model.

4. Conclusions

Several HDT approaches are currently being tested in a number of preclinical and clinical trials as adjuvants complementing conventional anti-TB treatment. Clinical trial results provided in the near future will present an important milestone for the implementation of HDT in routine clinical use. While representing a promising therapeutic approach in theory, most compounds targeting mycobacterial virulence factors lack in vivo proof of principle data.

Author Contributions: All of the authors participated in writing and reviewing the manuscript. All authors have read and agreed to the published version of the manuscript.

References

1. World Health Organization (WHO). *Global Tuberculosis Report 2019*; World Health Organization (WHO): Geneva, Switzerland, 2019.
2. Du Bruyn, E.; Peton, N.; Esmail, H.; Howlett, P.J.; Coussens, A.K.; Wilkinson, R.J. Recent progress in understanding immune activation in the pathogenesis in HIV-tuberculosis co-infection. *Curr. Opin. Hiv Aids* **2018**, *13*, 455–461. [CrossRef] [PubMed]
3. Ferlita, S.; Yegiazaryan, A.; Noori, N.; Lal, G.; Nguyen, T.; To, K.; Venketaraman, V. Type 2 Diabetes Mellitus and Altered Immune System Leading to Susceptibility to Pathogens, Especially Mycobacterium tuberculosis. *J. Clin. Med.* **2019**, *8*, 2219. [CrossRef] [PubMed]
4. World Health Organization (WHO). *The End-TB Strategy*; World Health Organization (WHO): Geneva, Switzerland, 2014.
5. Mabhula, A.; Singh, V. Drug-resistance in Mycobacterium tuberculosis: Where we stand. *MedChemComm* **2019**, *10*, 1342–1360. [CrossRef] [PubMed]
6. Pontali, E.; Raviglione, M.C.; Migliori, G.B. Regimens to treat multidrug-resistant tuberculosis: Past, present and future perspectives. *Eur. Respir. Rev. Off. J. Eur. Respir. Soc.* **2019**, *28*. [CrossRef] [PubMed]

7. Levine, B.; Mizushima, N.; Virgin, H.W. Autophagy in immunity and inflammation. *Nature* **2011**, *469*, 323–335. [CrossRef] [PubMed]
8. Gutierrez, M.G.; Master, S.S.; Singh, S.B.; Taylor, G.A.; Colombo, M.I.; Deretic, V. Autophagy is a defense mechanism inhibiting BCG and Mycobacterium tuberculosis survival in infected macrophages. *Cell* **2004**, *119*, 753–766. [CrossRef]
9. Watson, R.O.; Manzanillo, P.S.; Cox, J.S. Extracellular, M. tuberculosis DNA targets bacteria for autophagy by activating the host DNA-sensing pathway. *Cell* **2012**, *150*, 803–815. [CrossRef]
10. Rovetta, A.I.; Pena, D.; Hernandez Del Pino, R.E.; Recalde, G.M.; Pellegrini, J.; Bigi, F.; Musella, R.M.; Palmero, D.J.; Gutierrez, M.; Colombo, M.I.; et al. IFNG-mediated immune responses enhance autophagy against Mycobacterium tuberculosis antigens in patients with active tuberculosis. *Autophagy* **2014**, *10*, 2109–2121. [CrossRef]
11. Nguyen, L.S.; Vautier, M.; Allenbach, Y.; Zahr, N.; Benveniste, O.; Funck-Brentano, C.; Salem, J.E. Sirolimus and mTOR Inhibitors: A Review of Side Effects and Specific Management in Solid Organ Transplantation. *Drug Saf.* **2019**, *42*, 813–825. [CrossRef]
12. Raught, B.; Gingras, A.C.; Sonenberg, N. The target of rapamycin (TOR) proteins. *Proc. Natl. Acad. Sci. USA* **2001**, *98*, 7037–7044. [CrossRef]
13. Ravikumar, B.; Vacher, C.; Berger, Z.; Davies, J.E.; Luo, S.; Oroz, L.G.; Scaravilli, F.; Easton, D.F.; Duden, R.; O'Kane, C.J.; et al. Inhibition of mTOR induces autophagy and reduces toxicity of polyglutamine expansions in fly and mouse models of Huntington disease. *Nat. Genet.* **2004**, *36*, 585–595. [CrossRef] [PubMed]
14. Kuhn, B.; Jacobsen, W.; Christians, U.; Benet, L.Z.; Kollman, P.A. Metabolism of sirolimus and its derivative everolimus by cytochrome P450 3A4: Insights from docking, molecular dynamics, and quantum chemical calculations. *J. Med. Chem.* **2001**, *44*, 2027–2034. [CrossRef] [PubMed]
15. Gao, P.; Ascano, M.; Zillinger, T.; Wang, W.; Dai, P.; Serganov, A.A.; Gaffney, B.L.; Shuman, S.; Jones, R.A.; Deng, L.; et al. Structure-function analysis of STING activation by c[G(2′,5′)pA(3′,5′)p] and targeting by antiviral DMXAA. *Cell* **2013**, *154*, 748–762. [CrossRef] [PubMed]
16. Shoji-Kawata, S.; Sumpter, R.; Leveno, M.; Campbell, G.R.; Zou, Z.; Kinch, L.; Wilkins, A.D.; Sun, Q.; Pallauf, K.; MacDuff, D.; et al. Identification of a candidate therapeutic autophagy-inducing peptide. *Nature* **2013**, *494*, 201–206. [CrossRef]
17. Gupta, S.; Tyagi, S.; Almeida, D.V.; Maiga, M.C.; Ammerman, N.C.; Bishai, W.R. Acceleration of tuberculosis treatment by adjunctive therapy with verapamil as an efflux inhibitor. *Am. J. Respir. Crit. Care Med.* **2013**, *188*, 600–607. [CrossRef]
18. Cerni, S.; Shafer, D.; To, K.; Venketaraman, V. Investigating the Role of Everolimus in mTOR Inhibition and Autophagy Promotion as a Potential Host-Directed Therapeutic Target in Mycobacterium tuberculosis Infection. *J. Clin. Med.* **2019**, *8*, 232. [CrossRef]
19. Gupta, S.; Cohen, K.A.; Winglee, K.; Maiga, M.; Diarra, B.; Bishai, W.R. Efflux inhibition with verapamil potentiates bedaquiline in Mycobacterium tuberculosis. *Antimicrob. Agents Chemother.* **2014**, *58*, 574–576. [CrossRef]
20. Gupta, S.; Tyagi, S.; Bishai, W.R. Verapamil increases the bactericidal activity of bedaquiline against Mycobacterium tuberculosis in a mouse model. *Antimicrob. Agents Chemother.* **2015**, *59*, 673–676. [CrossRef]
21. Xu, J.; Tasneen, R.; Peloquin, C.A.; Almeida, D.V.; Li, S.Y.; Barnes-Boyle, K.; Lu, Y.; Nuermberger, E. Verapamil Increases the Bioavailability and Efficacy of Bedaquiline but Not Clofazimine in a Murine Model of Tuberculosis. *Antimicrob. Agents Chemother.* **2018**, *62*. [CrossRef]
22. Hahn, D.; Hodson, E.M.; Hamiwka, L.A.; Lee, V.W.; Chapman, J.R.; Craig, J.C.; Webster, A.C. Target of rapamycin inhibitors (TOR-I; sirolimus and everolimus) for primary immunosuppression in kidney transplant recipients. *Cochrane Database Syst. Rev.* **2019**, *12*, Cd004290. [CrossRef]
23. Paluri, R.K.; Sonpavde, G.; Morgan, C.; Rojymon, J.; Mar, A.H.; Gangaraju, R. Renal toxicity with mammalian target of rapamycin inhibitors: A meta-analysis of randomized clinical trials. *Oncol. Rev.* **2019**, *13*, 455. [CrossRef] [PubMed]
24. Yew, W.W.; Chang, K.C.; Chan, D.P.; Zhang, Y. Metformin as a host-directed therapeutic in tuberculosis: Is there a promise? *Tuberculosis (Edinb. Scotl.)* **2019**, *115*, 76–80. [CrossRef] [PubMed]
25. Singhal, A.; Jie, L.; Kumar, P.; Hong, G.S.; Leow, M.K.; Paleja, B.; Tsenova, L.; Kurepina, N.; Chen, J.; Zolezzi, F.; et al. Metformin as adjunct antituberculosis therapy. *Sci. Transl. Med.* **2014**, *6*, 263ra159. [CrossRef]

26. Dutta, N.K.; Pinn, M.L.; Karakousis, P.C. Metformin Adjunctive Therapy Does Not Improve the Sterilizing Activity of the First-Line Antitubercular Regimen in Mice. *Antimicrob. Agents Chemother.* **2017**, *61*. [CrossRef] [PubMed]
27. Lin, S.Y.; Tu, H.P.; Lu, P.L.; Chen, T.C.; Wang, W.H.; Chong, I.W.; Chen, Y.H. Metformin is associated with a lower risk of active tuberculosis in patients with type 2 diabetes. *Respirology (Carltonvic)* **2018**, *23*, 1063–1073. [CrossRef] [PubMed]
28. Marupuru, S.; Senapati, P.; Pathadka, S.; Miraj, S.S.; Unnikrishnan, M.K.; Manu, M.K. Protective effect of metformin against tuberculosis infections in diabetic patients: An observational study of south Indian tertiary healthcare facility. *Braz. J. Infect. Dis. Off. Publ. Braz. Soc. Infect. Dis.* **2017**, *21*, 312–316. [CrossRef] [PubMed]
29. Pan, S.W.; Yen, Y.F.; Kou, Y.R.; Chuang, P.H.; Su, V.Y.; Feng, J.Y.; Chan, Y.J.; Su, W.J. The Risk of TB in Patients With Type 2 Diabetes Initiating Metformin vs Sulfonylurea Treatment. *Chest* **2018**, *153*, 1347–1357. [CrossRef]
30. Shui, W.; Petzold, C.J.; Redding, A.; Liu, J.; Pitcher, A.; Sheu, L.; Hsieh, T.Y.; Keasling, J.D.; Bertozzi, C.R. Organelle membrane proteomics reveals differential influence of mycobacterial lipoglycans on macrophage phagosome maturation and autophagosome accumulation. *J. Proteome Res.* **2011**, *10*, 339–348. [CrossRef]
31. Romagnoli, A.; Etna, M.P.; Giacomini, E.; Pardini, M.; Remoli, M.E.; Corazzari, M.; Falasca, L.; Goletti, D.; Gafa, V.; Simeone, R.; et al. ESX-1 dependent impairment of autophagic flux by Mycobacterium tuberculosis in human dendritic cells. *Autophagy* **2012**, *8*, 1357–1370. [CrossRef]
32. Zhang, L.; Zhang, H.; Zhao, Y.; Mao, F.; Wu, J.; Bai, B.; Xu, Z.; Jiang, Y.; Shi, C. Effects of Mycobacterium tuberculosis ESAT-6/CFP-10 fusion protein on the autophagy function of mouse macrophages. *Dna Cell Biol.* **2012**, *31*, 171–179. [CrossRef]
33. Shin, D.M.; Jeon, B.Y.; Lee, H.M.; Jin, H.S.; Yuk, J.M.; Song, C.H.; Lee, S.H.; Lee, Z.W.; Cho, S.N.; Kim, J.M.; et al. Mycobacterium tuberculosis eis regulates autophagy, inflammation, and cell death through redox-dependent signaling. *PLoS Pathog.* **2010**, *6*, e1001230. [CrossRef] [PubMed]
34. An, X.; Tiwari, A.K.; Sun, Y.; Ding, P.R.; Ashby, C.R., Jr.; Chen, Z.S. BCR-ABL tyrosine kinase inhibitors in the treatment of Philadelphia chromosome positive chronic myeloid leukemia: A review. *Leuk. Res.* **2010**, *34*, 1255–1268. [CrossRef] [PubMed]
35. Bruns, H.; Stegelmann, F.; Fabri, M.; Dohner, K.; van Zandbergen, G.; Wagner, M.; Skinner, M.; Modlin, R.L.; Stenger, S. Abelson tyrosine kinase controls phagosomal acidification required for killing of Mycobacterium tuberculosis in human macrophages. *J. Immunol. (Baltimore Md. 1950)* **2012**, *189*, 4069–4078. [CrossRef] [PubMed]
36. Napier, R.J.; Rafi, W.; Cheruvu, M.; Powell, K.R.; Zaunbrecher, M.A.; Bornmann, W.; Salgame, P.; Shinnick, T.M.; Kalman, D. Imatinib-sensitive tyrosine kinases regulate mycobacterial pathogenesis and represent therapeutic targets against tuberculosis. *Cell Host Microbe* **2011**, *10*, 475–485. [CrossRef] [PubMed]
37. Stancu, C.; Sima, A. Statins: Mechanism of action and effects. *J. Cell. Mol. Med.* **2001**, *5*, 378–387. [CrossRef] [PubMed]
38. Pandey, A.K.; Sassetti, C.M. Mycobacterial persistence requires the utilization of host cholesterol. *Proc. Natl. Acad. Sci. USA* **2008**, *105*, 4376–4380. [CrossRef] [PubMed]
39. Parihar, S.P.; Guler, R.; Khutlang, R.; Lang, D.M.; Hurdayal, R.; Mhlanga, M.M.; Suzuki, H.; Marais, A.D.; Brombacher, F. Statin therapy reduces the mycobacterium tuberculosis burden in human macrophages and in mice by enhancing autophagy and phagosome maturation. *J. Infect. Dis.* **2014**, *209*, 754–763. [CrossRef] [PubMed]
40. Lobato, L.S.; Rosa, P.S.; Ferreira Jda, S.; Neumann Ada, S.; da Silva, M.G.; do Nascimento, D.C.; Soares, C.T.; Pedrini, S.C.; Oliveira, D.S.; Monteiro, C.P.; et al. Statins increase rifampin mycobactericidal effect. *Antimicrob. Agents Chemother.* **2014**, *58*, 5766–5774. [CrossRef] [PubMed]
41. Rivas-Santiago, B.; Hernandez-Pando, R.; Carranza, C.; Juarez, E.; Contreras, J.L.; Aguilar-Leon, D.; Torres, M.; Sada, E. Expression of cathelicidin LL-37 during Mycobacterium tuberculosis infection in human alveolar macrophages, monocytes, neutrophils, and epithelial cells. *Infect. Immun.* **2008**, *76*, 935–941. [CrossRef]
42. Kahlenberg, J.M.; Kaplan, M.J. Little peptide, big effects: The role of LL-37 in inflammation and autoimmune disease. *J. Immunol. (Baltimore Md. 1950)* **2013**, *191*, 4895–4901. [CrossRef]
43. Shin, D.M.; Jo, E.K. Antimicrobial Peptides in Innate Immunity against Mycobacteria. *Immune Netw.* **2011**, *11*, 245–252. [CrossRef]

44. Liu, P.T.; Stenger, S.; Li, H.; Wenzel, L.; Tan, B.H.; Krutzik, S.R.; Ochoa, M.T.; Schauber, J.; Wu, K.; Meinken, C.; et al. Toll-like receptor triggering of a vitamin D-mediated human antimicrobial response. *Science* **2006**, *311*, 1770–1773. [CrossRef] [PubMed]
45. Liu, P.T.; Stenger, S.; Tang, D.H.; Modlin, R.L. Cutting edge: Vitamin D-mediated human antimicrobial activity against Mycobacterium tuberculosis is dependent on the induction of cathelicidin. *J. Immunol. (Baltimore Md. 1950)* **2007**, *179*, 2060–2063. [CrossRef] [PubMed]
46. Yuk, J.M.; Shin, D.M.; Lee, H.M.; Yang, C.S.; Jin, H.S.; Kim, K.K.; Lee, Z.W.; Lee, S.H.; Kim, J.M.; Jo, E.K. Vitamin D3 induces autophagy in human monocytes/macrophages via cathelicidin. *Cell Host Microbe* **2009**, *6*, 231–243. [CrossRef] [PubMed]
47. Rook, G.A.; Steele, J.; Fraher, L.; Barker, S.; Karmali, R.; O'Riordan, J.; Stanford, J. Vitamin D3, gamma interferon, and control of proliferation of Mycobacterium tuberculosis by human monocytes. *Immunology* **1986**, *57*, 159–163.
48. Mily, A.; Rekha, R.S.; Kamal, S.M.; Arifuzzaman, A.S.; Rahim, Z.; Khan, L.; Haq, M.A.; Zaman, K.; Bergman, P.; Brighenti, S.; et al. Significant Effects of Oral Phenylbutyrate and Vitamin D3 Adjunctive Therapy in Pulmonary Tuberculosis: A Randomized Controlled Trial. *PLoS ONE* **2015**, *10*, e0138340. [CrossRef]
49. Musarurwa, C.; Zijenah, L.S.; Mhandire, D.Z.; Bandason, T.; Mhandire, K.; Chipiti, M.M.; Munjoma, M.W.; Mujaji, W.B. Higher serum 25-hydroxyvitamin D concentrations are associated with active pulmonary tuberculosis in hospitalised HIV infected patients in a low income tropical setting: A cross sectional study. *BMC Pulm. Med.* **2018**, *18*, 67. [CrossRef]
50. Sudfeld, C.R.; Mugusi, F.; Aboud, S.; Nagu, T.J.; Wang, M.; Fawzi, W.W. Efficacy of vitamin D3 supplementation in reducing incidence of pulmonary tuberculosis and mortality among HIV-infected Tanzanian adults initiating antiretroviral therapy: Study protocol for a randomized controlled trial. *Trials* **2017**, *18*, 66. [CrossRef]
51. Aibana, O.; Huang, C.C.; Aboud, S.; Arnedo-Pena, A.; Becerra, M.C.; Bellido-Blasco, J.B.; Bhosale, R.; Calderon, R.; Chiang, S.; Contreras, C.; et al. Vitamin D status and risk of incident tuberculosis disease: A nested case-control study, systematic review, and individual-participant data meta-analysis. *PLoS Med.* **2019**, *16*, e1002907. [CrossRef]
52. Crowle, A.J.; Ross, E.J. Inhibition by retinoic acid of multiplication of virulent tubercle bacilli in cultured human macrophages. *Infect. Immun.* **1989**, *57*, 840–844. [CrossRef]
53. Wheelwright, M.; Kim, E.W.; Inkeles, M.S.; De Leon, A.; Pellegrini, M.; Krutzik, S.R.; Liu, P.T. All-trans retinoic acid-triggered antimicrobial activity against Mycobacterium tuberculosis is dependent on NPC2. *J. Immunol. (Baltimore Md. 1950)* **2014**, *192*, 2280–2290. [CrossRef] [PubMed]
54. Yamada, H.; Mizuno, S.; Ross, A.C.; Sugawara, I. Retinoic acid therapy attenuates the severity of tuberculosis while altering lymphocyte and macrophage numbers and cytokine expression in rats infected with Mycobacterium tuberculosis. *J. Nutr.* **2007**, *137*, 2696–2700. [CrossRef] [PubMed]
55. Lawson, L.; Thacher, T.D.; Yassin, M.A.; Onuoha, N.A.; Usman, A.; Emenyonu, N.E.; Shenkin, A.; Davies, P.D.; Cuevas, L.E. Randomized controlled trial of zinc and vitamin A as co-adjuvants for the treatment of pulmonary tuberculosis. *Trop. Med. Int. Health Tm Ih* **2010**, *15*, 1481–1490. [CrossRef] [PubMed]
56. Visser, M.E.; Grewal, H.M.; Swart, E.C.; Dhansay, M.A.; Walzl, G.; Swanevelder, S.; Lombard, C.; Maartens, G. The effect of vitamin A and zinc supplementation on treatment outcomes in pulmonary tuberculosis: A randomized controlled trial. *Am. J. Clin. Nutr.* **2011**, *93*, 93–100. [CrossRef] [PubMed]
57. Steinmann, J.; Halldorsson, S.; Agerberth, B.; Gudmundsson, G.H. Phenylbutyrate induces antimicrobial peptide expression. *Antimicrob. Agents Chemother.* **2009**, *53*, 5127–5133. [CrossRef]
58. Van der Does, A.M.; Kenne, E.; Koppelaar, E.; Agerberth, B.; Lindbom, L. Vitamin D(3) and phenylbutyrate promote development of a human dendritic cell subset displaying enhanced antimicrobial properties. *J. Leukoc. Biol.* **2014**, *95*, 883–891. [CrossRef]
59. Rekha, R.S.; Rao Muvva, S.S.; Wan, M.; Raqib, R.; Bergman, P.; Brighenti, S.; Gudmundsson, G.H.; Agerberth, B. Phenylbutyrate induces LL-37-dependent autophagy and intracellular killing of Mycobacterium tuberculosis in human macrophages. *Autophagy* **2015**, *11*, 1688–1699. [CrossRef]
60. Jarczak, J.; Kosciuczuk, E.M.; Lisowski, P.; Strzalkowska, N.; Jozwik, A.; Horbanczuk, J.; Krzyzewski, J.; Zwierzchowski, L.; Bagnicka, E. Defensins: Natural component of human innate immunity. *Hum. Immunol.* **2013**, *74*, 1069–1079. [CrossRef]
61. Rivas-Santiago, B.; Schwander, S.K.; Sarabia, C.; Diamond, G.; Klein-Patel, M.E.; Hernandez-Pando, R.;

Ellner, J.J.; Sada, E. Human {beta}-defensin 2 is expressed and associated with Mycobacterium tuberculosis during infection of human alveolar epithelial cells. *Infect. Immun.* **2005**, *73*, 4505–4511. [CrossRef]

62. Miyakawa, Y.; Ratnakar, P.; Rao, A.G.; Costello, M.L.; Mathieu-Costello, O.; Lehrer, R.I.; Catanzaro, A. In vitro activity of the antimicrobial peptides human and rabbit defensins and porcine leukocyte protegrin against Mycobacterium tuberculosis. *Infect. Immun.* **1996**, *64*, 926–932. [CrossRef]
63. Moreira-Teixeira, L.; Mayer-Barber, K.; Sher, A.; O'Garra, A. Type I interferons in tuberculosis: Foe and occasionally friend. *J. Exp. Med.* **2018**, *215*, 1273–1285. [CrossRef]
64. Condos, R.; Rom, W.N.; Schluger, N.W. Treatment of multidrug-resistant pulmonary tuberculosis with interferon-gamma via aerosol. *Lancet (Lond. Engl.)* **1997**, *349*, 1513–1515. [CrossRef]
65. Koh, W.J.; Kwon, O.J.; Suh, G.Y.; Chung, M.P.; Kim, H.; Lee, N.Y.; Kim, T.S.; Lee, K.S. Six-month therapy with aerosolized interferon-gamma for refractory multidrug-resistant pulmonary tuberculosis. *J. Korean Med. Sci.* **2004**, *19*, 167–171. [CrossRef] [PubMed]
66. Suarez-Mendez, R.; Garcia-Garcia, I.; Fernandez-Olivera, N.; Valdes-Quintana, M.; Milanes-Virelles, M.T.; Carbonell, D.; Machado-Molina, D.; Valenzuela-Silva, C.M.; Lopez-Saura, P.A. Adjuvant interferon gamma in patients with drug—Resistant pulmonary tuberculosis: A pilot study. *BMC Infect. Dis.* **2004**, *4*, 44. [CrossRef] [PubMed]
67. Sakai, S.; Kauffman, K.D.; Sallin, M.A.; Sharpe, A.H.; Young, H.A.; Ganusov, V.V.; Barber, D.L. CD4 T Cell-Derived IFN-gamma Plays a Minimal Role in Control of Pulmonary Mycobacterium tuberculosis Infection and Must Be Actively Repressed by PD-1 to Prevent Lethal Disease. *PLoS Pathog.* **2016**, *12*, e1005667. [CrossRef] [PubMed]
68. Johnson, J.L.; Ssekasanvu, E.; Okwera, A.; Mayanja, H.; Hirsch, C.S.; Nakibali, J.G.; Jankus, D.D.; Eisenach, K.D.; Boom, W.H.; Ellner, J.J.; et al. Randomized trial of adjunctive interleukin-2 in adults with pulmonary tuberculosis. *Am. J. Respir. Crit. Care Med.* **2003**, *168*, 185–191. [CrossRef] [PubMed]
69. Thwaites, G.E.; Nguyen, D.B.; Nguyen, H.D.; Hoang, T.Q.; Do, T.T.; Nguyen, T.C.; Nguyen, Q.H.; Nguyen, T.T.; Nguyen, N.H.; Nguyen, T.N.; et al. Dexamethasone for the treatment of tuberculous meningitis in adolescents and adults. *N. Engl. J. Med.* **2004**, *351*, 1741–1751. [CrossRef]
70. Critchley, J.A.; Young, F.; Orton, L.; Garner, P. Corticosteroids for prevention of mortality in people with tuberculosis: A systematic review and meta-analysis. *Lancet Infect. Dis.* **2013**, *13*, 223–237. [CrossRef]
71. Dooley, D.P.; Carpenter, J.L.; Rademacher, S. Adjunctive corticosteroid therapy for tuberculosis: A critical reappraisal of the literature. *Clin. Infect. Dis.* **1997**, *25*, 872–887. [CrossRef]
72. Critchley, J.A.; Orton, L.C.; Pearson, F. Adjunctive steroid therapy for managing pulmonary tuberculosis. *Cochrane Database Syst. Rev.* **2014**, Cd011370. [CrossRef]
73. Lai, R.P.J.; Meintjes, G.; Wilkinson, K.A.; Graham, C.M.; Marais, S.; Van der Plas, H.; Deffur, A.; Schutz, C.; Bloom, C.; Munagala, I.; et al. HIV-tuberculosis-associated immune reconstitution inflammatory syndrome is characterized by Toll-like receptor and inflammasome signalling. *Nat. Commun.* **2015**, *6*, 8451. [CrossRef] [PubMed]
74. Tan, H.Y.; Yong, Y.K.; Shankar, E.M.; Paukovics, G.; Ellegard, R.; Larsson, M.; Kamarulzaman, A.; French, M.A.; Crowe, S.M. Aberrant Inflammasome Activation Characterizes Tuberculosis-Associated Immune Reconstitution Inflammatory Syndrome. *J. Immunol. (Baltimore Md. 1950)* **2016**, *196*, 4052–4063. [CrossRef] [PubMed]
75. Walker, N.F.; Stek, C.; Wasserman, S.; Wilkinson, R.J.; Meintjes, G. The tuberculosis-associated immune reconstitution inflammatory syndrome: Recent advances in clinical and pathogenesis research. *Curr. Opin. Hiv Aids* **2018**, *13*, 512–521. [CrossRef] [PubMed]
76. Coutinho, A.E.; Chapman, K.E. The anti-inflammatory and immunosuppressive effects of glucocorticoids, recent developments and mechanistic insights. *Mol. Cell. Endocrinol.* **2011**, *335*, 2–13. [CrossRef]
77. Grab, J.; Suarez, I.; van Gumpel, E.; Winter, S.; Schreiber, F.; Esser, A.; Holscher, C.; Fritsch, M.; Herb, M.; Schramm, M.; et al. Corticosteroids inhibit Mycobacterium tuberculosis-induced necrotic host cell death by abrogating mitochondrial membrane permeability transition. *Nat. Commun.* **2019**, *10*, 688. [CrossRef]
78. Kroesen, V.M.; Groschel, M.I.; Martinson, N.; Zumla, A.; Maeurer, M.; van der Werf, T.S.; Vilaplana, C. Non-Steroidal Anti-inflammatory Drugs As Host-Directed Therapy for Tuberculosis: A Systematic Review. *Front. Immunol.* **2017**, *8*, 772. [CrossRef]
79. Pinault, L.; Han, J.S.; Kang, C.M.; Franco, J.; Ronning, D.R. Zafirlukast inhibits complexation of Lsr2 with DNA and growth of Mycobacterium tuberculosis. *Antimicrob. Agents Chemother.* **2013**, *57*, 2134–2140. [CrossRef]

80. Tobin, D.M.; Roca, F.J.; Oh, S.F.; McFarland, R.; Vickery, T.W.; Ray, J.P.; Ko, D.C.; Zou, Y.; Bang, N.D.; Chau, T.T.; et al. Host genotype-specific therapies can optimize the inflammatory response to mycobacterial infections. *Cell* **2012**, *148*, 434–446. [CrossRef]
81. Tobin, D.M.; Roca, F.J.; Ray, J.P.; Ko, D.C.; Ramakrishnan, L. An enzyme that inactivates the inflammatory mediator leukotriene b4 restricts mycobacterial infection. *PLoS ONE* **2013**, *8*, e67828. [CrossRef]
82. Dallenga, T.; Repnik, U.; Corleis, B.; Eich, J.; Reimer, R.; Griffiths, G.W.; Schaible, U.E. M. tuberculosis-Induced Necrosis of Infected Neutrophils Promotes Bacterial Growth Following Phagocytosis by Macrophages. *Cell Host Microbe* **2017**, *22*, 519–530.e3. [CrossRef]
83. Remot, A.; Doz, E.; Winter, N. Neutrophils and Close Relatives in the Hypoxic Environment of the Tuberculous Granuloma: New Avenues for Host-Directed Therapies? *Front. Immunol.* **2019**, *10*, 417. [CrossRef]
84. Warnatsch, A.; Tsourouktsoglou, T.D.; Branzk, N.; Wang, Q.; Reincke, S.; Herbst, S.; Gutierrez, M.; Papayannopoulos, V. Reactive Oxygen Species Localization Programs Inflammation to Clear Microbes of Different Size. *Immunity* **2017**, *46*, 421–432. [CrossRef] [PubMed]
85. Braverman, J.; Stanley, S.A. Nitric Oxide Modulates Macrophage Responses to Mycobacterium tuberculosis Infection through Activation of HIF-1alpha and Repression of NF-kappaB. *J. Immunol. (Baltimore Md. 1950)* **2017**, *199*, 1805–1816. [CrossRef] [PubMed]
86. Amaral, E.P.; Costa, D.L.; Namasivayam, S.; Riteau, N.; Kamenyeva, O.; Mittereder, L.; Mayer-Barber, K.D.; Andrade, B.B.; Sher, A. A major role for ferroptosis in Mycobacterium tuberculosis-induced cell death and tissue necrosis. *J. Exp. Med.* **2019**, *216*, 556–570. [CrossRef] [PubMed]
87. Martin, C.J.; Booty, M.G.; Rosebrock, T.R.; Nunes-Alves, C.; Desjardins, D.M.; Keren, I.; Fortune, S.M.; Remold, H.G.; Behar, S.M. Efferocytosis is an innate antibacterial mechanism. *Cell Host Microbe* **2012**, *12*, 289–300. [CrossRef]
88. Andersson, A.M.; Larsson, M.; Stendahl, O.; Blomgran, R. Efferocytosis of Apoptotic Neutrophils Enhances Control of Mycobacterium tuberculosis in HIV-Coinfected Macrophages in a Myeloperoxidase-Dependent Manner. *J. Innate Immun.* **2019**, 1–13. [CrossRef]
89. Hosseini, R.; Lamers, G.E.; Soltani, H.M.; Meijer, A.H.; Spaink, H.P.; Schaaf, M.J. Efferocytosis and extrusion of leukocytes determine the progression of early mycobacterial pathogenesis. *J. Cell Sci.* **2016**, *129*, 3385–3395. [CrossRef]
90. Keane, J.; Gershon, S.; Wise, R.P.; Mirabile-Levens, E.; Kasznica, J.; Schwieterman, W.D.; Siegel, J.N.; Braun, M.M. Tuberculosis associated with infliximab, a tumor necrosis factor alpha-neutralizing agent. *N. Engl. J. Med.* **2001**, *345*, 1098–1104. [CrossRef]
91. Bourigault, M.L.; Vacher, R.; Rose, S.; Olleros, M.L.; Janssens, J.P.; Quesniaux, V.F.; Garcia, I. Tumor necrosis factor neutralization combined with chemotherapy enhances Mycobacterium tuberculosis clearance and reduces lung pathology. *Am. J. Clin. Exp. Immunol.* **2013**, *2*, 124–134.
92. Wallis, R.S.; Kyambadde, P.; Johnson, J.L.; Horter, L.; Kittle, R.; Pohle, M.; Ducar, C.; Millard, M.; Mayanja-Kizza, H.; Whalen, C.; et al. A study of the safety, immunology, virology, and microbiology of adjunctive etanercept in HIV-1-associated tuberculosis. *Aids (Lond. Engl.)* **2004**, *18*, 257–264. [CrossRef]
93. Schoeman, J.F.; Springer, P.; van Rensburg, A.J.; Swanevelder, S.; Hanekom, W.A.; Haslett, P.A.; Kaplan, G. Adjunctive thalidomide therapy for childhood tuberculous meningitis: Results of a randomized study. *J. Child. Neurol.* **2004**, *19*, 250–257. [CrossRef]
94. Subbian, S.; Koo, M.S.; Tsenova, L.; Khetani, V.; Zeldis, J.B.; Fallows, D.; Kaplan, G. Pharmacologic Inhibition of Host Phosphodiesterase-4 Improves Isoniazid-Mediated Clearance of Mycobacterium tuberculosis. *Front. Immunol.* **2016**, *7*, 238. [CrossRef] [PubMed]
95. Subbian, S.; Tsenova, L.; O'Brien, P.; Yang, G.; Koo, M.S.; Peixoto, B.; Fallows, D.; Dartois, V.; Muller, G.; Kaplan, G. Phosphodiesterase-4 inhibition alters gene expression and improves isoniazid-mediated clearance of Mycobacterium tuberculosis in rabbit lungs. *PLoS Pathog.* **2011**, *7*, e1002262. [CrossRef] [PubMed]
96. Sabir, N.; Hussain, T.; Mangi, M.H.; Zhao, D.; Zhou, X. Matrix metalloproteinases: Expression, regulation and role in the immunopathology of tuberculosis. *Cell Prolif.* **2019**, *52*, e12649. [CrossRef] [PubMed]
97. Andrade, B.B.; Pavan Kumar, N.; Amaral, E.P.; Riteau, N.; Mayer-Barber, K.D.; Tosh, K.W.; Maier, N.; Conceicao, E.L.; Kubler, A.; Sridhar, R.; et al. Heme Oxygenase-1 Regulation of Matrix Metalloproteinase-1 Expression Underlies Distinct Disease Profiles in Tuberculosis. *J. Immunol. (Baltimore Md. 1950)* **2015**, *195*, 2763–2773. [CrossRef]

98. Walker, N.F.; Clark, S.O.; Oni, T.; Andreu, N.; Tezera, L.; Singh, S.; Saraiva, L.; Pedersen, B.; Kelly, D.L.; Tree, J.A.; et al. Doxycycline and HIV infection suppress tuberculosis-induced matrix metalloproteinases. *Am. J. Respir. Crit. Care Med.* **2012**, *185*, 989–997. [CrossRef]
99. Xu, Y.; Wang, L.; Zimmerman, M.D.; Chen, K.Y.; Huang, L.; Fu, D.J.; Kaya, F.; Rakhilin, N.; Nazarova, E.V.; Bu, P.; et al. Matrix metalloproteinase inhibitors enhance the efficacy of frontline drugs against Mycobacterium tuberculosis. *PLoS Pathog.* **2018**, *14*, e1006974. [CrossRef]
100. Vaziri, F.; Brosch, R. ESX/Type VII Secretion Systems-An Important Way Out for Mycobacterial Proteins. *Microbiol. Spectr.* **2019**, *7*. [CrossRef]
101. Tiwari, S.; Casey, R.; Goulding, C.W.; Hingley-Wilson, S.; Jacobs, W.R., Jr. Infect and Inject: How Mycobacterium tuberculosis Exploits Its Major Virulence-Associated Type VII Secretion System, ESX-1. *Microbiol. Spectr.* **2019**, *7*. [CrossRef]
102. Rybniker, J.; Chen, J.M.; Sala, C.; Hartkoorn, R.C.; Vocat, A.; Benjak, A.; Boy-Rottger, S.; Zhang, M.; Szekely, R.; Greff, Z.; et al. Anticytolytic screen identifies inhibitors of mycobacterial virulence protein secretion. *Cell Host Microbe* **2014**, *16*, 538–548. [CrossRef]
103. Wassermann, R.; Gulen, M.F.; Sala, C.; Perin, S.G.; Lou, Y.; Rybniker, J.; Schmid-Burgk, J.L.; Schmidt, T.; Hornung, V.; Cole, S.T.; et al. Mycobacterium tuberculosis Differentially Activates cGAS- and Inflammasome-Dependent Intracellular Immune Responses through ESX-1. *Cell Host Microbe* **2015**, *17*, 799–810. [CrossRef] [PubMed]
104. Walters, S.B.; Dubnau, E.; Kolesnikova, I.; Laval, F.; Daffe, M.; Smith, I. The Mycobacterium tuberculosis PhoPR two-component system regulates genes essential for virulence and complex lipid biosynthesis. *Mol. Microbiol.* **2006**, *60*, 312–330. [CrossRef] [PubMed]
105. Lee, J.S.; Krause, R.; Schreiber, J.; Mollenkopf, H.J.; Kowall, J.; Stein, R.; Jeon, B.Y.; Kwak, J.Y.; Song, M.K.; Patron, J.P.; et al. Mutation in the transcriptional regulator PhoP contributes to avirulence of Mycobacterium tuberculosis H37Ra strain. *Cell Host Microbe* **2008**, *3*, 97–103. [CrossRef] [PubMed]
106. Frigui, W.; Bottai, D.; Majlessi, L.; Monot, M.; Josselin, E.; Brodin, P.; Garnier, T.; Gicquel, B.; Martin, C.; Leclerc, C.; et al. Control of M. tuberculosis ESAT-6 secretion and specific T cell recognition by PhoP. *PLoS Pathog.* **2008**, *4*, e33. [CrossRef]
107. Anil Kumar, V.; Goyal, R.; Bansal, R.; Singh, N.; Sevalkar, R.R.; Kumar, A.; Sarkar, D. EspR-dependent ESAT-6 Protein Secretion of Mycobacterium tuberculosis Requires the Presence of Virulence Regulator PhoP. *J. Biol. Chem.* **2016**, *291*, 19018–19030. [CrossRef]
108. Gonzalo Asensio, J.; Maia, C.; Ferrer, N.L.; Barilone, N.; Laval, F.; Soto, C.Y.; Winter, N.; Daffe, M.; Gicquel, B.; Martin, C.; et al. The virulence-associated two-component PhoP-PhoR system controls the biosynthesis of polyketide-derived lipids in Mycobacterium tuberculosis. *J. Biol. Chem.* **2006**, *281*, 1313–1316. [CrossRef]
109. Johnson, B.K.; Colvin, C.J.; Needle, D.B.; Mba Medie, F.; Champion, P.A.; Abramovitch, R.B. The Carbonic Anhydrase Inhibitor Ethoxzolamide Inhibits the Mycobacterium tuberculosis PhoPR Regulon and Esx-1 Secretion and Attenuates Virulence. *Antimicrob. Agents Chemother.* **2015**, *59*, 4436–4445. [CrossRef]
110. Wang, L.; Xu, M.; Southall, N.; Zheng, W.; Wang, S. A High-Throughput Assay for Developing Inhibitors of PhoP, a Virulence Factor of Mycobacterium tuberculosis. *Comb. Chem. High Throughput Screen* **2016**, *19*, 855–864. [CrossRef]
111. Koul, A.; Choidas, A.; Treder, M.; Tyagi, A.K.; Drlica, K.; Singh, Y.; Ullrich, A. Cloning and characterization of secretory tyrosine phosphatases of Mycobacterium tuberculosis. *J. Bacteriol.* **2000**, *182*, 5425–5432. [CrossRef]
112. Singh, R.; Rao, V.; Shakila, H.; Gupta, R.; Khera, A.; Dhar, N.; Singh, A.; Koul, A.; Singh, Y.; Naseema, M.; et al. Disruption of mptpB impairs the ability of Mycobacterium tuberculosis to survive in guinea pigs. *Mol. Microbiol.* **2003**, *50*, 751–762. [CrossRef]
113. Beresford, N.; Patel, S.; Armstrong, J.; Szoor, B.; Fordham-Skelton, A.P.; Tabernero, L. MptpB, a virulence factor from Mycobacterium tuberculosis, exhibits triple-specificity phosphatase activity. *Biochem. J.* **2007**, *406*, 13–18. [CrossRef]
114. Vickers, C.F.; Silva, A.P.G.; Chakraborty, A.; Fernandez, P.; Kurepina, N.; Saville, C.; Naranjo, Y.; Pons, M.; Schnettger, L.S.; Gutierrez, M.G.; et al. Structure-Based Design of MptpB Inhibitors That Reduce Multidrug-Resistant Mycobacterium tuberculosis Survival and Infection Burden in Vivo. *J. Med. Chem.* **2018**, *61*, 8337–8352. [CrossRef] [PubMed]
115. Vieira, O.V.; Botelho, R.J.; Rameh, L.; Brachmann, S.M.; Matsuo, T.; Davidson, H.W.; Schreiber, A.; Backer, J.M.; Cantley, L.C.; Grinstein, S. Distinct roles of class I and class III phosphatidylinositol 3-kinases in phagosome

formation and maturation. *J. Cell. Biol.* **2001**, *155*, 19–25. [CrossRef] [PubMed]

116. Fernandez-Soto, P.; Bruce, A.J.E.; Fielding, A.J.; Cavet, J.S.; Tabernero, L. Mechanism of catalysis and inhibition of Mycobacterium tuberculosis SapM, implications for the development of novel antivirulence drugs. *Sci. Rep.* **2019**, *9*, 10315. [CrossRef] [PubMed]
117. Master, S.S.; Rampini, S.K.; Davis, A.S.; Keller, C.; Ehlers, S.; Springer, B.; Timmins, G.S.; Sander, P.; Deretic, V. Mycobacterium tuberculosis prevents inflammasome activation. *Cell Host Microbe* **2008**, *3*, 224–232. [CrossRef]
118. Song, Y.; Xu, H.; Chen, W.; Zhan, P.; Liu, X. 8-Hydroxyquinoline: A privileged structure with a broad-ranging pharmacological potential. *Med. Chem. Commun.* **2015**, *6*, 61–74. [CrossRef]
119. Paolino, M.; Brindisi, M.; Vallone, A.; Butini, S.; Campiani, G.; Nannicini, C.; Giuliani, G.; Anzini, M.; Lamponi, S.; Giorgi, G.; et al. Development of Potent Inhibitors of the Mycobacterium tuberculosis Virulence Factor Zmp1 and Evaluation of Their Effect on Mycobacterial Survival inside Macrophages. *ChemMedChem* **2018**, *13*, 422–430. [CrossRef]
120. Mehra, S.; Foreman, T.W.; Didier, P.J.; Ahsan, M.H.; Hudock, T.A.; Kissee, R.; Golden, N.A.; Gautam, U.S.; Johnson, A.M.; Alvarez, X.; et al. The DosR Regulon Modulates Adaptive Immunity and Is Essential for Mycobacterium tuberculosis Persistence. *Am. J. Respir. Crit. Care Med.* **2015**, *191*, 1185–1196. [CrossRef]
121. Converse, P.J.; Karakousis, P.C.; Klinkenberg, L.G.; Kesavan, A.K.; Ly, L.H.; Allen, S.S.; Grosset, J.H.; Jain, S.K.; Lamichhane, G.; Manabe, Y.C.; et al. Role of the dosR-dosS two-component regulatory system in Mycobacterium tuberculosis virulence in three animal models. *Infect. Immun.* **2009**, *77*, 1230–1237. [CrossRef]
122. Zheng, H.; Williams, J.T.; Aleiwi, B.; Ellsworth, E.; Abramovitch, R.B. Inhibiting Mycobacterium tuberculosis DosRST Signaling by Targeting Response Regulator DNA Binding and Sensor Kinase Heme. *ACS Chem. Biol.* **2019**. [CrossRef]

8

Development of Macozinone for TB treatment

Vadim Makarov [1,*] and Katarína Mikušová [2]

1 Federal Research Center "Fundamentals of Biotechnology RAS", Leninsky prospect 33, bld. 2, 119071 Moscow, Russia
2 Department of Biochemistry, Faculty of Natural Sciences, Comenius University in Bratislava, Mlynská dolina, Ilkovičova 6, 84215 Bratislava, Slovakia; katarina.mikusova@uniba.sk
* Correspondence: makarov@inbi.ras.ru

Abstract: Macozinone, a piperazine-benzothiazinone PBTZ169, is currently undergoing Phase 1/2 clinical studies for the treatment of tuberculosis (TB). In this review we summarize the key findings that led to the development of this compound and to identification of its target, decaprenylphospohoryl ribose oxidase DprE1, which is involved in the synthesis of the essential arabinan polymers of the cell wall in a TB pathogen, *Mycobacterium tuberculosis*. We present the results of the pilot clinical studies, which raise optimism regarding its further development towards more efficient TB drug regimens.

Keywords: macozinone; DprE1 inhibitor; clinical studies

---

1. Introduction

Tuberculosis (TB) as both an acute and chronic infectious disease is still unbeaten and represents an important social, medical, and biological challenge for the healthcare worldwide [1]. The infection caused by *Mycobacterium tuberculosis* strains is most often located in the respiratory tract from which it is transmitted in the population by aerosols. At the same time, mycobacteria can be disseminated also to other organs. However, it is now well acknowledged that even in its primary location, the TB pathogen is present in different microenvironments and thus in various metabolic states, which substantially complicates the treatment [2]. According to the last Global Tuberculosis Report issued by the World Health Organization (WHO) [3], in 2018 the death rate was estimated to be about 1.45 million people. Among the estimated 10 million new cases of TB, 3.4% had multidrug-resistant TB or rifampicin-resistant TB (MDR/RR-TB). This number increased to 18% in previously treated cases, with the highest proportions (>50% in previously treated cases) in countries of the former Soviet Union. Although efficient TB treatment is available, only 7 million new cases were treated for the disease in 2018, while an estimated 3 million patients did not have access to quality care or were not reported, and only one in three people with drug-resistant TB accessed care [3].

In addition to interventions in the social area and point-of-care management of TB, one of the key challenges in making the fight against TB more effective is to improve treatment options. The current chemotherapy for the drug-sensitive TB takes about six months and requires administration of four different medicines (isoniazid, rifampicin, ethambutol, pyrazinamide) to avoid development of drug resistance. The length of the treatment and its adverse effects result in bad compliance and thus it is imperative to find novel drugs and regimens that would be less demanding on patients [4].

During recent years, three novel drugs against TB were approved. These are bedaquiline [5], delamanid [6] and pretomanid [7], which are currently undergoing several clinical trials aimed at treatment of the drug-resistant TB, as well as at shortening standard TB treatment [8]. The efforts and hope for better TB drugs are exemplified also by the pipeline of several new molecules, that are currently at different stages of clinical development. Among them there are inhibitors of protein synthesis from the oxazolidinone family (delpazolid, sutezolid, contezolid, TBI 223), inhibitor of leucyl-tRNA synthetase (GSK3036656), inhibitor of DNA gyrase B (SPR720), compounds interfering with the respiratory chain of a TB pathogen (telacebec, TBI-166), a cell wall inhibitor targeting MmpL3 transporter (SQ109) and four compounds targeting another cell wall target, DprE1. These are BTZ043, TBA-7371, OPC-167832, and macozinone (Figure 1) [4,8]. In this review we will present the key findings towards the discovery and development of macozinone, an optimized benzothiazinone, which currently appears to be the most advanced DprE1 inhibitor.

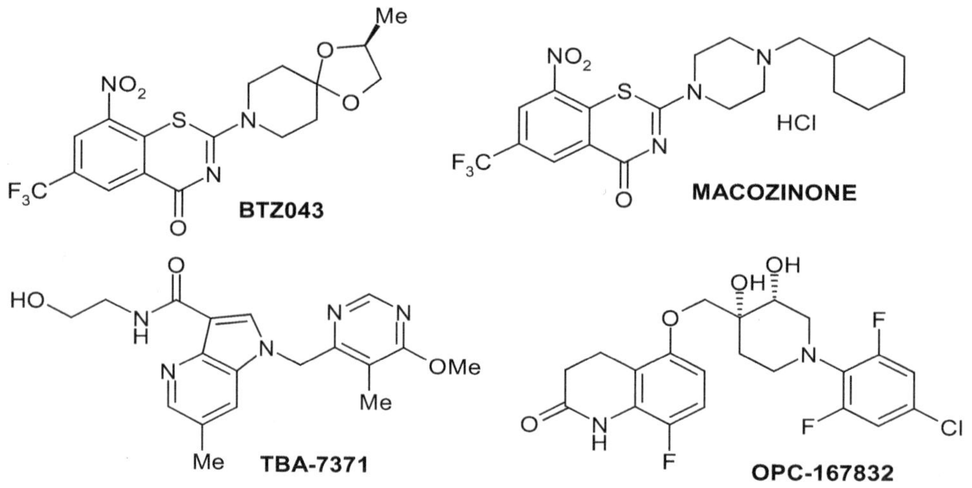

Figure 1. DprE1 inhibitors in clinical development.

2. Discovery of Benzothiazinones as Highly Potent Killers of *Mycobacterium Tuberculosis*

The very first scientific report on benzothiazinones (BTZs) with extremely high antimycobacterial activity was published in 2009 [9]. These compounds emerged as a result of several years of efforts focused on investigation of a family of ditiocarbamate (DTC) derivatives with antimicrobial properties, which was carried out at the Research Center for Antibiotics in Moscow and the Hans Knöll Institute in Jena [10]. DTCs gained their fame primarily as additives in industry and pesticides, which have been in use since 1930. However, some of them were tested as pharmacological agents for treatment of alcoholism, human immunodeficiency virus (HIV) or cancer [11]. It occurred that selected DTC derivatives had minimal inhibitory concentrations (MICs) between 3–30 μg/ml for *M. tuberculosis*, but were active also on several species of fast-growing mycobacteria and multiresistant staphylococci [10]. Thorough structure-activity studies focused on improvement of the activity and selectivity of these compounds for mycobacteria was performed. Selected compounds derived from the basic active ortho nitro-dialkyldithiocarbamate structure showed enhanced activity towards fast growing mycobacteria, with *M. vaccae* being the most sensitive reaching MICs 0.4–1.56 μg/ml [12]. In addition, 3 out of 7 tested molecules were efficient and well tolerated also in the mouse foot pad model of leprosy [12]. Nevertheless, it was clear that reactivity of DTCs poses a significant problem in further development of these compounds despite their activity and rather unexpected low level of toxicity as exemplified by studies in mice [12]. Consequently, a thorough investigation of the metabolic conversion of the most active DTCs containing spiroamine moiety, was undertaken. The drug was incubated with the non-pathogenic strain *M. smegmatis* and all isolated metabolites were tested for antimycobacterial activity. One of these metabolites was particularly active and its structure established by nuclear magnetic resonance (NMR) revealed the principal BTZ scaffold. A set of novel BTZ derivatives was synthesized and tested against both fast-growing and pathogenic mycobacteria in collaboration with Prof. Stewart Cole at Pasteur Institute in Paris [13]. Surprisingly, these compounds were highly active and selective against mycobacteria in vitro, with MIC values 0.195–1.56 μg/ml for *M. tuberculosis*, including the resistant strains. The lowest MIC value, 0.023 pg/ml, was obtained for *M. fortuitum* and 2,2-[2-methyl-1,4-dioxa-8-azaspiro[4.5]dec-8-yl]-8-nitro- 6-(trifluoromethyl)-4H-1,3-benzothiazin-4-one, later named BTZ038 [9]. The pilot in vivo studies with this compound revealed its potency in the murine model of TB, which was comparable to isoniazid used in the same dose of 25 mg/kg [13]. These encouraging results warranted further exploration of BTZs as perspective compounds for development of a new TB drug.

3. Mechanism of Action of Benzothiazinones

An investigation of mechanism of action of BTZ was carried out within the European Union (EU)-funded consortium New Medicines for Tuberculosis (NM4TB), which was formed in 2006 under the leadership of Prof. Stewart Cole. The compound BTZ038 was initially chosen as a lead molecule. Since it contains a chiral center, pure enantiomers BTZ043 (S) and BTZ044 (R) were prepared and subjected to MIC determination. Both forms showed comparable activities in vitro in *M. tuberculosis*. Accordingly, only one of them, BTZ043, was subjected to mechanistic studies [9].

Genetic experiments aimed at identification of the BTZ target were carried out by Prof. Giovanna Riccardi and her team at University of Pavia. The two approaches which were chosen for this purpose pointed out to the role of the gene *rv3790* in conferring resistance against the drug. In the first approach, *M. smegmatis* was transformed with a cosmid library containing DNA fragments from the same organism. An ortholog of the *rv3790* gene from *M. smegmatis* mc^{2}155, *MSMEG_6382*, was identified on a cosmid, which resulted in an increase in MICs towards BTZ043. In the second approach, BTZ-resistant strains of *M. smegmatis*, *M. bovis* BCG and *M. tuberculosis* were isolated and their resistance was traced to mutations in the same codon in *rv3790* and its orthologs. In all mutant strains codons corresponding to Cys387 in *rv3790* gene product were replaced by Ser or Gly, which increased the MICs of the resistant strains up to 10,000 times. Accordingly, the mycobacterial species *M. avium* and *M. aurum*, in which this position was occupied by Ala or Ser, respectively, were naturally resistant against BTZ, which supported identification of *rv3790* as a target [9]. Coincidentally, the function of the protein encoded by this gene was described only a short while before the data on the BTZ target became available. In the course of studies focused on the metabolism of arabinose in mycobacteria carried out by Prof. Michael McNeil with collaborators at Colorado State University in Fort Collins, the *rv3790* and *rv3791* gene products were proposed to be involved in a unique epimerisation of decaprenylphosphoryl ribose (DPR) to decaprenylphosphoryl arabinose (DPA) [14]. The latter molecule serves as a sole donor of arabinose residues for synthesis of the essential arabinan polymers of the mycobacterial cell wall [15]. It was shown that the conversion takes place via oxidation of the DPR substrate, followed by reduction of the resulting keto-intermediate and thus the two oxidoreductases, *rv3790* and *rv3791*, from the so-called arabinogalactan biosynthesis cluster [16] were ideal candidates to catalyse these reactions. However, at the time it was not possible to conclude which of the two is responsible for oxidation and which for the reduction step. Examination of the effects of BTZ043 on enzymatic conversion of DPR to DPA proved that the compound inhibited the oxidation step. Given the confirmed roles of Rv3790 and Rv3791 in epimerization of DPR, we named them DprE1 and DprE2, respectively (Figure 2) [9].

An important step towards understanding the mechanism of action of BTZs was isolation of a covalent adduct of BTZ043 and DprE1 by Trefzer et al. in 2010 [17]. The authors concluded that reduction of the nitro-group to nitroso derivative is critical for formation of the semimercaptal adduct of BTZ043 and DprE1 through the Cys387, which was verified by mass spectrometry. The following study proved that DprE1 itself is responsible for the reductive activation of DprE1. The electrons needed for the reaction are provided by the enzyme's prosthetic group, FAD, which gets reduced during the catalysis of DPR oxidation (Figure 2) [18]. Accordingly, BTZ represents a typical example of a suicide inhibitor. The proposed mechanism of action was confirmed by crystallographic studies in which structures of DprE1 from *M. smegmatis* were obtained in native and BTZ043-bound forms. As expected, the semimercaptal adduct was formed only in the presence of the substrate analog, farnesylphosphoryl ribose, which provided electrons for reduction of the FAD cofactor necessary for BTZ activation [19].

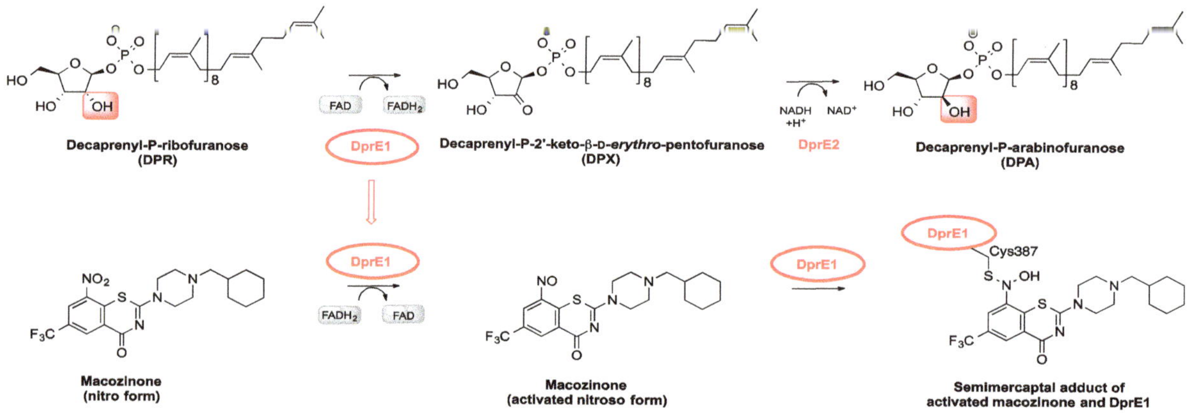

Figure 2. Mechanism of action of macozinone. *Upper line:* Reactions catalyzed by DprE1 and DprE2. *Bottom line:* Activation of macozinone and its covalent attachment to DprE1 from *M. tuberculosis* through Cys387 of the enzyme's active site. The scheme is based on mechanistic studies performed initially with benzothiazinone BTZ043 [17–19] and subsequently confirmed for piperazine-benzothiazinone PBTZ169 (macozinone) [20].

4. From BTZ043 to PBTZ169

At the time of its discovery, BTZ043 was the most efficient inhibitor of in vitro mycobacterial growth ever described. While MICs for first line drugs isoniazid or ethambutol for *M. tuberculosis* were 0.02–0.2 μg/ml or 1–5 μg/ml, respectively, the value for BTZ043 was just 1 ng/ml. The compound proved to be active also in intracellular *M. tuberculosis* infection in Raw 264.7 macrophages and in a mouse model of chronic tuberculosis and it did not show any signs of toxicity or mutagenicity in concentrations well above the amounts used for the experiments. Nevertheless, the extremely low MIC did not translate to comparably high efficiencies in animal studies [9].

In the effort to improve pharmacological properties of benzothiazinone series, structure-activity relationship (SAR) analysis was performed, with main focus on position 2 of BTZ scaffold [20]. It was previously shown that the rest of the positions harbor substituents critical for the antimycobacterial activity, e.g., replacement of 8-nitro-group with any other group, including hydroxylamino-, amino- and nitryl-, led to at least a 500-fold increase in the MIC against *M. tuberculosis* [9]. The new series contained a piperazine at the position 2 of the BTZ structure, which allowed extensive modifications of the N-4 position of this substituent. Evaluation of the 60 prepared piperazine-benzothiazinones (PBTZ) for in vitro activity on *M. tuberculosis* pointed to a strong correlation between the MICs and lipophilicity. The alkyl-PBTZ derivatives were most active and some of them reached the MICs between 0.19–0.75 ng/ml for *M. tuberculosis*. Five of these derivatives were tested in the chronic TB mouse model, which allowed for selection of PBTZ169 as the most promising candidate [20].

Comparison of BTZ043 with PBTZ169 confirmed superior properties of the latter in all tested parameters. It was three to seven times more active in vitro against *M. tuberculosis*, *M. bovis* BCG, *M. marinum*, *M. smegmatis*, *Corynebacterium diphtheriae* and *C. glutamicum* as established by resazurin microtiter assay (REMA). The molecule was also highly active against a panel of 9 MDR- and XDR-clinical isolates of *M. tuberculosis* [20]. Cross-resistance between BTZ043 and PBTZ169 was confirmed for BTZ-resistant strains of *M. tuberculosis*, *M. bovis* BCG and *M. smegmatis*, indicating the common mechanism of action. Interestingly, PBTZ169 was less susceptible to inactivation by nitro-reduction by the nitroreductase NfnB from *M. smegmatis* compared to BTZ043, as confirmed by the liquid chromatography-mass spectrometry analyses. This property could be critical for in vivo activity, due to inevitable actions of host nitroreductases or microbial nitroreductases in the digestive tract of the patients, which would potentially reduce the amount of the available active drug. Enzymologic studies confirmed that PBTZ169 is more efficient inhibitor of its DprE1 target than BTZ043; the enzyme was completely inactivated after 5 min of incubation with 5 μM PBTZ169, while four times higher concentration was needed to achieve the same result with BTZ043. The crystal structure of

M. tuberculosis DprE1 with covalently bound PBTZ169 showed similarities with the BTZ043-bound structure of the *M. smegmatis* enzyme. However, higher flexibility of the methyl-cyclohexyl group on piperazine, could account for better affinity of this drug for its target and explain its higher capacity to inactivate the enzyme [20].

Efficacies of PBTZ169 and BTZ043 were also evaluated against *M. marinum* in a zebrafish embryo model. Although after 5 days of treatment both drugs efficiently decreased the bacterial burden at concentrations of 25 nM and 50 nM, examination of BTZ043-treated embryos pointed to developmental defects. By contrast, application of PBTZ169 up to 10 μM did not cause any pathological changes. In vivo studies in the mouse chronic model of TB proved the superiority of PBTZ169 over BTZ043 in lowering colony forming unit counts in the spleen and lungs, which, however, could not be attributed to better pharmacokinetics, since the two compounds had similar properties except for faster uptake of PBTZ169 [20]. Aiming at the use of the novel PBTZ derivative in designing a new regimen for TB, combination studies with selection of approved and experimental drugs were performed. The combination of PBTZ169 and bedaquiline, which proved to be synergistic in the in vitro REMA assay, was tested in the mouse chronic model of TB. Simultaneous administration of PBTZ, bedaquiline and pyrazinamide was more efficient in reducing the mycobacterial counts both in the lungs and spleen compared to the standard mixture of isoniazid, rifampicin and pyrazinamide [20].

Among favorable properties of PBTZ169 over BTZ043 is the lack of the chiral center, which simplified the production of the drug and significantly decreased its price. This is critical for developing treatment for a disease greatly affecting low-income and middle-income countries in particular. Taken together, PBTZ169 was identified as a promising candidate for development as a novel TB medicine [20].

5. From PBTZ169 to Macozinone: First Results of the Clinical Studies

Establishment of a non-profit Innovative Medicines for Tuberculosis Foundation (iM4TB Foundation) at Ecole Polytechnique Fédérale de Lausanne (EPFL) in March 2014 was a principal milestone for the further development of PBTZ169 and its transformation from a valuable TB drug candidate to the compound reaching promising results in the pilot clinical studies (Figure 3) [21]. This approach was necessary to overcome the lack of interest from pharmaceutical companies to address the disease primarily affecting low-income countries. The mission of the foundation is "to develop better and faster-acting medicines to fight tuberculosis and bridge the gap between scientific discovery and the market in order to provide affordable TB treatment to anyone in the world". In July 2014 the foundation joined in this effort with the Russian pharmaceutical company Nearmedic Plus LLC, which bought a license covering the use of PBTZ169 in most countries of the former Soviet Union, while iM4TB retained the rights for the rest of the world. Investments of Nearmedic, along with funds raised by iM4TB, including the generous support of the Bill and Melinda Gates foundation, enabled performing all necessary pre-clinical trials with PBTZ169, such as ADME (absorption, distribution, metabolism, excretion) profiling, toxicology studies, as well as production of clinical supplies of the drug, and preparation of regulatory documents necessary for entering the first clinical trials [21,22].

Clinical studies were initiated by both iM4TB and Nearmedic. In the randomized, double-blind, placebo-controlled Phase 1a study performed in Switzerland (NCT03423030) [23] the aim was to assess safety, tolerability and pharmacokinetic profile of PBTZ169 formulated as a spray-dried dispersion versus a native crystal powder. In addition, antitubercular activity of single escalating doses of PBTZ169 ex vivo was evaluated. The study included 32 healthy male volunteers, grouped to 4 panels of 8 subjects, each undergoing 2 investigation periods, during which they received either single doses of PBTZ169 at increasing dose levels up to 320 mg or a matching placebo. Promising results of this study encouraged the iM4TB team to design of the Phase 1b trial (NCT03776500) [24] aimed at evaluation of the safety, tolerability and pharmacokinetics of PBTZ169 in multiple dosing up to 1200 mg/day in healthy volunteers (32 subjects grouped in 4 consecutive panels) receiving PBTZ169 for 14 consecutive days. An additional goal is to evaluate interactions of PBTZ169 with the human cytochrome P 450 enzyme family [24].

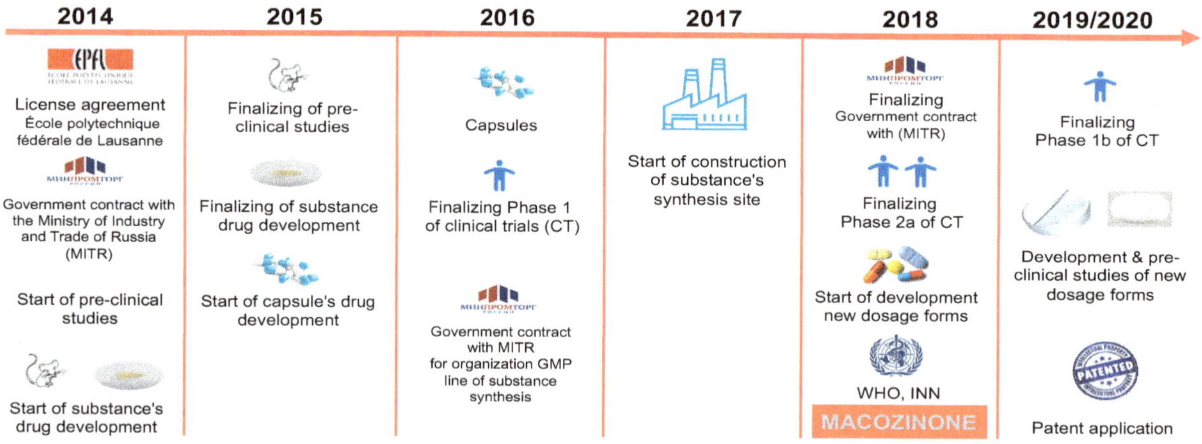

Figure 3. Pre-clinical and clinical development of macozinone.

The first Phase 1 clinical trial in Russia (Nearmedic Plus LLC) (NCT03036163, PBTZ169-Z00-C01-1) [25] with an official title "Open-label Prospective Non-comparative Study of Safety, Tolerability and Pharmacokinetics of PBTZ169 after Single and Multiple Fasting Oral Administration in Increasing Doses in Healthy Volunteers" was carried out between January and November 2016. The drug was administered in the form of capsules containing 40 mg of the drug. The study included single escalating doses (40, 80, 160, 320, and 640 mg) in fasting conditions, as well as multiple fasting doses (320 and 640 mg) for 14 days. Overall the study included 40 participants [22].

A completed open-label prospective Phase 1b study initiated by Nearmedic Plus LLC (NCT04150224, PBTZ169-Z00-C01-3) [26] was designed to assess the safety, tolerability, pharmacokinetics, and food effects on single, double, and multiple escalating doses in healthy volunteers. During the first part of the study, safety, tolerability, and pharmacokinetics of PBTZ169 in 80 mg capsules were studied in healthy volunteers who received single or double (twice daily) fasting doses, which increased sequentially (640, 960, and 1280 mg once a day and 640 mg twice a day). The food effects were studied for a single 640 mg dose. The second part of the study involved the safety, tolerability, and pharmacokinetics of PBTZ169 in 80 mg capsules in healthy volunteers who received 1280 mg daily in fed conditions, for 14 days. In total, 60 healthy volunteers (10 in each cohort) received the investigational drug and completed the study according to the protocol [22].

During these clinical trials, safety and tolerability of PBTZ169 in capsules were studied, including assessment of adverse effects, vital signs (blood pressure, heart rate, body temperature, respiratory rate), laboratory and instrumental parameters (hematology, blood chemistry, coagulation parameters, urinalysis, electrocardiography) and physical examination. In these studies (NCT03036163 and NCT04150224), good tolerability and favorable safety profile were demonstrated for PBTZ169 in the studied dose range. One event of dose-limiting toxicity (increase in the glucose level 2 hours after the drug administration) was documented after a single 80 mg dose of PBTZ169 in 40 mg capsules (NCT03036163). There were no other cases of dose-limiting toxicity in healthy volunteers in these studies. There were no serious adverse effects. There was no increase in the frequency of adverse effects associated with increased dose or with the administration regimen (fasting or in fed conditions), for single or multiple doses. Changes in some mean vital signs, laboratory, instrumental parameters, or physical examination data were not associated with a trend to increase with a growing dose [22].

Efficacy of PBTZ169 based on the early bactericidal activity (EBA), was studied in a Phase 2a clinical trial (PBTZ169-A15-C2A-1, NCT03334734) [27] by Nearmedic Plus LLC in patients with newly diagnosed smear-positive tuberculosis of the respiratory tract, with preserved sensitivity to isoniazid and rifampicin. Although the trial was terminated early because of slow enrollment, relevant information was obtained from 16 patients who participated in the study. The drug was administered in 80 mg capsules, orally as a monotherapy for 14 days, as follows: 160 mg/day dose—4 patients; 320 mg/day dose—4 patients; 640 mg/day dose—7 patients. Isoniazid tablets were used as a control treatment at 600 mg/day dose in one patient.

The primary efficacy of the treatment was evaluated by two methods:

(i) According to quantification of colony forming units in sputum by its inoculation on agar plates, in the group of patients receiving PBTZ169 in the 640 mg dose, EBA 0–14 (mean of the two measurements) and EBA 0–14 (the higher of the two measurements) were 0.071 log10 cells/ml/day [95% confidence interval (CI) 0; 0.143] and 0.080 log10 cells/ml/day [95% CI 0.002; 0.158], respectively.

(ii) According to quantitative polymerase chain reaction, in the same group of patients, EBA 0–14 (mean of the two measurements) and EBA 0–14 (the higher of the two measurements) were 0.098 log10 cells/ml/day [95% CI 0.021; 0.175] and 0.100 log10 cells/ml/day[95% CI 0.021; 0.180], respectively.

Thus, the analysis of efficacy based on the data obtained in a pilot Phase 2a clinical study revealed statistically significant early bactericidal activity of PBTZ169 14 days after the start of monotherapy (EBA0-14) in the group of PBTZ169 with the 640 mg dose. During this clinical study, there were no cases of death or severe adverse effects related to the PBTZ169. No adverse effects were considered as definitely related to the drug and, at the study completion, all adverse effects were resolved. There was no increase in adverse effects frequency with growing dose [22].

During the clinical studies it was confirmed that PBTZ169 after single, double, or multiple doses was detectable in the blood plasma of all volunteers and patients who had received the drug. However, it should be noted that pharmacokinetic studies in animals and in healthy volunteers (in Phase 1 clinical studies) demonstrated that PBTZ169, being more soluble in an acidic environment, is absorbed primarily in the stomach. These data agree with the results of in vitro studies, which were conducted by Nearmedic Plus LLC, assessing cellular permeability and solubility in biorelevant media, which mimicked native gastric and intestinal juices. They confirmed that the highest solubility of PBTZ169 is observed at the pH range of 1 to 2, which coincides with the pH in the lower part of the stomach, and its solubility gradually decreases with the growing pH. In the media with pH higher than 5, PBTZ169 was virtually insoluble. According to the test of solubility in biorelevant media, the drug level in the gastric juice was much higher than in the intestinal juice. So, one of the possible methods to increase bioavailability and exposure of PBTZ169 is to prolong its presence in the stomach.

After a single fasting dose, PBTZ169 absorbed rapidly, and the speed of absorption was independent of the administered dose (median T_{max} was 1.5–2.5 hours for the dose range 40–640 mg (NCT03036163), and 1.5–1.75 hours for the dose range 640–1280 mg (NCT04150224). Meantime of retention of the drug in the body was 13.02–19.30 hours and was independent of the administered dose (NCT03036163) [22].

According to the obtained pharmacokinetic data, dose proportionality of C_{max} and $AUC_{0\text{-}t}$ was demonstrated for single, as well as for multiple administrations of the investigational drug in the dose range 40–640 mg (NCT03036163, NCT03334734). After single fasting escalating doses (640, 960, and 1280 mg), C_{max}, $AUC_{0\text{-}24}$, $AUC_{0\text{-}\infty}$ were less than dose proportional. Thus, it can be concluded that there is a trend for linear pharmacokinetics for single and multiple doses up to 640 mg.

When pharmacokinetics of different administration regimens for 1280 mg daily dose was studied (640 mg twice daily or 1280 mg once in fasting conditions), the pharmacokinetic parameters $AUC_{0\text{-}\infty}$ and $AUC_{0\text{-}t}$ increased 1.5–1.6-fold (NCT04150224). The relation of mean $AUC_{0\text{-}\infty}$ and $AUC_{0\text{-}t}$ in cohorts receiving the investigational drug as 640 mg twice a day and 1280 mg once a day, was 153.68% and 160.32%. For C_{max}, a slight decrease (1.1-fold) was observed for the 640 mg twice a day (the relation of means was 90.84%). All observed differences were statistically significant.

According to the results of analysis of relative bioavailability and relative degree of absorption, the main pharmacokinetic parameters of PBTZ169 substantially and statistically significantly increased when 640 mg dose was administered in fed conditions: $AUC_{0\text{-}\infty}$increased 3.45-fold, $AUC_{0\text{-}t}$ (f′) increased 3.50-fold, C_{max} increased 2.29-fold. The drug absorbed and cleared from the body significantly more slowly, when it was administered in fed conditions compared to the fasting conditions (median T_{max}

increased 2-fold, mean $T_{1/2}$ increased 1.44-fold). These data allow to conclude that it is preferable to administer PBTZ169 in fed conditions [22].

In October 2018, the international non-proprietary name "macozinone" was given to PBTZ169 by WHO [28]. In addition to the clinical studies, macozinone is undergoing further in vitro and in vivo testing focused on improvement of its pharmacological properties by structure-based design [29], or on the interactions with anti-TB drugs [30]. Importantly, an efficient method for monitoring metabolism of macozinone in human plasma was recently developed. It enables simultaneous measurement of concentrations of macozinone and its five active metabolites in the clinical samples, which is important for comprehensive pharmacokinetic/pharmacodynamic analyses [31].

6. Other DprE1 Inhibitors under Active Clinical Development

Following the discovery of DprE1 as a target of BTZ043, numerous molecules acting on this enzyme emerged, particularly from the whole-cell based phenotypic screening campaigns (for a recent review see [32]). As a result, DprE1 was given an unflattering attribute—a promiscuous target [33]. Nevertheless, DprE1 remains to be one of the best understood and the most vulnerable novel targets. One of the reasons for its high sensitivity against a number of different pharmacophores could be its periplasmic localization, which makes it easily accessible for the drugs [34]. Consequently, in addition to macozinone, there are currently three other DprE1 inhibitors progressing down the clinical studies pipeline. BTZ043, sponsored by the University of Munich; the Hans Knöll Institute, Jena; and the German Center for Infection Research, successfully completed a single dose escalation Phase 1 study (NCT03590600) [35] and is currently recruiting for a combined Phase 1 and 2 study, which will evaluate safety, tolerability, pharmacokinetics and early bactericidal activity of the multiple ascending doses (NCT04044001) [36]. A non-covalent DprE1 inhibitor, TBA-7371 [37] developed by TB Alliance, Bill and Melinda Gates Medical Research Institute and Foundation for Neglected Disease Research, completed a Phase 1 study (NCT03199339) [38]—a partially blind, placebo-controlled study of (i) a combined single ascending dose with a food effect cohort, (ii) multiple ascending dose group, and (iii) a cohort to investigate interactions between TBA-7371 with midazolam and bupropion. Currently, recruitment of adult patients with rifampicin-sensitive pulmonary tuberculosis is taking place for the participation in a Phase 2 study (NCT04176250) [39] to assess safety, early bactericidal activity, and pharmacokinetics of escalating doses of TBA-7371. A combined Phase 1 and 2 study of OPC-167832 by Otsuka is in progress (NCT03678688) [40], aimed at evaluation of the safety, tolerability, pharmacokinetics, and efficacy of multiple oral doses of the drug in patients with uncomplicated drug-sensitive pulmonary tuberculosis with a positive smear. In a parallel group, low dose or high dose OPC-167832 will be combined with delamanid and compared to delamanid only, or standard treatment with isoniazid, rifampin, pyrazinamide, and ethambutol.

7. Conclusions

The ultimate goal of the TB drug-development efforts is a design of new, more effective regimen, which could replace the current combination therapy. One of the most promising DprE1 inhibitors is macozinone. Its safety and tolerability profiles, pharmacokinetics, and efficacy in terms of early bactericidal activity were evaluated in the course of three clinical trials conducted by Nearmedic Plus LLC in the Russian Federation, two clinical trials by iM4TB foundation are in progress. High tolerability and a favorable safety profile of the drug in the studied dose range were demonstrated both in healthy volunteers and in patients with newly diagnosed pulmonary tuberculosis with bacterial excretion and preserved sensitivity to isoniazid and rifampicin. The main pharmacokinetics parameters of macozinone after single and multiple administration in the dosage range up to 1280 mg were studied, and a statistically significant efficacy of the drug after monotherapy at a dose of 640 mg a day was established, which allowed the preferred regimen of its intake to be determined.

A thorough study aimed at interactions of macozinone with a spectrum of clinically used and experimental TB drugs was recently performed [30]. It revealed that macozinone does not have synergistic or antagonistic interactions with the tested first-line (rifampin, isoniazid, ethambutol) or second-line (amikacin, levofloxacin, moxifloxacin, D-cycloserin, ethionamide, *para*-aminosalicyc acid) drugs. Among the tested re-purposed or new drugs, clarithromycin, delamanid, lansoprazole sulfide, linezolid, meropenem or sutezolid did not show synergistic effects, when tested individually with macozinone by the checkerboard assay. Synergism was observed for macozinone and clofazimine or bedaquiline, confirming previous findings [20,41]. At the same time, enumeration of colony forming units after drug exposure revealed the next two potentially synergistic candidates—delamanid and sutezolid. In the mouse model of TB, the combination of macozinone-delamanid-sutezolid was more active in the lungs of *M. tuberculosis*-infected animals compared to the regimen of rifampin-isoniazid-pyrazinamide, while the bacterial burden in spleen remained comparable. However, increased toxicity of the combination for HepG2 cells was observed, so further studies are needed to evaluate the potential of this drug combination [30]. Nevertheless, neither antagonism nor increased toxicity was found for most combinations, which paves the way for using macozinone in the development of more efficient TB regimens [30].

Author Contributions: Both authors contributed to writing of the paper. All authors have read and agreed to the published version of the manuscript.

Acknowledgments: Authors would like to thank Nearmedic Plus LLC, and personally to R. Bolgarin for information concerning clinical trials and preclinical studies including unpublished data.

References

1. Bloom, B.R.; Atun, R.; Cohen, T.; Dye, C.; Fraser, H.; Gomez, G.B.; Knight, G.; Murray, M.; Nardell, E.; Rubin, E.; et al. Chapter 11. Tuberculosis. In *Major Infectious Diseases. Disease Control Priorities*, 3rd ed.; Holmes, K.K., Bertozzi, S., Bloom, B., Jha, P., Eds.; World Bank: Washington, DC, USA, 2017; Volume 6, pp. 233–313.
2. Baer, C.E.; Rubin, E.J.; Sassetti, C.M. New insights into TB physiology suggest untapped therapeutic opportunities. *Immunol. Rev.* **2015**, *264*, 327–343. [CrossRef]
3. *Global TB Report 2019*; WHO: Geneva, Switzerland, 2019; Available online: https://apps.who.int/iris/bitstream/handle/10665/329368/9789241565714-eng.pdf?ua=1 (accessed on 20 February 2020).
4. Tiberi, S.; du Plessis, N.; Walzl, G.; Vjecha, M.J.; Rao, M.; Ntoumi, F.; Mfinanga, S.; Kapata, N.; Mwaba, P.; McHugh, T.D.; et al. Tuberculosis: Progress and advances in development of new drugs, treatment regimens, and host-directed therapies. *Lancet Infect. Dis.* **2018**, *18*, e183–e198. [CrossRef]
5. Andries, K.; Verhasselt, P.; Guillemont, J.; Gohlmann, H.W.; Neefs, J.M.; Winkler, H.; Van Gestel, J.; Timmerman, P.; Zhu, M.; Lee, E.; et al. A diarylquinoline drug active on the ATP synthase of *Mycobacterium tuberculosis*. *Science* **2005**, *307*, 223–227. [CrossRef] [PubMed]
6. Matsumoto, M.; Hashizume, H.; Tomishige, T.; Kawasaki, M.; Tsubouchi, H.; Sasaki, H.; Shimokawa, Y.; Komatsu, M. OPC-67683, a nitro-dihydro-imidazooxazole derivative with promising action against tuberculosis in vitro and in mice. *PLoS Med.* **2006**, *3*, e466. [CrossRef] [PubMed]
7. Stover, C.K.; Warrener, P.; VanDevanter, D.R.; Sherman, D.R.; Arain, T.M.; Langhorne, M.H.; Anderson, S.W.; Towell, J.A.; Yuan, Y.; McMurray, D.N.; et al. A small-molecule nitroimidazopyran drug candidate for the treatment of tuberculosis. *Nature* **2000**, *405*, 962–966. [CrossRef] [PubMed]
8. WGND Global TB Drug Pipeline. Available online: https://www.newtbdrugs.org/pipeline/clinical (accessed on 20 February 2020).
9. Makarov, V.; Manina, G.; Mikusova, K.; Mollmann, U.; Ryabova, O.; Saint-Joanis, B.; Dhar, N.; Pasca, M.R.; Buroni, S.; Lucarelli, A.P.; et al. Benzothiazinones kill *Mycobacterium tuberculosis* by blocking arabinan synthesis. *Science* **2009**, *324*, 801–804. [CrossRef] [PubMed]
10. Makarov, V.; Moellmann, U. New Dithiocarbamate Derivatives, Useful as Antibacterial Agents, for Treating e.g., Tuberculosis and Infections Caused by Mycobacteria and Staphylococci. U.S. Patent WO2003042186-A, 22 May 2003.
11. Szolar, O.H. Environmental and pharmaceutical analysis of dithiocarbamates. *Anal. Chim. Acta* **2007**, *582*, 191–200. [CrossRef] [PubMed]
12. Makarov, V.; Riabova, O.B.; Yuschenko, A.; Urlyapova, N.; Daudova, A.; Zipfel, P.F.; Mollmann, U. Synthesis

and antileprosy activity of some dialkyldithiocarbamates. *J. Antimicrob. Chemother.* **2006**, *57*, 1134–1138. [CrossRef]

13. Makarov, V.A.; Cole, S.T.; Moellmann, U. New Benzothiazinone Derivatives Useful for the Treatment of Tuberculosis Infection or Leprosy Infection in Mammals. U.S. Patent WO2007134625-A1, 29 November 2007.
14. Mikusova, K.; Huang, H.; Yagi, T.; Holsters, M.; Vereecke, D.; D'Haeze, W.; Scherman, M.S.; Brennan, P.J.; McNeil, M.R.; Crick, D.C. Decaprenylphosphoryl arabinofuranose, the donor of the D-arabinofuranosyl residues of mycobacterial arabinan, is formed via a two-step epimerization of decaprenylphosphoryl ribose. *J. Bacteriol.* **2005**, *187*, 8020–8025. [CrossRef]
15. Wolucka, B.A.; McNeil, M.R.; de Hoffmann, E.; Chojnacki, T.; Brennan, P.J. Recognition of the lipid intermediate for arabinogalactan/arabinomannan biosynthesis and its relation to the mode of action of ethambutol on mycobacteria. *J. Biol. Chem.* **1994**, *269*, 23328–23335.
16. Belanger, A.E.; Inamine, J.M. Genetics of Cell Wall Biosythesis. In *Molecular Genetics of Mycobacteria*; Hatfull, G.F., Jacobs, W.R., Jr., Eds.; ASM Press: Washington, DC, USA, 2000; pp. 191–202.
17. Trefzer, C.; Rengifo-Gonzalez, M.; Hinner, M.J.; Schneider, P.; Makarov, V.; Cole, S.T.; Johnsson, K. Benzothiazinones: Prodrugs that covalently modify the decaprenylphosphoryl-beta-D-ribose 2′-epimerase DprE1 of *Mycobacterium tuberculosis*. *J. Am. Chem. Soc.* **2010**, *132*, 13663–13665. [CrossRef] [PubMed]
18. Trefzer, C.; Skovierova, H.; Buroni, S.; Bobovska, A.; Nenci, S.; Molteni, E.; Pojer, F.; Pasca, M.R.; Makarov, V.; Cole, S.T.; et al. Benzothiazinones are suicide inhibitors of mycobacterial decaprenylphosphoryl-beta-D-ribofuranose 2′-oxidase DprE1. *J. Am. Chem. Soc.* **2012**, *134*, 912–915. [CrossRef] [PubMed]
19. Neres, J.; Pojer, F.; Molteni, E.; Chiarelli, L.R.; Dhar, N.; Boy-Rottger, S.; Buroni, S.; Fullam, E.; Degiacomi, G.; Lucarelli, A.P.; et al. Structural basis for benzothiazinone-mediated killing of *Mycobacterium tuberculosis*. *Sci. Transl. Med.* **2012**, *4*, 150ra121. [CrossRef]
20. Makarov, V.; Lechartier, B.; Zhang, M.; Neres, J.; van der Sar, A.M.; Raadsen, S.A.; Hartkoorn, R.C.; Ryabova, O.B.; Vocat, A.; Decosterd, L.A.; et al. Towards a new combination therapy for tuberculosis with next generation benzothiazinones. *EMBO Mol. Med.* **2014**, *6*, 372–383. [CrossRef] [PubMed]
21. Innovative Medicines for Tuberculosis. Available online: http://im4tb.org (accessed on 24 February 2020).
22. Mariandyshev, A.O.; Khokhlov, A.L.; Smerdin, S.V.; Shcherbakova, V.S.; Igumnova, O.V.; Ozerova, I.V.; Bolgarina, A.A.; Nikitina, N.A. The main results of clinical trials of the efficacy, safety and pharmacokinetics of the perspective anti-tuberculosis drug Macozinone (PBTZ169). *Terapevt. Arkh.* **2020**, *92*, 61–72.
23. Study to Evaluate the Safety, Tolerability, Pharmacokinetics and Ex-Vivo Antitubercular Activity of PBTZ169 Formulation. Available online: https://clinicaltrials.gov/ct2/show/NCT03423030 (accessed on 25 February 2020).
24. Study to Evaluate the Safety, Tolerability and Pharmacokinetics of PBTZ169 in Multiple Dosing. Available online: https://clinicaltrials.gov/ct2/show/NCT03776500 (accessed on 25 February 2020).
25. Phase 1 Study of PBTZ169. Available online: https://clinicaltrials.gov/ct2/show/NCT03036163 (accessed on 25 February 2020).
26. Safety, Tolerability, Pharmacokinetics and Food Effects Study of PBTZ169. Available online: https://clinicaltrials.gov/ct2/show/study/NCT04150224 (accessed on 25 February 2020).
27. Phase 2a Study of PBTZ169. Available online: https://clinicaltrials.gov/ct2/show/NCT03334734 (accessed on 25 February 2020).
28. WHO Drug Information Volume 32, N° 3. 2018. Available online: https://www.who.int/medicines/publications/druginformation/issues/DrugInformation2018_Vol32-3/en/ (accessed on 25 February 2020).
29. Piton, J.; Vocat, A.; Lupien, A.; Foo, C.S.; Riabova, O.; Makarov, V.; Cole, S.T. Structure-Based drug design and characterization of sulfonyl-piperazine benzothiazinone inhibitors of DprE1 from *Mycobacterium tuberculosis*. *Antimicrob. Agents Chemot.* **2018**, *62*. [CrossRef] [PubMed]
30. Lupien, A.; Vocat, A.; Foo, C.S.; Blattes, E.; Gillon, J.Y.; Makarov, V.; Cole, S.T. Optimized background regimen for treatment of active tuberculosis with the next-generation benzothiazinone macozinone (PBTZ169). *Antimicrob. Agents Chemot.* **2018**, *62*, e00840-18. [CrossRef]
31. Spaggiari, D.; Desfontaine, V.; Cruchon, S.; Guinchard, S.; Vocat, A.; Blattes, E.; Pitteloud, J.; Ciullini, L.; Bardinet, C.; Ivanyuk, A.; et al. Development and validation of a multiplex UHPLC-MS/MS method for the determination of the investigational antibiotic against multi-resistant tuberculosis macozinone (PBTZ169) and five active metabolites in human plasma. *PLoS ONE* **2019**, *14*, e0217139. [CrossRef]

32. Degiacomi, G.; Belardinelli, J.M.; Pasca, M.R.; De Rossi, E.; Riccardi, G.; Chiarelli, L.R. Promiscuous targets for antitubercular drug discovery: The paradigm of DprE1 and MmpL3. *Appl. Sci.* **2020**, *10*, 623. [CrossRef]
33. Lechartier, B.; Rybniker, J.; Zumla, A.; Cole, S.T. Tuberculosis drug discovery in the post-post-genomic era. *EMBO Mol. Med.* **2014**, *6*, 158–168. [CrossRef]
34. Brecik, M.; Centarova, I.; Mukherjee, R.; Kolly, G.S.; Huszar, S.; Bobovska, A.; Kilacskova, E.; Mokosova, V.; Svetlikova, Z.; Sarkan, M.; et al. DprE1 is a vulnerable tuberculosis drug target due to its cell wall localization. *ACS Chem. Biol.* **2015**, *10*, 1631–1636. [CrossRef] [PubMed]
35. A Single Ascending Dose Study of BTZ043. Available online: https://clinicaltrials.gov/ct2/show/NCT03590600 (accessed on 25 February 2020).
36. BTZ-043—Multiple Ascending Dose (MAD) to Evaluate Safety, Tolerability and Early Bactericidal Activity (EBA). Available online: https://clinicaltrials.gov/ct2/show/NCT04044001 (accessed on 25 February 2020).
37. Chatterji, M.; Shandil, R.; Manjunatha, M.R.; Solapure, S.; Ramachandran, V.; Kumar, N.; Saralaya, R.; Panduga, V.; Reddy, J.; Prabhakar, K.R.; et al. 1,4-azaindole, a potential drug candidate for treatment of tuberculosis. *Antimicrob. Agents Chemother.* **2014**, *58*, 5325–5331. [CrossRef] [PubMed]
38. A Phase 1 Study to Evaluate Safety, Tolerability, PK, and PK Interactions of TBA-7371. Available online: https://clinicaltrials.gov/ct2/show/NCT03199339 (accessed on 25 February 2020).
39. Early Bactericidal Activity of TBA-7371 in Pulmonary Tuberculosis. Available online: https://clinicaltrials.gov/ct2/show/NCT04176250 (accessed on 25 February 2020).
40. A Phase 1/2 Trial of Multiple oral Doses of OPC-167832 for Uncomplicated Pulmonary Tuberculosis. Available online: https://clinicaltrials.gov/ct2/show/NCT03678688 (accessed on 25 February 2020).
41. Lechartier, B.; Cole, S.T. Mode of action of clofazimine and combination therapy with benzothiazinones against *Mycobacterium tuberculosis*. *Antimicrob. Agents Chemother.* **2015**, *59*, 4457–4463. [CrossRef] [PubMed]

9

TB Elimination Requires Discovery and Development of Transformational Agents

Christian Lienhardt [1] and Mario C. Raviglione [2,*]

[1] Unité Mixte Internationale TransVIHMI (UMI 233 IRD–U1175 INSERM, Université de Montpellier)-Institut de Recherche pour le Développement (IRD), 34000 Montpellier, France; christian.lienhardt@ird.fr

[2] Centre for Multidisciplinary Research in Health Science (MACH), Università di Milano, Milan, Italy and Global Studies Institute, Université de Genève, 1211 Genève, Switzerland

* Correspondence: mario.raviglione@unimi.it

Abstract: The World Health Organization (WHO) End Tuberculosis (TB) Strategy has set ambitious targets to reduce 2015 TB incidence and deaths by 80% and 90%, respectively, by the year 2030. Given the current rate of TB incidence decline (about 2% per year annually), reaching these targets will require new transformational tools and innovative ways to deliver them. In addition to improved tests for early and rapid detection of TB and universal drug-susceptibility testing, as well as novel vaccines for improved prevention, better, safer, shorter and more efficacious treatments for all forms of TB are needed. Only a handful of new drugs are currently in phase II or III clinical trials, and a few combination regimens are being tested, mainly for drug-resistant TB. In this article, capitalising on an increasingly rich medicine pipeline and taking advantage of new methodological designs with great potential, the main areas where progress is needed for a transformational improvement of treatment of all forms of TB are described.

Keywords: tuberculosis treatment; biomarkers; drug combination; clinical trial

---

On 14 May 2014, the 67th World Health Assembly (WHA) endorsed a resolution detailing the global strategy to control and eliminate tuberculosis (TB) in the 2015–2030 Sustainable Development Goal (SDG) era [1]. The 3-pillar strategy was branded as the "End TB Strategy" [2]. Additional to two pillars devoted to patient-centred care and to health system policies, a third pillar is fully devoted to research and the need of innovations. This pillar and its components are fundamental in reaching ambitious international targets set as part of the new strategy to "End TB": to reduce 2015 TB incidence and deaths by 80% and 90%, respectively, by the year 2030. The simple projection model underpinning such figures, presented at the 67th WHA, is based on previous empirical experiences showing the plausibility of declining trends conducive to those targets. The large-scale interventions promoted by the End TB Strategy would be able to reduce TB incidence at a much higher annual rate than the current 1.5–2% per year [3]. For instance, it is known that in the Netherlands, United Kingdom, Germany and other western European countries, TB incidence was declining at 8%–10% per year during the late 1950s and 1960s thanks to wide access to diagnosis and effective chemotherapy, screening of people at risk, affordable care and social protection mechanisms [4]. It is also known that additional intensive interventions, including large-scale preventive therapy, were associated with even faster declines reaching 17% per year among the small Inuit populations of Alaska and North-Western Territory of Canada [5]. However, while these declines could in theory be achieved with optimal implementation of existing diagnostic and treatment tools—which are better than those available 70 years ago—the needed acceleration towards 15%–20% incidence decline per year to reach the 2030 targets will require new transformational tools and innovative ways to deliver them. These tools need to cover all aspects of TB care and its cascade, as well as prevention.

1. Which New Tools Are Necessary to End the Tuberculosis (TB) Epidemic?

First of all, achieving the End TB targets will require improved tests for early and rapid detection of TB and for universal drug-susceptibility testing (DST) to reach more patients when they first seek care so that one can cut transmission early and accelerate the decline in TB incidence and mortality. Diagnostics must be rapid, precise, connectable, available at the point-of-care and effective in detecting both active disease and latent infection [6]. Molecular diagnostics and sequencing technology available today are powerful tools, but still need relatively sophisticated laboratory capacity, and are not offering a point of care solution thus limiting their efficacy in the field.

Second, we need better, safer, shorter and more efficacious treatment for all forms of TB. The current research and development pipeline—although the most populated seen in the past few decades—still shows only less than 10 new agents in phase 1 trials, a handful of new drugs in phase 2 or 3 trials, and a few combination regimens being tested mainly for drug-resistant TB [7]. Completely new classes of anti-TB compounds are scarce, and potential synergistic combinations still unknown. Furthermore, targeting better treatment of active TB towards elimination goals is clearly not enough, as the reservoir of latent TB infection needs to be tackled as well. Mathematical models show that elimination may not be possible without targeting simultaneously latent infection and active disease [8]. Thus, addressing the vast pool of at-risk individuals among the estimated 1.7 billion people who may be latently infected is paramount, and solutions must be found that are simple and can be implemented safely among those at the highest risk of disease. Currently, the pipeline for treatment of latent infection includes a few trials using essentially known drugs such as isoniazid, rifampicin and rifapentine in different combinations, dosage and duration.

Lastly, a vaccine would be the ultimate solution if found to be highly effective, safe, able to prevent pre-exposure infection as well as reactivation. However, at the moment, the most advanced and promising vaccine candidate among the 14 in the current pipeline offers at best a 50% protection among those with latent infection, and this still needs confirmation [9]. A fully effective potent vaccine is not envisaged for several years, and will certainly not be available on time to allow reaching the 2030 targets.

Notwithstanding the importance of new, rapid diagnostics and efficacious vaccines, efforts to populate the pipeline and accelerate anti-TB drug research are a top priority for investors and researchers alike. Lately, after several years of stagnation, financial investments have been growing slowly passing 800 million US$ in 2019 [10]. However, this is far from sufficient to truly accelerate research toward new agents and regimens. The modest target of 2 billion US$/year, promoted within an existing international plan [11], is not at reach at the moment.

At the same time, efforts in drug research begun in the early 2000s resulted in some successes with the discovery and development of agents such as bedaquiline and delamanid that are recommended for the treatment of drug-resistant TB. Recently, the combination of two new drugs—pretomanid and bedaquiline—with a re-purposed agent, linezolid, has resulted in unprecedented high rates of cure among advanced forms of multidrug-resistant TB (MDR-TB) and of extensively drug-resistant TB (XDR-TB) (Nix-TB trial) [12]. The demonstrated 90% cure rates observed in a single-arm, open-label trial in South Africa has prompted approval by the US Food and Drug Administration (FDA), despite the high frequency of adverse events, including bone marrow suppression and peripheral neuropathy, due to linezolid. These advances show that with wise investments and a well-thought strategy that pursues development of a full regimen composed of new and existing or re-purposed drugs rather than of individual new drugs-as promoted by the WHO Target Regimen Profiles [13] -may be conducive to success despite the obvious challenges that TB research poses. This now needs to be consolidated and accelerated, so that we can hope to obtain a shorter and safer novel regimen that can treat TB irrespective of pre-existing drug resistance (and thus with reduced need for drug-resistance testing).

2. Which New Drugs and Regimens?

First, further progress would require improving molecules of known classes. The Nix-TB trial has raised much hope for the development of a short fully oral regimen for the treatment of severe drug-resistant TB. The use of the tested regimen may, however, be limited in clinical practice due to severe side-effects caused by linezolid. While a trial is on-going to test lower dose of linezolid, [14] new oxazolidinones are being developed to try and reduce toxic effects. Four oxazolidinones are now in early phases of the clinical development pipeline, i.e., contezolid, delpazolid, sutezolid and TBI-223 [7]. Similarly, the use of clofazimine, another important component of the therapeutic armamentarium against drug-resistant TB, is hampered by potential undesirable skin pigmentation. Novel riminophenazine derivatives are being developed with the goal of maintaining potent anti-tuberculosis activity while lowering side effects–such as TBI-166, a compound currently in clinical development in China [15].

The second requirement is that of developing new agents or, better classes of anti-TB drugs.

While improving existing classes has the advantage of initiating the risky discovery process with a well-characterized, validated compound, some level fast adaptation of bacterial populations can be expected. Ideally, therefore, research and development should produce entirely new classes, targets and modes of action to avoid cross-resistance to existing antibiotics. Thus, in parallel with improvements in existing drug and regimen models, innovative approaches, including discovery of novel chemical scaffolds and identification of new targets, are urgently needed.

The discovery of bedaquiline opened the way to investigating the possibility to alter the energy metabolism in mycobacteria, in particular the oxidative phosphorylation pathway, as a novel target pathway in drug discovery, leading to the depletion of ATP synthesis of *M. tuberculosis*. New classes of antibacterial drugs interfering with elements of this pathway have been shown to be highly active in combating latent mycobacterial infections. The discovery of Q203, a candidate drug targeting the cytochrome bc1 complex in the respiratory chain, has highlighted the importance of this new target pathway. Inhibiting the bacterial energy metabolism might be a key feature of novel and sterilizing drug combinations for the treatment of TB [16]. Furthermore, Q203 was shown to have good synergy with bedaquiline in the murine chronic infection model, indicating promising potential for new treatment regimens [17]. Thus, the combination of drugs targeting various elements of the oxidative phosphorylation pathway could lead to a completely new regimen for drug-susceptible and multi-drug resistant tuberculosis.

A series of new compounds are currently developed that focus on newly identified targets. Four of these inhibit DprE1 (decaprenylphosphoryl-β-D-ribose 2-epimerase), a flavoenzyme that catalyses a key step in the synthesis of the complex cell wall of *M. tuberculosis*: macozinone, BTZ-043, OPC-167832 and TBA-7371 [7]. Another compound targets the leucyl-tRNA synthetase (LeuRS), which is essential for protein synthesis (GSK3036656).

The third approach is to identify efficient and seamless development processes to accelerate testing of novel treatment regimens. The current TB treatment development pathway is complex, lengthy and costly, partly due to the fact that some drugs are still being developed individually, and partly due to the lack of reliable surrogate markers of treatment outcomes and the lack of predictive quantitative relationships between Phase II and Phase III outcomes [18]. Currently, Phase II TB drug development includes 14-day early bactericidal activity monotherapy studies to identify the maximally efficacious dose for a new chemical entity (Phase IIA), followed by 2-month serial sputum colony count studies (Phase IIB), in which the efficacy of treatment combinations is usually studied with time-to-sputum-culture-conversion as the primary endpoint. In addition to long duration, this approach suffers multiple weaknesses, including an inadequate exploration of dose-response, the lack of means to determine early the optimal combination of drugs to be tested and the optimal duration of therapy, as well as the inability to study multiple regimens in parallel [19].

Research is needed to identify biomarkers that could predict relapse and guide selection of suitable drug combination(s) and treatment duration(s) so as to accelerate drug development in TB. Novel approaches are being explored to identify early and streamline suitable drug combinations to advance from early to late phases of development taking into account new developments in pharmacokinetic and pharmacodynamic methodology and modelling [20], as well as novel adaptive designs [21]. The "multi-arm multi-stage" (MAMS) design, initially used in oncology, allows testing a broad range of combinations and dose levels without requiring a large sample size, dropping early arms that do not meet pre-specified efficacy threshold [22]. Recently, a newer approach has been proposed that combines Phase II and Phase III features. In this design, named "selection trial with extended post-treatment follow-up" (STEP), limited long-term follow-up data on relapse are collected, together with data on culture conversion, permitting estimation of a Bayesian prediction interval for the likely results of a future Phase III trial [23]. Such Phase IIB/C studies, with arms testing different doses and durations, coupled with the use of novel biomarkers for sterilising cures—these being either RNA expression, cytokine, bacterial or radiological markers—would strengthen and accelerate the process for identifying candidate regimens likely to succeed in Phase III [24], as well as prospectively validating novel biomarkers against the relapse endpoint.

3. Conclusions

We are now at a crossroads in new anti-tuberculosis drug and regimen development. New initiatives, such as the the European Union (EU) Innovative Medicines Initiative IMI2 call and the Gates Medical Research Institute alliance, have the potential to accelerate research and synergize with existing efforts carried out by academia, public-private partnerships, such as the TB Alliance, and industry. If researchers collaborate and join forces towards the common aim of innovative regimens, there is a possibility of pursuing effectively a transformational improvement of treatment of all forms of TB [25]. If, however, such initiatives compete for limited resources and resist cooperation, the targets expressed at the time of the Moscow Conference in late 2017 and subsequently at the United Nations General Assembly in 2018 may remain a dream.

Author Contributions: The two authors contributed equally to the writing of the article. All authors have read and agreed to the published version of the manuscript.

References

1. World Health Organization. *Sixty-Seventh World Health Assembly WHA67.1*; World Health Organization: Geneva, Switzerland, 2014.
2. World Health Organization. *Global Strategy and Targets for Tuberculosis Prevention, Care and Control after 2015*; Agenda item 12.1, 21 May 2014; World Health Organization: Geneva, Switzerland, 2014.
3. Uplekar, M.; Weil, D.; Lönnroth, K.; Jaramillo, E.; Lienhardt, C.; Dias, H.M.; Falzon, D.; Floyd, K.; Gargioni, G.; Getahun, H.; et al. WHO's End TB Strategy. *Lancet* **2015**, *385*, 1799–1801. [CrossRef]
4. World Health Organization. *Global Tuberculosis Report 2019*; World Health Organization: Geneva, Switzerland, 2019.
5. Styblo, K. *Epidemiology of Tuberculosis*; The Royal Netherlands Tuberculosis Association (KNCV): The Hague, The Netherlands, 1991.
6. Grzybowski, S.; Styblo, K.; Dorken, E. Tuberculosis in Eskimos. *Tubercle* **1976**, *57*, 1–58. [CrossRef]
7. Walzl, G.; McNerney, R.; du Plessis, N.; Bates, M.; McHugh, T.D.; Chegou, N.N.; Zumla, A. Tuberculosis: Advances and challenges in development of new diagnostics and biomarkers. *Lancet Infect Dis.* **2018**, *18*, e199–e210. [CrossRef]
8. Stop TB Partnership's Working Group on New TB Drugs Clinical Pipeline. Available online: https://www.newtbdrugs.org/pipeline/clinical (accessed on 30 March 2020).
9. Dye, C.; Williams, B.G. Eliminating human tuberculosis in the 21st century. *J. R. Soc. Interface* **2008**, *5*, 653–662. [CrossRef] [PubMed]
10. Tait, D.R.; Hatherill, M.; Van Der Meeren, O.; Ginsberg, A.M.; Van Brakel, E.; Salaun, B.; Scriba, T.J.; Akite, E.J.; Ayles, H.M.; Bollaerts, A.; et al. Final Analysis of a Trial of M72/AS01$_E$ Vaccine to Prevent Tuberculosis. *N. Engl. J. Med.* **2019**, *381*, 2429–2439. [CrossRef]
11. Treatment Action Group. *Tuberculosis Research Funding Trends 2005–2018*; Treatment Action Group: New York, NY, USA, 2019; ISBN 978-0-9983966-8-2.

10. Tait, D.R.; Hatherill, M.; Van Der Meeren, O.; Ginsberg, A.M.; Van Brakel, E.; Salaun, B.; Scriba, T.J.; Akite, E.J.; Ayles, H.M.; Bollaerts, A.; et al. Final Analysis of a Trial of M72/AS01$_E$ Vaccine to Prevent Tuberculosis. *N. Engl. J. Med.* **2019**, *381*, 2429–2439. [CrossRef]
11. Treatment Action Group. *Tuberculosis Research Funding Trends 2005–2018*; Treatment Action Group: New York, NY, USA, 2019; ISBN 978-0-9983966-8-2.
12. The Lancet Commission on TB. Building a Tuberculosis-Free World: The Lancet Commission on Tuberculosis. *Lancet* **2019**. [CrossRef]
13. Conradie, F.; Diacon, A.H.; Ngubane, N.; Howell, P.; Everitt, D.; Crook, A.M.; Mendel, C.M.; Egizi, E.; Moreira, J.; Timm, J.; et al. Treatment of Highly Drug-Resistant Pulmonary Tuberculosis. *N. Engl. J. Med.* **2020**, *382*, 893–902. [CrossRef]
14. World Health Organization. *Target Regimen Profiles for TB Treatment: Candidates: rifampicin-Susceptible, Rifampicinresistant and pan-TB Treatment Regimens*; World Health Organization: Geneva, Switzerland, 2016.
15. Zhang, D.; Liu, Y.; Zhang, C.; Zhang, H.; Wang, B.; Xu, J.; Fu, L.; Yin, D.; Cooper, C.B.; Ma, Z.; et al. Synthesis and biological evaluation of novel 2-methoxypyridylamino-substituted riminophenazine derivatives as antituberculosis agents. *Molecules* **2014**, *19*, 4380–4394. [CrossRef]
16. Bald, D.; Villellas, C.; Lu, P.; Koul, A. Targeting energy metabolism in *Mycobacterium tuberculosis*, a new paradigm in antimycobacterial drug discovery. *mBio* **2017**, *8*, e00272-17. [CrossRef]
17. Shi-Yan Foo, C.; Pethe, K.; Lupien, A. Oxidative Phosphorylation—an Update on a New, Essential Target Space for Drug Discovery in Mycobacterium tuberculosis. *Appl. Sci.* **2020**, *10*, 2339. [CrossRef]
18. Ginsberg, A.M.; Spigelman, M. Challenges in tuberculosis drug research and development. *Nat Med.* **2007**, *13*, 290–294. [CrossRef]
19. Lienhardt, C.; Nahid, P. Advances in clinical trial design for development of new TB treatments: A call for innovation. *PLoS Med.* **2019**, *16*, e1002769. [CrossRef]
20. Dooley, K.E.; Hanna, D.; Mave, V.; Eisenach, K.; Savic, R.M. Advancing the development of new tuberculosis treatment regimens: The essential role of translational and clinical pharmacology and microbiology. *PLoS Med.* **2019**, *16*, e1002842. [CrossRef] [PubMed]
21. Davies, G.R.; Phillips, P.P.J.; Jaki, T. Adaptive clinical trials in tuberculosis: Applications, challenges and solutions. *Int. J. Tuberc. Lung Dis.* **2015**, *19*, 626–634. [CrossRef]
22. Boeree, M.J.; Heinrich, N.; Aarnoutse, R.; Diacon, A.H.; Dawson, R.; Rehal, S.; Kibiki, G.S.; Churchyard, G.; Sanne, I.; Ntinginya, N.E.; et al. High-dose rifampicin, moxifloxacin, and SQ109 for treating tuberculosis: A multi-arm, multi-stage randomised controlled trial. *Lancet Infect Dis.* **2017**, *17*, 39–49. [CrossRef]
23. Phillips, P.P.J.; Dooley, K.E.; Gillespie, S.H.; Heinrich, N.; Stout, J.E.; Nahid, P.; Diacon, A.H.; Aarnoutse, R.E.; Kibiki, G.S.; Boeree, M.J.; et al. A new trial design to accelerate tuberculosis drug development: The Phase IIC Selection Trial with Extended Post treatment follow-up (STEP). *BMC Med.* **2016**, *14*, 51. [CrossRef] [PubMed]
24. Davies, G.; Hoelscher, M.; Boeree, M.; Hermann, D. Accelerating the transition of new tuberculosis drug combinations from Phase II to Phase III trials: New technologies and innovative designs. *PLoS Med.* **2019**, *16*, e1002851. [CrossRef]
25. Lienhardt, C.; Nunn, A.; Chaisson, R.; Vernon, A.A.; Zignol, M.; Nahid, P.; Delaporte, E.; Kasaeva, T. Advances in clinical trial design: Weaving tomorrow's TB treatments. *PLoS Med.* **2020**, *17*, e1003059. [CrossRef]

10

Model-Informed Drug Discovery and Development Strategy for the Rapid Development of Anti-Tuberculosis Drug Combinations

Rob C. van Wijk [1], Rami Ayoun Alsoud [1], Hans Lennernäs [2] and Ulrika S. H. Simonsson [1,*]

1 Department of Pharmaceutical Biosciences, Uppsala University, Uppsala 75123, Sweden; rob.vanwijk@farmbio.uu.se (R.C.v.W.); rami.alsoud@farmbio.uu.se (R.A.A.)
2 Department of Pharmacy, Uppsala University, Uppsala 75123, Sweden; hans.lennernas@farmaci.uu.se
* Correspondence: ulrika.simonsson@farmbio.uu.se.

Featured Application: Model-informed drug discovery and development (MID3) is proposed to be applied throughout the preclinical to clinical phases to provide an informative prediction of drug exposure and efficacy in humans in order to select novel anti-tuberculosis drug combinations for the treatment of tuberculosis.

Abstract: The increasing emergence of drug-resistant tuberculosis requires new effective and safe drug regimens. However, drug discovery and development are challenging, lengthy and costly. The framework of model-informed drug discovery and development (MID3) is proposed to be applied throughout the preclinical to clinical phases to provide an informative prediction of drug exposure and efficacy in humans in order to select novel anti-tuberculosis drug combinations. The MID3 includes pharmacokinetic-pharmacodynamic and quantitative systems pharmacology models, machine learning and artificial intelligence, which integrates all the available knowledge related to disease and the compounds. A translational *in vitro-in vivo* link throughout modeling and simulation is crucial to optimize the selection of regimens with the highest probability of receiving approval from regulatory authorities. *In vitro-in vivo* correlation (IVIVC) and physiologically-based pharmacokinetic modeling provide powerful tools to predict pharmacokinetic drug-drug interactions based on preclinical information. Mechanistic or semi-mechanistic pharmacokinetic-pharmacodynamic models have been successfully applied to predict the clinical exposure-response profile for anti-tuberculosis drugs using preclinical data. Potential pharmacodynamic drug-drug interactions can be predicted from *in vitro* data through IVIVC and pharmacokinetic-pharmacodynamic modeling accounting for translational factors. It is essential for academic and industrial drug developers to collaborate across disciplines to realize the huge potential of MID3.

Keywords: tuberculosis; MID3; pharmacokinetics; pharmacodynamics; drug-drug interactions; *in vitro*; *in vivo*; drug development

---

1. Introduction

Drug discovery and development is a challenging, lengthy, and costly process. The costs of a novel drug reaching the market can be as much as 2–3 billion dollars [1]. In the early discovery phase, libraries consisting of thousands of compounds can be synthesized chemically and tested for efficacy *in vitro* at a relatively low cost. The largest expenditures are in the late preclinical and clinical phases of drug development, where the efficacy and safety of treatment are assessed. Smart decisions need to be made regarding which compounds and regimens should progress through the preclinical phase and subsequently into clinical trials. Early characterization of each compound's exposure-response relationship, i.e., pharmacokinetic (PK)-pharmacodynamic (PD) relationship and potential interactions within regimens and with commonly co-administered drugs, can allow for informative decision making throughout preclinical development and into clinical development [2].

Tuberculosis (TB) is the leading cause of adult mortality through infectious diseases and 10 million new cases are reported globally every year [3]. Sensitive TB is currently treated with a six-month regimen of antibiotics, consisting of isoniazid, pyrazinamide, rifampicin and ethambutol, which was developed in the mid-twentieth century. This therapy is believed to be suboptimal and was not developed using modern approaches for drug development, thereby lacking important information on the PK-PD relationship. Therefore, clinical trials have recently been conducted in order to define the relationship between exposure and efficacy, as well as safety, where statistically significant exposure-response relationships for rifampicin have been identified, in order to support a higher dose of rifampicin [4–7]. Almost one in five patients will acquire multidrug-resistant tuberculosis (MDR-TB) or rifampicin-resistant tuberculosis (RR-TB) [3]. Recently, the new anti-TB drugs bedaquiline, delamanid and pretomanid were conditionally approved against MDR-TB, which led to updates to the World Health Organization (WHO) treatment guideline for MDR-TB [8]. Bedaquiline is a diarylquinoline, a new class of antibiotics. It is an inhibitor of the membrane-bound adenosine triphosphate (ATP)-synthase enzyme, therefore blocking mycobacterial ATP formation and energy metabolism. Bedaquiline is therefore bactericidal for dormant mycobacteria as well, a preferable feature for the shortening of treatment duration and prevention of relapse [9]. Delamanid is a nitroimidazole and affects the mycobacterial cell wall, thereby also improving drug penetration into the mycobacterium. It is the most potent TB drug and is active against replicating and dormant mycobacteria as well [9]. The combination of delamanid with bedaquiline is, however, not recommended, due to QT-prolongation-related cardiotoxicity [10]. Pretomanid belongs to the same class of antibiotics as delamanid [9]. Pretomanid was developed as part of a drug combination together with bedaquiline and linezolid, an oxazolidinone-class otherwise used for the treatment of pneumonia and skin infection. There is a clear need for the additional development of new effective drug combinations. The European Medical Agency (EMA) drug development guideline for TB specifies that efforts should be made to develop entirely new regimens to treat TB, rather than focusing on single drugs [11]. Due to the burden of polypharmacy for the patients and the increased risk of side effects, the focus should be on developing new regimens instead of the development of single agents as an add-on to a current regimen which was recommended in the earlier EMA TB drug development guideline [12]. Of the three new drugs against TB, only pretomanid is approved as a new combination regimen, while bedaquiline and delamanid were developed as add-ons to existing therapy [13]. The development of new combination regimens is the way forward, the acceleration of which is the objective of the new Innovative Medicines Initiative (IMI)-funded consortium European Regimen Accelerator for Tuberculosis (ERA4TB). It is important to assess drug-drug interactions (DDI), with respect to both PK and PD, to understand how the different drugs behave in certain combinations and doses in order to maximize the efficacy and potentially learn how the efficacy of the combination varies with time and concentration. The development of drug combinations is, however, challenging. It is difficult to demonstrate the contribution of an individual drug to a regimen regarding efficacy or safety [14]. The duration of treatment is lengthy, especially when considering follow-up to ensure no relapse. Moreover, the design and execution of preclinical experiments and clinical trials are complex, as the number of treatments to test grows exponentially with every added drug or dose, leading to longer development times and higher costs. Tuberculosis drug development, which focuses on regimens rather than unique drugs as an add-on treatment, thus challenges our methods to assess and identify optimal regimens. Therefore, smart experimental designs and optimized data analysis are essential. Data from larger scale *in vitro* preclinical experiments, with different drug regimens that explore the PD interaction space in order to investigate the synergism and/or antagonism of the interacting drugs, should be used to select the best regimens to determine the exposure range *in vivo*. Based on the exposure-response relationship in animals, and/or pure *in vitro* predictions, the first in-human (FIH) and early bactericidal activity (EBA) trials can be designed. These steps all require a mathematical translational approach, taking into account the PK-PD and translational factors to account for differences between preclinical species and patients [15,16].

The European Medicines Agency/European Federation of Pharmaceutical Industries and Associations (EFPIA) Modeling and Simulation joint workshop held in 2011 assembled scientists from the pharmaceutical industry, academia and regulatory authorities from across Europe, the USA and Japan to consider the future role of modeling and simulation in drug development and regulatory assessment. As a follow up to the workshop, one of the EFPIA groups' commitment to EMA was to generate a "good practice" manuscript covering aspects of planning, conduct and documentation of a variety of quantitative approaches for modeling and simulation methods where the concept of Model-Informed Drug Discovery and Development (MID3) was defined [17]. The aim of MID3 is to enable more efficient and robust research and development and regulatory decisions using an integrated model-based drug development approach [17,18]. The MID3 strategy for the development of drugs in any therapeutic area is supported by the EMA [19].

The MID3 framework has been defined as a "quantitative framework for prediction and extrapolation, centered on knowledge and inference generated from integrated models of compound, mechanism and disease level data and aimed at improving the quality, efficiency and cost effectiveness of decision making" [17]. The MID3 framework should be applied in the development of new TB drug regimens and is necessary for the reliable prediction of the optimal selection of novel TB drug combination therapies based on pre-clinical information, and subsequent decisions on which combinations to evaluate in clinical trials in order to confirm their efficacy and safety. The framework integrates all available data and information on the disease and the compounds.

In addition to PK and PD models, systems biology or systems pharmacology models [18] and machine learning based on, for example, imaging data [20] or even artificial intelligence (AI) [21,22] are important tools. Figure 1 shows the proposed MID3 strategy for the rapid development of anti-TB regimens through the prediction of human-concentration-time relationships (PK), exposure-response relationships (PK-PD) and DDIs to select FIH doses, as well as the prediction of Phase II and Phase III drug regimens. Initially in a drug development program, preclinical data is mostly available. The impact of modeling and simulation increases towards the prediction of human exposure-response. With this input efficient decision can be made about the optimal combination of different drugs, and the right dose for each drug in the combination. Currently, limited modeling and simulation are required for market approval, which relies more on statistical comparison between treatment groups after phase III [23].

However, modeling and simulation can have a role in the analysis of Phase III data in order to define the relationship between exposure and clinical endpoint, evaluate PK DDI and simulate alternative potential regimens in certain subgroups, for example, patients with renal impairment [24]. A key step for successful TB drug development is to use modeling and simulation to predict the efficacy of combinations, including DDIs, for, for example, synergy. We will review the necessary steps from this perspective for the successful MID3 application to the preclinical to clinical translation of efficacious TB drug combinations, regarding the optimal doses of drugs in complex regimens.

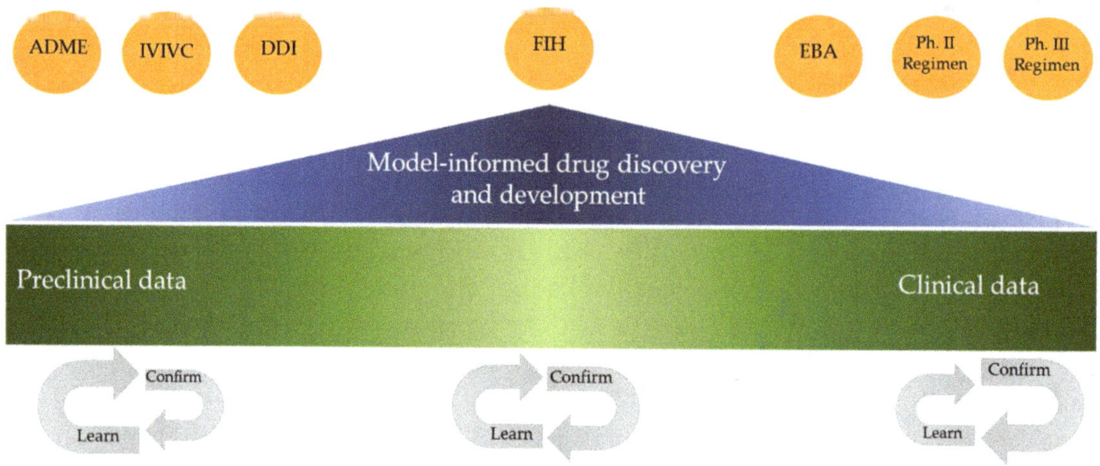

Figure 1. Illustration of the role of Model-Informed Drug Discovery and Development (MID3) and the application across preclinical to clinical drug development.

MID3, with modeling and simulation as key tools, is suggested to be applied throughout the pre-clinical to clinical drug development phases in order to optimize and inform decision making with respect to clinical trial design and the selection of drugs and doses to be carried forward from the preclinical phase and into clinical trial programs. The prediction of human-concentration-time relationships (PK), exposure-response relationships (PK-PD) in monotherapy and combination therapy, as well as drug-drug interactions, (DDI), requires the application of MID3 techniques and integration of all available data. In early preclinical drug development, preclinical data is used for predictions using, for example, *in vitro-in vivo* correlation (IVIVC), physiology-based pharmacokinetics (PBPK) and a biopharmaceutics drug disposition classification system (BDDCS) in order to define absorption, distribution, metabolism, and excretion (ADME) properties. Further down the developmental process, MID3 becomes more important in order to define exposure-response relationships and pharmacodynamic (PD) interactions using preclinical data for optimal design of first-in-human (FIH) and early bactericidal activity (EBA) trials. The need to define the optimal combination regimen using preclinical information data is evident, as the necessary number of clinical trial arms/experimental groups grow exponentially with the number of drugs within a regimen. Techniques using optimal design and simulation studies are essential and part of the MID3 framework. Throughout the process, the precision of human predictions increases. Different important drug development decision steps (circles) are subject to learn-and-confirm cycles, for example, early EBA clinical studies where the earlier defined exposure-response relationship using pre-clinical data (learning phase) is confirmed (confirming phase).

2. Model-Informed Drug Discovery and Development

Model-informed drug discovery and development is given by a quantitative framework for prediction and extrapolation, aimed at improving the quality, efficiency and cost-effectiveness of decision making in drug development [17]. It can also be utilized in early drug discovery through target identification and validation, and in describing the PK-PD and toxicological properties of the candidate drug. In addition, it increases the efficiency of trials and reduces the cost through facilitating dose and sample size selection [17]. Because of the great potential of MID3, it has been received well and implemented by drug developers [18,25]. The EMA supports MID3 and has built competence to meet the increasing modeling and simulation work in the dossiers submitted to EMA through the implementation of the modeling and Simulation Working Group (MSWG). Further, the EMA stresses that, in order to benefit from the full potential of MID3, stand-alone applications of modeling and simulation, dissociated from clinical decisions with respect to the design and objectives of clinical trials, should be avoided [19]. This is also pointed out in the MID3 white paper [17], where the implementation process is described as very important, and where the modeling and simulation work should be clearly motivated in the analysis, with clear objectives that are relevant and understandable for the entire development team. To realize the full potential of MID3, it needs to be integrated into the development plan rather than being seen as an ad-hoc activity [23]. The FDA has implemented a new Model-Informed Drug Development Paired Meeting Pilot Program which refers to the application of a wide range of quantitative approaches in drug development to facilitate the decision-making process, such as dose optimization, supportive evidence for efficacy, clinical trial design, and informing policy [26]. Despite the recent efforts within academia, EFPIA and regulatory agencies, MID3 has not been utilized to its full potential within TB drug development, where the need is great due to the complex development of new drug regimens consisting of at least three drugs.

Model-informed drug discovery and development builds upon pharmacometrics, the discipline that applies mathematical and statistical methods to understand, quantify, translate, and predict PK and PD behavior, including uncertainty in that behavior [27,28]. Pharmacometric population PK and PK-PD modeling can quantify these processes to better predict the concentration-time and exposure-response relationships of anti-TB drugs as compared to non-modeling techniques, such as non-compartmental analyses (NCA) for PK or traditional statistical analysis of, for example, the relationship between dose and baseline-reduced response at the end of treatment [29] The advantage of pharmacometric modeling is that it takes the inter-individual and inter-occasion variabilities into account. Once a population model has been developed and evaluated, various simulation techniques can be used, e.g., Monte Carlo simulations where virtual patients are drawn from the earlier quantified variance of variability in the population. Pharmacokinetic models are usually nonlinear mixed-effects models with unique parameters for fixed effects and random effects. Pharmacodynamic models can consist of a statistical method suitable for the biomarker or endpoint where time-to-positivity and relapse would be described with a time-to-event model, while colony forming unit (CFU) is a continuous variable and, as such, can be described with similar nonlinear mixed effects modeling.

Model-informed drug discovery and development is likely most impactful in the translation from preclinical to clinical, where the understanding and extrapolation of the exposure-response from preclinical to clinical is crucial. Model-informed drug discovery and development is also very important in the early clinical phases of anti-TB drug development, specifically phase II EBA trials, as it is difficult to investigate all drug combinations and associated PD interactions in clinical trials. The majority of the knowledge about the potential PD interaction space needs to come from preclinical information. Additionally, MID3 can be used to design the next preclinical or clinical study in order to optimize the likelihood of collecting informative data. A crucial step in drug development is the prediction of FIH design and associated doses. Model-informed drug discovery and development strategies and methods can be used to scale preclinical information to humans to design the FIH trial. Pharmacometric techniques have been shown to reduce the sample size needed in comparison to traditional statistical methods [29–31], while MID3 has been reported to save significant costs through its impact on decision making [17]. Preclinical experiments should be designed to be able to quantify the exposure-response relationship, including quantitative biomarkers relative to the interspecies' translation thereof [32]. An MID3 framework integrates all relevant preclinical and clinical information, and can therefore be used to back-translate results from the clinic to improve the preclinical understanding of the pathophysiology and pharmacology [33]. Even failed translations to humans are valuable in correcting the preclinical methods used. An iterative forward- and reverse-translational cycle has the potential to continuously enhance confidence in preclinical models [34]. The availability of large clinical datasets from, for example, electronic medical records accelerates reverse translation and improves the preclinical modeling of clinical manifestations [35]. Additionally, data from veterinary medicine can be utilized to guide human medicine development [36]. For this framework to really have an impact, data repositories and common languages are essential for application across different disciplines, disease areas, or stages of development [23,37]. In addition, to ensure that modeling and simulation adds value through an MID3 approach, pharmacometricians must communicate with their project teams before any data analysis starts to understand the key strategic development questions, clinical context, available data, assumptions, and decision criteria [23].

The prediction of efficacy and safety in new drug combinations with new or unknown mechanisms of action will benefit from the next paradigm in drug development and MID3, namely quantitative systems pharmacology (QSP). This is the pharmacological perspective on a systems' modeling, a body-system-wide characterization of the health and disease of an organism based on a mechanistic and molecular understanding of the individual components in the context of the holistic network [38]. QSP is the middle-out interface between systems biology and pharmacometrics, describing the pharmacological perturbation within the studied context [39]. It accounts for differences in (molecular) mechanisms of a disease [40], which is very relative for TB with its heterogeneous pathophysiology of acute, chronic, and latent infections. Because of its mathematical description of all the relevant elements of the pharmacological and pathophysiological pathways, and their differences between species, it becomes key to translational medicine [41]. Because of this quantitative understanding of the network, the prediction of the effects of drugs with new mechanisms of action improves significantly [42]. The development of QSP models in the preclinical phase is, however, uncommon, and the dedicated acquisition of experimental data like transcriptomics or metabolomics for the development of QSP models is rare [43,44]. Quantitative systems pharmacology models are intended to be applied to a wider scale than the individual questions or problems they were originally developed for [45]. For TB specifically, this could mean a systems model of the *M. tuberculosis* infection in the human context of macrophage infiltration, granuloma formation and pulmonary lesion development, with all relevant pathways and drug targets quantitatively described. The effect of new combinations, including drugs with novel mechanism of actions, can be predicted.

3. Prediction of Human Pharmacokinetics

In silico ADME-PK (absorption, distribution, metabolism, excretion, and pharmacokinetics) is the use of computer modeling to understand structure–property relationships and to predict DMPK (drug metabolism and pharmacokinetics) properties from compound structure. This is related to but distinct from physiologically based pharmacokinetic (PBPK) modeling, which strives to provide accurate predictions of the PK profile of drug candidates [46]. The focus of *in silico* ADME-PK is to guide the design of novel compounds with superior ADME properties. Most often a quantitative structure–property relationship (QSPR) approach is used to relate a compound's structure to the chemical property in question (e.g., cell permeability or metabolic clearance) measured in an *in vitro* assay. Related terms are also quantitative-structure-activity relationships (QSAR), when a set of predictor variables is related to the potency of the drug.

Orally administered products are subject to a sequence of transport and enzymatic barriers in enterohepatic systems affecting bioavailability, including extraction in the intestinal and liver tissues, which could impact the fraction of the orally administered dose that reaches the systemic circulation and thereby the site of action. Bioavailability is mainly dependent on three general and rather complex serial processes: the fraction of the oral dose that is absorbed (F_{abs}), the first-pass extraction of the drug in the gut wall (E_G), and the first-pass extraction of the drug in the liver (E_H) [47]. In general, oral products with a low F (<25%–35%) have a higher inter- and intra-individual variability in plasma exposure (coefficient of variation >60%–120%) [48]. Drugs with high degree of F_{abs} show sufficiently high solubility of the active pharmaceutical ingredient (API), no luminal degradation, and absorption along the small and/or large intestine [49,50]. The regulatory framework Biopharmaceutics Classification System (BCS) of drugs provides information relevant to understanding and predicting GI drug absorption and bioavailability in general, which is relevant to the absorption potential in the small and large intestine [51]. After the drug is absorbed, it passes to the liver, which expresses a broader range of different enzymes compared to the intestine [52], such as the family of CYP enzymes [53]. Other enzymes such as microsomal uridine 5′-diphospho-glucuronosyltransferases (UGTs), sulfotransferases, and glutathione S-transferases are found in great amounts in the human liver [54]. Humans show large inter-individual variation in the amount of different enzymes, which accounts, in part, for the large inter-individual variation reported for E_H and CL. A considerable large inter-individual variation in the expression of the different CYP isoforms has also been observed, ranging from 20-(CYP2E1 and CYP3A4) to >1000-fold (CYP2D6). The liver is also the major organ for glucuronidation in the body. Glucuronide conjugates have molecular characteristics that are associated with biliary excretion of a compound, i.e., a high molecular weight, ionized and the presence of polar groups [55].

The identification and quantification of the important PK processes described above can be investigated in relevant *in vitro* models, and predictions of PK properties like regional intestinal permeability can be made early [56]. Most importantly, an estimate of human drug clearance will determine how fast a drug is eliminated, and conversely define the dose range to study in FIH [57]. Several different models have been suggested for the prediction of oral absorption for the biopharmaceutical design of oral drug delivery systems [58,59]. The proposed BDDCS has been shown to be useful in predicting some crucial ADME parameters and especially the transport/absorption/elimination interplay [60]. Preclinical data can then be translated through *in vitro-in vivo* extrapolation, or even through PBPK modeling to generate basic PK parameters such as fraction of dose absorbed, bioavailability, clearance (CL), volume of distribution, and terminal half-life. Furthermore, the accuracy of the QSAR predictions of effective intestinal permeability (P_{eff}), is significantly improved when based on a combination of molecular physicochemical descriptors and molecular dynamics simulations from *in vitro* data [61]. Molecular simulations have been successfully used to predict the effects of cholesterol in the lipid membrane fluidity [62]. Additionally, molecular simulations have been reported to be useful as they are comparable to experimental data [63]. Among the molecular descriptors evaluated by Lipinski (e.g., polar surface area, hydrogen bond donors (HBDs)/acceptors, Log D), the number of HBDs is the most restrictive when it comes to intestinal membrane transport/absorption [64,65]. Two drugs violating this rule (i.e., >5 HBDs and low intestinal P_{eff} and F_{abs}), one of which is rifampicin, have been investigated thoroughly and offered a potential explanation for drug absorption beyond the Lipinski Rule-of-five [66]. Based on a liposomal permeation assay, it has been proposed that drug molecules with more than five HBD can be sufficiently absorbed in the intestine by passive lipoidal diffusion [66]. Some drugs are absorbed by passive lipoidal diffusion despite their unfavorable physicochemical properties. It is therefore necessary to find more complex descriptions of the molecular interaction by applying a combination of experimental data and molecular dynamic modeling and simulation to further improve the accuracy in predicting general membrane transport across the cellular membrane barrier and not only in the GI-tract [66–69].

Physiologically based pharmacokinetic modeling is considered to assist drug product development by providing quantitative predictions through a systems approach [70]. A mechanism-based model, like that of the PBPK approach, separates drug-specific from system-specific elements, which allows for the interspecies translation of the time course of the drug [41]. Physiologically based pharmacokinetic models divide the body into anatomically and physiologically meaningful compartments, including the gastrointestinal tract for absorption, the eliminating organs, and non-eliminating tissue compartments [71]. In addition, compound-specific parameters such as physicochemical and biochemical parameters (e.g., tissue/blood partitioning and metabolic CL) are incorporated into the model to predict the plasma and tissue concentration versus the time profiles of a compound in an *in vivo* system following intravenous or oral administration. Translation between species, special populations, or disease states, are the result of changing these physiological parameters accordingly. Several variations are in use, including a whole-body PBPK model describing the complete organism, and hybrid PBPK models, combining PBPK elements with empirical compartmental PK to simplify the model [72]. An important element in the physiologically based translation of PK is binding of the drug of interest to proteins in the plasma, mainly albumin, lipo- or glycoproteins, or globulins. Protein binding differs between experimental settings (*in vitro*) and species (*in vivo*) and should be taken into account because it influences tissue penetration and the free drug that can interact with its target [73]. Physiologically based pharmacokinetic modeling predictions are a valuable tool in the pharmaceutical industry due to the possibility of combining all the available and relevant information that is generated during the preclinical stage, which helps improve decision making during the selection process [74]. For instance, biorelevant dissolution-absorption PBPK modeling and simulation has been reported as applied in 88% of early drug development processes [75]. Moreover, PBPK modeling provides a powerful tool to study potential PK DDIs through incorporating the drug's physicochemical properties, PK properties, human physiological variables, and inter-individual variability estimates.

Predictions of PK parameters use information from preclinical studies in animals to transition to clinical trials, i.e., FIH studies, when no clinical information is available to guide the decision of the starting dose. Thus, the estimation of the starting dose in human subjects relies on the PK knowledge of the drug from different species. It is essential to have preclinical PK data based on blood, plasma, and/or tissue sampled longitudinally to optimally capture the complete drug profile during a dosing interval. A model-based approach to the starting dose often uses allometric scaling to predict human drug clearance and distribution volumes. Allometric scaling is based on the assumption that physiological similarities exist between different species arising from anatomical similarities, specifically similarities in body weights and body surface areas [76]. Historically, a maximum dose for FIH studies was based on the no observed adverse effect level (NOAEL) in preclinical experiments, an arbitrary safety factor, and allometric scaling. This approach is empirical by nature and therefore limited. When more mechanistic data and models are available, a minimal anticipated biological effect level (MABEL) can be estimated [42]. For example, preclinical PK-PD and interspecies differences in the target can be utilized to estimate the MABEL for a FIH trial [77]. This has the benefit of being driven by pharmacology, where FIH trials will answer pharmacological questions on PK and PD, rather than being driven by toxicology or tolerability. Taking into account MABEL and safety factors, a first study with single ascending doses (SAD study) will quantify the PK and ensure safety and tolerability. A second study with multiple administered doses (MAD) can subsequently be designed accordingly [78].

In addition to allometric scaling, the use of IVIVC has markedly increased [79–82]. It is suggested that animal PBPK models should be used as part of a stepwise approach, in which the first step uses animal data to understand the processes and verify the predictive power of *in vitro* systems, and the second step is about forecasting human PK from *in vitro* data and *in silico* methods (learn-and-confirm) [82]. The first step in predicting drug CL using IVIVC is to obtain intrinsic CL (CL_{int}) from *in vitro* data [83,84]. *In vitro* CL_{int} values determined from various systems including hepatocytes, cell transport models, liver or intestinal microsomes, or recombinant CYPs, either by substrate depletion or metabolite formation, are normalized for cell, microsomal protein or enzyme concentration. The next step consists of scaling the activity determined *in vitro* to the whole liver by the use of a scaling factor, to account for incomplete microsomal recovery from the tissue to obtain *in vivo* CL_{int}. Finally, the third step involves the use of a liver model which incorporates the effects of hepatic blood flow, plasma protein-binding and blood cell partitioning to convert the estimated *in vivo* CL_{int} into a hepatic CL (CL_H). The well-stirred liver model is most commonly used, but the dispersion model or the parallel tube model is also available [84].

Using high doses of oral anti-TB drugs may result in high plasma concentrations, leading to an increased risk of adverse effects [85] while not ensuring adequate concentrations at the site of action [85,86]. This has prompted investigation into the use of the pulmonary route to deliver anti-TB drugs directly to the site of action in the lungs. Administering anti-TB drugs as inhaled formulations ensures the delivery of the drug directly to the target organ, avoiding any unwanted systemic side effects, thereby improving patient compliance [87]. Optimal pulmonary drug delivery for locally acting drugs includes a high local lung concentration, extended lung residence time and low systemic concentration [88]. A fundamental understanding of pulmonary dissolution, residence time, and lung absorption processes is key for the successful development of inhaled products [89,90]. However, inhaled formulations have many challenges, including formulation stability, pulmonary distribution, lung toxicity, and additives safety [91]. Furthermore, dosing of inhaled drugs is more complicated than other routes of administration as their absorption in the lung is highly variable [91]. Thus, many *in vitro* and *in vivo* models have been developed to study the PK of inhaled anti-TB drugs, specifically their absorption and distribution, in order to evaluate the efficacy and safety of anti-TB drugs in the lungs. These models, while allowing a reduction in biological complexity, still face many challenges, and can be demanding to build [92]. *In vivo* animal models are the gold standard regarding the assessment of drug clearance, systemic side effects and PK after pulmonary administration [92]. However, animal models are not always able to mimic human pulmonary anatomy and physiology, or TB disease progression in humans, and they do not exhibit extrapulmonary dissemination similar to humans [86]. Translation from animal data to the clinic has been recognized as challenging [93]. Understanding the pulmonary exposure is important, and animal data can contribute specific information about the lesion to plasma ratio [94], as similar lung distribution ratios can be obtained in human. However, little is known about the factors that influence drug distribution from plasma into the range of tissues, nodules and cavities that are inhabited by the TB pathogen. Pulmonary TB lesions consist of a diversity of cell types, tissue structures and vascular architectures which suggests that the distribution of the drug is not only governed by passive equilibration between unbound drug concentration in plasma and tissue [95]. MALDI mass spectrometry imaging (MALD-MSI) is a new technique to study the distribution of small molecules in the various compartments of pulmonary lesions [96]. Information from such studies not only provides knowledge of regional differences in drug exposure, but also confirms a high exposure in regions where a high density of persistent TB bacteria is found.

4. Prediction of Human Pharmacokinetic-Pharmacodynamic Relationship

In order to translate drug effects from preclinical information to the clinical phase of drug development, defining a drug exposure-response relationship using preclinical information is of importance. The PK-PD relationship is quantitative, predictive, and reproducible and is valid in all disease models [57,58]. Thus, characterizing this relationship is of great benefit in preclinical PK-PD studies to help guide dose selection and study design in humans. Exhaustive reviews of preclinical experimental methods that quantify exposure-response relationships have previously been performed [97,98]. These methods, such as classical time-kill experiments, hollow-fiber system (HF), different murine models, rabbits and guinea pig, all mimic elements of the human pathology to a certain extent, but all have their limitations. Here, the focus is on their informativeness of the exposure-response relationship for translation to human prediction.

In vitro determination of the minimum inhibitory concentration (MIC) is informative about the sensitivity of the bacterial strain to the compound. This is especially the case when the target sizes of the *M. tuberculosis* infection, macrophages, are utilized as environmental context [97]. The MIC is a measure of the net effect of the drug on bacterial growth and survival. However, it is very crude and undynamic as it is measured at a specific concentration and after a fixed time, which might cause it to deviate from the true MIC [99]. The MIC is also limited because the resolution is determined by the chosen dilution steps, and bigger dilution steps increase the risk of under- or overestimating the MIC. In addition, the determination of MIC is based on visual inspection which makes it prone to subjective error [99]. Mouton et al. have studied the variability between MIC measurements in *Staphylococcus aureus* treated with linezolid and have concluded that over half of the variability in the MIC measurements is either due to systemic and significant inter-laboratory differences or differences between strains [100]. The other half can be explained by assay variation and different environmental conditions, such as the media used and incubation temperature [100].

Several preclinical animal models for TB are in use. The advantage of an animal model over *in vitro* systems is the holistic environment of a whole organism, including a functioning immune system, physiological feedback systems and (drug) disposition. This results in more variability in the determination of the exposure-response relationship and requires more effort to elucidate drug effect from, for example, the immune system. The most emphasis is placed on murine models of

TB [101], although there are arguments that the mouse is not a good model for TB in humans [102]. Mice can be housed in the required biosafety laboratories with ease, blood and tissue sampling is well established, and both chronic and latent infections have been successfully used [103]. However, the mice have a low susceptibility to *M. tuberculosis* and show only loosely organized granulomas, and are therefore limited when considering lesion-specific treatment. Granuloma formation in guinea pigs and rabbits is more representative of human granulomas, including caseous necrosis [102]. Guinea pigs are highly susceptible to *M. tuberculosis* which makes infection as straightforward as exposure to exhaustion from TB patients [103]. Rabbits are also utilized to study a slower response to treatment, disease relapse, and resistance development due to lung cavities, and their size makes studying drug distribution to TB lesions more feasible [98]. The experimental toolbox regarding immunologic reagents and genetic techniques is, however, more restricted in these animals, and both need more difficult and expensive husbandry. Granuloma formation can also be studied non-invasively in the zebrafish, a relatively new disease model organism in drug discovery and development [103]. Because of their transparency and easy genetic modification, fluorescence microscopy of pathogen and immune cells can be leveraged to follow infection and treatment [104]. With the small size and high fecundity of the zebrafish, high-throughput assays are available to test large numbers of compounds in short amounts of time with enough statistical power [105]. Methods to quantify internal drug exposure have also been established [106–108]. Recently, an exposure-response relationship has been developed for isoniazid in the zebrafish, which translated well to humans [109]. In general, non-invasive imaging of lesion pathology by computed tomography (CT) and positron emission tomography (PET) has the potential to improve the comparison between preclinical and clinical measurements of disease progression and treatment [102]. Ordonez et al have demonstrated this by using dynamic [^{11}C]rifampicin PET-CT imaging in patients newly diagnosed with pulmonary TB and rabbits infected with cavitary TB to noninvasively measure intralesional drug concentration-time profiles and, consequently, time to bacterial extinction [110]. They also employed integrated modeling of the PET-captured concentration-time profiles in hollow-fiber bacterial kill curve experiments to predict the rifampicin dose required to achieve a cure in 4 months, which has a huge potential in antimicrobial drug development to shorten TB treatments [110]. It is clear that no single animal model represents a heterogeneous disease such as TB. A mechanistic understanding of TB in humans will identify which elements are characterized best by which animal model [103]. Independently of which preclinical experimental method is utilized, the sampling design of both PK (e.g., drug and/or metabolite concentration) and PD (e.g., infection, bacterial burden) biomarkers is of the utmost importance. The careful selection of datapoints over the duration of the experiment and at different drug concentrations is essential for a reliable quantification of the exposure-response relationship.

Regulatory agencies suggest determining PK/PD indices based on preclinical data for antibiotics, e.g., the area under the concentration curve over MIC (AUC/MIC), the maximum concentration (C_{max}) over MIC (C_{max}/MIC), and the percent of a 24-hour time period that the drug concentration is above MIC (T > MIC), for the establishment of the PK-PD profile of antimicrobials and for deciding the most optimal dosing regimens. PK/PD indices are based on preclinical studies that describe the PK-PD relationships of antimicrobials [111]. However, PK/PD indices suffer from several clear limitations, some of which are inherent to their use of MIC, the limitations of which are discussed above. Using PK/PD indices ignores information about the time-course of individual PK and PD processes [112]. As summary endpoints, they lack the ability to track the changes in the bacterial load over time [113]. Furthermore, when using AUC/MIC as a PK/PD index, the rate of drug administration is ignored, while, when using C_{max}/MIC, bacterial killing is assumed to depend solely on the maximum drug concentration, ignoring drug half-life and infusion duration [99]. Using T > MIC assumes that the maximal drug effect has been reached when MIC is reached, regardless of whether higher concentrations were given [99]. Additionally, the colony-forming units (CFU) versus PK/PD indices profile shows great variability in the CFU observations for the same PK/PD indices value [99]. These PK/PD indices are selected and predicted as PD targets using HFS-TB to quantify a more realistic *in vitro* exposure-response relationship that is translatable to *in vivo* [98,99,114]. However, despite EMA's qualification of the preclinical HFS-TB to be used to complement existing methodologies, it still suffers from a number of limitations. The EMA advises caution when interpreting HFS-TB results, as many instances of over- and under-estimates of the drug's anti-TB activity have been reported [115]. In addition, HFS-TB cannot replace animal models or clinical studies [116], while the reproducibility of the method by other laboratories has not yet been assessed [115].

Mechanistic, or semi-mechanistic, PK-PD models in TB based on preclinical data allow for the description of the multiple mycobacterial populations present. A mechanism-based PK-PD model by Hollow-fiber systems for TB has the advantage of being able to mimic dynamic PK in comparison to more traditional static time-kill experiments. A semi-mechanistic PK-PD model can be derived using HTS data [117–119]. Khan et al. describes susceptible, resting, and non-colony-forming bacterial populations [120]. The multistate tuberculosis pharmacometric (MTP) model is a semi-mechanistic mathematical model that can describe and identify the exposure-response profile of a drug towards three bacterial subpopulations: fast-, slow-, and non-multiplying bacteria. It has been successfully applied to describe *in vitro* [121], mouse [122], and clinical data [123]. In addition, the MTP model has been successfully used in an MID3 approach, to predict observations from early clinical studies using clinical dose-response forecasting from preclinical *in vitro* studies of rifampicin and in combination with isoniazid [15,16]. This model has been selected by *The Impact and Influence Initiative* of the Quantitative Pharmacology (QP) Network of the American society of Clinical Pharmacology and Therapeutics (ASCPT) to highlight the most impactful examples of QP applications where the role of quantitative translational pharmacology has bridged science and practice to make better, faster, and more efficient decisions in drug discovery and development [25]. Another mechanism-based model is the Magombedze et al. model that mimics the disease state in TB patients by describing the mycobacterial population as logarithmic growth-phase, semi-dormant, and persister bacilli [117]. In addition, a pulmonary PK-PD model of isoniazid has been developed to better characterize the relationship between its PK and its anti-TB effects in the lungs [124].

5. Prediction of Human Drug-Drug Interactions

Tuberculosis requires a combination therapy of three different antibiotics or more, which increases the risk of DDIs. Drug-drug interactions between drugs that are intended to be used in combination should be considered as early as possible. The prediction of DDIs from preclinical data will improve the ability to predict the total efficacy of the combination in relation to the drugs in monotherapy, as well as compared to expected additivity, i.e., the sum of all effects from the drugs when given alone. DDIs that result in less efficacy in the combination than in a combination with one less drug should be avoided. However, combinations that result in an efficacy less than the expected additivity, but still result in more efficacy than when one drug is omitted, can be considered. Drug-drug interactions can relate to both PK interactions, i.e., one drug (the perpetrator) impacting the absorption, distribution, metabolism, or excretion of another drug (the victim), or PD interactions, i.e., the perpetrator impacting the potency or efficacy of the victim drug.

Regulatory guidelines on the investigation of DDIs are brief about the use of *in vitro* data, while in an MID3 context, knowledge on the relevant mechanisms of, e.g., metabolism combined with *in vitro* data can be leveraged to decide on suitable combinations of drugs without extensive experimentation [125]. Both *in vitro* studies as well as animal experiments can be utilized to assess the potential for PK DDIs [126]. *In vitro* studies make use of metabolically active hepatocytes or cells overexpressing drug transporters to determine the PK interaction potential of a new drug [127]. When studying DDIs in preclinical species, the between-species differences in transporters or enzymes should be taken into account [128]. Pharmacokinetic DDIs mostly impact drug clearance by the induction or inhibition of metabolic enzymes like those from the CYP family and, to some extent, ABC and transport proteins. Such an interaction by the perpetrator drug will greatly enhance or reduce the exposure of the victim drug. For example, rifampicin induces bedaquiline clearance 5-fold, and should therefore not be combined for therapy [129]. Because bedaquiline has a very long terminal half-life, potential DDIs are difficult to identify using traditional methods, whereas properly designed experiments and quantitative modeling are necessary to elucidate such interactions [130]. Drug distribution can also be impacted because of the induction or inhibition of drug transporters like the permeability glycoprotein (P-gp), which is present on the canalicular membrane and blood-brain barrier, among others. Physiology based pharmacokinetic modeling can be very successful to predict metabolic DDIs, and specific DDI studies can be assisted by modeling and simulations [131]. Some anti-TB drugs are reported to be substrates for different hepatic enzymes or known to be inducers or inhibitors of metabolic enzymes. Rifampicin is well known as a CYP3A4 modulator [132,133], as well as an inducer of P-gp [134]. Additionally, even though the effect of clofazimine on CYP3A4 and P-gp is still unclear, clofazimine has been shown to delay the time taken to reach C_{max} of rifampicin [135]. Horita et al. studied the effects of anti-TB and antiretroviral drugs on CYP3A4 and P-gp, and they found that clofazimine exhibits weak inductive effects on CYP3A4 [136]. Furthermore, the co-administration of bedaquiline and clofazimine has been reported to increase the risk of QT prolongation [137,138]. As described above, these potential DDIs can be predicted from *in vitro* data through, for example, *in vitro-in vivo* scaling [139] or PBPK [140]. A transcription/translation model and a PBPK model have been developed to predict rifampicin-induced DDIs with reasonable accuracy [141].

In contrast to PK interactions, due to clearly defined processes of absorption, distribution, metabolism, and excretion, PD interactions are harder to investigate and quantify. This is because, since a clinical DDI study has to study the drugs both alone and in combination, the number of arms in the study will substantially increase when studying three or more interacting drugs. The Greco model [142], which is derived from Loewe additivity, was developed to assess PD interactions. However, such a model suffers from being limited to interactions between only two drugs. On the other hand, the general pharmacodynamic interaction (GPDI) model overcomes this limitation, in addition to being flexible to different drug interaction data without requiring knowledge on the modes of action of the studied drugs [143]. The GPDI model-based approach proposes a PD interaction to be quantifiable, as multidirectional shifts in drug efficacy (E_{max}) or potency (EC_{50}) and explicates the drugs' role as victim, perpetrator or even both at the same time. The GPDI model has been utilized along with the MTP model [121] to develop a model-informed preclinical approach for the prediction of PD interactions [144]. The MTP-GPDI model has been further employed to successfully evaluate and quantify the PD interactions of anti-TB drug combinations in mice [145]. Furthermore, it has been demonstrated that the GPDI model outperforms conventional methods in the evaluation of PD interactions for TB drugs [146].

It is clear that the need for a combination therapy of TB could potentially result in DDIs in the clinic. It is therefore essential to quantitatively understand the DDIs, both PK- and PD-interactions, as early as possible in drug development. Utilizing data from *in vitro* combination experiments combined with preclinical *in vivo* data on the exposure-response relationships of the drugs in combination and early clinical data, will inform on which combinations of drugs at which doses are efficacious and safe for patients. This quantitative integration of data and translation to the clinic is possible through the MID3 model-informed framework.

6. Conclusions

The development of new combinations of anti-TB drugs is both promising and challenging. Novel drug combinations and drug delivery routes require novel and innovative techniques. Model-informed drug discovery and development is an integrated framework of preclinical and clinical data through translational models that show great promise in selecting and predicting which drug regimens to carry forward to be evaluated in clinical trials. The MID3 framework supports decision making in drug development in relation to the prediction of efficacious and safe combinations of new drugs and translates this to the clinic. It is essential for drug developers to collaborate across disciplines, and academic and industry borders and train a new type of scientist in experimental and computational innovation.

Author Contributions: All authors contributed to conceptualization of this work. All authors contributed to original draft preparation, review and editing. All authors have read and agreed to the published version of the manuscript.

References

1. DiMasi, J.A.; Grabowski, H.G.; Hansen, R.W. Innovation in the Pharmaceutical Industry: New Estimates of R & D Costs. *J. Health Econ.* **2016**, *47*, 20–33. [CrossRef]
2. Bellanti, F.; Van Wijk, R.C.; Danhof, M.; Della Pasqua, O. Integration of PKPD Relationships into Benefit-Risk Analysis. *Br. J. Clin. Pharmacol.* **2015**, *80*, 979–991. [CrossRef] [PubMed]
3. World Health Organization. *Global Tuberculosis Report 2019*; World Health Organization: Geneva, Sweitzerland, 2019.
4. Boeree, M.J.; Diacon, A.H.; Dawson, R.; Narunsky, K.; Du Bois, J.; Venter, A.; Phillips, P.P.J.; Gillespie, S.H.; McHugh, T.D.; Hoelscher, M.; et al. A Dose-Ranging Trial to Optimize the Dose of Rifampin in the Treatment of Tuberculosis. *Am. J. Respir. Crit. Care Med.* **2015**, *191*, 1058–1065. [CrossRef] [PubMed]
5. Svensson, E.M.; Svensson, R.J.; Te Brake, L.H.M.; Boeree, M.J.; Heinrich, N.; Konsten, S.; Churchyard, G.; Dawson, R.; Diacon, A.H.; Kibiki, G.S.; et al. The Potential for Treatment Shortening with Higher Rifampicin Doses: Relating Drug Exposure to Treatment Response in Patients with Pulmonary Tuberculosis. *Clin. Infect. Dis.* **2018**, *67*, 34–41. [CrossRef] [PubMed]
6. Svensson, R.J.; Svensson, E.M.; Aarnoutse, R.E.; Diacon, A.H.; Dawson, R.; Gillespie, S.H.; Moodley, M.; Boeree, M.J.; Simonsson, U.S.H. Greater Early Bactericidal Activity at Higher Rifampicin Doses Revealed by Modeling and Clinical Trial Simulations. *J. Infect. Dis.* **2018**, *218*, 991–999. [CrossRef]
7. Susanto, B.O.; Svensson, R.J.; Svensson, E.M.; Aarnoutse, R.; Boeree, M.J.; Simonsson, U.S.H. Rifampicin Can Be given as Flat-Dosing Instead of Weight-Band Dosing. *Clin. Infect. Dis.* **2019**. [CrossRef]
8. WHO. *Consolidated Guidelines on Drug-Resistant Tuberculosis Treatment*; Licence: CC BY-NC-SA 3.0 IGO; World Health Organization: Geneva, Sweitzerland, 2019.
9. Bahuguna, A.; Rawat, D.S. An Overview of New Antitubercular Drugs, Drug Candidates, and Their Targets. *Med. Res. Rev.* **2020**, *40*, 263–292. [CrossRef]
10. Pontali, E.; Sotgiu, G.; Tiberi, S.; Tadolini, M.; Visca, D.; D'Ambrosio, L.; Centis, R.; Spanevello, A.; Migliori, G.B. Combined Treatment of Drug-Resistant Tuberculosis with Bedaquiline and Delamanid: A Systematic Review. *Eur. Respir. J.* **2018**, *52*. [CrossRef]
11. European Medicines Agency. *Addendum to the Guideline on the Evaluation of Medicinal Products Indicated for Treatment of Bacterial Infections to Address the Clinical Development of New Agents to Treat Pulmonary Disease Due to Mycobacterium Tuberculosis*; European Medicines Agency: London, UK, 2017.
12. European Medicines Agency. *Addendum to the Note for Guidance on Evaluation of Medicinal Products Indicated for Treatment of Bacterial Infections to Specifically Address the Clinical Development of New Agents to Treat Disease Due to Mycobacterium Tuberculosis*; European Medicines Agency: London, UK, 2010.
13. Dheda, K.; Gumbo, T.; Maartens, G.; Dooley, K.E.; Murray, M.; Furin, J.; Nardell, E.A.; Warren, R.M.; Esmail, A.; Nardell, E.; et al. The Lancet Respiratory Medicine Commission: 2019 Update: Epidemiology, Pathogenesis, Transmission, Diagnosis, and Management of Multidrug-Resistant and Incurable Tuberculosis. *Lancet Respir. Med.* **2019**, *7*, 820–826. [CrossRef]
14. European Medicines Agency. *Guideline on Strategies to Identify and Mitigate Risks for First-in-Human and Early Clinical Trials with Investigational Medicinal Products*; European Medicines Agency: London, UK, 2017.
15. Wicha, S.G.; Clewe, O.; Svensson, R.J.; Gillespie, S.H.; Hu, Y.; Coates, A.R.M.; Simonsson, U.S.H. Forecasting Clinical Dose-Response From Preclinical Studies in Tuberculosis Research: Translational Predictions With Rifampicin. *Clin. Pharmacol. Ther.* **2018**, *104*, 1208–1218. [CrossRef]

16. Susanto, B.O.; Wicha, S.G.; Hu, Y.; Coates, A.R.M.; Simonsson, U.S.H.; Biosciences, P.; Pharmacy, C.; Kingdom, U.; Simonsson, U.S.H.; Biosciences, P.; et al. Translational Model-Informed Approach for Selection of Tuberculosis Drug Combination Regimens in Early Clinical Development. *Clin. Pharmacol. Ther.* **2020**. [CrossRef] [PubMed]

17. Marshall, S.F.; Burghaus, R.; Cosson, V.; Cheung, S.; Chenel, M.; DellaPasqua, O.; Frey, N.; Hamrén, B.; Harnisch, L.; Ivanow, F.; et al. Good Practices in Model-Informed Drug Discovery and Development: Practice, Application, and Documentation. *CPT Pharmacomet. Syst. Pharmacol.* **2016**, *5*, 93–122. [CrossRef]

18. Marshall, S.; Madabushi, R.; Manolis, E.; Krudys, K.; Staab, A.; Dykstra, K.; Visser, S.A.G. Model-Informed Drug Discovery and Development: Current Industry Good Practice and Regulatory Expectations and Future Perspectives. *CPT Pharmacomet. Syst. Pharmacol.* **2019**, *8*, 87–96. [CrossRef]

19. Manolis, E.; Brogren, J.; Cole, S.; Hay, J.L.; Nordmark, A.; Karlsson, K.E.; Lentz, F.; Benda, N.; Wangorsch, G.; Pons, G.; et al. Commentary on the MID3 Good Practices Paper. *CPT Pharmacomet. Syst. Pharmacol.* **2017**, *6*, 416–417. [CrossRef]

20. Goulooze, S.C.; Zwep, L.B.; Vogt, J.E.; Krekels, E.H.J.; Hankemeier, T.; Van den Anker, J.N.; Knibbe, C.A.J. Beyond the Randomized Clinical Trial: Innovative Data Science to Close the Pediatric Evidence Gap. *Clin. Pharmacol. Ther.* **2020**. [CrossRef]

21. Ribba, B. Model-Informed Artificial Intelligence: Reinforcement Learning for Precision Dosing. *Clin. Pharmacol. Ther.* **2020**. [CrossRef]

22. Harrer, S.; Shah, P.; Antony, B.; Hu, J. Artificial Intelligence for Clinical Trial Design. *Trends Pharmacol. Sci.* **2019**, *40*, 577–591. [CrossRef]

23. Krishnaswami, S.; Austin, D.; Della Pasqua, O.; Gastonguay, M.R.; Gobburu, J.; van der Graaf, P.H.; Ouellet, D.; Tannenbaum, S.; Visser, S.A.G. MID3: Mission Impossible or Model-Informed Drug Discovery and Development? Point-Counterpoint Discussions on Key Challenges. *Clin. Pharmacol. Ther.* **2020**. [CrossRef]

24. Marshall, S.F.; Hemmings, R.; Josephson, F.; Karlsson, M.O.; Posch, M.; Steimer, J.L. Modeling and Simulation to Optimize the Design and Analysis of Confirmatory Trials, Characterize Risk-Benefit, and Support Label Claims. *CPT Pharmacomet. Syst. Pharmacol.* **2013**, *2*, 3–5. [CrossRef]

25. Gupta, N.; Bottino, D.; Simonsson, U.S.H.; Musante, C.J.; Bueters, T.; Rieger, T.R.; Macha, S.; Chenel, M.; Fancourt, C.; Kanodia, J.; et al. Transforming Translation Through Quantitative Pharmacology for High-Impact Decision Making in Drug Discovery and Development. *Clin. Pharmacol. Ther.* **2019**, 1–5. [CrossRef]

26. Wang, Y.; Zhu, H.; Madabushi, R.; Liu, Q.; Huang, S.M.; Zineh, I. Model-Informed Drug Development: Current US Regulatory Practice and Future Considerations. *Clin. Pharmacol. Ther.* **2019**, *105*, 899–911. [CrossRef] [PubMed]

27. Gieschke, R.; Steimer, J.L. Pharmacometrics: Modelling and Simulation Tools to Improve Decision Making in Clinical Drug Development. *Eur. J. Drug Metab. Pharmacokinet.* **2000**, *25*, 49–58. [CrossRef] [PubMed]

28. Ette, E.I.; Williams, P.J. Pharmacometrics: The Science of Quantitative Pharmacology. John Wiley & Sons, Inc.: Hoboken, NJ, USA, 2007; ISBN 978-0-471-67783-3.

29. Svensson, R.J.; Gillespie, S.H.; Simonsson, U.S.H. Improved Power for TB Phase IIa Trials Using a Model-Based Pharmacokinetic-Pharmacodynamic Approach Compared with Commonly Used Analysis Methods. *J. Antimicrob. Chemother.* **2017**, *72*, 2311–2319. [CrossRef] [PubMed]

30. Karlsson, K.E.; Vong, C.; Bergstrand, M.; Jonsson, E.N.; Karlsson, M.O. Comparisons of Analysis Methods for Proof-of-Concept Trials. *CPT Pharmacomet. Syst. Pharmacol.* **2013**, *2*. [CrossRef] [PubMed]

31. Chen, C.; Ortega, F.; Alameda, L.; Ferrer, S.; Simonsson, U.S.H. Population Pharmacokinetics, Optimised Design and Sample Size Determination for Rifampicin, Isoniazid, Ethambutol and Pyrazinamide in the Mouse. *Eur. J. Pharm. Sci.* **2016**, *93*, 319–333. [CrossRef]

32. Muliaditan, M.; Davies, G.R.; Simonsson, U.S.H.; Gillespie, S.H.; Della Pasqua, O. The Implications of Model-Informed Drug Discovery and Development for Tuberculosis. *Drug Discov. Today* **2017**, *22*, 481–486. [CrossRef]

33. Visser, S.A.G.; Aurell, M.; Jones, R.D.O.; Schuck, V.J.A.; Egnell, A.C.; Peters, S.A.; Brynne, L.; Yates, J.W.T.; Jansson-Löfmark, R.; Tan, B.; et al. Model-Based Drug Discovery: Implementation and Impact. *Drug Discov. Today* **2013**, *18*, 764–775. [CrossRef]

34. Kasichayanula, S.; Venkatakrishnan, K. Reverse Translation: The Art of Cyclical Learning. *Clin. Pharmacol. Ther.* **2018**, *103*, 152–159. [CrossRef]

35. Li, L. Reverse Translational Pharmacology Research Is Driven by Big Data. *CPT Pharmacomet. Syst. Pharmacol.* **2018**, *7*, 63–64. [CrossRef]
36. Schneider, B.; Balbas-Martinez, V.; Jergens, A.E.; Troconiz, I.F.; Allenspach, K.; Mochel, J.P. Model-Based Reverse Translation Between Veterinary and Human Medicine: The One Health Initiative. *CPT Pharmacometrics Syst. Pharmacol.* **2017**. [CrossRef]
37. Van der Graaf, P.H.; Benson, N. The Role of Quantitative Systems Pharmacology in the Design of First-in-Human Trials. *Clin. Pharmacol. Ther.* **2018**, *104*, 797. [CrossRef] [PubMed]
38. van der Greef, J.; McBurney, R.N. Rescuing Drug Discovery: In Vivo Systems Pathology and Systems Pharmacology. *Nat. Rev. Drug Discov.* **2005**, *4*, 961–967. [CrossRef] [PubMed]
39. Vicini, P.; Van der Graaf, P.H. Systems Pharmacology for Drug Discovery and Development: Paradigm Shift or Flash in the Pan? *Clin. Pharmacol. Ther.* **2013**, *93*, 379–381. [CrossRef] [PubMed]
40. Danhof, M.; Klein, K.; Stolk, P.; Aitken, M.; Leufkens, H. The Future of Drug Development: The Paradigm Shift towards Systems Therapeutics. *Drug Discov. Today* **2018**, *23*, 1990–1995. [CrossRef] [PubMed]
41. Sorger, P.K.; Allerheiligen, S.R.B.; Abernethy, D.R.; Altmann, R.B.; Brouwer, K.L.R.; Califano, A.; D'Argenio, D.Z.; Iyengar, R.; Jusko, W.J.; Lalonde, R.; et al. Quantitative and Systems Pharmacology in the Post-Genomic Era: New Approaches to Discovering Drugs and Understanding Therapeutic Mechanisms (White Paper). In *An NIH White Paper by the QSP Workshop Group*; Bethesda: Rockville, MD, USA, 2011; Volume 48.
42. Visser, S.A.G.; Manolis, E.; Danhof, M.; Kerbusch, T. Modeling and Simulation at the Interface of Nonclinical and Early Clinical Drug Development. *CPT Pharmacomet. Syst. Pharmacol.* **2013**, *2*, 8–10. [CrossRef]
43. Nijsen, M.J.; Wu, F.; Bansal, L.; Bradshaw-Pierce, E.; Chan, J.R.; Liederer, B.M.; Mettetal, J.T.; Schroeder, P.; Schuck, E.; Tsai, A.; et al. Preclinical QSP Modeling in the Pharmaceutical Industry: An IQ Consortium Survey Examining the Current Landscape. *CPT Pharmacomet. Syst. Pharmacol.* **2018**, *7*, 135–146. [CrossRef]
44. Schulthess, P.; Van Wijk, R.C.; Krekels, E.H.J.; Yates, J.W.T.; Spaink, H.P.; Van der Graaf, P.H. Outside-in Systems Pharmacology Combines Innovative Computational Methods with High-Throughput Whole Vertebrate Studies. *CPT Pharmacomet. Syst. Pharmacol.* **2018**, *7*, 285–287. [CrossRef]
45. Van der Graaf, P.H. Pharmacometrics and/or Systems Pharmacology. *CPT Pharmacomet. Syst. Pharmacol.* **2019**, *8*, 331–332. [CrossRef]
46. Lombardo, F.; Desai, P.V.; Arimoto, R.; Desino, K.E.; Fischer, H.; Keefer, C.E.; Petersson, C.; Winiwarter, S.; Broccatelli, F. In Silico Absorption, Distribution, Metabolism, Excretion, and Pharmacokinetics (ADME-PK): Utility and Best Practices. An Industry Perspective from the International Consortium for Innovation through Quality in Pharmaceutical Development. *J. Med. Chem.* **2017**, *60*, 9097–9113. [CrossRef]
47. Wu, C.Y.; Benet, L.Z.; Hebert, M.F.; Gupta, S.K.; Rowland, M.; Gomez, D.Y.; Wacher, V.J. Differentiation of Absorption and First-Pass Gut and Hepatic Metabolism in Humans: Studies with Cyclosporine. *Clin. Pharmacol. Ther.* **1995**, *58*, 492–497. [CrossRef]
48. Hellriegel, E.T.; Bjornsson, T.D.; Hauck, W.W. Interpatient Variability in Bioavailability Is Related to the Extent of Absorption: Implications for Bioavailability and Bioequivalence Studies. *Clin. Pharmacol. Ther.* **1996**, *60*, 601–607. [CrossRef]
49. Amidon, G.L.; Lennernäs, H.; Shah, V.P.; Crison, J.R. A Theoretical Basis for a Biopharmaceutic Drug Classification: The Correlation of in Vitro Drug Product Dissolution and in Vivo Bioavailability. *Pharm. Res.* **1995**, *12*, 413–420. [CrossRef] [PubMed]
50. Dahlgren, D.; Roos, C.; Lundqvist, A.; Abrahamsson, B.; Tannergren, C.; Hellström, P.M.; Sjögren, E.; Lennernäs, H. Regional Intestinal Permeability of Three Model Drugs in Human. *Mol. Pharm.* **2016**, *13*, 3013–3021. [CrossRef] [PubMed]
51. Tannergren, C.; Bergendal, A.; Lennernäs, H.; Abrahamsson, B. Toward an Increased Understanding of the Barriers to Colonic Drug Absorption in Humans: Implications for Early Controlled Release Candidate Assessment. *Mol. Pharm.* **2009**, *6*, 60–73. [CrossRef]
52. Shimada, T.; Yamazaki, H.; Mimura, M.; Inui, Y.; Guengerich, F.P. Interindividual Variations in Human Liver Cytochrome P-450 Enzymes Involved in the Oxidation of Drugs, Carcinogens and Toxic Chemicals: Studies with Liver Microsomes of 30 Japanese and 30 Caucasians. *J. Pharmacol. Exp. Ther.* **1994**, *270*, 414–423.
53. Rendic, S. Summary of Information on Human CYP Enzymes: Human P450 Metabolism Data. *Drug Metab. Rev.* 2002. [CrossRef]

54. Zamek-Gliszczynski, M.J.; Hoffmaster, K.A.; Nezasa, K.; Tallman, M.N.; Brouwer, K.L.R. Integration of Hepatic Drug Transporters and Phase II Metabolizing Enzymes: Mechanisms of Hepatic Excretion of Sulfate, Glucuronide, and Glutathione Metabolites. *Eur. J. Pharm. Sci.* **2006**, *27*, 447–486. [CrossRef]
55. Luo, G.; Johnson, S.; Hsueh, M.M.; Zheng, J.; Cai, H.; Xin, B.; Chong, S.; He, K.; Harper, T.W. In Silico Prediction of Biliary Excretion of Drugs in Rats Based on Physicochemical Properties. *Drug Metab. Dispos.* **2010**, *38*, 422–430. [CrossRef]
56. Roos, C.; Dahlgren, D.; Tannergren, C.; Abrahamsson, B.; Sjögren, E.; Lennernas, H. Regional Intestinal Permeability in Rats: A Comparison of Methods. *Mol. Pharm.* **2017**, *14*, 4252–4261. [CrossRef]
57. Gumbo, T.; Lenaerts, A.J.; Hanna, D.; Romero, K.; Nuermberger, E. Nonclinical Models for Antituberculosis Drug Development: A Landscape Analysis. *J. Infect. Dis.* **2015**, *211*, S83–S95. [CrossRef]
58. Yu, L.X.; Lipka, E.; Crison, J.R.; Amidon, G.L. Transport Approaches to the Biopharmaceutical Design of Oral Drug Delivery Systems: Prediction of Intestinal Absorption. *Adv. Drug Deliv. Rev.* **1996**, *19*, 359–376. [CrossRef]
59. Heimbach, T.; Suarez-Sharp, S.; Kakhi, M.; Holmstock, N.; Olivares-Morales, A.; Pepin, X.; Sjögren, E.; Tsakalozou, E.; Seo, P.; Li, M. Dissolution and Translational Modeling Strategies Toward Establishing an In Vitro-In Vivo Link—A Workshop Summary Report. *AAPS J.* **2019**, *21*, 29. [CrossRef]
60. Wu, C.Y.; Benet, L.Z. Predicting Drug Disposition via Application of BCS: Transport/Absorption/ Elimination Interplay and Development of a Biopharmaceutics Drug Disposition Classification System. *Pharm. Res.* **2005**, *22*, 11–23. [CrossRef]
61. Bennion, B.J.; Be, N.A.; McNerney, M.W.; Lao, V.; Carlson, E.M.; Valdez, C.A.; Malfatti, M.A.; Enright, H.A.; Nguyen, T.H.; Lightstone, F.C. Predicting a Drug's Membrane Permeability: A Computational Model Validated with in Vitro Permeability Assay Data. *J. Phys. Chem. B* **2017**, *121*, 5228–5237. [CrossRef]
62. Awoonor-Williams, E.; Rowley, C.N. Molecular Simulation of Nonfacilitated Membrane Permeation. *Biochim. Biophys. Acta Biomembr.* **2016**, *1858*, 1672–1687. [CrossRef]
63. Orsi, M.; Essex, J.W. Permeability of Drugs and Hormones through a Lipid Bilayer: Insights from Dual-Resolution Molecular Dynamics. *Soft Matter* **2010**, *6*, 3797–3808. [CrossRef]
64. Lipinski, C.A.; Lombardo, F.; Dominy, B.W.; Feeney, P.J. Experimental and Computational Approaches to Estimate Solubility and Permeability in Drug Discovery and Development Settings. *Adv. Drug Deliv. Rev.* **1997**, *23*, 3–25. [CrossRef]
65. Bickerton, G.R.; Paolini, G.V.; Besnard, J.; Muresan, S.; Hopkins, A.L. Quantifying the Chemical Beauty of Drugs. *Nat. Chem.* **2012**, *4*, 90. [CrossRef]
66. Krämer, S.D.; Aschmann, H.E.; Hatibovic, M.; Hermann, K.F.; Neuhaus, C.S.; Brunner, C.; Belli, S. When Barriers Ignore the "Rule-of-Five". *Adv. Drug Deliv. Rev.* **2016**, *101*, 62–74. [CrossRef]
67. Bemporad, D.; Luttmann, C.; Essex, J.W. Behaviour of Small Solutes and Large Drugs in a Lipid Bilayer from Computer Simulations. *Biochim. Biophys. Acta Biomembr.* **2005**, *1718*, 1–21. [CrossRef]
68. Kuhn, B.; Mohr, P.; Stahl, M. Intramolecular Hydrogen Bonding in Medicinal Chemistry. *J. Med. Chem.* **2010**, *53*, 2601–2611. [CrossRef] [PubMed]
69. Alex, A.; Millan, D.S.; Perez, M.; Wakenhut, F.; Whitlock, G.A. Intramolecular Hydrogen Bonding to Improve Membrane Permeability and Absorption in beyond Rule of Five Chemical Space. *MedChemComm* **2011**, *2*, 669–674. [CrossRef]
70. Agoram, B.; Woltosz, W.S.; Bolger, M.B. Predicting the Impact of Physiological and Biochemical Processes on Oral Drug Bioavailability. *Adv. Drug Deliv. Rev.* **2001**, *50*, S41–S67. [CrossRef]
71. Rowland, M.; Peck, C.; Tucker, G. Physiologically-Based Pharmacokinetics in Drug Development and Regulatory Science. *Annu. Rev. Pharmacol. Toxicol.* **2011**, *51*, 45–73. [CrossRef]
72. Zhou, Q.; Gallo, J.M. The Pharmacokinetic/Pharmacodynamic Pipeline: Translating Anticancer Drug Pharmacology to the Clinic. *AAPS J.* **2011**, *13*, 111–120. [CrossRef]
73. Woo, J.; Cheung, W.; Chan, R.; Chan, H.S.; Cheng, A.; Chan, K. In Vitro Protein Binding Characteristics of Isoniazid, Rifampicin, and Pyrazinamide to Whole Plasma, Albumin, and α-1-Acid Glycoprotein. *Clin. Biochem.* **1996**, *29*, 175–177. [CrossRef]
74. Lavé, T.; Parrott, N.; Grimm, H.P.; Fleury, A.; Reddy, M. Challenges and Opportunities with Modelling and Simulation in Drug Discovery and Drug Development. *Xenobiotica* **2007**, *37*, 1295–1310. [CrossRef]

75. Flanagan, T.; Van Peer, A.; Lindahl, A. Use of Physiologically Relevant Biopharmaceutics Tools within the Pharmaceutical Industry and in Regulatory Sciences: Where Are We Now and What Are the Gaps? *Eur. J. Pharm. Sci.* **2016**, *91*, 84–90. [CrossRef]
76. Mahmood, I. Application of Allometric Principles for the Prediction of Pharmacokinetics in Human and Veterinary Drug Development. *Adv. Drug Deliv. Rev.* **2007**, *59*, 1177–1192. [CrossRef]
77. Teitelbaum, Z.; Lave, T.; Freijer, J.; Cohen, A.F. Risk Assessment in Extrapolation of Pharmacokinetics from Preclinical Data to Humans. *Clin. Pharmacokinet.* **2010**, *49*, 619–632. [CrossRef]
78. Gumbo, T.; Angulo-Barturen, I.; Ferrer-Bazaga, S. Pharmacokinetic-Pharmacodynamic and Dose-Response Relationships of Antituberculosis Drugs: Recommendations and Standards for Industry and Academia. *J. Infect. Dis.* **2015**, *211*, S96–S106. [CrossRef] [PubMed]
79. Jones, H.M.; Parrott, N.; Jorga, K.; Lavé, T. A Novel Strategy for Physiologically Based Predictions of Human Pharmacokinetics. *Clin. Pharmacokinet.* **2006**, *45*, 511–542. [CrossRef] [PubMed]
80. Pelkonen, O.; Turpeinen, M. In Vitro-in Vivo Extrapolation of Hepatic Clearance: Biological Tools, Scaling Factors, Model Assumptions and Correct Concentrations. *Xenobiotica* **2007**, *37*, 1066–1089. [CrossRef] [PubMed]
81. Houston, J.; Galetin, A. Methods for Predicting In Vivo Pharmacokinetics Using Data from In Vitro Assays. *Curr. Drug Metab.* **2008**. [CrossRef] [PubMed]
82. Lavé, T.; Chapman, K.; Goldsmith, P.; Rowland, M. Human Clearance Prediction: Shifting the Paradigm. *Expert Opin. Drug Metab. Toxicol.* **2009**. [CrossRef]
83. Ito, K.; Houston, J.B. Prediction of Human Drug Clearance from in Vitro and Preclinical Data Using Physiologically Based and Empirical Approaches. *Pharm. Res.* **2005**, *22*, 103–112. [CrossRef]
84. Rostami-Hodjegan, A.; Tucker, G.T. Simulation and Prediction of in Vivo Drug Metabolism in Human Populations from in Vitro Data. *Nat. Rev. Drug Discov.* **2007**, *6*, 140–148. [CrossRef]
85. Aït Moussa, L.; El Bouazzi, O.; Serragui, S.; Soussi Tanani, D.; Soulaymani, A.; Soulaymani, R. Rifampicin and Isoniazid Plasma Concentrations in Relation to Adverse Reactions in Tuberculosis Patients: A Retrospective Analysis. *Ther. Adv. Drug Saf.* **2016**, *7*, 239–247. [CrossRef]
86. Muttil, P.; Wang, C.; Hickey, A.J. Inhaled Drug Delivery for Tuberculosis Therapy. *Pharm. Res.* **2009**, *26*, 2401–2416. [CrossRef]
87. Pandey, R.; Khuller, G.K. Antitubercular Inhaled Therapy: Opportunities, Progress and Challenges. *J. Antimicrob. Chemother.* **2005**, *55*, 430–435. [CrossRef]
88. Patton, J.S.; Byron, P.R. Inhaling Medicines: Delivering Drugs to the Body through the Lungs. *Nat. Rev. Drug Discov.* **2007**, *6*, 67–74. [CrossRef] [PubMed]
89. Bäckman, P.; Arora, S.; Couet, W.; Forbes, B.; de Kruijf, W.; Paudel, A. Advances in Experimental and Mechanistic Computational Models to Understand Pulmonary Exposure to Inhaled Drugs. *Eur. J. Pharm. Sci.* **2018**, *113*, 41–52. [CrossRef] [PubMed]
90. Eriksson, J.; Sjögren, E.; Thörn, H.; Rubin, K.; Bäckman, P.; Lennernäs, H. Pulmonary Absorption-Estimation of Effective Pulmonary Permeability and Tissue Retention of Ten Drugs Using an Ex Vivo Rat Model and Computational Analysis. *Eur. J. Pharm. Biopharm.* **2018**, *124*, 1–12. [CrossRef] [PubMed]
91. Scheuch, G.; Kohlhaeufl, M.J.; Brand, P.; Siekmeier, R. Clinical Perspectives on Pulmonary Systemic and Macromolecular Delivery. *Adv. Drug Deliv. Rev.* **2006**, *58*, 996–1008. [CrossRef]
92. Hittinger, M.; Juntke, J.; Kletting, S.; Schneider-Daum, N.; de Souza Carvalho, C.; Lehr, C.-M. Preclinical Safety and Efficacy Models for Pulmonary Drug Delivery of Antimicrobials with Focus on in Vitro Models. *Adv. Drug Deliv. Rev.* **2015**, *85*, 44–56. [CrossRef]
93. McGonigle, P.; Ruggeri, B. Animal Models of Human Disease: Challenges in Enabling Translation. *Biochem. Pharmacol.* **2014**, *87*, 162–171. [CrossRef]
94. Kjellsson, M.C.; Via, L.E.; Goh, A.; Weiner, D.; Low, K.M.; Kern, S.; Pillai, G.; Barry, C.E.; Dartois, V. Pharmacokinetic Evaluation of the Penetration of Antituberculosis Agents in Rabbit Pulmonary Lesions. *Antimicrob. Agents Chemother.* **2012**, *56*, 446–457. [CrossRef]
95. Dartois, V. The Path of Anti-Tuberculosis Drugs: From Blood to Lesions to Mycobacterial Cells. *Nat. Rev. Microbiol.* **2014**, *12*, 159–167. [CrossRef]
96. Prideaux, B.; Dartois, V.; Staab, D.; Weiner, D.M.; Goh, A.; Via, L.E.; Barry III, C.E.; Stoeckli, M. High-Sensitivity MALDI-MRM-MS Imaging of Moxifloxacin Distribution in Tuberculosis-Infected Rabbit Lungs and Granulomatous Lesions. *Anal. Chem.* **2011**, *83*, 2112–2118. [CrossRef]

97. Franzblau, S.G.; Degroote, M.A.; Cho, S.H.; Andries, K.; Nuermberger, E.; Orme, I.M.; Mdluli, K.; Angulo-Barturen, I.; Dick, T.; Dartois, V.; et al. Comprehensive Analysis of Methods Used for the Evaluation of Compounds against Mycobacterium Tuberculosis. *Tuberculosis* **2012**, *92*, 453–488. [CrossRef]
98. Nuermberger, E.L. Preclinical Efficacy Testing of New Drug Candidates. *Microbiol. Spectr.* **2017**, *5*. [CrossRef]
99. Nielsen, E.I.; Friberg, L.E. Pharmacokinetic-Pharmacodynamic Modeling of Antibacterial Drugs. *Pharmacol. Rev.* **2013**, *65*, 1053–1090. [CrossRef] [PubMed]
100. Mouton, J.W.; Meletiadis, J.; Voss, A.; Turnidge, J. Variation of MIC Measurements: The Contribution of Strain and Laboratory Variability to Measurement Precision. *J. Antimicrob. Chemother.* **2018**, *73*, 2374–2379. [CrossRef] [PubMed]
101. Singh, A.K.; Gupta, U.D. Animal Models of Tuberculosis: Lesson Learnt. *Indian J. Med. Res.* **2018**, *147*, 456–463. [CrossRef] [PubMed]
102. Young, D. Animal Models of Tuberculosis. *Eur. J. Immunol.* **2009**, *39*, 2011–2014. [CrossRef]
103. Myllymäki, H.; Niskanen, M.; Oksanen, K.E.; Rämet, M. Animal Models in Tuberculosis Research-Where Is the Beef? *Expert Opin. Drug Discov.* **2015**, *10*, 871–883. [CrossRef]
104. Meijer, A.H. Protection and Pathology in TB: Learning from the Zebrafish Model. *Semin. Immunopathol.* **2016**, *38*, 261–273. [CrossRef]
105. Carvalho, R.; de Sonneville, J.; Stockhammer, O.W.; Savage, N.D.L.; Veneman, W.J.; Ottenhoff, T.H.M.; Dirks, R.P.; Meijer, A.H.; Spaink, H.P. A High-Throughput Screen for Tuberculosis Progression. *PLoS ONE* **2011**, *6*, e16779. [CrossRef]
106. Kantae, V.; Krekels, E.H.; Ordas, A.; Gonzalez, O.; Van Wijk, R.C.; Harms, A.C.; Racz, P.I.; Van Der Graaf, P.H.; Spaink, H.P.; Hankemeier, T. Pharmacokinetic Modeling of Paracetamol Uptake and Clearance in Zebrafish Larvae: Expanding the Allometric Scale in Vertebrates with Five Orders of Magnitude. *Zebrafish* **2016**, *13*, 504–510. [CrossRef]
107. Van Wijk, R.C.; Krekels, E.H.J.; Kantae, V.; Harms, A.C.; Hankemeier, T.; Van der Graaf, P.H.; Spaink, H.P. Impact of Post-Hatching Maturation on the Pharmacokinetics of Exogenous Compounds in Zebrafish Larvae. *Sci. Rep.* **2018**, *9*, 2149. [CrossRef]
108. Van Wijk, R.C.; Krekels, E.H.J.; Kantae, V.; Ordas, A.; Kreling, T.; Harms, A.C.; Hankemeier, T.; Spaink, H.P.; van der Graaf, P.H. Mechanistic and Quantitative Understanding of Pharmacokinetics in Zebrafish Larvae through Nanoscale Blood Sampling and Metabolite Modelling of Paracetamol. *J. Pharmacol. Exp. Ther.* **2019**, *371*, 15–24. [CrossRef] [PubMed]
109. Van Wijk, R.C.; Krekels, E.H.J.; Hu, W.; Van der Sar, A.M.; Dijkema, S.M.; Van den Berg, D.-J.; Bahi, R.; Liu, J.; Verboom, T.; Verbeek, F.J.; et al. Translational quantitative systems pharmacology; crossing borders between experimental and computational drug development using zebrafish as model organism. *PAGE* **2021**, *29*, 9455.
110. Ordonez, A.A.; Wang, H.; Magombedze, G.; Ruiz-Bedoya, C.A.; Srivastava, S.; Chen, A.; Tucker, E.W.; Urbanowski, M.E.; Pieterse, L.; Fabian Cardozo, E.; et al. Dynamic Imaging in Patients with Tuberculosis Reveals Heterogeneous Drug Exposures in Pulmonary Lesions. *Nat. Med.* **2020**, 1–6. [CrossRef] [PubMed]
111. Committee for Human Medicinal Products (CHMP). Guideline on the Use of Pharmacokinetics and Pharmacodynamics in the Development of Antibacterial Medicinal Products. (EMA/CHMP/594085/2015). *Eur. Med. Agency* **2016**, *44*, 1–21.
112. Nielsen, E.I.; Cars, O.; Friberg, L.E. Pharmacokinetic/Pharmacodynamic (PK/PD) Indices of Antibiotics Predicted by a Semimechanistic PKPD Model: A Step toward Model-Based Dose Optimization. *Antimicrob. Agents Chemother.* **2011**, *55*, 4619–4630. [CrossRef]
113. Khan, D.D.; Friberg, L.E.; Nielsen, E.I. A Pharmacokinetic-Pharmacodynamic (PKPD) Model Based on in Vitro Time-Kill Data Predicts the in Vivo PK/PD Index of Colistin. *J. Antimicrob. Chemother.* **2016**, *71*, 1881–1884. [CrossRef]
114. Pasipanodya, J.G.; Nuermberger, E.; Romero, K.; Hanna, D.; Gumbo, T. Systematic Analysis of Hollow Fiber Model of Tuberculosis Experiments. *Clin. Infect. Dis.* **2015**, *61* (Suppl. 1), S10–S17. [CrossRef]
115. European Medicines Agency. *Qualification Opinion In-Vitro Hollow Fiber System Model of Tuberculosis (HSF-TB)*; European Medicines Agency: London, UK, 2015.
116. Chilukuri, D.; McMaster, O.; Bergman, K.; Colangelo, P.; Snow, K.; Toerner, J.G. The Hollow Fiber System Model in the Nonclinical Evaluation of Antituberculosis Drug Regimens. *Clin. Infect. Dis.* **2015**, *61*, S32–S33. [CrossRef]

117. Magombedze, G.; Pasipanodya, J.G.; Srivastava, S.; Deshpande, D.; Visser, M.E.; Chigutsa, E.; McIlleron, H.; Gumbo, T. Transformation Morphisms and Time-to-Extinction Analysis That Map Therapy Duration from Preclinical Models to Patients with Tuberculosis: Translating from Apples to Oranges. *Clin. Infect. Dis.* **2018**, *67*, S349–S358. [CrossRef]
118. Deshpande, D.; Magombedze, G.; Srivastava, S.; Bendet, P.; Lee, P.S.; Cirrincione, K.N.; Martin, K.R.; Dheda, K.; Gumbo, T. Once-a-Week Tigecycline for the Treatment of Drug-Resistant TB. *J. Antimicrob. Chemother.* **2019**, *74*, 1607–1617. [CrossRef]
119. Srivastava, S.; Deshpande, D.; Magombedze, G.; van Zyl, J.; Cirrincione, K.; Martin, K.; Bendet, P.; Berg, A.; Hanna, D.; Romero, K.; et al. Duration of Pretomanid/Moxifloxacin/Pyrazinamide Therapy Compared with Standard Therapy Based on Time-to-Extinction Mathematics. *J. Antimicrob. Chemother.* **2020**, *75*, 392–399. [CrossRef]
120. Khan, D.D.; Lagerbäck, P.; Cao, S.; Lustig, U.; Nielsen, E.I.; Cars, O.; Hughes, D.; Andersson, D.I.; Friberg, L.E. A Mechanism-Based Pharmacokinetic/Pharmacodynamic Model Allows Prediction of Antibiotic Killing from MIC Values for WT and Mutants. *J. Antimicrob. Chemother.* **2015**, *70*, 3051–3060. [CrossRef] [PubMed]
121. Clewe, O.; Aulin, L.; Hu, Y.; Coates, A.R.M.; Simonsson, U.S.H. A Multistate Tuberculosis Pharmacometric Model: A Framework for Studying Anti-Tubercular Drug Effects in Vitro. *J. Antimicrob. Chemother.* **2016**, *71*, 964–974. [CrossRef] [PubMed]
122. Chen, C.; Ortega, F.; Rullas, J.; Alameda, L.; Angulo-Barturen, I.; Ferrer, S.; Simonsson, U.S. The Multistate Tuberculosis Pharmacometric Model: A Semi-Mechanistic Pharmacokinetic-Pharmacodynamic Model for Studying Drug Effects in an Acute Tuberculosis Mouse Model. *J. Pharmacokinet. Pharmacodyn.* **2017**, *44*, 133–141. [CrossRef] [PubMed]
123. Svensson, R.J.; Simonsson, U.S.H. Application of the Multistate Tuberculosis Pharmacometric Model in Patients with Rifampicin-Treated Pulmonary Tuberculosis. *CPT Pharmacomet. Syst. Pharmacol.* **2016**, *5*, 264–273. [CrossRef]
124. Lalande, L.; Bourguignon, L.; Bihari, S.; Maire, P.; Neely, M.; Jelliffe, R.; Goutelle, S. Population Modeling and Simulation Study of the Pharmacokinetics and Antituberculosis Pharmacodynamics of Isoniazid in Lungs. *Antimicrob. Agents Chemother.* **2015**, *59*, 5181–5189. [CrossRef]
125. European Medicines Agency. *Guideline on the Investigation of Drug Interactions*; European Medicines Agency: Lonon, UK, 2012. [CrossRef]
126. Kuhlmann, J.; Mück, W. Clinical-Pharmacological Strategies to Assess Drug Interaction Potential during Drug Development. *Drug Saf.* **2001**, *24*, 715–725. [CrossRef]
127. Barton, H.A.; Lai, Y.; Goosen, T.C.; Jones, H.M.; El-Kattan, A.F.; Gosset, J.R.; Lin, J.; Varma, M.V. Model-Based Approaches to Predict Drug-Drug Interactions Associated with Hepatic Uptake Transporters: Preclinical, Clinical and Beyond. *Expert Opin. Drug Metab. Toxicol.* **2013**, *9*, 459–472. [CrossRef]
128. Chu, X.; Bleasby, K.; Evers, R. Species Differences in Drug Transporters and Implications for Translating Preclinical Findings to Humans. *Expert Opin. Drug Metab. Toxicol.* **2013**, *9*, 237–252. [CrossRef]
129. McIlleron, H.; Chirehwa, M.T. Current Research toward Optimizing Dosing of First-Line Antituberculosis Treatment. *Expert Rev. Anti. Infect. Ther.* **2019**, *17*, 27–38. [CrossRef]
130. Svensson, E.M.; Acharya, C.; Clauson, B.; Dooley, K.E.; Karlsson, M.O. Pharmacokinetic Interactions for Drugs with a Long Half-Life—Evidence for the Need of Model-Based Analysis. *AAPS J.* **2016**, *18*, 171–179. [CrossRef] [PubMed]
131. Margolskee, A.; Darwich, A.S.; Pepin, X.; Pathak, S.M.; Bolger, M.B.; Aarons, L.; Rostami-Hodjegan, A.; Angstenberger, J.; Graf, F.; Laplanche, L.; et al. IMI-Oral Biopharmaceutics Tools Project-Evaluation of Bottom-up PBPK Prediction Success Part 1: Characterisation of the OrBiTo Database of Compounds. *Eur. J. Pharm. Sci.* **2017**, *96*, 598–609. [CrossRef]
132. Chen, J.; Raymond, K. Roles of Rifampicin in Drug-Drug Interactions: Underlying Molecular Mechanisms Involving the Nuclear Pregnane X Receptor. *Ann. Clin. Microbiol. Antimicrob.* **2006**, *5*. [CrossRef] [PubMed]
133. Chattopadhyay, N.; Kanacher, T.; Kanacher, T.; Frechen, S.; Ligges, S.; Zimmermann, T.; Rottmann, A.; Ploeger, B.; Höchel, J.; Schultze-Mosgau, M.H. CYP3A4-Mediated Effects of Rifampicin on the Pharmacokinetics of Vilaprisan and Its UGT1A1-Mediated Effects on Bilirubin Glucuronidation in Humans. *Br. J. Clin. Pharmacol.* **2018**, *84*, 2857–2866. [CrossRef] [PubMed]

134. Greiner, B.; Eichelbaum, M.; Fritz, P.; Kreichgauer, H.P.; Von Richter, O.; Zundler, J.; Kroemer, H.K. The Role of Intestinal P-Glycoprotein in the Interaction of Digoxin and Rifampin. *J. Clin. Invest.* **1999**, *104*, 147–153. [CrossRef] [PubMed]
135. Mehta, J.; Gandhit, I.S.; Sanet, S.B.; Wamburkart, M.N. Effect of Clofazimine and Dapsone on Rifampicin (Lositril) Pharmacokinetics in Multibacillary and Paucibacillary Leprosy Cases. *Lepr. Rev.* **1986**, *57*, 67–76. [CrossRef]
136. Horita, Y.; Doi, N. Comparative Study of the Effects of Antituberculosis Drugs and Antiretroviral Drugs on Cytochrome P450 3a4 and P-Glycoprotein. *Antimicrob. Agents Chemother.* **2014**, *58*, 3168–3176. [CrossRef]
137. Dannemann, B.; Bakare, N.; De Marez, T.; Lounis, N.; Van Heeswijk, R.P.G.; Meyvisch, P.; Haxaire-Theeuwes, M.; Andries, K.; Everitt, D.; Upton, A. Corrected QT Interval (QTcF) Prolongation in a Phase 2 Open-Label Trial of TMC207 plus Background Regimen as Treatment for MDR-TB: Effect of Co-Administration with Clofazimine. In Proceedings of the Abstract at 52nd Interscience Conference on Antimicrobial Agents and Chemotherapy, San Francisco, CA, USA, 9–12 September 2012.
138. Pym, A.S.; Diacon, A.H.; Tang, S.J.; Conradie, F.; Danilovits, M.; Chuchottaworn, C.; Vasilyeva, I.; Andries, K.; Bakare, N.; De Marez, T.; et al. Bedaquiline in the Treatment of Multidrug- and Extensively Drugresistant Tuberculosis. *Eur. Respir. J.* **2016**, *47*, 564–574. [CrossRef]
139. Iwatsubo, T.; Suzuki, H.; Shimada, N.; Chiba, K.; Ishizaki, T.; Green, C.E.; Tyson, C.A.; Yokoi, T.; Kamataki, T.; Sugiyama, Y. Prediction of in Vivo Hepatic Metabolic Clearance of YM796 from in Vitro Data by Use of Human Liver Microsomes and Recombinant P-450 Isozymes. *J. Pharmacol. Exp. Ther.* **1997**, *282*, 909–919.
140. Zhao, P.; Zhang, L.; Grillo, J.A.; Liu, Q.; Bullock, J.M.; Moon, Y.J.; Song, P.; Brar, S.S.; Madabushi, R.; Wu, T.C.; et al. Applications of Physiologically Based Pharmacokinetic (PBPK) Modeling and Simulation during Regulatory Review. *Clin. Pharmacol. Ther.* **2011**, *89*, 259–267. [CrossRef]
141. Yamashita, F.; Sasa, Y.; Yoshida, S.; Hisaka, A.; Asai, Y.; Kitano, H.; Hashida, M.; Suzuki, H. Modeling of Rifampicin-Induced CYP3A4 Activation Dynamics for the Prediction of Clinical Drug-Drug Interactions from In Vitro Data. *PLoS ONE* **2013**, *8*. [CrossRef] [PubMed]
142. Greco, W.R.; Park, H.S.; Rustum, Y.M. Application of a New Approach for the Quantitation of Drug Synergism to the Combination of Cis-Diamminedichloroplatinum and 1-θ-d-Arabinofuranosylcytosine. *Cancer Res.* **1990**, *50*, 5318–5327. [PubMed]
143. Wicha, S.G.; Chen, C.; Clewe, O.; Simonsson, U.S.H. A General Pharmacodynamic Interaction Model Identifies Perpetrators and Victims in Drug Interactions. *Nat. Commun.* **2017**, *8*. [CrossRef] [PubMed]
144. Clewe, O.; Wicha, S.G.; de Vogel, C.P.; de Steenwinkel, J.E.M.; Simonsson, U.S.H. A Model-Informed Preclinical Approach for Prediction of Clinical Pharmacodynamic Interactions of Anti-TB Drug Combinations. *J. Antimicrob. Chemother.* **2018**, *73*, 437–447. [CrossRef]
145. Chen, C.; Wicha, S.G.; De Knegt, G.J.; Ortega, F.; Alameda, L.; Sousa, V.; De Steenwinkel, J.E.M.; Simonsson, U.S.H. Assessing Pharmacodynamic Interactions in Mice Using the Multistate Tuberculosis Pharmacometric and General Pharmacodynamic Interaction Models. *CPT Pharmacomet. Syst. Pharmacol.* **2017**, *6*, 787–797. [CrossRef]
146. Chen, C.; Wicha, S.G.; Nordgren, R.; Simonsson, U.S.H. Comparisons of Analysis Methods for Assessment of Pharmacodynamic Interactions Including Design Recommendations. *AAPS J.* **2018**, *20*, 1–12. [CrossRef]

11

Promiscuous Targets for Antitubercular Drug Discovery: The Paradigm of DprE1 and MmpL3

Giulia Degiacomi [1,†], Juan Manuel Belardinelli [2,†], Maria Rosalia Pasca [1], Edda De Rossi [1], Giovanna Riccardi [1,*] and Laurent Roberto Chiarelli [1,*]

1 Department of Biology and Biotechnology "Lazzaro Spallanzani", University of Pavia, 27100 Pavia, Italy; giulia.degiacomi@unipv.it (G.D.); mariarosalia.pasca@unipv.it (M.R.P.); edda.derossi@unipv.it (E.D.R.)

2 Mycobacteria Research Laboratories, Department of Microbiology, Immunology and Pathology, Colorado State University, Fort Collins, CO 80523-1682, USA; juan.belardinelli@colostate.edu

* Correspondence: giovanna.riccardi@unipv.it (G.R.); laurent.chiarelli@unipv.it (L.R.C.).

† These authors contributed equally to this work.

Abstract: The development and spread of *Mycobacterium tuberculosis* multi-drug resistant strains still represent a great global health threat, leading to an urgent need for novel anti-tuberculosis drugs. Indeed, in the last years, several efforts have been made in this direction, through a number of high-throughput screenings campaigns, which allowed for the identification of numerous hit compounds and novel targets. Interestingly, several independent screening assays identified the same proteins as the target of different compounds, and for this reason, they were named "promiscuous" targets. These proteins include DprE1, MmpL3, QcrB and Psk13, and are involved in the key pathway for *M. tuberculosis* survival, thus they should represent an Achilles' heel which could be exploited for the development of novel effective drugs. Indeed, among the last molecules which entered clinical trials, four inhibit a promiscuous target. Within this review, the two most promising promiscuous targets, the oxidoreductase DprE1 involved in arabinogalactan synthesis and the mycolic acid transporter MmpL3 are discussed, along with the latest advancements in the development of novel inhibitors with anti-tubercular activity.

Keywords: mycobacteria; tuberculosis; multi-drug resistance; drug discovery; promiscuous targets

---

1. The Added Value of Promiscuous Targets for Antitubercular Drug Discovery

One of the biggest problems in fighting *Mycobacterium tuberculosis* (Mtb), the etiologic agent of tuberculosis (TB), is the development and spread of multi-drug resistant strains [1]. Therefore, there is an urgent need to identify novel druggable targets for the development of more efficient anti-TB agents [2,3]. In this context, the medicinal chemistry efforts made in the last years led to the discovery of new antimycobacterial compounds, and the identification of novel targets [3–5].

High-throughput screenings (HTS), based on Mtb whole cells, were developed to identify hit compounds with potent inhibitory activity, and consequently, new targets emerged. The HTS had the merit of fueling the scarce TB drug development pipeline, since many molecules under preclinical and clinical development came out from this approach. Indeed, the first new TB drug, Bedaquiline, approved by the Food and Drug Administration (FDA) since 1971, was discovered in a whole-cell HTS campaign [6], and the same origin had both Delamanid [7] and Pretomanid [8], other two drugs recently approved for multidrug resistant tuberculosis (MDR-TB) and extensively drug-resistant tuberculosis (XDR-TB) treatment [9,10].

Curiously, an unforeseen outcome of many phenotypic screens against Mtb is the finding that the same targets have been frequently found in many different screening assays, despite the use of different compound libraries [11]. These targets were named "promiscuous" targets, for their nonspecific susceptibility to being inhibited by different scaffolds [2,12]. Although this term was initially given with a negative connotation, the value of these potential pharmacological targets has been reevaluated. Indeed, the high vulnerability of these essential targets, reflecting the biggest vulnerabilities of Mtb, can provide new opportunities to be explored for the development of TB drugs [12]. Among them, there are DprE1, MmpL3, QcrB and Psk13 [3,13].

DprE1 is an enzyme that works in concert with DprE2 to synthesize the unique arabinose precursor for lipoarabinomannan and arabinogalactan, essential building blocks of the mycobacterial cell-wall [14]. To date, more than 15 pharmacophores were found to inhibit DprE1 activity.

MmpL3 is the only Mtb transporter of trehalose monomycolate, required for the formation of the mycolic acid layer of the cell wall [15], and has been found to be affected by several molecules. Recently, direct inhibition of MmpL3 by BM212, the first compound found to hit MmpL3, was shown using spheroplasts [15], while the dissipation of proton motive force is the proposed mechanism for the other molecules [16].

QcrB encodes the *b* subunit of ubiquinol cytochrome C reductase, involved in the electron transport. Among the other compounds, Q203 is a promising clinical candidate, which blocks Mtb cell growth by targeting the respiratory cytochrome bc1 complex [17,18].

Finally, polyketide synthase Psk13, essential for the formation of the mycolic acid precursors, has been targeted by thiophenes and benzofuran containing molecules [19,20].

It is noteworthy that several research groups independently identified these promiscuous targets. These proteins are embedded in pathways that have key roles for Mtb growth and survival under the screening conditions, but even more important during infection. Their essentiality represents an Mtb Achilles' heel that is important to exploit for the development of new effective drug regimens able to shorten the TB treatment. Interestingly, all these promiscuous targets are localized within the cell envelope, emphasizing that the cell wall still represents a fruitful source of drug targets.

In recent years, several innovative strategies have been implemented to avoid the rediscovery of promiscuous targets [17,21–23]. Nevertheless, it is noteworthy that promiscuous targets proved to be successful in medicinal chemistry: four inhibitors Q203 (QcrB), SQ-109 (MmpL3), Macozinone (MCZ) and TBA-7371 (DprE1) entered clinical trials [24–29]. Thus, in parallel, a rational exploitation of already available promiscuous targets could lead to optimized scaffolds that retain the ability to attack the most vulnerable weakness of tubercle bacilli.

2. The First Discovery of DprE1 and MmpL3 as Drug Target

Dr. Vadim Makarov and collaborators, including our Laboratory, published in 2009 the first report in which DprE1 was described as the target of 1,3-benzothiazin-4-ones (BTZ), a new class of agents endowed with antimycobacterial activity [30]. To find the BTZ target, two genetic approaches were performed in parallel using both a *Mycobacterium smegmatis* cosmid library for resistance to BTZ, and the selection and characterization of *M. smegmatis*, *Mycobacterium bovis* BCG and *M. tuberculosis* spontaneous resistant mutants. Both methods revealed that *dprE1* gene was responsible for BTZ resistance. It is noteworthy that all the mutants carried mutations in the same codon of *dprE1*, leading to the replacement of Cys387 with a Ser or Gly residue [30]. DprE1 was known to be involved in the arabinogalactan biosynthesis, a key precursor required for the synthesis of the cell-wall [14,31], and it was demonstrated that its inhibition abolishes the formation of decaprenylphosphoryl arabinose (DPA), thus provoking cell lysis and bacterial death [30]. Later, new antimycobacterial compounds targeting DprE1 were identified by independent whole cell-based screens, like dinitrobenzamides (DNB) and bromoquinoxaline (VI-9376) [32,33], and afterward, numerous DprE1 inhibitors have come out since that groundbreaking report in 2009.

In this context, it has been demonstrated that DprE1 is essential for mycobacterial cell growth and survival [34,35]. Moreover, using *M. tuberculosis* conditional knockdown mutants, it has been shown that depletion of the DprE1 mRNA and protein level leads to a rapid cell death in vitro and ex vivo, suggesting that some enzymatic reactions are more sensitive to inhibition [35], providing the proof-of-principle of why it is so successful hitting DprE1 enzyme.

MmpL3 was firstly identified in our laboratory as the cellular target of BM212, the hit compound of a pyrrole-derivative class of antimycobacterial agents by screening the *M. smegmatis* cosmid library for BM212 resistance, as well as the selection and characterization of spontaneous resistant mutants [36]. MmpL3 is a transporter belonging to the mycobacterial membrane protein large (MmpL) family, specific for Actinobacteria. Since MmpL3 protein belongs to the resistance-nodulation-cell division (RND) permease superfamily, involved mainly in drug efflux, there was concern that the BM212 resistance could have been due to an enhanced efflux of the drug. Using efflux pump inhibitors, the authors provided evidence that mutations in *mmpL3* gene were instead responsible for resistance to BM212 per se and did not mediate resistance to BM212 via drug efflux [36]. Moreover, *M. smegmatis* spheroplasts assay showed that BM212 inhibits the MmpL3 transport activity, corroborating the evidence that MmpL3 was the BM212 cellular target [15].

Immediately after this first publication, MmpL3 was demonstrated to be the target of SQ109, an antitubercular in clinical trials, for which the mechanism of action was still unclear, and adamantyl urea AU1235, a compound displaying potent bactericidal activity against Mtb [37,38]. Genetic and biochemical studies indicated a clear effect of inhibiting MmpL3 on the translocation of trehalose monomycolate (TMM) in Mtb, thus abolishing the trehalose dimycolate (TDM) formation and mycolic acid transfer onto arabinogalactan [37,38]. Subsequently, several papers have reported the discovery of new MmpL3 inhibitors.

MmpL3 is essential for both mycobacterial growth and intracellular survival [16,39]. Strikingly, its broad promiscuity can be explained not only for its essentiality for tubercle bacilli, but also because the proton motive force needed to TMM transport across the membrane is dissipated by different MmpL3 inhibitors [16], a possible indirect mechanism.

The importance of these promiscuous targets can be exemplified by the numerous papers that report novel compound(s) able to exert antimycobacterial activity targeting these proteins, but the presence of drug candidates in the antitubercular pipeline better highlight the relevance of promiscuous targets. Indeed, among the new drug candidates, Macozinone (MCZ), BTZ-043 and TBA-7371 (or AZ 7371), present in Phase I or II, inhibit DprE1, while SQ109, hitting MmpL3, has completed Phase IIb study. Moreover, the Phase IIa of telacebec (Q203) has given positive results: telacebec has a high specificity for the cytochrome bc1 complex of Mtb, particularly for QcrB, another promiscuous target.

3. DprE1: The Hot TB Target of the Moment

3.1. Why DprE1 Is a Promiscuous Target

DprE1 (Decaprenylphosphoryl-β-D-ribofuranose 2-oxidoreductase, EC 1.1.98.3), is involved along with DprE2 (Decaprenylphosphoryl-2-keto-β-D-erythro-pentose reductase, EC 1.1.1.333), in the two-step epimerization of decaprenylphosphoribose (DPR) to decaprenylphosphoarabinose (DPA), a key arabinosyl donor essential for the biosynthesis of cell-wall arabinan polymers [40].

As a flavoprotein, after the first half-reaction in which DPR is oxidized into decaprenylphosphorylerythropentose (DPX), DprE1 needs to reoxidize the reduced flavin to begin a new catalytic cycle, thus, to complete this half-reaction the enzyme must use an electron acceptor. Initially, DprE1 was considered an oxidase, which uses molecular oxygen as an electron acceptor [41]. However, the enzyme was found to utilize more efficiently organic compounds, including bacterial membrane-embedded quinones, such as menaquinone, which was postulated as a physiological electron acceptor [41]. For this reason, the enzyme should be more precisely defined as an oxidoreductase.

In this context, DprE1 was found to have a very broad specificity for the electron acceptor, being able to use several compounds belonging to very different chemical classes. Indeed, the enzyme can reduce not only quinones, but also indophenols such as 2,6-dichlorophenolindophenol, or the phenoxazine moiety of resazurin, both compounds used in DprE1 activity assays [41,42], as well as different nitroaromatic moieties that characterize several covalent inhibitors of this enzyme [30,32,33,43,44].

To date, more than 15 chemical classes of compounds inhibiting DprE1 have been reported. These classes encompass both covalent and noncovalent inhibitors, and although the covalent ones are the most successful, several noncovalent inhibitors with significant antitubercular activity have actually been described [45,46].

The success of DprE1 covalent inhibitors in antitubercular drug discovery partly resides in this peculiar reactivity of the enzyme with the nitroaromatic moiety. Indeed, the most potent class of these inhibitors, the benzothiazinones, has been demonstrated to be suicide prodrugs that need activation to covalently bind DprE1 [47]. This activation consists of the reduction of the nitro group to nitroso, which rapidly forms a semimercaptal covalent adduct with a cysteine residue, located in a pocket just in front of the flavin cofactor. In this way, since the electron acceptor site is occupied, the enzyme is unable to reoxidize the flavin cofactor, resulting in being irreversibly inhibited [41,48] (Figure 1).

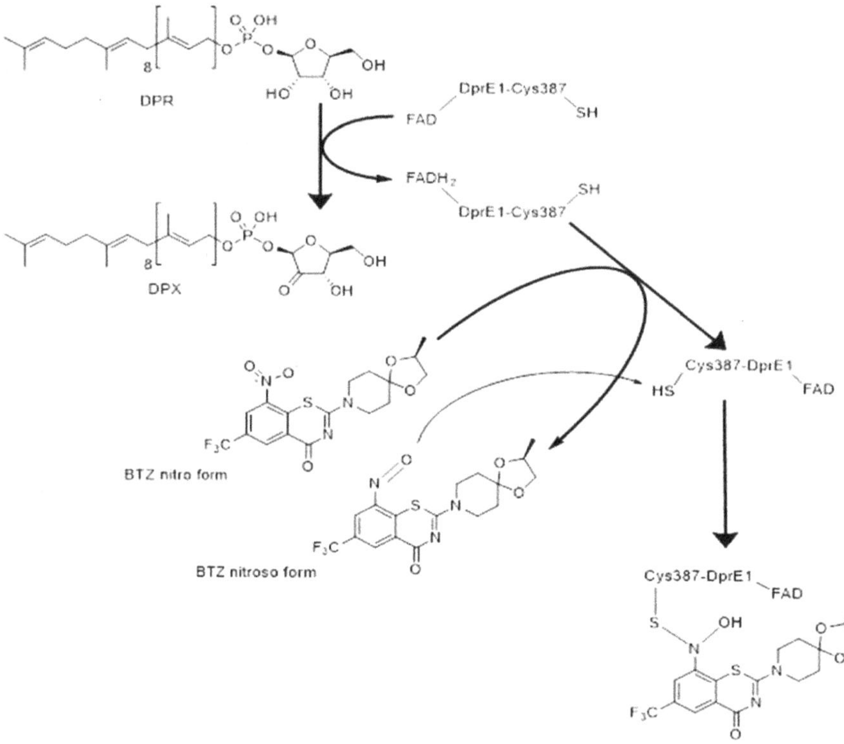

Figure 1. Mechanism of activation of the BTZ043 suicide inhibitor of DprE1.

This mechanism of action has been demonstrated for benzothiazinones and benzothiazinone analogs [41,43,49,50]. However, other different classes of nitro-compounds have been identified as potent DprE1 inhibitors, including dinitrobenzamides [32], nitroquinoxalines [33] and nitroimidazoles [51], that conceivably share the same mechanism of action of benzothiazinones [52].

Currently, 33 DprE1 structures from *M. tuberculosis* or *M. smegmatis* have been deposited in the Protein Data Bank, as apoenzyme [41,53] or in complex with both covalent [41,43,44,49,54] and noncovalent inhibitors [43,50,55–58]. The enzyme is characterized by the two-domain topology of the vanillyl-alcohol oxidase family of oxidoreductases, which includes a flavin adenine dinucleotide (FAD)-binding domain and the substrate-binding domain [41]. The isoalloxazine ring of FAD is located at the interface of the substrate-binding domain and the cofactor-binding domain, where are located in two disordered loops, which have been supposed to be involved in interactions with the DPR substrate, or with other proteins involved in the DPA biosynthesis [42].

In all structures of DprE1 in complex with inhibitors, all molecules showed binding sites that are significantly overlapped (Figure 2). This binding pocket, which conceivably constitutes the binding site of the physiological electron acceptor of DprE1, shows a very broad specificity, thus explaining the promiscuity of DprE1 for inhibitors.

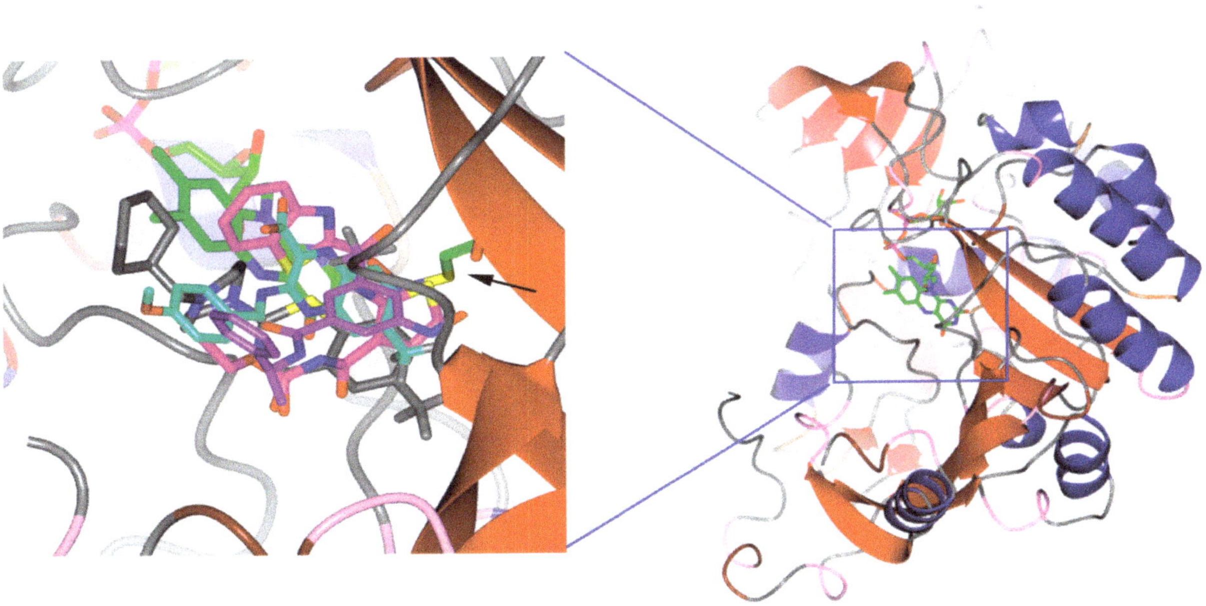

Figure 2. Crystal structure of *Mycobacterium tuberculosis* (Mtb) DprE1 and detail of the inhibitor binding sites. The superimposition of the structures of DprE1, cocrystallized with both covalent and noncovalent inhibitors (PBTZ-169, PDB: 4NCR [49] with carbon atoms in grey; Ty38c, PDB: 4P8K [58] with carbon atoms in cyan; TCA1, PDB: 4KWS [55] with carbon atoms in magenta; CT325, PDB: 4FF6 [43] with carbon atoms in violet), shows how the compounds have significantly overlapping binding sites, located in front of the isoalloxazine ring of the FAD cofactor (with carbon atoms in green). The black arrow points to the Cys387 side chain.

A broad specificity for inhibitors is a necessary but not sufficient condition for a target, to be considered promiscuous. Indeed, as promiscuous targets usually emerge during phenotypic screening, this implies that the inhibitors identified have antitubercular activity, so they can reach the cellular compartment in which the target resides. It is noteworthy that among the obstacles for the antitubercular drug discovery process, there is the difficulty of the compounds to cross the cell wall and the cellular membranes. Moreover, the presence of efflux pumps that can extrude the compounds outside the cells, and potential cytosolic inactivation processes of drugs lead to a lack of activity. In this context, it is noteworthy that one of the most successful pathways for antitubercular discovery is the cell wall compartment [59].

Recently, it was demonstrated that DPA biosynthesis partly occurs also outside the cytosolic membrane, and in particular, DprE1 was localized into the periplasm [60]. How DprE1 can reach the periplasmic compartment is still not clear, despite this protein, as well as its partner DprE2, do not possess any export signal for the translocation across the cytosolic membrane [60]. Anyhow, this localization allows drugs against DprE1 not only to easily reach the target, but also to escape several resistance mechanisms such as efflux pump or potential cytoplasmic inactivating enzymes.

3.2. DprE1 Inhibitors, Which Are the Current Status and Future Perspectives

Currently, at least 11 different scaffolds have been reported as effective DprE1 inhibitors, either covalent and noncovalent, showing different efficacy in vitro, ex vivo and in vivo [46]. It is noteworthy that the majority of these compounds have been identified through phenotypic screening, then subjected to optimization processes. The most representative compounds are reported in Table 1.

Table 1. Main covalent and not covalent DprE1 inhibitors showing antitubercular activity.

Chemical Class	Compound	Structure	*M. tuberculosis* MIC	Ref.
		Covalent inhibitors		
Benzothiazinones	BTZ043	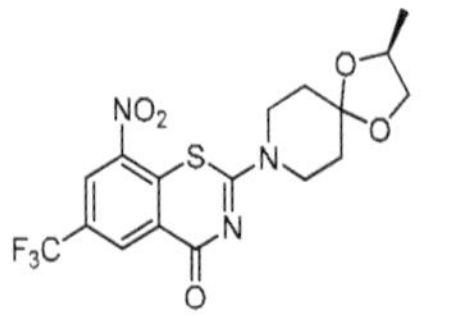	0.0023 μM	[30]
	PBTZ169	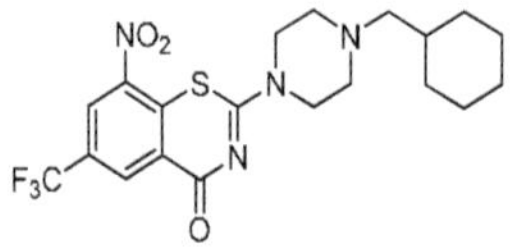	0.001 μM	[49]
Dinitrobenzamides	DNB1	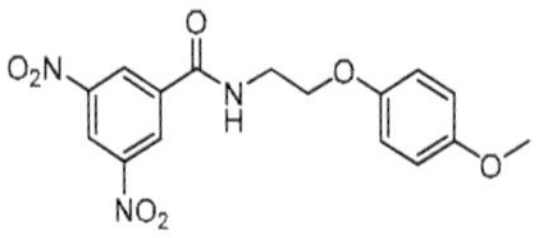	0.69 μM	[32]
Nitro-quinoxalines	VI-9376	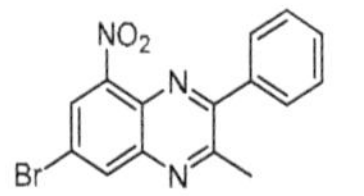	3.1 μM	[33]
Triazoles	377790	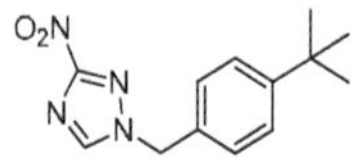	0.48 μM	[51]
		Noncovalent inhibitors		
Benzothiazoles	TCA1	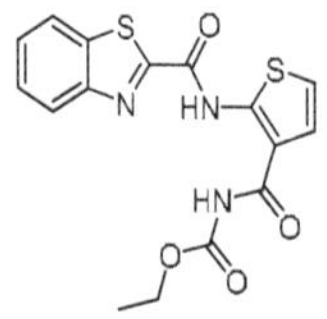	0.51 μM	[55]
	7a	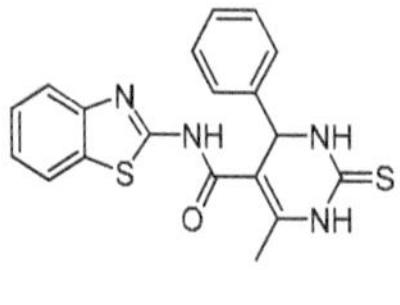	0.08 μM	[61]
Thiadiazoles	GSK-710	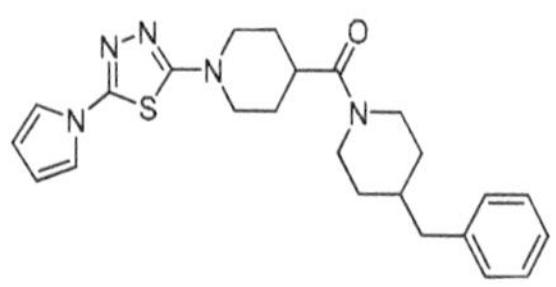	4 μM	[42]
Carboxy-quinoxalines	Ty38c	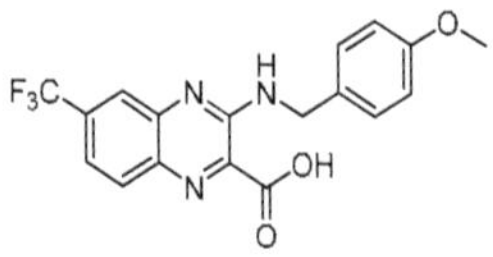	3.1 μM	[58]
Aminoquinolones	3	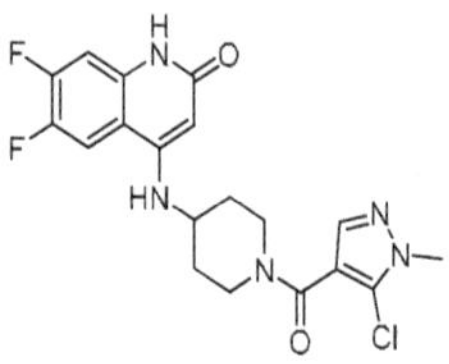	0.8 μM	[62]

Table 1. *Cont.*

Chemical Class	Compound	Structure	*M. tuberculosis* MIC	Ref.
Pyrazolopyridones	19	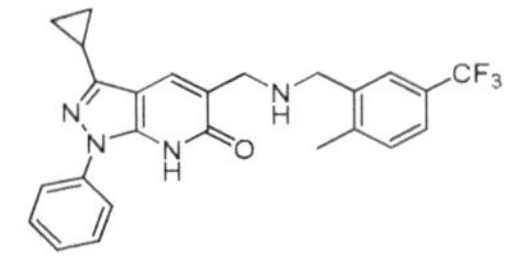	0.1 μM	[63]
Azaindoles	TBA-7371	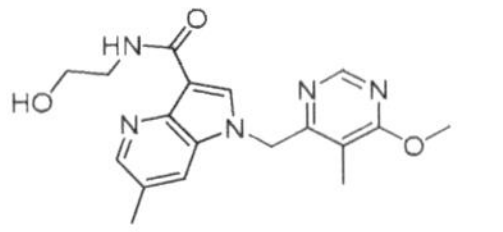	0.01 μM	[64]

The first DprE1 inhibitors identified is the BTZ043, belonging to the class of the benzothiazinones [30]. Moreover, nearly in the same period other classes of compounds, such as dinitrobenzamides, nitroquinoxaline and triazoles, have been described as covalent inhibitors [32,33,51].

As above reported, all these compounds possess a nitro group, that is converted to nitroso through the oxidation of the $FADH_2$ cofactor of DprE1, allowing the formation of a covalent bond with a cysteine residue. However, an alternative and similarly probable mechanism of formation of the nitroso group has been proposed. In this model, the thiol group of the cysteine is able to start the redox reaction which converts the nitro group into nitroso similarly to the von Richter reaction [65].

Despite BTZ043 was extremely potent against *M. tuberculosis* with an MIC of 1 ng/mL (2.3 nM) [30], its great efficacy was not translated into a mouse model, probably due to its relatively high lipophilicity, and low pharmacokinetic properties. Several attempts were then done to improve this class of compounds, and in particular, a structure activity relationship (SAR) study of piperazine benzothiazinone derivatives afforded the PBTZ-169 [49]. This compound, bearing a cyclohexylmethyl substituted piperazine showed improved in vitro and in vivo potency, and resulted in being less susceptible to the attack of nitroreductases [66]. PBTZ-169 is currently in a clinical trial under the name macozinone (MCZ) [29].

Although the nitro group is essential for the activity of the benzothiazinones [30,66], although potentially mutagenic, several attempts to substitute it, for instance by a pyrrole ring, or by an azide group were performed [67,68]. However, all these attempts led to noncovalent inhibitors, with much-reduced efficacy.

Also, noncovalent inhibitors, although less potent in vitro, can show in-vivo efficacy. For instance, the first discovered noncovalent inhibitor was the benzothiazole TCA1. This compound showed a relatively high MIC against *M. tuberculosis* of 0.5 μM, nevertheless, it proved to be effective in mice, both in acute and chronic infection models [55]. A series of pyrimidine conjugate of the benzothiazole give a further improvement of this compound, with the best derivatives showing MIC of 0.08–0.09 μM [61]. More recently a new class of inhibiting DprE1 benzothiazoles, benzothiazole-N-oxides, have been identified through a whole cells screening [44], but despite their promising bactericidal activity they showed toxicity issues.

The high vulnerability of DprE1 as an antitubercular drug target was confirmed by the number of screening campaigns that identified effective noncovalent inhibitors, including thiadiazoles [42], carboxy-quinoxalines [58], aminoquinolones [62], pyrazolopyridones [63], and azaindoles [69,70].

The latter are the most promising drug candidates among the noncovalent DprE1 inhibitors, the best inhibitor showing potent antitubercular activity in vitro and in in vivo chronic infection models, low toxicity and no antagonistic activity with other TB drugs [64]. Currently, the azaindole TBA-7371 has started phase I clinical trials [27], further confirming the great potential of DprE1 inhibitors in anti-tubercular drug discovery.

3.3. DprE2: A Promising Target for Future Drug Discovery

As above reported, the conversion of DPR to DPA is a two steps reaction, in which the product of DprE1 decaprenyl-phospho-2′-keto-D-arabinose must be reduced to finalize the epimerization of the substrate. This second step is catalyzed by the enzyme DprE2 (decaprenylphosphoryl-2-keto-β-D-erythro-pentose reductase) [14]. As DprE1, also DprE2 is essential for mycobacterial growth [35]. Moreover, the two enzymes have been supposed to strongly interact, and sometimes they were considered two subunits of a single enzyme named decaprenylphosphoryl-β-D-ribofuranose 2-epimerase. Indeed, DprE1 and DprE2 interaction in *Corynebacterium glutamicum*, strongly related to mycobacteria, have been demonstrated by a bacterial two-hybrid system [71]. An in silico study using homology modeling, protein threading and molecular dynamics proposed a model in which DprE1 and DprE2 form a complex [72], but currently, no structural and functional data on DprE2 have been reported yet. Anyhow, to fulfill their reactions it is conceivable that the two enzymes must work in concert, thus, reasonably a strong interaction occurs. In this context, the elucidation of the structural and functional behavior of the full decaprenylphosphoryl-β-D-ribofuranose 2-epimerase complex should be a useful tool for the development of further antitubercular inhibitors [73].

4. Mmpl3 Transporter: The Other Hot TB Target of the Moment

4.1. MmpL3: A Mycolic Acid Transporter

MmpL3 is a membrane protein, member of the resistance-nodulation-cell division (RND) superfamily of transporters. In mycobacteria, MmpL transporters have specialized in the export of several lipids and glycolipids across the plasma membrane to the cell surface, namely, trehalose monomycolates (TMM), di- and poly-acyltrehaloses, sulfolipids, phthiocerol dimycocerosates, monomycolyldiacylglycerol, glycopeptidolipids and mycobactins [38,74–78]. Genetic studies with transposon mutant libraries and the inability to knock-out the gene using different strategies suggested that MmpL3 was essential for the survival of *M. tuberculosis* [38,79]. An alternative strategy, utilizing knock-down strains both in vitro and in vivo had confirmed that MmpL3 is indeed essential for survival. Silencing of MmpL3 in mice, both during the acute or persistence phase of infection, led to a complete clearance of bacteria from lungs and spleens. These studies not only reinforce the idea of MmpL3 as an attractive drug target but also the potential of MmpL3 inhibitors to shorten TB treatment [80].

MmpL3 contains 12 transmembrane segments with two periplasmic loops and one C-terminal cytoplasmic domain. The periplasmic loops are essential for the MmpL3 function and are involved in substrate binding. On the other hand, the cytoplasmic loop, which is only present in MmpL3 and MmpL11 but not in other members of the MmpL family, is not essential for MmpL3 transport activity [81]. The exact role of the C-terminal domain is still not clear but it has been proposed to act as a signal for polar localization of the protein, since its removal caused MmpL3 to be more diffuse across the cells in contrast to the typical subpolar localization of the full protein [82]. In addition to that, this domain was shown to be involved in protein–protein interactions with itself as well as with other proteins, pointing to a role in oligomerization and/or coordination of synthesis of other cell wall components [83]. MmpL3 transports TMM across the cell membrane to the periplasmic space where it serves as a mycolic acid donor to another TMM molecule to form TDM, or to arabinogalactan as part of the mAGP core. Both of these reactions are catalyzed by the Ag85 family of enzymes. Mycolic acids are essential components of the mycobacterial cell wall and its biosynthesis has been shown as an effective drug target in mycobacteria, with several antibiotics targeting this pathway. The best example of this is isoniazid, which inhibits the FASII enoyl-ACP reductase InhA, and is one of the pillars in tuberculosis treatment [84].

MmpL3 relies on the proton motive force as an energy source to drive TMM transport. Thus, the flux of protons across the transmembrane region of MmpL3 would drive the conformational changes necessary for the translocation of TMM. This is evidenced by mutagenesis studies showing that charged residues lying on the transmembrane region are essential for MmpL3 function and are most likely involved in this proton relay pathway. The mechanism and extent of TMM transport mediated by MmpL3 is still not fully understood. Spheroplasts assays have suggested that MmpL3 acts as a flippase [15]. This conclusion was derived from the accumulation of TMM in the inner leaflet of the plasma membrane after MmpL3 inhibition. Although this would point to MmpL3 acting as a flippase, there is the possibility that MmpL3 inhibition would affect also other proteins acting upstream in the transport pathway and/or TMM biosynthetic enzymes. This holds true for other MmpL transporters where disruption of the transport leads to the accumulation of biosynthetic precursors and, in some cases, the complete abolition of the synthesis of the substrate [74,78,85,86].

The recently solved crystal structure of MmpL3 has shed some light as to the possible mechanism of TMM translocation [25,87]. Crystals of MmpL3 from *M. smegmatis* were diffracted to a 2.59 Å resolution. Surprisingly, the 3D structure of this transporter is different from other RND transporters like AcrB, MexB, CusA, MtrD, CmeB and HpnN. The structure shows that the *N*-terminal and *C*-terminal halves are assembled in a twofold pseudo symmetrical fashion and the two periplasmic domains (PD1 and PD2) interact with each other and are also flexible. MmpL3 possesses a cavity that extends from the outer leaflet of the inner membrane up to the periplasmic domain. This cavity is large enough to fit a TMM molecule. Fortuitously, MmpL3 co-purified with n-dodecyl-β-D-maltoside (the detergent used for solubilization) and phosphatidylethanolamine (PE) bound to it. The former was found in the hydrophobic pocket created by TMs 7–10 while the latter was bound to the periplasmic domain within the large space between PD1 and PD2. These results reinforce the idea of MmpL3 channeling its substrate from the outer leaflet of the inner membrane up to the periplasmic space. The authors further demonstrated that TMM binds to purified MmpL3 with a K_d of 3.7 ± 1.3 μM while there was no binding when TDM was assayed. In addition to PE and TMM, both phosphatidylglycerol and cardiolipin interacted with MmpL3. Whether these phospholipids act as substrates for MmpL3 in whole cells remains to be determined.

Native mass spectra, Small-angle X-ray scattering (SAXS) data and Blue-Native PAGE of the purified MmpL3 transporter indicate that it is a monomer in detergent solution [25,87]. It has to be noted that in both cases MmpL3 was purified devoid of the C-terminal domain due to its instability in solution and this domain was shown to be important for MmpL3 oligomerization [83]. This is in contrast to the quaternary structure of CmpL1, a *Corynebacterium glutamicum* ortholog, which has been shown to possess a trimeric quaternary structure [81]. There is a great variety of quaternary structures among the RND superfamily of transporters, while the efflux subfamily of RND transporters, namely, AcrB [88], MexB [89] and MtrD [90] exist as trimers, the hopanoid biosynthesis-associated transporter (HpnN) from *Burkholderia multivorans* is a dimer [91] and human NPC1 is a monomer [92]. Due to this high variability, we cannot rule out that MmpL3 has a higher oligomerization state in native conditions found in the mycobacterial cell membrane.

4.2. MmpL3: The Achilles Heel of Mycobacterium Tuberculosis

In recent years, a diversity of scaffolds have been reported to inhibit MmpL3 (Table 2): SQ109 (diamine), DA5 (SQ109 related compound), BM212 (diarylpyrrole), Au1235 (adamantyl urea), C215 (benzimidazole), NITD-349 (indolecarboxamides), THP P (tetrathydropyrazolo pyrimidine), Spiro (*N*-benzyl-6′,7′-dihydrospiro[piperidine-4,4′-thieno[3,2-c]pyrans]), PIPD1 (piperidinol), E11 (acetamide) and HC2091 (carboxamide) [36–38,51,93–97].

Table 2. Main MmpL3 inhibitors showing antitubercular activity.

Chemical Class	Compound	Structure	*M. tuberculosis* MIC	Ref.
Diarylpyrroles	BM212	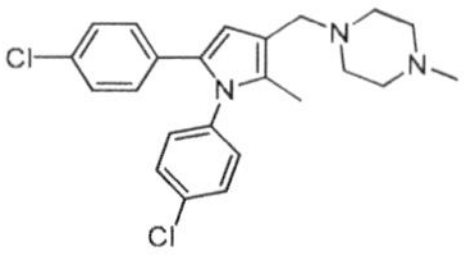	3.6 μM	[36]
1,2-diamine derivatives	DA5	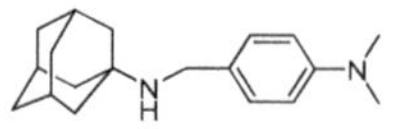	9.97 μM	[37]
	SQ109	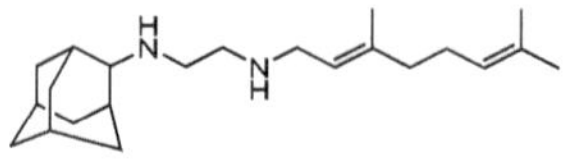	0.78 μM	[37]
Adamantyl urea	AU1235	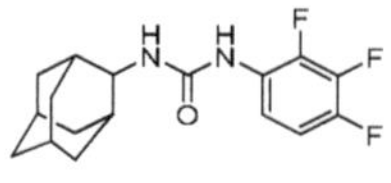	0.3 μM	[38]
Benzimidazoles	C215	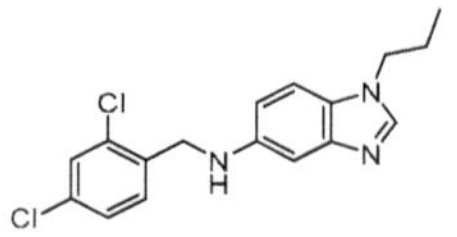	16.0 μM	[51]
Indolcarboxamides	NIDT349	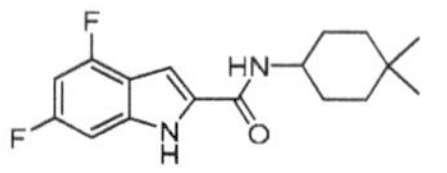	0.023 μM	[93]
Tetrahydropyrazolo pyrimidine	THP P	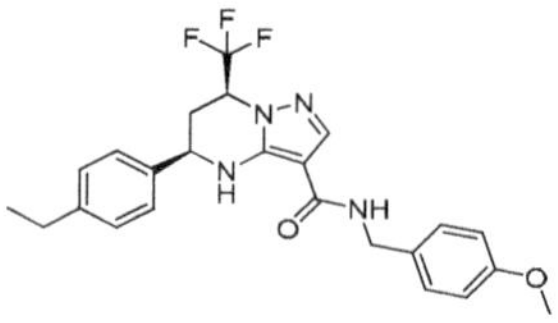	0.3 μM	[94]
Dihydrospiro[piperidine-4,4′-thieno[3,2-c]pyrans]	Spiro	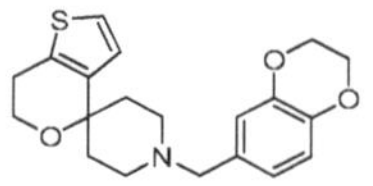	0.3 μM	[94]
Piperidinols	PIPD1	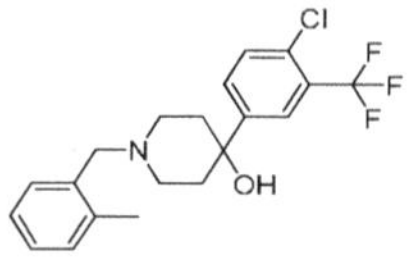	1.28 μM	[95]
Acetamides	E11	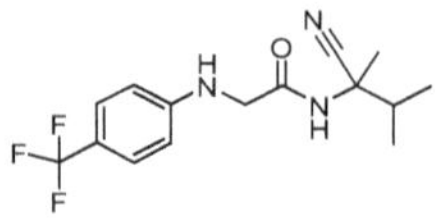	8.0 μM	[96]
Carboxamides	HC2091	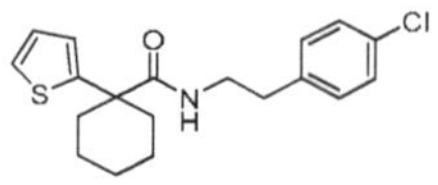	19.3 μM	[97]

Among these compounds, SQ109 is the most advanced in the TB drug pipeline and has completed Phase I clinical trials in the US and Phase II clinical trials in Africa. SQ109 was identified originally from a combinatorial library screening based on the 1,2-ethylenediamine structure of ethambutol. However, other structural dissimilarities between SQ109 and ethambutol, the significant activity of SQ109 against drug-resistant strains of *M. tuberculosis*, including those that were ethambutol-resistant, suggested that SQ109 had a different target than its parent molecule [98]. SQ109 showed bactericidal activity against *M. tuberculosis* in vitro, including MDR and XDR-TB. Furthermore, it had activity against intracellular bacilli as well as an extremely low spontaneous resistance rate [37]. In addition to that, it showed synergistic activity with isoniazid and rifampicin and additive effects with streptomycin in vitro [99].

SQ109 also increases the activity of the new TB drug bedaquiline in vitro [100]. Replacement of ethambutol by SQ109 in the standard regimen in mice led to a 1.5 n log decrease in colony-forming units (CFUs) [101]. Furthermore, SQ109 was safe and well-tolerated in Phase I and Phase IIa clinical trials [102].

MmpL3 seems to be a promiscuous target since a plethora of compounds with dissimilar scaffolds have been shown to affect its activity and every new library screening seems to lead to novel scaffolds targeting the same enzyme. However, the reason for this extreme susceptibility is not clear. One possibility is that the compounds, due to their high hydrophobicity, get vastly enriched in the membrane where they can bind readily to MmpL3. This, in addition to the extreme vulnerability of MmpL3, would explain the variety of compounds targeting MmpL3.

There has been some controversy as to the direct or indirect inhibition of these compounds against MmpL3, it has been suggested that some compounds may act indirectly on MmpL3 by disrupting the pH gradient and/or membrane potential which will disrupt the proton relay needed by MmpL3 to pump out TMM. Indeed, while SQ109 and BM212 display a broad spectrum of activity and are active against non-replicating Mtb bacilli, some others specifically target mycobacteria and do not kill nonreplicating bacilli [16,103,104]. In order to solve this controversy and to shed more light on the mechanism of action of these inhibitors, Li et al. have recently developed assays both in vitro and in whole cells to identify direct inhibitors of MmpL3. Their use of fluorescent competition assays and surface plasmon resonance experiments with MmpL3 purified protein has shown that SQ109, BM212, Au1235, NITD304, NITD349 and THPP1 all bind to MmpL3. The authors also showed that only SQ109 and BM212 dissipated both ΔpH and $\Delta\Psi$ (although the latter only at high concentrations). These assays could be a great tool for assessing the specificity of new and previously identified drugs that are believed to act against MmpL3 [105].

Recently, the crystal structure of *M. smegmatis* MmpL3 alone and in complex with four TB drug candidates has been solved [25]. Analysis of the transmembrane region has shown the existence of two pairs of hydrophilic residues (D256-Y646 and Y257-D645) on TM4 and TM 10 which links these two helices by forming hydrogen bonds. These residues are similar to the Asp-Asp-Lys triad found in AcrB and the Asp-Asp-Thr triad in SecDF, which are known to be involved in the proton relay pathway [106,107]. Consistently with this, three out of four of these residues have been shown to be essential for MmpL3 activity [81]. Furthermore, this catalytic tetrad is conserved in most MmpL transporters, with the exception of MmpL7, so it is likely that all MmpL transporters use the same mechanism to drive its substrate translocation [81].

The crystal structure of MmpL3 bound to SQ109, Au1235 and ICA38 has shown that these MmpL3 inhibitors bind to the same pocket in the center of the transmembrane region of the protein (Figure 3A), inducing conformational changes which in turn disrupt the interaction of the two Asp-Tyr pairs involved in proton translocation (Figure 3B,C). Furthermore, molecular docking assays with six other compounds (BM212, NITD-349, GSK2200150A, C215, PIPD1 and HC2091) showed that they can fit the same binding pocket within MmpL3. Thus, MmpL3 inhibitors seem to have an identical mechanism of action, binding to the same pocket and blocking the proton translocation relay pathway that is essential for substrate transport. This is also supported by the fact that the majority of resistance mutations found in MmpL3 lie in the TM region, close to the binding pocket. Zhang et al. purified 12 different mutant versions of MmpL3 and showed that most of the mutations affected the binding of the inhibitors to the pocket by disrupting hydrophobic/electrostatic interactions, inducing conformational changes or causing steric hindrance which leads to a decrease or abolition of the binding. On the other hand, there is still no clear evidence as to how mutations located further for the binding pocket induce resistance. Although MmpL3 is the only essential MmpL protein in *M. tuberculosis*, several other MmpL proteins have been shown to be required for virulence and/or drug efflux [108,109]. The fact that all inhibitors act by disrupting the proton relay pathway, a conserved feature of all MmpL transporters, opens the avenue for the development of molecules that target not only MmpL3 but all the MmpL family of transporters and thus affect virulence and resistance to other drugs.

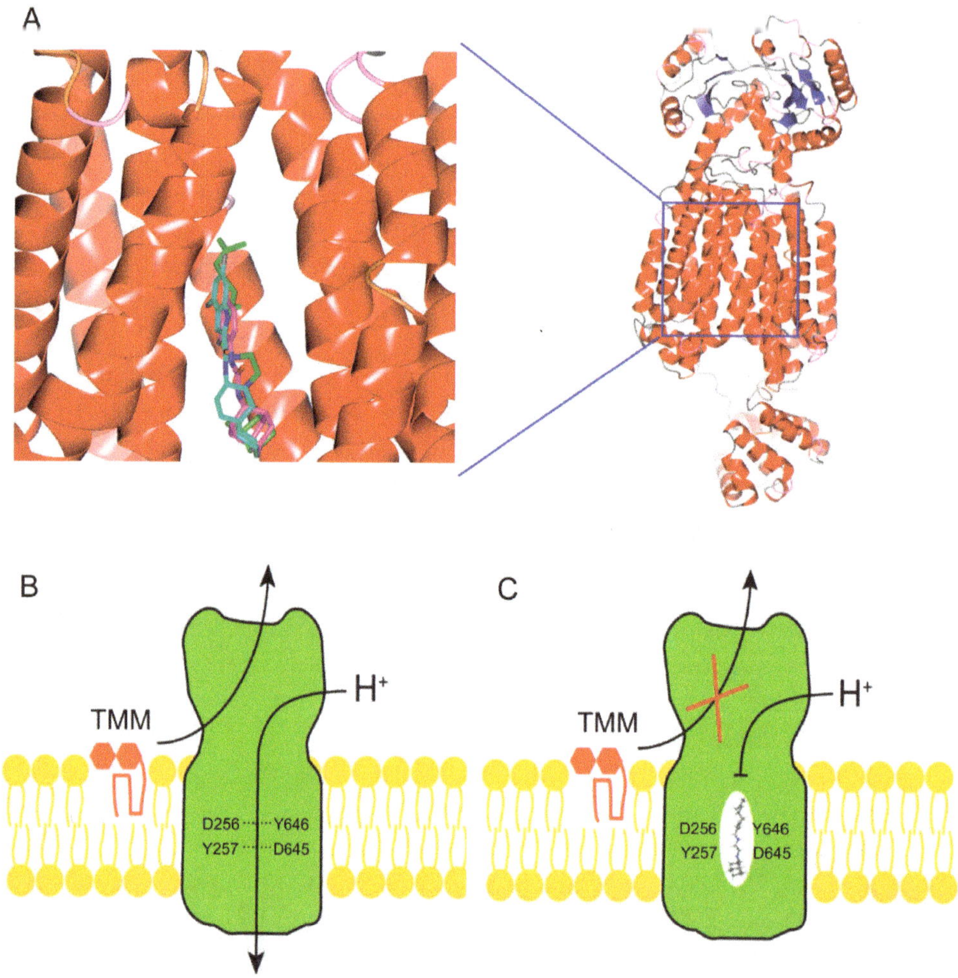

Figure 3. (**A**) Crystal structure of Mtb MmpL3 and detail of the inhibitors binding site (SQ109, PDB: 6AJG with carbon atoms in green; AU1235, PDB: 6AJH with carbon atoms in magenta; ICA38 PDB: 6AJJ with carbon atoms in cyan [25]). (**B**) Mechanism of transport of MmpL3: The flow of protons through charged residues in the transmembrane region of MmpL3 drives conformational changes that lead to the transport of TMM from the membrane to the periplasmic space. (**C**) MmpL3 inhibitors bind to a pocket in the transmembrane region of MmpL3, disrupting the electrostatic interactions between D256 and Y257 with Y646 and D645, respectively. This blocks the proton relay pathway and ultimately TMM translocation.

In summary, these findings will lead to a new era in MmpL3 inhibitor drug discovery since structure-guided molecules can now be designed with better anti-tubercular efficacy and pharmacokinetic/pharmacodynamic (PK/PD) properties.

5. Future Perspectives for DprE1 and MmpL3 Inhibitors in Clinical Therapy

Promiscuous targets could be an obstacle in the discovery of novel antitubercular drug targets, being recurrently found in HTS [110], nevertheless, they have been proven really useful for the development of novel drug candidates. This is well demonstrated by the fact that five compounds currently in clinical trials inhibit these targets, with DprE1 inhibitors TBA-7379, BTZ043 and Macozinone in Phase I, while the QcrB inhibitor Telacebec, the MmpL3 inhibitor SQ109 and again the Macozinone are in Phase II [26–29].

In particular, Macozinone has completed a dose-escalation phase I study in healthy male volunteers and a multiple ascending dose study in Russia, which demonstrated the good safety profile of the compound. Moreover, in 2018 it completed a Phase IIa Early Bactericidal Activity (EBA) study in Russia and Belarus in drug sensitive-TB (DS-TB) patients, confirming the safety and efficacy of the drug. In parallel, a Phase I clinical study has been initiated in Switzerland, by the nonprofit Innovative Medicines for Tuberculosis (iM4TB) foundation [24].

The MmpL3 inhibitor SQ109 has completed a Phase 2b study in Russia which demonstrated its efficacy in MDR-TB patients, with a good tolerability profile [111]. Furthermore, SQ109 was demonstrated to enhance the activity of isoniazid, rifampicin and bedaquiline and shortened clearance of TB in a mice model. The drug now has also completed three Phase I studies in the USA and two Phase II studies in Africa in DS-TB patients.

These studies thus demonstrate the great potential of these targets for the development of a new drug to reach the objective to eradicate TB.

Author Contributions: Conceptualization, G.R. and L.R.C.; writing, G.D., J.M.B. and L.R.C., review and editing, M.R.P., E.D.R., G.R. and L.R.C.; visualization, J.M.B. and L.R.C.; project administration, G.R. All authors have read and agreed to the published version of the manuscript.

References

1. World Health Organization. Global Tuberculosis Report 2019. Available online: https://www.who.int/tb/publications/global_report/en/ (accessed on 7 January 2020).
2. Lechartier, B.; Rybniker, J.; Zumla, A.; Cole, S.T. Tuberculosis drug discovery in the post-post-genomic era. *EMBO Mol. Med.* **2014**, *6*, 158–168. [CrossRef]
3. Chiarelli, L.R.; Mori, G.; Esposito, M.; Orena, B.S.; Pasca, M.R. New and old hot drug targets in tuberculosis. *Curr. Med. Chem.* **2016**, *23*, 3813–3846. [CrossRef]
4. Meneghetti, F.; Villa, S.; Gelain, A.; Barlocco, D.; Chiarelli, L.R.; Pasca, M.R.; Costantino, L. Iron acquisition pathways as targets for antitubercular drugs. *Curr. Med. Chem.* **2016**, *23*, 4009–4026. [CrossRef]
5. Mori, M.; Sammartino, J.C.; Costantino, L.; Gelain, A.; Meneghetti, F.; Villa, S.; Chiarelli, L.R. An Overview on the Potential Antimycobacterial Agents Targeting Serine/Threonine Protein Kinases from *Mycobacterium tuberculosis*. *Curr. Top. Med. Chem.* **2019**, *19*, 646–661. [CrossRef] [PubMed]
6. Andries, K.; Verhasselt, P.; Guillemont, J.; Göhlmann, H.W.; Neefs, J.M.; Winkler, H.; Van Gestel, J.; Timmerman, P.; Zhu, M.; Lee, E.; et al. A diarylquinoline drug active on the ATP synthase of *Mycobacterium tuberculosis*. *Science* **2005**, *307*, 223–227. [CrossRef] [PubMed]
7. Matsumoto, M.; Hashizume, H.; Tomishige, T.; Kawasaki, M.; Tsubouchi, H.; Sasaki, H.; Shimokawa, Y.; Komatsu, M. OPC-67683, a nitro-dihydro-imidazooxazole derivative with promising action against tuberculosis in vitro and in mice. *PLoS Med.* **2006**, *3*, e466. [CrossRef] [PubMed]
8. Stover, C.K.; Warrener, P.; VanDevanter, D.R.; Sherman, D.R.; Arain, T.M.; Langhorne, M.H.; Anderson, S.W.; Towell, J.A.; Yuan, Y.; McMurray, D.N.; et al. A small-molecule nitroimidazopyran drug candidate for the treatment of tuberculosis. *Nature* **2000**, *405*, 962–966. [CrossRef] [PubMed]
9. Ryan, N.J.; Lo, J.H. Delamanid: First global approval. *Drugs* **2014**, *74*, 1041–1045. [CrossRef] [PubMed]
10. Keam, S.J. Pretomanid: First Approval. *Drugs* **2019**, *79*, 1797–1803. [CrossRef]
11. Cole, S.T. Inhibiting Mycobacterium tuberculosis within and without. *Philos. Trans. R. Soc. Lond. B Biol. Sci.* **2016**, *371*, 20150506. [CrossRef]
12. Lee, B.S.; Pethe, K. Therapeutic potential of promiscuous targets in *Mycobacterium tuberculosis*. *Curr. Opin. Pharmacol.* **2018**, *42*, 22–26. [CrossRef] [PubMed]
13. Campaniço, A.; Moreira, R.; Lopes, F. Drug discovery in tuberculosis. New drug targets and antimycobacterial agents. *Eur. J. Med. Chem.* **2018**, *150*, 525–545. [CrossRef] [PubMed]
14. Mikusová, K.; Huang, H.; Yagi, T.; Holsters, M.; Vereecke, D.; D'Haeze, W.; Scherman, M.S.; Brennan, P.J.; McNeil, M.R.; Crick, D.C. Decaprenylphosphoryl arabinofuranose, the donor of the D-arabinofuranosyl residues of mycobacterial arabinan, is formed via a two-step epimerization of decaprenylphosphoryl ribose. *J. Bacteriol.* **2005**, *187*, 8020–8025. [CrossRef] [PubMed]

15. Xu, Z.; Meshcheryakov, V.A.; Poce, G.; Chng, S.S. MmpL3 is the flippase for mycolic acids in mycobacteria. *Proc. Natl. Acad. Sci. USA* **2017**, *114*, 7993–7998. [CrossRef] [PubMed]
16. Li, W.; Upadhyay, A.; Fontes, F.L.; North, E.J.; Wang, Y.; Crans, D.C.; Grzegorzewicz, A.E.; Jones, V.; Franzblau, S.G.; Lee, R.E.; et al. Novel insights into the mechanism of inhibition of MmpL3, a target of multiple pharmacophores in *Mycobacterium tuberculosis*. *Antimicrob. Agents Chemother.* **2014**, *58*, 6413–6423. [CrossRef] [PubMed]
17. Abrahams, K.A.; Cox, J.A.; Spivey, V.L.; Loman, N.J.; Pallen, M.J.; Constantinidou, C.; Fernández, R.; Alemparte, C.; Remuiñán, M.J.; Barros, D.; et al. Identification of novel imidazo[1,2-a]pyridine inhibitors targeting *M. tuberculosis* QcrB. *PLoS ONE* **2012**, *7*, e52951. [CrossRef]
18. Pethe, K.; Bifani, P.; Jang, J.; Kang, S.; Park, S.; Ahn, S.; Jiricek, J.; Jung, J.; Jeon, H.K.; Cechetto, J.; et al. Discovery of Q203, a potent clinical candidate for the treatment of tuberculosis. *Nat. Med.* **2013**, *19*, 1157–1160. [CrossRef]
19. Wilson, R.; Kumar, P.; Parashar, V.; Vilchèze, C.; Veyron-Churlet, R.; Freundlich, J.S.; Barnes, S.W.; Walker, J.R.; Szymonifka, M.J.; Marchiano, E.; et al. Antituberculosis thiophenes define a requirement for Pks13 in mycolic acid biosynthesis. *Nat. Chem. Biol.* **2013**, *9*, 499–506. [CrossRef]
20. Aggarwal, A.; Parai, M.K.; Shetty, N.; Wallis, D.; Woolhiser, L.; Hastings, C.; Dutta, N.K.; Galaviz, S.; Dhakal, R.C.; Shrestha, R.; et al. Development of a Novel Lead that Targets *M. tuberculosis* Polyketide Synthase 13. *Cell* **2017**, *170*, 249–259. [CrossRef]
21. Grant, S.S.; Kawate, T.; Nag, P.P.; Silvis, M.R.; Gordon, K.; Stanley, S.A.; Kazyanskaya, E.; Nietupski, R.; Golas, A.; Fitzgerald, M.; et al. Identification of novel inhibitors of nonreplicating *Mycobacterium tuberculosis* using a carbon starvation model. *ACS Chem. Biol.* **2013**, *8*, 2224–2234. [CrossRef]
22. Bonnett, S.A.; Dennison, D.; Files, M.; Bajpai, A.; Parish, T. A class of hydrazones are active against non-replicating *Mycobacterium tuberculosis*. *PLoS ONE* **2018**, *13*, e0198059. [CrossRef] [PubMed]
23. Boldrin, F.; Degiacomi, G.; Serafini, A.; Kolly, G.S.; Ventura, M.; Sala, C.; Provvedi, R.; Palù, G.; Cole, S.T.; Manganelli, R. Promoter mutagenesis for fine-tuning expression of essential genes in *Mycobacterium tuberculosis*. *Microb. Biotechnol.* **2018**, *11*, 238–247. [CrossRef] [PubMed]
24. Lupien, A.; Vocat, A.; Foo, C.S.; Blattes, E.; Gillon, J.Y.; Makarov, V.; Cole, S.T. Optimized background regimen for treatment of active tuberculosis with the next-generation benzothiazinone Macozinone (PBTZ169). *Antimicrob. Agents Chemother.* **2018**, *62*, e00840-18. [CrossRef] [PubMed]
25. Zhang, B.; Li, J.; Yang, X.; Wu, L.; Zhang, J.; Yang, Y.; Zhao, Y.; Zhang, L.; Cheng, X.; Liu, Z.; et al. Crystal structures of membrane transporter MmpL3, an anti-TB drug target. *Cell* **2019**, *176*, 636–648. [CrossRef] [PubMed]
26. Available online: https://www.newtbdrugs.org/pipeline/compound/sq109 (accessed on 4 December 2019).
27. Available online: https://www.newtbdrugs.org/pipeline/compound/tba-7371 (accessed on 4 December 2019).
28. Available online: https://www.newtbdrugs.org/pipeline/trials/phase-2-telacebec-q203-eba (accessed on 4 December 2019).
29. Available online: https://www.newtbdrugs.org/pipeline/compound/macozinone-mcz-pbtz-169 (accessed on 4 December 2019).
30. Makarov, V.; Manina, G.; Mikusova, K.; Möllmann, U.; Ryabova, O.; Saint-Joanis, B.; Dhar, N.; Pasca, M.R.; Buroni, S.; Lucarelli, A.P.; et al. Benzothiazinones kill *Mycobacterium tuberculosis* by blocking arabinan synthesis. *Science* **2009**, *324*, 801–804. [CrossRef] [PubMed]
31. Wolucka, B.A. Biosynthesis of D-arabinose in mycobacteria—A novel bacterial pathway with implications for antimycobacterial therapy. *FEBS J.* **2008**, *275*, 2691–2711. [CrossRef]
32. Christophe, T.; Jackson, M.; Jeon, H.K.; Fenistein, D.; Contreras-Dominguez, M.; Kim, J.; Genovesio, A.; Carralot, J.P.; Ewann, F.; Kim, E.H.; et al. High content screening identifies decaprenyl-phosphoribose 2′ epimerase as a target for intracellular antimycobacterial inhibitors. *PLoS Pathog.* **2009**, *5*, e1000645. [CrossRef]
33. Magnet, S.; Hartkoorn, R.C.; Székely, R.; Pató, J.; Triccas, J.A.; Schneider, P.; Szántai-Kis, C.; Orfi, L.; Chambon, M.; Banfi, D.; et al. Leads for antitubercular compounds from kinase inhibitor library screens. *Tuberculosis* **2010**, *90*, 354–360. [CrossRef]
34. Matsoso, L.G.; Kana, B.D.; Crellin, P.K.; Lea-Smith, D.J.; Pelosi, A.; Powell, D.; Dawes, S.S.; Rubin, H.; Coppel, R.L.; Mizrahi, V. Function of the cytochrome bc1-aa3 branch of the respiratory network in mycobacteria and network adaptation occurring in response to its disruption. *J. Bacteriol.* **2005**, *187*, 6300–6308. [CrossRef]

35. Kolly, G.S.; Boldrin, F.; Sala, C.; Dhar, N.; Hartkoorn, R.C.; Ventura, M.; Serafini, A.; McKinney, J.D.; Manganelli, R.; Cole, S.T. Assessing the essentiality of the decaprenyl-phospho-d-arabinofuranose pathway in *Mycobacterium tuberculosis* using conditional mutants. *Mol. Microbiol.* **2014**, *92*, 194–211. [CrossRef]
36. La Rosa, V.; Poce, G.; Canseco, J.O.; Buroni, S.; Pasca, M.R.; Biava, M.; Raju, R.M.; Porretta, G.C.; Alfonso, S.; Battilocchio, C.; et al. MmpL3 is the cellular target of the antitubercular pyrrole derivative BM212. *Antimicrob. Agents Chemother.* **2012**, *56*, 324–331. [CrossRef] [PubMed]
37. Tahlan, K.; Wilson, R.; Kastrinsky, D.B.; Arora, K.; Nair, V.; Fischer, E.; Barnes, S.W.; Walker, J.R.; Alland, D.; Barry, C.E.; et al. SQ109 targets MmpL3, a membrane transporter of trehalose monomycolate involved in mycolic acid donation to the cell wall core of *Mycobacterium tuberculosis*. *Antimicrob. Agents Chemother.* **2012**, *56*, 1797–1809. [CrossRef] [PubMed]
38. Grzegorzewicz, A.E.; Pham, H.; Gundi, V.A.; Scherman, M.S.; North, E.J.; Hess, T.; Jones, V.; Gruppo, V.; Born, S.E.; Korduláková, J.; et al. Inhibition of mycolic acid transport across the Mycobacterium tuberculosis plasma membrane. *Nat. Chem. Biol.* **2012**, *8*, 334–341. [CrossRef]
39. Degiacomi, G.; Benjak, A.; Madacki, J.; Boldrin, F.; Provvedi, R.; Palù, G.; Kordulakova, J.; Cole, S.T.; Manganelli, R. Essentiality of mmpL3 and impact of its silencing on *Mycobacterium tuberculosis* gene expression. *Sci. Rep.* **2017**, *7*, 43495. [CrossRef] [PubMed]
40. Riccardi, G.; Pasca, M.R.; Chiarelli, L.R.; Manina, G.; Mattevi, A.; Binda, C. The DprE1 enzyme, one of the most vulnerable targets of *Mycobacterium tuberculosis*. *Appl. Microbiol. Biotechnol.* **2013**, *97*, 8841–8848. [CrossRef]
41. Neres, J.; Pojer, F.; Molteni, E.; Chiarelli, L.R.; Dhar, N.; Boy-Rottger, S.; Buroni, S.; Fullam, E.; Degiacomi, G.; Lucarelli, A.P.; et al. Structural basis for benzothiazinone-mediated killing of *Mycobacterium tuberculosis*. *Sci. Trans. Med.* **2012**, *4*, 150ra121. [CrossRef]
42. Batt, S.M.; Cacho Izquierdo, M.; Castro Pichel, J.; Stubbs, C.J.; Del Peral, L.V.-G.; Pérez-Herrán, E.; Dhar, N.; Mouzon, B.; Rees, M.; Hutchinson, J.P.; et al. Whole cell target engagement identifies novel inhibitors of *Mycobacterium tuberculosis* decaprenylphosphoryl-β-D-ribose oxidase. *ACS Infect. Dis* **2015**, *1*, 615–626. [CrossRef]
43. Batt, S.M.; Jabeen, T.; Bhowruth, V.; Quill, L.; Lund, P.A.; Eggeling, L.; Alderwick, L.J.; Fütterer, K.; Besra, G.S. Structural basis of inhibition of *Mycobacterium tuberculosis* DprE1 by benzothiazinone inhibitors. *Proc. Natl. Acad. Sci. USA* **2012**, *109*, 11354–11359. [CrossRef]
44. Landge, S.; Mullick, A.B.; Nagalapur, K.; Neres, J.; Subbulakshmi, V.; Murugan, K.; Ghosh, A.; Sadler, C.; Fellows, M.D.; Humnabadkar, V.; et al. Discovery of benzothiazoles as antimycobacterial agents: Synthesis, structure-activity relationships and binding studies with *Mycobacterium tuberculosis* decaprenylphosphoryl-β-D-ribose 2′-oxidase. *Bioorg. Med. Chem.* **2015**, *23*, 7694–7710. [CrossRef]
45. Piton, J.; Foo, C.S.; Cole, S.T. Structural studies of *Mycobacterium tuberculosis* DprE1 interacting with its inhibitors. *Drug Discov. Today* **2017**, *22*, 526–533. [CrossRef]
46. Chikhale, R.V.; Barmade, M.A.; Murumkar, P.R.; Yadav, M.R. Overview of the development of dpre1 inhibitors for combating the menace of tuberculosis. *J. Med. Chem.* **2018**, *61*, 8563–8593. [CrossRef] [PubMed]
47. Mori, G.; Chiarelli, L.R.; Riccardi, G.; Pasca, M.R. New prodrugs against tuberculosis. *Drug Discov. Today* **2017**, *22*, 519–525. [CrossRef] [PubMed]
48. Trefzer, C.; Škovierová, H.; Buroni, S.; Bobovská, A.; Nenci, S.; Molteni, E.; Pojer, F.; Pasca, M.R.; Makarov, V.; Cole, S.T.; et al. Benzothiazinones are suicide inhibitors of mycobacterial decaprenylphosphoryl-β-D-ribofuranose 2′-oxidase DprE1. *J. Am. Chem. Soc.* **2012**, *134*, 912–915. [CrossRef] [PubMed]
49. Makarov, V.; Lechartier, B.; Zhang, M.; Neres, J.; van der Sar, A.M.; Raadsen, S.A.; Hartkoorn, R.C.; Ryabova, O.B.; Vocat, A.; Decosterd, L.A.; et al. Towards a new combination therapy for tuberculosis with next generation benzothiazinones. *EMBO Mol. Med.* **2014**, *6*, 372–383. [CrossRef]
50. Richter, A.; Rudolph, I.; Möllmann, U.; Voigt, K.; Chung, C.W.; Singh, O.M.P.; Rees, M.; Mendoza-Losana, A.; Bates, R.; Ballell, L.; et al. Novel insight into the reaction of nitro, nitroso and hydroxylamino benzothiazinones and of benzoxacinones with *Mycobacterium tuberculosis* DprE1. *Sci. Rep.* **2018**, *8*, 13473. [CrossRef]
51. Stanley, S.A.; Grant, S.S.; Kawate, T.; Iwase, N.; Shimizu, M.; Wivagg, C.; Silvis, M.; Kazyanskaya, E.; Aquadro, J.; Golas, A.; et al. Identification of novel inhibitors of *M. tuberculosis* growth using whole cell based high-throughput screening. *ACS Chem. Biol.* **2012**, *7*, 1377–1384. [CrossRef]

52. De Jesus Lopes Ribeiro, A.L.; Degiacomi, G.; Ewann, F.; Buroni, S.; Incandela, M.L.; Chiarelli, L.R.; Mori, G., Kim, J.; Contreras-Dominguez, M.; Park, Y.-S.; et al. Analogous mechanisms of resistance to benzothiazinones and dinitrobenzamides in *Mycobacterium smegmatis*. *PLoS ONE* **2011**, *6*, e26675. [CrossRef]

53. Li, H.; Jogl, G. Crystal structure of decaprenylphosphoryl-β-D-ribose 2′-epimerase from *Mycobacterium smegmatis*. *Proteins* **2013**, *81*, 538–543. [CrossRef]

54. Landge, S.; Ramachandran, V.; Kumar, A.; Neres, J.; Murugan, K.; Sadler, C.; Fellows, M.D.; Humnabadkar, V.; Vachaspati, P.; Raichurkar, A.; et al. Nitroarenes as antitubercular agents: Stereoelectronic modulation to mitigate mutagenicity. *ChemMedChem* **2016**, *11*, 331–339. [CrossRef]

55. Wang, F.; Sambandan, D.; Halder, R.; Wang, J.; Batt, S.M.; Weinrick, B.; Ahmad, I.; Yang, P.; Zhang, Y.; Kim, J.; et al. Identification of a small molecule with activity against drug-resistant and persistent tuberculosis. *Proc. Natl. Acad. Sci. USA* **2013**, *110*, E2510–E2517. [CrossRef]

56. Liu, R.; Lyu, X.; Batt, S.M.; Hsu, M.H.; Harbut, M.B.; Vilchèze, C.; Cheng, B.; Ajayi, K.; Yang, B.; Yang, Y.; et al. Determinants of the inhibition of DprE1 and CYP2C9 by antitubercular thiophenes. *Angew. Chem. Int. Ed. Engl.* **2017**, *56*, 13011–13015. [CrossRef] [PubMed]

57. Piton, J.; Vocat, A.; Lupien, A.; Foo, C.S.; Riabova, O.; Makarov, V.; Cole, S.T. Structure-based drug design and characterization of sulfonyl-piperazine benzothiazinone inhibitors of DprE1 from *Mycobacterium tuberculosis*. *Antimicrob. Agents Chemother.* **2018**, *62*, e00681-18. [CrossRef] [PubMed]

58. Neres, J.; Hartkoorn, R.C.; Chiarelli, L.R.; Gadupudi, R.; Pasca, M.R.; Mori, G.; Venturelli, A.; Savina, S.; Makarov, V.; Kolly, G.S.; et al. 2-carboxyquinoxalines kill *Mycobacterium tuberculosis* through noncovalent inhibition of DprE1. *ACS Chem. Biol.* **2015**, *10*, 705–714. [CrossRef] [PubMed]

59. Abrahams, K.A.; Besra, G.S. Mycobacterial cell wall biosynthesis: A multifaceted antibiotic target. *Parasitology* **2018**, *145*, 116–133. [CrossRef] [PubMed]

60. Brecik, M.; Centárová, I.; Mukherjee, R.; Kolly, G.S.; Huszár, S.; Bobovská, A.; Kilacsková, E.; Mokošová, V.; Svetlíková, Z.; Šarkan, M.; et al. DprE1 is a vulnerable tuberculosis drug target due to its cell wall localization. *ACS Chem. Biol.* **2015**, *10*, 1631–1636. [CrossRef] [PubMed]

61. Chikhale, R.; Menghani, S.; Babu, R.; Bansode, R.; Bhargavi, G.; Karodia, N.; Rajasekharan, M.V.; Paradkar, A.; Khedekar, P. Development of selective DprE1 inhibitors: Design, synthesis, crystal structure and antitubercular activity of benzothiazolylpyrimidine-5-carboxamides. *Eur. J. Med. Chem.* **2015**, *96*, 30–46. [CrossRef]

62. Naik, M.; Humnabadkar, V.; Tantry, S.J.; Panda, M.; Narayan, A.; Guptha, S.; Panduga, V.; Manjrekar, P.; Jena, L.K.; Koushik, K.; et al. 4-Aminoquinolone piperidine amides: Noncovalent inhibitors of DprE1 with long residence time and potent antimycobacterial activity. *J. Med. Chem.* **2014**, *57*, 5419–5434. [CrossRef]

63. Panda, M.; Ramachandran, S.; Ramachandran, V.; Shirude, P.S.; Humnabadkar, V.; Nagalapur, K.; Sharma, S.; Kaur, P.; Guptha, S.; Narayan, A.; et al. Discovery of pyrazolopyridones as a novel class of noncovalent DprE1 inhibitor with potent anti-mycobacterial activity. *J. Med. Chem.* **2014**, *57*, 4761–4771. [CrossRef]

64. Chatterji, M.; Shandil, R.; Manjunatha, M.R.; Solapure, S.; Ramachandran, V.; Kumar, N.; Saralaya, R.; Panduga, V.; Reddy, J.; Prabhakar, K.R.; et al. 1,4-azaindole, a potential drug candidate for treatment of tuberculosis. *Antimicrob. Agents Chemother.* **2014**, *58*, 5325–5331. [CrossRef]

65. Tiwari, R.; Moraski, G.C.; Krchňák, V.; Miller, P.A.; Colon-Martinez, M.; Herrero, E.; Oliver, A.G.; Miller, M.J. Thiolates chemically induce redox activation of BTZ043 and related potent nitroaromatic anti-tuberculosis agents. *J. Am. Chem. Soc.* **2013**, *135*, 3539–3549. [CrossRef]

66. Manina, G.; Bellinzoni, M.; Pasca, M.R.; Neres, J.; Milano, A.; De Jesus Lopes Ribeiro, A.L.; Buroni, S.; Skovierová, H.; Dianišková, P.; Mikušová, K.; et al. Biological and structural characterization of the *Mycobacterium smegmatis* nitroreductase NfnB, and its role in benzothiazinone resistance. *Mol. Microbiol.* **2010**, *77*, 1172–1185. [CrossRef] [PubMed]

67. Makarov, V.; Neres, J.; Hartkoorn, R.C.; Ryabova, O.B.; Kazakova, E.; Šarkan, M.; Huszár, S.; Piton, J.; Kolly, G.S.; Vocat, A.; et al. The 8-Pyrrole-Benzothiazinones Are Noncovalent Inhibitors of DprE1 from Mycobacterium tuberculosis. *Antimicrob. Agents Chemother.* **2015**, *59*, 4446–4452. [CrossRef] [PubMed]

68. Tiwari, R.; Miller, P.A.; Chiarelli, L.R.; Mori, G.; Šarkan, M.; Centárová, I.; Cho, S.; Mikusová, K.; Franzblau, S.G.; Oliver, A.G.; et al. Design, syntheses, and anti-tb activity of 1,3-benzothiazinone azide and click chemistry products inspired by BTZ043. *ACS Med. Chem. Lett.* **2016**, *7*, 266–270. [CrossRef] [PubMed]

69. Shirude, P.S.; Shandil, R.; Sadler, C.; Naik, M.; Hosagrahara, V.; Hameed, S.; Shinde, V.; Bathula, C.; Humnabadkar, V.; Kumar, N.; et al. Azaindoles: Noncovalent DprE1 inhibitors from scaffold morphing efforts, kill *Mycobacterium tuberculosis* and are efficacious in vivo. *J. Med. Chem.* **2013**, *56*, 9701–9708. [CrossRef]
70. Shirude, P.S.; Shandil, R.K.; Manjunatha, M.R.; Sadler, C.; Panda, M.; Panduga, V.; Reddy, J.; Saralaya, R.; Nanduri, R.; Ambady, A.; et al. Lead optimization of 1,4-azaindoles as antimycobacterial agents. *J. Med. Chem.* **2014**, *57*, 5728–5737. [CrossRef]
71. Jankute, M.; Byng, C.V.; Alderwick, L.J.; Besra, G.S. Elucidation of a protein-protein interaction network involved in *Corynebacterium glutamicum* cell wall biosynthesis as determined by bacterial two-hybrid analysis. *Glycoconj. J.* **2014**, *31*, 475–483. [CrossRef]
72. Bhutani, I.; Loharch, S.; Gupta, P.; Madathil, R.; Parkesh, R. Structure, dynamics, and interaction of *Mycobacterium tuberculosis* (Mtb) DprE1 and DprE2 examined by molecular modeling, simulation, and electrostatic studies. *PLoS ONE* **2015**, *10*, e0119771. [CrossRef]
73. Gawad, J.; Bonde, C. Decaprenyl-phosphoryl-ribose 2′-epimerase (DprE1): Challenging target for antitubercular drug discovery. *Chem. Cent. J.* **2018**, *12*, 72. [CrossRef]
74. Camacho, L.R.; Constant, P.; Raynaud, C.; Laneelle, M.A.; Triccas, J.A.; Gicquel, B.; Daffe, M.; Guilhot, C. Analysis of the phthiocerol dimycocerosate locus of *Mycobacterium tuberculosis*. Evidence that this lipid is involved in the cell wall permeability barrier. *J. Biol. Chem.* **2001**, *276*, 19845–19854. [CrossRef]
75. Converse, S.E.; Mougous, J.D.; Leavell, M.D.; Leary, J.A.; Bertozzi, C.R.; Cox, J.S. MmpL8 is required for sulfolipid-1 biosynthesis and *Mycobacterium tuberculosis* virulence. *Proc. Natl. Acad. Sci. USA* **2003**, *100*, 6121–6126. [CrossRef]
76. Pacheco, S.A.; Hsu, F.F.; Powers, K.M.; Purdy, G.E. MmpL11 protein transports mycolic acid-containing lipids to the mycobacterial cell wall and contributes to biofilm formation in *Mycobacterium smegmatis*. *J. Biol. Chem.* **2013**, *288*, 24213–24222. [CrossRef] [PubMed]
77. Wells, R.M.; Jones, C.M.; Xi, Z.; Speer, A.; Danilchanka, O.; Doornbos, K.S.; Sun, P.; Wu, F.; Tian, C.; Niederweis, M. Discovery of a siderophore export system essential for virulence of *Mycobacterium tuberculosis*. *PLoS Pathog.* **2013**, *9*, e1003120. [CrossRef] [PubMed]
78. Belardinelli, J.M.; Larrouy-Maumus, G.; Jones, V.; de Carvalho, L.P.S.; McNeil, M.R.; Jackson, M. Biosynthesis and translocation of unsulfated acyltrehaloses in *Mycobacterium tuberculosis*. *J. Biol. Chem.* **2014**, *289*, 27952–27965. [CrossRef] [PubMed]
79. Domenech, P.; Reed, M.B.; Barry, C.E. Contribution of the *Mycobacterium tuberculosis* MmpL protein family to virulence and drug resistance. *Infect. Immun.* **2005**, *73*, 3492–3501. [CrossRef]
80. Li, W.; Obregón-Henao, A.; Wallach, J.B.; North, E.J.; Lee, R.E.; Gonzalez-Juarrero, M.; Schnappinger, D.; Jackson, M. Therapeutic potential of the *Mycobacterium tuberculosis* mycolic acid transporter, MmpL3. *Antimicrob. Agents Chemother.* **2016**, *60*, 5198–5207. [CrossRef]
81. Belardinelli, J.M.; Yazidi, A.; Yang, L.; Fabre, L.; Li, W.; Jacques, B.; Angala, S.K.; Rouiller, I.; Zgurskaya, H.I.; Sygusch, J.; et al. Structure-function profile of MmpL3, the essential mycolic acid transporter from *Mycobacterium tuberculosis*. *ACS Infect. Dis.* **2016**, *2*, 702–713. [CrossRef]
82. Carel, C.; Nukdee, K.; Cantaloube, S.; Bonne, M.; Diagne, C.T.; Laval, F.; Daffé, M.; Zerbib, D. Mycobacterium tuberculosis proteins involved in mycolic acid synthesis and transport localize dynamically to the old growing pole and septum. *PLoS ONE* **2014**, *9*, e97148. [CrossRef]
83. Belardinelli, J.M.; Stevens, C.M.; Li, W.; Tan, Y.Z.; Jones, V.; Mancia, F.; Zgurskaya, H.I.; Jackson, M. The MmpL3 interactome reveals a complex crosstalk between cell envelope biosynthesis and cell elongation and division in mycobacteria. *Sci. Rep.* **2019**, *9*, 10728. [CrossRef]
84. Vilchèze, C.; Jacobs, W.R. The mechanism of isoniazid killing: Clarity through the scope of genetics. *Annu. Rev. Microbiol.* **2007**, *61*, 35–50. [CrossRef]
85. Medjahed, H.; Reyrat, J.M. Construction of *Mycobacterium abscessus* defined glycopeptidolipid mutants: Comparison of genetic tools. *Appl. Environ. Microbiol.* **2009**, *75*, 1331–1338. [CrossRef]
86. Seeliger, J.C.; Holsclaw, C.M.; Schelle, M.W.; Botyanszki, Z.; Gilmore, S.A.; Tully, S.E.; Niederweis, M.; Cravatt, B.F.; Leary, J.A.; Bertozzi, C.R. Elucidation and chemical modulation of sulfolipid-1 biosynthesis in *Mycobacterium tuberculosis*. *J. Biol. Chem.* **2012**, *287*, 7990–8000. [CrossRef] [PubMed]

87. Su, C.C.; Klenotic, P.A.; Bolla, J.R.; Purdy, G.E.; Robinson, C.V.; Yu, E.W. MmpL3 is a lipid transporter that binds trehalose monomycolate and phosphatidylethanolamine. *Proc. Natl. Acad. Sci. USA* **2019**, *116*, 11241–11246. [CrossRef] [PubMed]

88. Murakami, S.; Nakashima, R.; Yamashita, E.; Yamaguchi, A. Crystal structure of bacterial multidrug efflux transporter AcrB. *Nature* **2002**, *419*, 587–593. [CrossRef]

89. Sennhauser, G.; Bukowska, M.A.; Briand, C.; Grütter, M.G. Crystal structure of the multidrug exporter MexB from *Pseudomonas aeruginosa*. *J. Mol. Biol.* **2009**, *389*, 134–145. [CrossRef] [PubMed]

90. Bolla, J.R.; Su, C.C.; Do, S.V.; Radhakrishnan, A.; Kumar, N.; Long, F.; Chou, T.H.; Delmar, J.A.; Lei, H.T.; Rajashankar, K.R.; et al. Crystal structure of the *Neisseria gonorrhoeae* MtrD inner membrane multidrug efflux pump. *PLoS ONE* **2014**, *9*, e97903. [CrossRef] [PubMed]

91. Kumar, N.; Su, C.C.; Chou, T.H.; Radhakrishnan, A.; Delmar, J.A.; Rajashankar, K.R.; Yu, E.W. Crystal structures of the *Burkholderia multivorans* hopanoid transporter HpnN. *Proc. Natl. Acad. Sci. USA* **2017**, *114*, 6557–6562. [CrossRef]

92. Gong, X.; Qian, H.; Zhou, X.; Wu, J.; Wan, T.; Cao, P.; Huang, W.; Zhao, X.; Wang, X.; Wang, P.; et al. Structural insights into the Niemann-Pick C1 (NPC1)-mediated cholesterol transfer and ebola infection. *Cell* **2016**, *165*, 1467–1478. [CrossRef]

93. Rao, S.P.; Lakshminarayana, S.B.; Kondreddi, R.R.; Herve, M.; Camacho, L.R.; Bifani, P.; Kalapala, S.K.; Jiricek, J.; Ma, N.L.; Tan, B.H.; et al. Indolcarboxamide is a preclinical candidate for treating multidrug-resistant tuberculosis. *Sci. Transl. Med.* **2013**, *5*, 214ra168. [CrossRef]

94. Remuiñán, M.J.; Pérez-Herrán, E.; Rullás, J.; Alemparte, C.; Martínez-Hoyos, M.; Dow, D.J.; Afari, J.; Mehta, N.; Esquivias, J.; Jiménez, E.; et al. Tetrahydropyrazolo[1,5-a]pyrimidine-3-carboxamide and *N*-benzyl-6′,7′-dihydrospiro[piperidine-4,4′-thieno[3,2-c]pyran] analogues with bactericidal efficacy against *Mycobacterium tuberculosis* targeting MmpL3. *PLoS ONE* **2013**, *8*, e60933. [CrossRef]

95. Dupont, C.; Viljoen, A.; Dubar, F.; Blaise, M.; Bernut, A.; Pawlik, A.; Bouchier, C.; Brosch, R.; Guérardel, Y.; Lelièvre, J.; et al. A new piperidinol derivative targeting mycolic acid transport in Mycobacterium abscessus. *Mol. Microbiol.* **2016**, *101*, 515–529. [CrossRef]

96. Shetty, A.; Xu, Z.; Lakshmanan, U.; Hill, J.; Choong, M.L.; Chng, S.S.; Yamada, Y.; Poulsen, A.; Dick, T.; Gengenbacher, M. Novel acetamide indirectly targets mycobacterial transporter MmpL3 by proton motive force disruption. *Front. Microbiol.* **2018**, *9*, 2960. [CrossRef] [PubMed]

97. Zheng, H.; Williams, J.T.; Coulson, G.B.; Haiderer, E.R.; Abramovitch, R.B. HC2091 Kills *Mycobacterium tuberculosis* by targeting the MmpL3 mycolic acid transporter. *Antimicrob. Agents Chemother.* **2018**, *62*, e02459-17. [CrossRef] [PubMed]

98. Protopopova, M.; Hanrahan, C.; Nikonenko, B.; Samala, R.; Chen, P.; Gearhart, J.; Einck, L.; Nacy, C.A. Identification of a new antitubercular drug candidate, SQ109, from a combinatorial library of 1,2-ethylenediamines. *J. Antimicrob. Chemother.* **2005**, *56*, 968–974. [CrossRef] [PubMed]

99. Chen, P.; Gearhart, J.; Protopopova, M.; Einck, L.; Nacy, C.A. Synergistic interactions of SQ109, a new ethylene diamine, with front-line antitubercular drugs in vitro. *J. Antimicrob. Chemother.* **2006**, *58*, 332–337. [CrossRef] [PubMed]

100. Reddy, V.M.; Einck, L.; Andries, K.; Nacy, C.A. In vitro interactions between new antitubercular drug candidates SQ109 and TMC207. *Antimicrob. Agents Chemother.* **2010**, *54*, 2840–2846. [CrossRef] [PubMed]

101. Nikonenko, B.V.; Protopopova, M.; Samala, R.; Einck, L.; Nacy, C.A. Drug therapy of experimental tuberculosis (TB): Improved outcome by combining SQ109, a new diamine antibiotic, with existing TB drugs. *Antimicrob. Agents Chemother.* **2007**, *51*, 1563–1565. [CrossRef]

102. Heinrich, N.; Dawson, R.; du Bois, J.; Narunsky, K.; Horwith, G.; Phipps, A.J.; Nacy, C.A.; Aarnoutse, R.E.; Boeree, M.J.; Gillespie, S.H.; et al. Early phase evaluation of SQ109 alone and in combination with rifampicin in pulmonary TB patients. *J. Antimicrob. Chemother.* **2015**, *70*, 1558–1566. [CrossRef]

103. Veiga-Santos, P.; Li, K.; Lameira, L.; de Carvalho, T.M.; Huang, G.; Galizzi, M.; Shang, N.; Li, Q.; Gonzalez-Pacanowska, D.; Hernandez-Rodriguez, V.; et al. SQ109, a new drug lead for Chagas disease. *Antimicrob. Agents Chemother.* **2015**, *59*, 1950–1961. [CrossRef]

104. García-García, V.; Oldfield, E.; Benaim, G. Inhibition of *Leishmania mexicana* growth by the tuberculosis drug SQ109. *Antimicrob. Agents Chemother.* **2016**, *60*, 6386–6389. [CrossRef]

105. Li, W.; Stevens, C.M.; Pandya, A.N.; Darzynkiewicz, Z.; Bhattarai, P.; Tong, W.; Gonzalez-Juarrero, M.; North, E.J.; Zgurskaya, H.I.; Jackson, M. Direct inhibition of MmpL3 by novel antitubercular compounds. *ACS Infect. Dis.* **2019**, *5*, 1001–1012. [CrossRef]
106. Seeger, M.A.; Diederichs, K.; Eicher, T.; Brandstätter, L.; Schiefner, A.; Verrey, F.; Pos, K.M. The AcrB efflux pump: Conformational cycling and peristalsis lead to multidrug resistance. *Curr. Drug Targets* **2008**, *9*, 729–749. [CrossRef]
107. Tsukazaki, T.; Mori, H.; Echizen, Y.; Ishitani, R.; Fukai, S.; Tanaka, T.; Perederina, A.; Vassylyev, D.G.; Kohno, T.; Maturana, A.D.; et al. Structure and function of a membrane component SecDF that enhances protein export. *Nature* **2011**, *474*, 235–238. [CrossRef] [PubMed]
108. Lamichhane, G.; Tyagi, S.; Bishai, W.R. Designer arrays for defined mutant analysis to detect genes essential for survival of *Mycobacterium tuberculosis* in mouse lungs. *Infect. Immun.* **2005**, *73*, 2533–2540. [CrossRef] [PubMed]
109. Hartkoorn, R.C.; Uplekar, S.; Cole, S.T. Cross-resistance between clofazimine and bedaquiline through upregulation of MmpL5 in *Mycobacterium tuberculosis*. *Antimicrob. Agents Chemother.* **2014**, *58*, 2979–2981. [CrossRef]
110. Oh, S.; Park, Y.; Engelhart, C.A.; Wallach, J.B.; Schnappinger, D.; Arora, K.; Manikkam, M.; Gac, B.; Wang, H.; Murgolo, N.; et al. Discovery and structure-activity-relationship study of N-Alkyl-5-hydroxypyrimidinone carboxamides as novel antitubercular agents targeting decaprenylphosphoryl-β-D-ribose 2′-oxidase. *J. Med. Chem.* **2018**, *61*, 9952–9965. [CrossRef] [PubMed]
111. Borisov, S.E.; Bogorodskaya, E.M.; Volchenkov, G.V.; Kulchavenya, E.V.; Maryandyshev, A.O.; Skornyakov, S.N.; Talibov, O.B.; Tikhonov, A.M.; Vasilyeva, I.A. Efficiency and safety of chemotherapy regimen with SQ109 in those suffering from multiple drug resistant tuberculosis. *Tuberc. Lung Dis.* **2018**, *96*, 6–18. [CrossRef]

12

A Physical Cure for Tuberculosis: Carlo Forlanini and the Invention of Therapeutic Pneumothorax

Paolo Mazzarello

Department of Brain and Behavioral Sciences and University Museum System, University of Pavia, 27100 Pavia, Italy; paolo.mazzarello@unipv.it.

Abstract: Carlo Forlanini (1847–1918), a medical doctor professor at the universities of Turin and Pavia, was the inventor of artificial pneumothorax, a method that allowed a first significant victory in the long war of medicine against pulmonary tuberculosis. The article outlines a portrait of this important clinician and focuses on the therapeutic innovation he introduced for the treatment of this infectious disease.

Keywords: Carlo Forlanini; tuberculosis; artificial pneumothorax

---

1. Annus Mirabilis

Sometimes it seems that, at certain moments, the lines of history converge in determining radical changes in scientific thought and practice. The year 1882 was certainly one of these for the history of infectious diseases. On March 24 of that year, Robert Koch announced the isolation and identification of *Mycobacterium tuberculosis* as the causative agent of tuberculosis. The session of the Berlin Physiological Society, during which the German medical doctor gave the report on the discovery of this new microorganism, was one of the most dramatic moments in the history of medicine: finally, the elusive nature of one of the main 19th-century scourges found a unitary etiological explanation. Paul Ehrlich (who would be awarded the Nobel Prize for medicine in 1908), present at the time of the conference, always remembered that evening as "the most important scientific experience of my life" [1]. Against all those who still rejected the contagious nature of tuberculosis, invoking constitutional, degenerative, food or toxic explanations, Koch advanced his overwhelming evidence. When the work was published a few weeks later, it quickly became a source of methodological inspiration for new microbiological investigations.

The year 1882 was also a milestone in the history of tuberculosis for a second important contribution, the publication of a revolutionary therapeutic proposal for the cure of pulmonary phthisis, that would have great importance until the discovery of the treatment of the disease with streptomycin: the "therapeutic" or "artificial pneumothorax" conceived by the Italian medical doctor Carlo Forlanini [2–5] in Figure 1.

Formulated at first only as a theoretical hypothesis (one of the few cases in medicine in which the public hypothetical prediction precedes the practical realization), it would go on to become, in the hands of its proponents during the first half of the twentieth century, an invention generally applied to treat many selected cases of phthisis, the wasting disease due to tuberculosis of the lungs. The method was also destined to be depicted by an important literary figure. In Thomas Mann's "Magic Mountain", set in the years immediately preceding the First World War, the group of patients who underwent this treatment—which was at the time the main effective direct therapy—consider themselves as part of a special club. In Mann's words: "They have formed a group, for of course a thing like the pneumothorax brings people together. They call themselves the Half-Lung Club" [6,7]. The novel by the Scottish doctor-writer Archibald Cronin, "The Citadel", also dedicates, from a descriptive point of view, an important and precise space to the treatment with artificial pneumothorax.

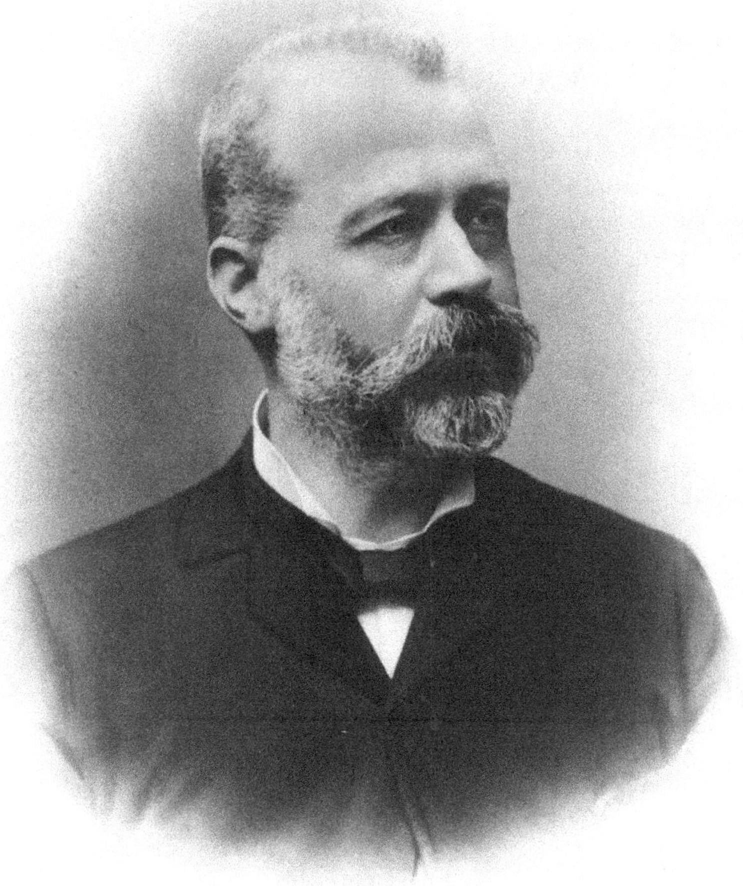

Figure 1. Carlo Forlanini. University Museum System, University of Pavia, Italy.

The cure continued to be the primary one until the discovery of streptomycin, the first effective antibiotic therapy for tuberculosis infection, introduced in 1943 by the microbiologists Selman Abraham Waksman, Albert Schatz and Elizabeth Bugie. However, pneumothorax did not immediately disappear from the therapeutic possibilities and continued to be used until the 1970s, in those cases where the presence of large lung cavities made patients easily susceptible to stagnation of infectious processes.

2. The Path to an Invention

Born in Milan on 11 June 1847, Carlo Forlanini, as the son of a doctor, had breathed medicine since childhood. Tuberculosis was also present early in his life, because his mother was killed by pulmonary phthisis. After high school studies, Forlanini enrolled in the medical faculty of the University of Pavia in 1864 as a pupil of the prestigious Borromeo College. It was a time of great scientific and political enthusiasm because the University of Pavia was at the forefront in the applications of new theories on diseases based on Rudolf Virchow's book "Die Cellularpathologie" and, at the same time, the young students were enthusiastic about the revolutionary movements led by Giuseppe Garibaldi, who in a few years would have brought about the unification of Italy. In 1866 Forlanini was a voluntary fighter in the Garibaldi ranks, in the battles of Monte Suello and Bezzecca. Back in Pavia he published his first scientific work in 1868 and linked himself to a fraternal friendship with Camillo Golgi, who was at the beginning of his stellar scientific career [8]. In 1870 he graduated in medicine under the guidance of the ophthalmologist Antonio Quaglino; the following year, Forlanini was at work in the chronically ill division of the Ospedale Maggiore in Milan. Meanwhile, he began to develop a great interest in the study of lung diseases by starting to conceive devices that could increase lung ventilation. In these endeavors he found help from his younger brother, Enrico, a gifted engineer who was one of the pioneers of air flight (the Milan Linate airport of 1937 is named after him). In 1875, Carlo Forlanini founded the Pneumotherapy Society and the Pneumatic Institute of Milan, and from 1881, he was also chief physician for skin diseases. Meanwhile, he began a series of attempts to treat tuberculosis and lung diseases with forced respiratory movements and with aerotherapy to increase blood flow and air supply to the lung. With the scientific collaboration of his brother Enrico, he would also build some of the first hyperbaric chambers in Figure 2.

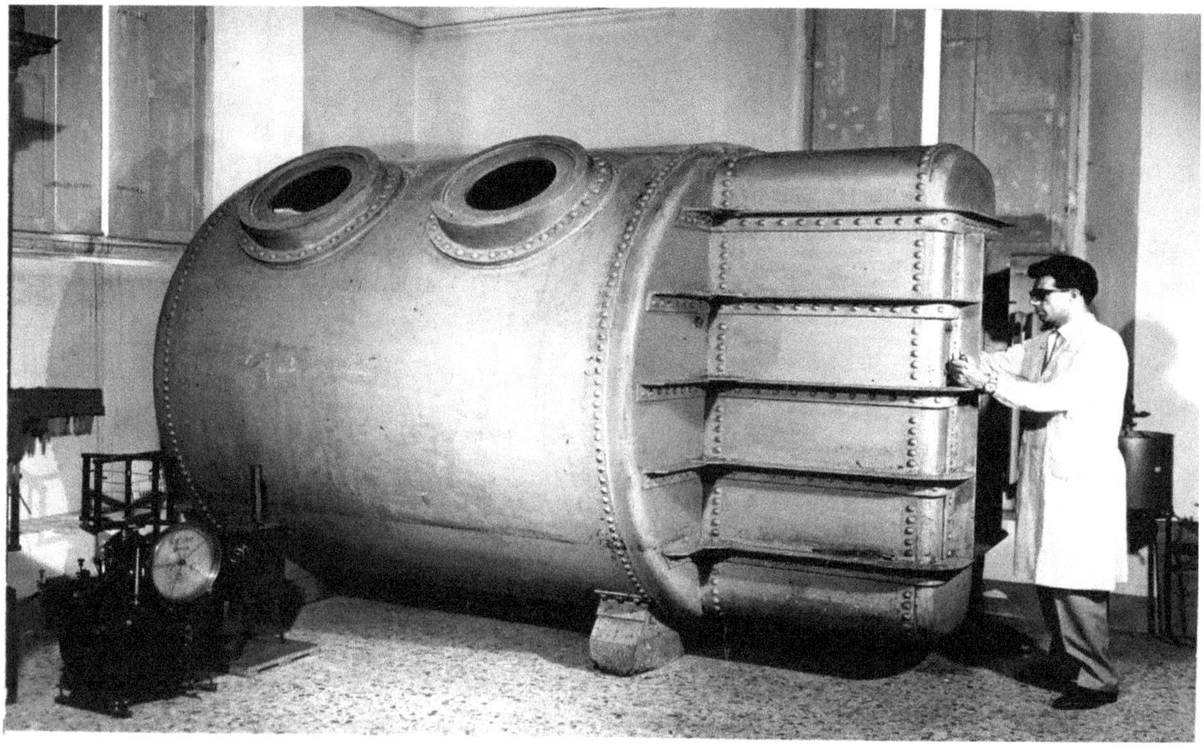

Figure 2. Hyperbaric chamber. Museum for the History of the University of Pavia.

He observed some positive results in the treatment of pulmonary emphysema and also some mild improvement in phthisis. Soon, however, Forlanini began to develop opposite therapeutic considerations for pulmonary tuberculosis. It was not the respiratory act of advantage to the sick lung, but rest. In fact, a lesion in the pulmonary tissue, as in the case of tuberculosis, could have worsened with its movements up to the formation and the subsequent development of the cavities, which then became continuously enlarged during each respiratory act. From this consideration, he was convinced that the proper therapy to stop and block the progress of pulmonary disease was to put the lungs to rest through their artificial collapse. In fact, there had already been occasional previous observations that correlated the blockage of the movement of a lung, due to a spontaneous pneumothorax, with the improvement of a tuberculous process there.

In 1822, a British doctor, James Carson, after some experiments on rats, had also made attempts to cure pulmonary tuberculosis by causing pneumothorax on humans, but the attempt had failed [9]. However, other doctors, such as the French physicians Emile Toussaint in 1880 and Hippolyte Hérard in 1881, had reported improvement of the pulmonary tuberculosis process after lung collapse following spontaneous pneumothorax or hydro-pneumothorax [4,10,11]. Forlanini's studies on the mechanism of development of the tuberculosis process in the lung and the careful reading of previous studies, in particular Toussaint's observations, made him think of an articulated therapeutic suggestion: to make a gas penetrate the pleural cavity (interpleural space), causing the collapse of the lung below. In July 1882, Forlanini proposed his method [10], which he applied only in 1888 with his first intervention of artificial pneumothorax. Two years later, in an article by two of his collaborators, we find the first reference to four patients treated with the method [12].

Forlanini's great merit was to propose a technology through which to achieve the purpose of resting a collapsed lung, allowing the drainage and obliteration of tubercular cavity and then the scarring of the underlying lesions. The improvement of the patient became not only local, but also general, because the lung mechanical constriction of artificial pneumothorax reduced the pulmonary inflammatory source of the disease state, and perhaps could improve the body's overall immune reaction to the pathological process. It was also proposed that the method decreased the absorption of toxic factors released by the tuberculosis lesion. Forlanini observed a reduction and disappearance of the cough; the reduction and disappearance of sputum; the fall of fever and sweating; and the disappearance of asthenia. The patient became euphoric, increased his state of nutrition and had the reduction or the disappearance of the toxic-infectious state. Forlanini also noted favorable effects on the other lung, if affected by phthisis, as a consequence of the general improvement [13]. Finally, he argued that there was also an indirect therapeutic effect on initial laryngeal and intestinal tuberculosis.

To develop the appropriate technique for a repetitive injection of a small amount of gas into the pleural cavity (200–250 mL) through a large hypodermic needle, he asked for help and advice from his brother Enrico. Thus, medical expertise combined with the technological skills of the creative engineer, and the result was the new apparatus. At first, Forlanini made several attempts with atmospheric air, but then he realized that the oxygen component of this gas was being reabsorbed too quickly and so he switched to nitrogen [14,15].

In this way, the lung was immobilized for longer. To carry out the pneumothorax, Forlanini made use of two apparatuses, one for the production of nitrogen, the second for administering under pressure (controlled by a pressure gauge) the gas in the interpleural space. The production of nitrogen in the first apparatus took place through a chemical reaction by means of pyrogallic-acid which avidly absorbs the oxygen of the air. The nitrogen was then transferred to the second apparatus connected to a needle, which was introduced very slowly into the previously selected intercostal space in Figure 3.

With preliminary experiments on animals and corpses, Forlanini had come to the conclusion that, once the parietal pleura was perforated, as soon as the tip of the needle touched the visceral pleura, the underlying elastic tissue retracted, dragging the visceral pleura with it, while the gas entered the interpleural space. In this way, if the introduction was slow, the visceral pleura and the underlying lung were not pierced. Forlanini usually started the treatment by introducing around 200 cc, and never more than 400 cc (to avoid the risk of subcutaneous emphysema, i.e., the passage of gas into the tissues of the chest wall) or less than 100 cc. [14]. After a few days, nitrogen was administered again to achieve a complete lung collapse. Then, pneumothorax was repeated every 15–20 days and continued for many months, usually up to two years or more.

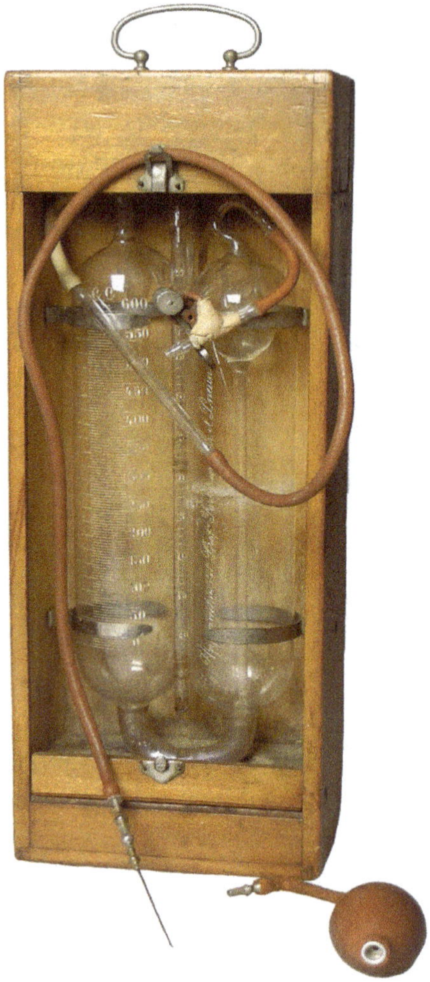

Figure 3. Artificial pneumothorax: Forlanini's apparatus for the injection of nitrogen into the pleural cavity. Museum for the History of the University of Pavia.

3. Success and Difficulty

In 1884, Forlanini began his university career at the University of Turin and obtained the position of "extraordinarius" professor of "Clinica medica preparatoria" (preparatory medical clinic). Soon after, he reached the peak of his university career, becoming full professor of special medical pathology. Among Forlanini's pupils at the University of Turin, the most important was Scipione Riva Rocci, who, under the supervision of the master, developed the pneumatic cuff sphygmomanometer, which soon became a worldwide symbol of practical medicine. In 1898, Forlanini returned to Pavia, first on a provisional teaching of special medical demonstrative pathology and, from 1900, in the prestigious position of full professor of medical clinic. Here a school of talented doctors gathered around him, like Riva Rocci, who moved to Pavia from Turin, Umberto Carpi De Resmini and Eugenio Morelli [5].

Meanwhile, Forlanini made his operation known in Figure 4 with a report held on 2 April 1894 to the eleventh international medical congress of Rome [16] and, the following year, with a lecture to the Italian congress of internal medicine [17]. However, the reaction by the medical community was not very lively and artificial pneumothorax also found oppositions and objections. With the spread of the operation and its application by physicians who did not know the method very well, and who used inadequate criteria for the selection of candidate patients, the number of serious and even fatal complications greatly increased [18]. This is despite the fact that the security of the method steadily improved in the first decades of the new century. Among the complications, those reported and also discussed by Forlanini included empyema, emphysema and cerebral embolism, especially gaseous. A further complication was pleural eclampsia, i.e., a syncope whose symptoms Forlanini described in this way: "the patient falls, suddenly, in abandonment on the bed, unconscious, with his head bent to one side, or back; the eye wide open, the bulbs fixed at the front or rotated up or to one side; the pupil of maximum amplitude, rigid; the face of an extreme pallor, sometimes cyanotic, cold, with bluish streaks in the neck, chest, limbs; clenched teeth; stiff trunk and limbs; breathless and imperceptible pulse rhythm;-in short, an impressive syndrome, for the real impotence of the symptoms, for the suddenness, for the thought that the accident follows an operational act and can be fatal" [14]. Moreover, artificial pneumothorax was sometimes ineffective due to pleural adhesions that prevented lung collapse. To overcome these difficulties, the Swedish physician Hans Christian Jacobaeus introduced the section of endopleural adhesions using a thoracoscope and a cautery [19]. Some alternative methods to artificial pneumothorax for treatment of pulmonary tuberculosis were also developed. An attempt to put the lung at rest to limit diaphragm excursions was made in 1913 by Ernst Sauerbruch, who introduced phrenicotomy [20]. In the years preceding the First World War, the foundations of pulmonary tuberculosis surgery were also laid. Already in 1891, Theodore Tuffier removed the pulmonary apex in a case of cavitated tuberculosis; in 1893 David Lawson introduced pneumonectomy; and two years later, William Macewen removed a left lung for tuberculosis (the patient was still alive in 1940). In 1908 Ludolph Brauer published the first radical thoracoplasty and in the following twenty years, lung surgery for pulmonary tuberculosis continuously developed [21–24]. However, artificial pneumothorax remained the first choice when an intervention to treat the disease had to be considered.

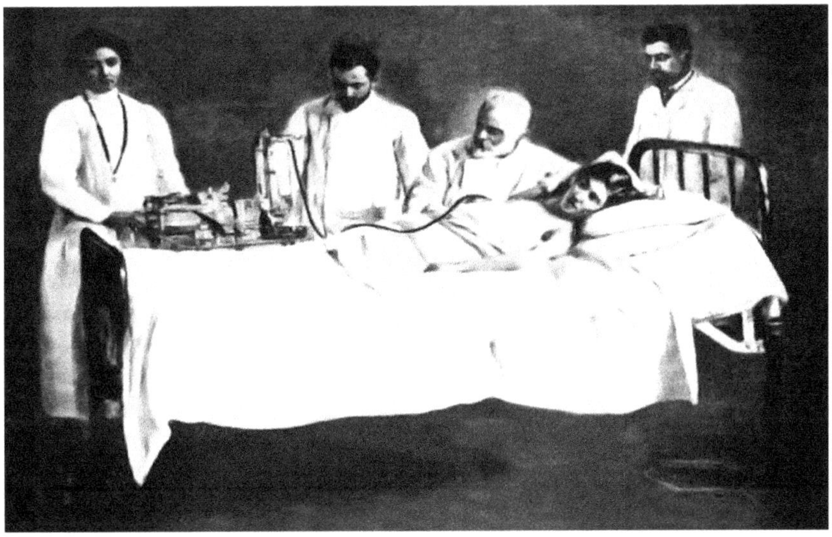

Figure 4. Carlo Forlanini while practicing artificial pneumothorax. Museum for the History of the University of Pavia.

4. Disputes and Diffusion

A bad surprise caught Forlanini when, in 1906, he read an article by Ludolph Brauer of Marburg, published in an authoritative German journal, in which the invention of the method was attributed to the important American surgeon John Benjamin Murphy [25]. The latter had developed a version of the operation, presumably without knowing the work of the Italian, and had described it in 1898 at the meeting of the American Medical Association [26–28]. Murphy was the first to adopt the new x-ray technology (Wilhelm Roentgen had discovered x-ray in 1895) to control pneumothorax therapy results. Forlanini immediately reacted to Brauer's article and published in another authoritative German journal the results obtained by him in 25 cases of pulmonary tuberculosis, also to claim the priority of the invention [29]. Moreover he criticized Murphy's treatment modalities, as they involved an incision of the skin and the chest muscles (and not a single puncture as he did) and again the large amount of nitrogen introduced (1000–3000 mL) by the American surgeon, which led to excessive compression of the lung. Forlanini's article contributed to the diffusion of his invention in the German medical world and therefore in transalpine Europe. From this moment on, Forlanini promoted the method, also with conferences for doctors. In 1906–1907, there was a technological development that made the apparatus more applicable, when Christian Saugman, of the Vejlefjord sanatorium in Denmark, perfected it by inserting in the pneumothorax instrument a water pressure monitor, which allowed a precise control of the gas introduced. Moreover, in 1912, Maurizio Ascoli proposed a partial collapse therapy that allowed a bilateral pneumothorax to treat cases of involvement of the two lungs in the pathological process.

On April 1912, Forlanini held a memorable lecture in Rome entitled "Artificial pneumothorax in the treatment of pulmonary phthisis", at the seventh international congress on tuberculosis [30]. The presentation obtained a great ovation and, after thirty years of studies on pneumothorax, Forlanini at last obtained full international recognition.

In England, the method was not used before 1911; subsequently, it achieved considerable success. In 1917, the doctor Clive Riviere wrote in his textbook "The pneumothorax treatment of pulmonary tuberculosis": "No more hopeful ray of sunshine has ever come to illuminate the dark kingdoms of disease than that introduced into the path of the consumptive through the discovery of artificial pneumothorax" [31]. Riviere confirmed this judgment ten years later in the "British Journal of Tuberculosis" [32]. Other British doctors expressed an overall positive opinion on the treatment [33–47], which was also applied to children [48]. Its level of popularization is also demonstrated by the fact that one of the important episodes in the novel "The Citadel" (1937) by the Scottish writer Archibald Joseph Cronin concerns precisely the description of an artificial pneumothorax operation. However, the spread of the method, after 1912, reached all European countries and, with some delay, also the United States. In Imperial Russia, the therapeutic pneumothorax was already used in 1910 by Arkadij N. Rubel who, two years later, published the first monograph on the topic, contributing to its knowledge in the country [18,49]. In the 1930s, in Stalinist Russia, the application of this method took on political connotations. The treatment was considered an "aristocratic therapy", therefore counter-revolutionary, and in the end the pneumothorax device was attacked by propaganda as a "killing machine". One of the leading Russian physicians advocating pneumothorax therapy, Volf S. Kholtsman, director of the Moscow Oblast Tuberculosis Institute, was arrested in 1939 during the Stalinist purges and then executed two years later.

5. The Battle and the War

In 1912, with the success at the Seventh International Congress of Rome, Forlanini became a famous scientist worldwide. In that same year he was proposed for the first time to the Nobel Prize for Medicine and, over the following years, Forlanini was unsuccessfully nominated for this award at least twenty times. His friend and fellow professor at the University of Pavia, Camillo Golgi (Nobel Prize winner for 1906), proposed him three times with the motivation that the invention of pneumothorax was "of great benefit to humanity", a phrase that underlined the consonance of the candidate's merits with the will of Alfred Nobel. However, the Nobel Prize was not awarded in the years of the First World War between 1915 and 1918, and in this last year Forlanini died. The Italian doctor thus had the possibility of winning the prize only in the three years between 1912 and 1914. There were, however, some reasons analyzed in detail by Hansson and Polianski [18] that probably prevented him from being awarded in this short period of time. In fact, all the nominations came from Italian scientists; the method had not yet reached the safety standards that it would obtain a few years later; and there were other alternative surgical operations, less successful, but used in the treatment of pulmonary tuberculosis.

In 1913, Forlanini was nominated senator of the kingdom and member of the council of public education in Figure 5. During the years of the First World War, his health gradually declined. However, he had the satisfaction of seeing his invention widely used in clinics all over the world. Forlanini died in Nervi, on the Ligurian Riviera, on 25 May 1918. Immediately after his death, Golgi published a very heartfelt obituary [50].

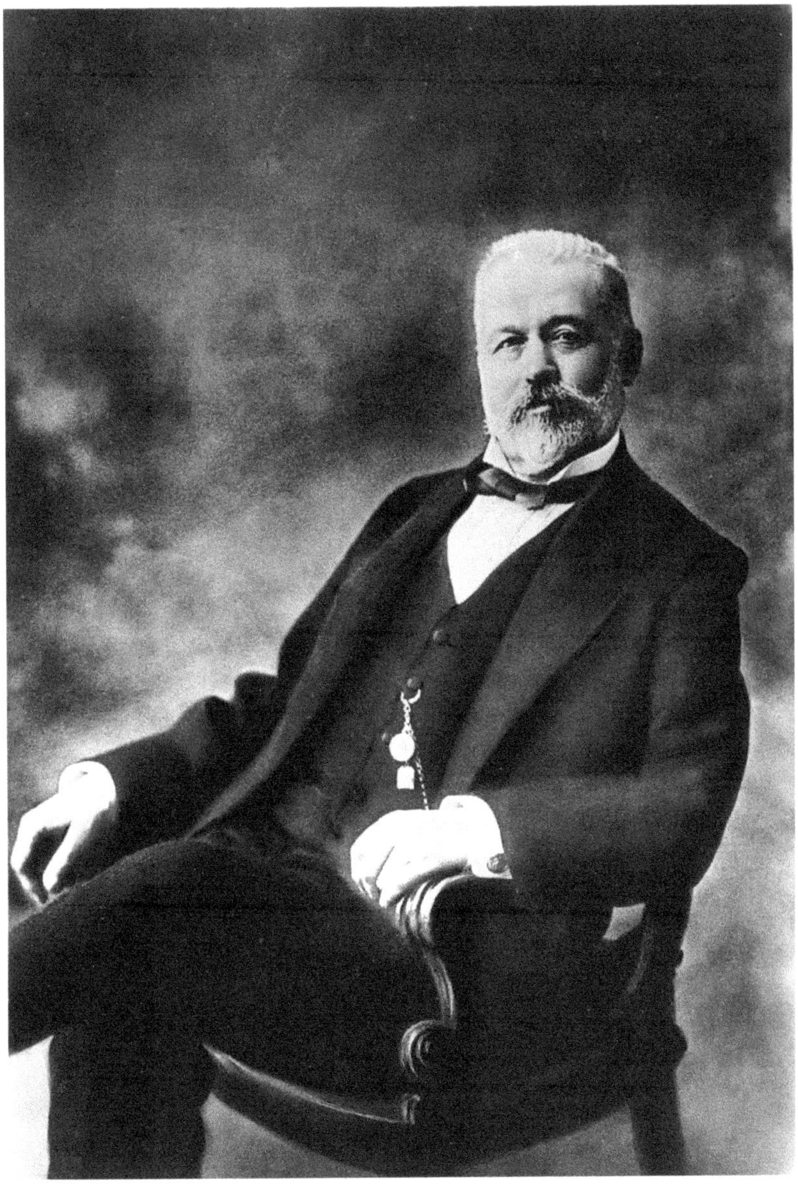

Figure 5. Carlo Forlanini in the last years of his life. Museum for the History of the University of Pavia.

This great physician won his battle against tuberculosis, the first of a series that will follow with other protagonists. His invention has not completely disappeared from medical practice and is still used in special cases, for example in pre-thoracoscopic artificial pneumothorax [51], a fact that would have pleased Forlanini. Unfortunately, however, the war against tuberculosis is still going on and the final victory has not yet been achieved.

References

1. Gradmann, C. *Laboratory Disease. Robert Koch's Medical Bacterology*; The Johns Hopkins University Press: Baltimore, MD, USA, 2009; p. 69.
2. Bottero, A. *Carlo Forlanini Inventore del Pneumotorace Artificiale*; Ulrico Hoepli: Milano, Italy, 1947.
3. Spina, G. Carlo Forlanini: Storia di una invenzione geniale, il pneumotorace terapeutico. *Med. Torac.* **1982**, *4*, 473–479.
4. Sakula, A. Carlo Forlanini, inventor of artificial pneumothorax for treatment of pulmonary tuberculosis. *Thorax* **1983**, *38*, 326–332. [CrossRef] [PubMed]
5. Porro, A.; Franchini, A.F. Forlanini Carlo. In *Dizionario Biografico degli Italiani*; Istituto della Enciclopedia Italiana: Roma, Italy, 1997; Volume 49, pp. 3–7.

6. Mann, T. *The Magic Mountain*; Alfred, A., Ed.; Knopf: New York, NY, USA, 1949; pp. 50–51.
7. Garbarino, M.C.; Cani, V.; Mazzarello, P. A century ago: Carlo Forlanini and the first successful treatment of tuberculosis. *Lancet* **2018**, *392*, 475. [CrossRef]
8. Mazzarello, P. *Golgi. A Biography of the Founder of Modern Neuroscience*; Oxford University Press: New York, NY, USA, 2010; pp. 35–70.
9. Keers, R.Y. Two forgotten pioneers. James Carson and George Bodington. *Thorax* **1980**, *35*, 483–489. [CrossRef] [PubMed]
10. Forlanini, C. A contribuzione della terapia chirurgica della tisi polmonare. Ablazione del polmone? Pneumotorace artificiale? In *Scritti di Carlo Forlanini*; L. Cappelli Editore: Roma, Italy, 1928; pp. 400–432.
11. Rist, É. *25 Portraits de Médecins Français 1900–1950*; Masson: Paris, France, 1955.
12. Cavallero, G.; Riva Rocci, S. La funzione respiratoria negli individui affetti da riduzione di area polmonare respirante. *G. Internazionale Sci. Med.* **1890**, *12*, 361–390.
13. Forlanini, C. Cura della tisi polmonare col pneumotorace prodotto artificialmente. In *Scritti di Carlo Forlanini*; L. Cappelli Editore: Roma, Italy, 1928; pp. 486–505.
14. Forlanini, C. Pneumotorace artificiale (nella tisi). Indicazioni, tecnica dell'atto operative, suoi accidenti. In *Scritti di Carlo Forlanini*; L. Cappelli Editore: Roma, Italy, 1928; pp. 579–619.
15. Forlanini, C. Riassunto, con note originali, dell'articolo "Sulla cura della tubercolosi polmonare mediante il pneumotorace artificiale" del Prof. Chr. Saugmann. In *Scritti di Carlo Forlanini*; L. Cappelli Editore: Roma, Italy, 1928; pp. 539–578.
16. Forlanini, C. Primi tentativi di pneumotorace artificiale nella tisi polmonare. *Gazz. Medica Torino* **1894**, *45*, 381–384, 401–403.
17. Forlanini, C. Primo caso di tisi polmonare monolaterale avanzato curato felicemente col pneumotorace artificiale. In *Scritti di Carlo Forlanini*; L. Cappelli Editore: Roma, Italy, 1928; pp. 469–471.
18. Hansson, N.; Polianski, I.J. Therapeutic pneumothorax and the Nobel Prize. *Ann. Thorac. Surg.* **2015**, *100*, 761–765. [CrossRef]
19. Jacobaeus, H.C. Endopleurale Operationen unter der Leitung des Thorakoskops. *Beitr. Klin. Tuberk.* **1916**, *35*, 1–35. [CrossRef]
20. Sauerbruch, E.F. Die Beeinflussung von Lungenerkrankungen durch Künstliche Lähmung des Zwerchfells (phrenikotomie). *Munch. Med. Wochenschr.* **1913**, *60*, 625–626.
21. Lowson, D. A case of pneumonectomy. *British. Med. J.* **1893**, *1*, 1152–1154. [CrossRef]
22. Tuffier, T. Résection du sommet du poumon droit pour tuberculose au début. Résultat éloigné (18 mois). *Bull. Soc. Chir.* **1892**, *18*, 726–727.
23. Tuffier, T. *Chirurgie du Poumon en Particulier Dans les Cavernes Tuberculeuses et la Gangrène Pulmonaire*; Masson & Cie: Paris, France, 1897.
24. Mann, R. Tuberculosis. *Int. J. STD AIDS* **1991**, *2*, 13–19. [CrossRef] [PubMed]
25. Brauer, L. Die Behandlung der einseitigen Lungenphthisis mit künstlichem Pneumothorax (nach Murphy). *Münch. Med. Woch.* **1906**, *53*, 338–339.
26. Murphy, J.B. Surgery of the lungs. *JAMA* **1898**, *31*, 151–165, 208–216, 281–297, 341–356. [CrossRef]
27. Murphy, J.B. *The Story of Clinical Pulmonary Tuberculosis*; Brown, L., Ed.; Williams & Wilkins: Baltimore, MD, USA, 1941; pp. 261–265.
28. Papagiannis, A.; Lazaridis, G.; Zarogoulidis, K.; Papaiwannou, A.; Karavergou, A.; Lampaki, S.; Baka, S.; Mpoukovinas, I.; Karavasilis, V.; Kioumis, I.; et al. Pneumothorax: An up to date "Introduction". *Ann. Transl. Med.* **2015**, *3*, 53.
29. Forlanini, C. Zur Behandlung der Lungenschwindsucht durch künstlich erzeugten Pneumothorax. *Dtsch. Med. Woch.* **1906**, *32*, 1401–1405. [CrossRef]
30. Forlanini, C. Le pneumothorax artificiel dans le traitement de la phtisie pulmonaire. In *Scritti di Carlo Forlanini*; L. Cappelli Editore: Roma, Italy, 1928; pp. 999–1012.
31. Riviere, C. *The Pneumothorax Treatment of Pulmonary Tuberculosis*; Frowde, H., Ed.; Hodder & Stoughton: London, UK, 1917.
32. Riviere, C. Artificial pneumothorax in the treatment of pulmonary tuberculosis. *Br. J. Tuberc.* **1927**, *21*, 123–124.
33. Horton-Smith Hartley, P. Artificial pneumothorax in the treatment of pulmonary tuberculosis. *Br. J. Tuberc.* **1927**, *21*, 121–123.

34. Pearson, S.V. Artificial pneumothorax in the treatment of pulmonary tuberculosis. *Br. J. Tuberc.* **1927**, *21*, 124–125.
35. Burrell, L.S.T. Artificial pneumothorax in the treatment of pulmonary tuberculosis. *Br. J. Tuberc.* **1927**, *21*, 125–126.
36. Wynn, W.H. Artificial pneumothorax in the treatment of pulmonary tuberculosis. *Br. J. Tuberc.* **1927**, *21*, 126.
37. Morriston Davies, H. Artificial pneumothorax in the treatment of pulmonary tuberculosis. *Br. J. Tuberc.* **1927**, *21*, 126–127.
38. De Carle Woodcock, H. Artificial pneumothorax in the treatment of pulmonary tuberculosis. *Br. J. Tuberc.* **1927**, *21*, 127–128. [CrossRef]
39. Hudson, B. Artificial pneumothorax in the treatment of pulmonary tuberculosis. *Br. J. Tuberc.* **1927**, *21*, 128–129.
40. Haef, F.R.G. Artificial pneumothorax in the treatment of pulmonary tuberculosis. *Br. J. Tuberc.* **1927**, *21*, 129–131. [CrossRef]
41. Morland, A. Artificial pneumothorax in the treatment of pulmonary tuberculosis. *Br. J. Tuberc.* **1927**, *21*, 131.
42. Wingfield, R.C. Artificial pneumothorax in the treatment of pulmonary tuberculosis. *Br. J. Tuberc.* **1927**, *21*, 132.
43. Johnston, J.M. Artificial pneumothorax in the treatment of pulmonary tuberculosis. *Br. J. Tuberc.* **1927**, *21*, 133.
44. Tattersall, N. Artificial pneumothorax in the treatment of pulmonary tuberculosis. *Br. J. Tuberc.* **1927**, *21*, 133–134.
45. Ford, A.P. Artificial pneumothorax in the treatment of pulmonary tuberculosis. *Br. J. Tuberc.* **1927**, *21*, 134–135.
46. Allon Pask, E.H. Artificial pneumothorax in the treatment of pulmonary tuberculosis. *Br. J. Tuberc.* **1927**, *21*, 135–136.
47. Hutchinson, R.C. Artificial pneumothorax in the treatment of pulmonary tuberculosis. *Br. J. Tuberc.* **1927**, *21*, 136.
48. Soltau, E. Artificial pneumothorax in the treatment of pulmonary tuberculosis. *Br. J. Tuberc.* **1927**, *21*, 137.
49. Polianski, I.J. Bolshevik disease and Stalinist terror: On the historical casuistry of artificial pneumothorax. *Med. Hist.* **2015**, *59*, 32–43. [CrossRef] [PubMed]
50. Golgi, C. *Carlo* Forlanini. *Rendiconti R. Istituto Lombardo* **1918**, *51* (Suppl. 2), 654–658.
51. Faurschou, P.; Viskum, K. Artificial pneumothorax by the Veress cannula: Efficacy and safety. *Resp. Med.* **1997**, *91*, 402–405. [CrossRef]

13

Development of Delpazolid for the Treatment of Tuberculosis

Young Lag Cho [1] and Jichan Jang [2,*]

[1] LegoChem Biosciences, Inc., 8-26 Munoyeongseo-ro, Daedeok-gu, Daejeon 34302, Korea; young@legochembio.com
[2] Molecular Mechanisms of Antibiotics, Division of Life Science, Research Institute of Life Sciences, Gyeongsang National University, Jinju 52828, Korea
* Correspondence: jichanjang@gnu.ac.kr.

Abstract: A novel oxazolidinone with cyclic amidrazone, delpazolid (LCB01-0371), was synthesized by LegoChem BioSciences, Inc. (Daejeon, Korea). Delpazolid can improve the minimum bactericidal concentration of *Mycobacterium tuberculosis* H37Rv and significantly reduce resistance rates, especially of multi-drug-resistant tuberculosis (MDR-TB) isolates, compared with linezolid. Therefore, delpazolid can be used to treat MDR-TB. The safety, tolerability, and pharmacokinetics of delpazolid have been evaluated in a phase 1 clinical trial, which revealed that it does not cause adverse events such as myelosuppression even after three weeks of repeated dosing. Interim efficacy and safety results, particularly those from a clinical phase 2a early bactericidal activity trial including patients with drug-susceptible tuberculosis, were reported and the findings will be further analyzed to guide phase 2a studies.

Keywords: *Mycobacterium tuberculosis*; delpazolid; drug discovery; multi-drug resistance

---

1. Linezolid, the First Oxazolidinone Antibacterial Agent

Oxazolidinone is a heterocyclic organic compound containing both nitrogen and oxygen in a 5-membered ring and is mainly used as an antimicrobial agent. This class of antimicrobials is active against a large spectrum of Gram-positive bacteria, including methicillin-resistant *Staphylococcus aureus* (MRSA), vancomycin-resistant enterococci (VRE), vancomycin-intermediate strains, and penicillin-resistant pneumococci, and acts via inhibiting protein synthesis [1,2].

Linezolid is the first oxazolidinone antimicrobial to be developed; it exhibits a high degree of in vitro activity against various Gram-positive pathogens [3]. Linezolid exhibits bactericidal activity against *Mycobacterium tuberculosis* and has been used to treat rifampicin-resistant tuberculosis (RR-TB) or multi-drug-resistant tuberculosis (MDR-TB) [4]. Although the integration of linezolid into RR-TB or MDR-TB treatment can improve outcomes, prolonged administration is often limited by long-term side effects, including reversible myelosuppression, potentially irreversible optic neuropathy, and peripheral neuropathy [5]. Therefore, safety and tolerability are critical issues to consider when prescribing these antibiotics [6]. Less toxic alternatives are under development for diseases that require long-term therapy such as tuberculosis.

2. Development of Delpazolid (LCB01-0371)

LegoChem Biosciences (Daejeon, Korea) is a company that develops effective and safe drugs using legochemistry technology, which enables the manipulation of substances by attaching and detaching compounds around scaffold-like Lego blocks. LegoChem Biosciences searches for novel candidate substances based on the concept that a good scaffold with novel blocks, based on medicinal chemistry, can accelerate the process of improving previous scaffolds with weak activity or have side effects. Delpazolid (code No: LCB01-0371), a derivative of oxazolidinone, is the first candidate antibiotic substance identified by LegoChem Biosciences.

Delpazolid is an antibiotic that targets Gram-positive bacteria (MRSA, VRE) including *M. tuberculosis*. It is currently undergoing a phase 2 clinical trial for oral (PO) administration and a phase 1 trial for intravenous (IV) administration to treat Gram-positive (MRSA, VRE) bacteraemia. Cyclic amidrazone blocks were applied to the key scaffold of delpazolid (Figure 1). In general, after a drug is absorbed, it must be dissolved well to ensure proper secretion. Most small molecules with suboptimal pharmacokinetic (PK) profiles tend to have low solubility. In general, small-molecule ligands that bind their targets with high efficiency are more hydrophobic, and hydrophobic interactions are essential for increased ligand efficiency [7]. Hydrophobicity not only increases target binding efficacy, but also decreases the solubility of a small molecule. The cyclic amidrazone (Figure 1) on the side chain of delpazolid maintains its hydrophobicity to some extent and has a slightly basic pH similar to that of carboxylate. Therefore, it can be charged by obtaining a proton from carboxylic acid under human physiological conditions, which enhances the solubility and PK profile. Therefore, the drug is accumulated slowly and excreted well, and can be administered over the long-term with minimal side effects.

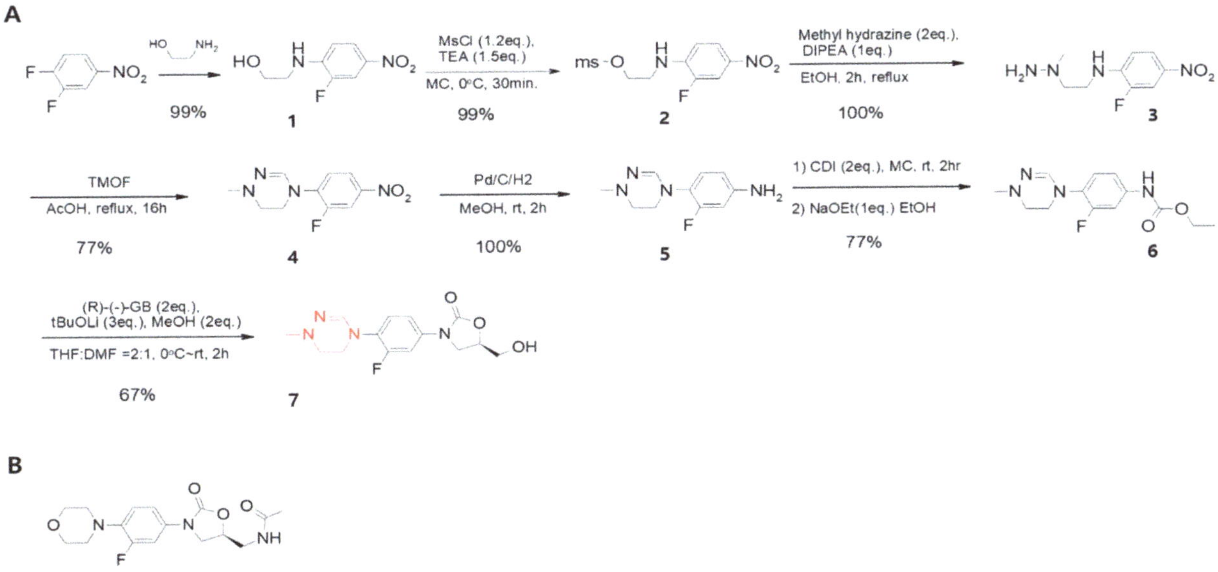

Figure 1. (**A**). Synthetic scheme showing that delpazolid can be synthesised in only seven steps with difluoro-nitrobenzene as the starting material. Each step shows a high yield and the products are easily purified without chromatography. The red color indicates cyclic amidrazone. (**B**). Chemical structure of linezolid.

3. Safety Evaluation in the Phase 1 Clinical Trial as PO

The greatest advantage associated with delpazolid is its safety. In phase 1a of a phase 1 clinical trial to evaluate its safety, as illustrated in Table 1, 64 subjects were divided into eight groups, six of whom were administered delpazolid and two who were administered the placebo. The study was the first double-blind, randomized human trial of delpazolid. To deliver single-ascending-doses (SADs), delpazolid was administered in a step-wise manner from 50 mg up to 3200 mg. Only mild adverse events were observed up to 2400 mg. At a delpazolid dose of 3200 mg, gastrointestinal (GI) tract-related adverse events were noted. In the 3200 mg dose group, volunteers had to ingest 16 tablets of 200 mg delpazolid tablets at once, resulting in GI tract-related adverse events. Therefore, the maximum tolerated dose of delpazolid was determined to be 2400 mg per day.

Table 1. Summary of phase 1a/b and 2a dose-escalation study to assess the safety, tolerability, and pharmacokinetics of delpazolid as a single agent.

Clinical Trial Phase	Experimental Design and Adverse Effects Reported
Phase 1a [9] (SAD)	Study design: Double blind, randomized, placebo control, first-in-human design
	N=64, 8 subject per group (6 active + 2 placebo)
	Doses: 50, 100, 200, 400, 800, 1,600, 2,400, and 3,200 mg
	MTD: 2,400 mg (Up to 2,400 mg, only mild adverse events were reported)
Phase 1b [8] (MAD-7 days)	Study design: Double blind, randomized, placebo control
	N=32, 8 subject per group (6 active + 2 placebo)
	Doses: 400, 800, 1,200, 1,600 mg BID for 7 days
	MTD: 1,200 mg BID (Up to 2,400 mg/day, only mild adverse events were reported)
Phase 1b [6] (MAD-21 days)	Study design: Double blind, randomized, placebo control
	N=36, 12 subject per group (10 active + 2 placebo)
	Doses: 800 mg QD and BID, 1,200 mg BID for 21 days
	MTD: 1,200 mg BID (Up to 2,400mg/day, No SAE reported)
Phase 2a [a] (EBA Trial)	Study design: Open label, randomized
	N=80, 16 subject per delpazolid group; 8 patients in active control groups, HRZE and linezolid
	Doses: Delpazolid 400 mg BID, 800 mg QD, 800 mg BID, 1,200 mg QD, HRZE and linezolid 600 mg BID for 14 days

Dose-escalation process consisted of a single-ascending-dose phase (SAD) and multiple-ascending-dose phase (MAD). MTD, maximum tolerated dose; QD, quaque die (daily); BID, bis in die (twice per day); SAE, serious adverse event; EBA, early bactericidal activity; HRZE, isoniazid (H), rifampin (R), pyrazinamide (Z), and ethambutol (E). [a] Results were not yet published.

A phase 1b study was conducted based on multiple-ascending-doses (MADs) over seven days. Thirty-two subjects were divided into eight groups, six of whom were administered delpazolid and two of whom were administered the placebo. Subjects were given delpazolid in MADs from 400 mg BID (bis in die, twice a day) up to 1600 mg BID over seven days. Doses up to 1200 mg BID for seven days were well-tolerated with no specific adverse events observed. After the 7-day MAD study, a 21-day MAD study was conducted to evaluate bone marrow toxicity, which is one of the most critical side effects of linezolid [8]. Subjects administered 800 mg once a day (QD) to 1200 mg BID delpazolid were monitored for up to three weeks to more accurately assess adverse events such as myelosuppression, as signs such as decreased platelet count may be observed even after two weeks. As illustrated in Table 1, serious adverse events were not observed under the MAD-21-day condition. In summary, no myelosuppression-related adverse events or serious adverse events were observed in phase 1a with SADs up to 2400 mg and in phase 1b with MAD up to 1200 mg BID (2400 mg per day) for 21 days. Therefore, delpazolid does not appear to exhibit adverse events associated with repeated dosing. In addition, delpazolid did not cause CYP-mediated metabolism and cardiac repolarisation issues [6,9–11].

4. Poor PK Profiles but Safe for Humans

The underlying antibacterial mechanism of delpazolid is similar to that of oxazolidinone in that it inhibits bacterial protein synthesis, which kills or inhibits the growth of bacteria [12]. However, protein synthesis also occurs in the mitochondria of eukaryotes, although mitochondria use independent protein-synthesis machinery that differs from nuclear-encoded protein synthesis in the cytoplasm. In humans, 13 genes are translated into proteins through this process, all of which participate in synthesizing membrane proteins associated with oxidative phosphorylation [13].

However, oxazolidinones uniformly inhibit human mitochondrial protein synthesis [14]. Similarly, linezolid, an oxazolidinone analogue used to treat TB, inhibits mitochondrial protein synthesis with potentially severe clinical consequences [15]. Therefore, the inhibition of protein synthesis by oxazolidinone intended to kill bacteria can impair mitochondria inside eukaryotic cells. Furthermore, myelosuppression may be a product of linezolid inhibition of mitochondrial protein synthesis [16].

As shown in Table 2, delpazolid showed a greater inhibitory effect than linezolid towards *Escherichia coli* at a 5-fold lower concentration (0.8 μg/mL).

Table 2. Antibiotic properties of oxazolidinones on bacterial and mitochondrial protein synthesis.

Compound	Bacteria	Human Mitochondria (IC_{50})		Animal Mitochondria [14]
	Escherichia coli	K562 cell	AC16 cell	Rat, Rabbit (liver & heart)
Delpazolid	2.6 μM (0.8 μg/mL)	4.8 μM (1.5 μg/mL)	10.9 μM (3.4 μg/mL)	NA
Linezolid	11.6 μM (3.9 μg/mL)	3.1 μM (1.0 μg/mL)	10.0 μM (3.4 μg/mL)	12.8 μM

In addition, in a study of human cells (immortalised myelogenous leukaemia cell line K562 and human cardiomyocyte cell line AC16), delpazolid showed inhibitory effects on mitochondrial protein synthesis similar to those of linezolid. Although delpazolid exhibited activity superior to that of linezolid in prokaryotic protein synthesis inhibition, it had similar negative effects on mitochondrial protein synthesis. Therefore, delpazolid doses lower than linezolid doses would be adequate for the treatment of Gram-positive bacteria, including TB. A lower dose would effectively inhibit bacterial protein synthesis, with relatively fewer adverse effects on human mitochondrial protein synthesis.

The association between delpazolid and myelosuppression, one of the most serious side effects of linezolid, was also tested. Healthy subjects were administered delpazolid and linezolid, and the plasma area under the concentration–time curve (AUC) was determined. As shown in Figure 2, subjects were administered delpazolid at doses ranging from 400 to 1200 mg, and 600 mg linezolid as the comparator.

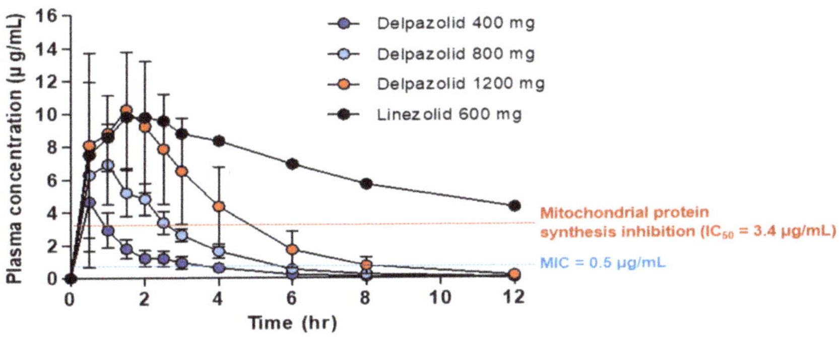

Figure 2. Mean plasma concentrations of linezolid and delpazolid in adults following oral dosing (mean ± standard deviation, $n = 6$).

As shown in Table 2, the IC_{50} values of delpazolid and linezolid at which mitochondrial protein synthesis in the two human cell-lines (K562 and AC16) were similar at 3.4 μg/mL indicated that these agents killed approximately 50% of human cells at 3.4 μg/mL. Thus, 3.4 μg/mL of delpazolid and linezolid is the mitochondrial damage limit. At higher concentrations, mitochondrial protein synthesis is affected severely, leading to cell death. Therefore, considering 3.4 μg/mL as the reference value at which toxicity of the two drugs occurs, a phase 1 trial based on linezolid 600 mg BID revealed that the linezolid plasma concentration was maintained at above the IC_{50} (3.4 μg/mL) for 12 h. However, delpazolid 800 mg maintained the IC_{50} above the mitochondrial damage limit for only 3 h, after which it was cleared rapidly from the blood. Therefore, delpazolid provides ample time for mitochondria to recover its protein synthesis function. In addition, increasing the delpazolid dose to 1200 mg raises the IC_{50}

to above 3,4 μg/mL for only 5 h, after which it also clears from the blood. Therefore, the low AUC with rapid clearance in delpazolid ironically minimizes cellular toxicity. Consequently, repeated BID dosing of delpazolid results in much lower levels of myelosuppression because of the lower mitochondrial protein synthesis inhibition compared to linezolid [9,10]. Therefore, the side effects of delpazolid were much milder than those of linezolid. The difference in side effects despite the similar structure of the two drugs may be due to differences in their chemical structures. The cyclic amidrazone side chain of delpazolid facilitates more rapid clearance and prevents accumulation in the plasma compared to linezolid. Thus, rapid clearance has been demonstrated as a key advantage that reduces myelosuppression compared to linezolid. Therefore, delpazolid may replace linezolid for MDR-TB for long-term treatment [11].

5. Toxicology

In vivo animal toxicity tests on delpazolid did not reveal specific toxicity profiles for six months in rats and for nine months in dogs. Furthermore, genetic toxicity tests, including the Ames test, in vitro chromosomal aberration test, and rat micronucleus test, as well as pharmacological safety tests including the hERG safety test, cardiovascular, respiratory and neurobehavioral tests, and reproductive toxicity tests were conducted, none of which revealed a specific toxicity profile (Table 3).

Table 3. Toxicology summary (PO: per oral /IV: intravenous). The general toxicity of delpazolid in animals lasted up to six months in rats and nine months in dogs, and no unusual findings after long-term treatment [a].

General Toxicity	**Status**	**PO**	**IV**
Single dose acute toxicity study in rats	Completed	MTD = 2000 mpk	MTD = 1000 mpk
Single dose acute toxicity study in dogs	Completed	MTD = 1000 mpk	MTD = 500 mpk
4- week toxicity study in rats with 4 -week recovery	Completed	NOAEL = 60 mpk	NOAEL = 120 mpk
4- week toxicity study in dogs with 4 -week recovery	Completed	NOAEL (male = 20 mpk, female=10 mpk)	NOAEL = 15 mpk
26- week(6 months) toxicity study in rats with 4 -week recovery	Completed	NOAEL (male = 10 mpk, female=100→75 mpk)	-
39- week (9 months) toxicity study in dogs with 4 -week recovery	Completed	NOAEL = 10 mpk	-
Genetic Toxicity			
Ames test	Completed	Negative	
In vitro chromosomal aberration test	Completed	Negative	
Rat micronucleus test	Completed	Negative	
Safety Pharmacology			
Assessment of blockage of hERG potassium channels	Completed	Negative(IC_{50}> 100μM)	
Cardiovascular telemetry study in beagle dogs	Completed	Negative	
Respiratory (Pulmonary) study in rats	Completed	Negative	
Neurobehavioral safety evaluation in rats	Completed	Negative	
Reproductive Toxicity		**PO**	
Fertility and Embryonic Development to Implantation toxicity in rat	Completed	NOAEL (male = 15 mpk, female=60 mpk)	
Embryo-Fetal Development toxicity in rat	Completed	NOAEL = 15 mpk	

MTD; maximum tolerated dose, NOAEL; no-observed-adverse-effect level. [a] Results were not yet published.

In a human bioavailability study, the bioavailability of the PO form was 99–100% (800 mg) of that of the IV form. Considering that the PK profiles between the IV and PO forms are similar, conversion would be relatively easy in the future. Because delpazolid is slightly polar, it exhibits low protein binding (37% in human), rapid clearance with no accumulation, and no food-related effects (Table 4).

Table 4. Phase 1 study: summary of delpazolid pharmacokinetic parameters. IV infusion 400 mg and PO 800 mg, cross-over study IV administration of delpazolid was generally safe and well-tolerated 800 mg (PO): Bioavailability was approximately 99% switchable between the PO and IV, with no dose adjustment.

Pharmacokinetic Parameter [a]	IV Infusion; 200 mg (n=6)	IV Infusion; 400 mg (n=8)	PO; 800 mg (n=8)
C_{max} (μg/mL)	2.92 ± 0.46	5.25 ± 0.96	8.20 ± 3.47
T_{max} (hr)	0.83 ± 0.13	0.84 ± 0.13	1.22 ± 0.98
$T_{1/2}$ (hr)	1.70 ± 0.26	1.48 ± 0.16	1.64 ± 0.48
$AUC_{0\text{-}24h}$ (μg·hr/mL)	5.59 ± 0.98	9.39 ± 1.46	18.65 ± 4.88
AUC_{inf} (μg·hr/mL)	5.63 ± 1.00	9.42 ± 1.47	18.86 ± 4.99
V_{ss}, V_z/F (L/kg)	0.90 ± 0.06	1.05 ± 0.20	1.67 ± 0.79
CL, Cl/F (L/hr/kg)	0.56 ± 0.10	0.67 ± 0.10	0.69 ± 0.18
MRT_{last} (hr)	1.55 ± 0.21	1.53 ± 0.14	2.87 ± 0.92
$C_{max,\ norm}$ (μg/mL)	0.95 ± 0.15	0.85 ± 0.16	0.67 ± 0.28
$AUC_{inf,\ norm}$ (μg·hr/mL)	1.83 ± 0.33	1.53 ± 0.24	1.53 ± 0.40
F (%)	-	-	99.8 ± 20.6

[a] Values are the means ± standard deviation (range). C_{max}, maximal drug concentration; T_{max}, time to reach C_{max}; $T_{\frac{1}{2}}$, half-life; $AUC_{0\text{-}24}$, area under the concentration-24-h curve; AUC_{inf}, AUC from time zero extrapolated to infinity; V_{ss}, steady-state volume of distribution; V_z/F, apparent volume of distribution; CL, clearance; Cl/F, apparent oral clearance; MRT_{last}, mean residence time when the drug concentration is based on values up to and including the last measured concentration; $C_{max,\ norm}$, C_{max} divided by dose per body weight; $AUC_{inf,\ norm}$, weight-normalised AUC_{inf}; F, bioavailability.

6. Activity Against TB and Combination Study of Delpazolid with Other Anti-TB Agents

Studies of the early development of delpazolid focused on Gram-positive bacteria. The efficacy of delpazolid on Gram-positive bacteria was similar or slightly better than that of linezolid. For example, in animal studies of systemic infection [17], soft tissue infection, lung infection, and thigh infection models in mice, delpazolid showed greater efficacy than linezolid (data not shown).

To evaluate the efficacy of delpazolid in TB, an in vitro susceptibility test was conducted for *M. tuberculosis* H37Rv. Compared to linezolid, the minimum inhibitory concentration (MIC) for *M. tuberculosis* H37Rv was similar to that under delpazolid; however, the minimum bactericidal concentration was more than 4-fold lower under delpazolid (Table 5).

Table 5. Drug activities and resistance rates of linezolid and delpazolid.

Drug Activities / Resistant Rate [a]	Linezolid	Delpazolid
MIC value for *M. tuberculosis* H37Rv (μg/mL)	0.5	0.5
MBC_{99} value for *M. tuberculosis* H37Rv (μg/mL)	>16	4
MDR-TB MIC_{90} (μg/mL)	1	0.5
XDR-TB MIC_{90} (μg/mL)	0.25	1
ECOFFs (epidemiological cutoff values) (μg/mL)	1.0	2.0
Resistant rate of MDR-TB (%)	6. 7	0.8
Resistant rate of XDR-TB (%)	4.2	4.2

[a] A total of 240 *M. tuberculosis* isolates were tested for ECOFFS and resistant rates, including 120 MDR-TB isolates and 120 XDR-TB samples in China.

The MIC_{90} values of delpazolid for MDR/extensively drug resistant (XDR) TB isolates were 0.25 and 1 μg/mL, respectively. However, an in vitro study of MDR/XDR TB isolates from China showed that the resistance rate varied considerably. The resistance of MDR-TB to linezolid was 6.7%, whereas that to delpazolid was 0.8%, suggesting higher potential efficacy of delpazolid in the treatment of MDR-TB, although no significant difference in resistance rates was observed between linezolid and delpazolid among XDR-TB isolates [18]. Therefore, delpazolid has been considered as a targeted application for MDR-TB treatment. Considering the significantly lower resistance rate of MDR-TB against delpazolid despite its similar structure to linezolid, further studies are needed to investigate structural variations in delpazolid to evaluate the correlations between the structures of various delpazolid derivatives and their resistance rates. In addition, intracellular MICs of delpazolid that can inhibit the growth of intracellular *M. tuberculosis* H37Rv revealed efficacy levels similar to those of linezolid under low concentrations, whereas delpazolid had greater efficacy at higher concentrations (Figure 3).

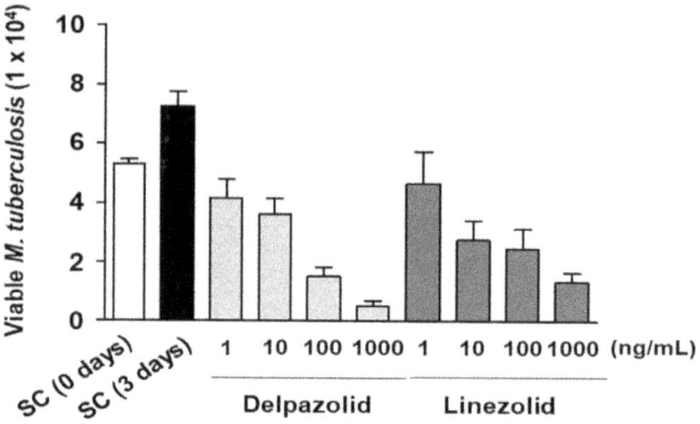

Figure 3. Intracellular activity of delpazolid. The activity of delpazolid on intracellular *M. tuberculosis* was compared to linezolid in bone marrow-derived macrophages (BMDMs) at three days after infection. The experiment was performed in triplicate, and the results are shown as the mean ± standard error of the mean (SEM). SC, solvent control.

The treatment of tuberculosis requires a combination of several antimicrobial agents and long-term therapy [19]. Therefore, evaluating synergy with other anti-TB agents is a crucial step in finding drugs that can be co-administered with delpazolid. As indicated in Table 6, a checkerboard assay was performed to identify pre-existing anti-TB medications with potential synergistic effects with delpazolid.

Table 6. MICs of selected anti-tuberculosis compounds against *M. tuberculosis* H37Rv and corresponding interaction profiles with delpazolid assessed by checkerboard.

Ref. Drug	MIC (μg/mL)	Tested TB Drugs	MIC (μg/mL)	FIC index	Activity [a]
Delpazolid	1	Isoniazid	0.13	1.13	I
		Rifampicin	0.06	0.75	Ad
		Rifapentine	0.01	0.75	Ad
		Ethambutol	0.50	1.02	I
		Cycloserine	4.0	1.02	I
		Amikacin	0.04	1.02	I
		Streptomycin	0.25	1.02	I
		Capreomycin	0.31	1.02	I
		Moxifloxacin	0.06	0.75	Ad
		Levofloxacin	0.25	0.75	Ad
		Clofazimine	0.25	0.52	pS
		Bedaquiline	0.25	0.53	pS
		Delamanid	0.02	0.75	Ad
		Ethionamide	0.5	1.03	I
		p-aminosalicylic acid	0.02	1	I
		Pyrazinamide [b]	200	0.63	pS

[a] S: synergy, pS: partial synergy, Ad: additive, I: indifference. [b] Tested in acidic condition (pH 5.2)

The assay revealed that delpazolid has partial synergism with clofazimine, bedaquiline, and pyrazinamide. Based on the results, in vitro time-kill kinetics tests were conducted by combining delpazolid with clofazimine and bedaquiline (Figure 4).

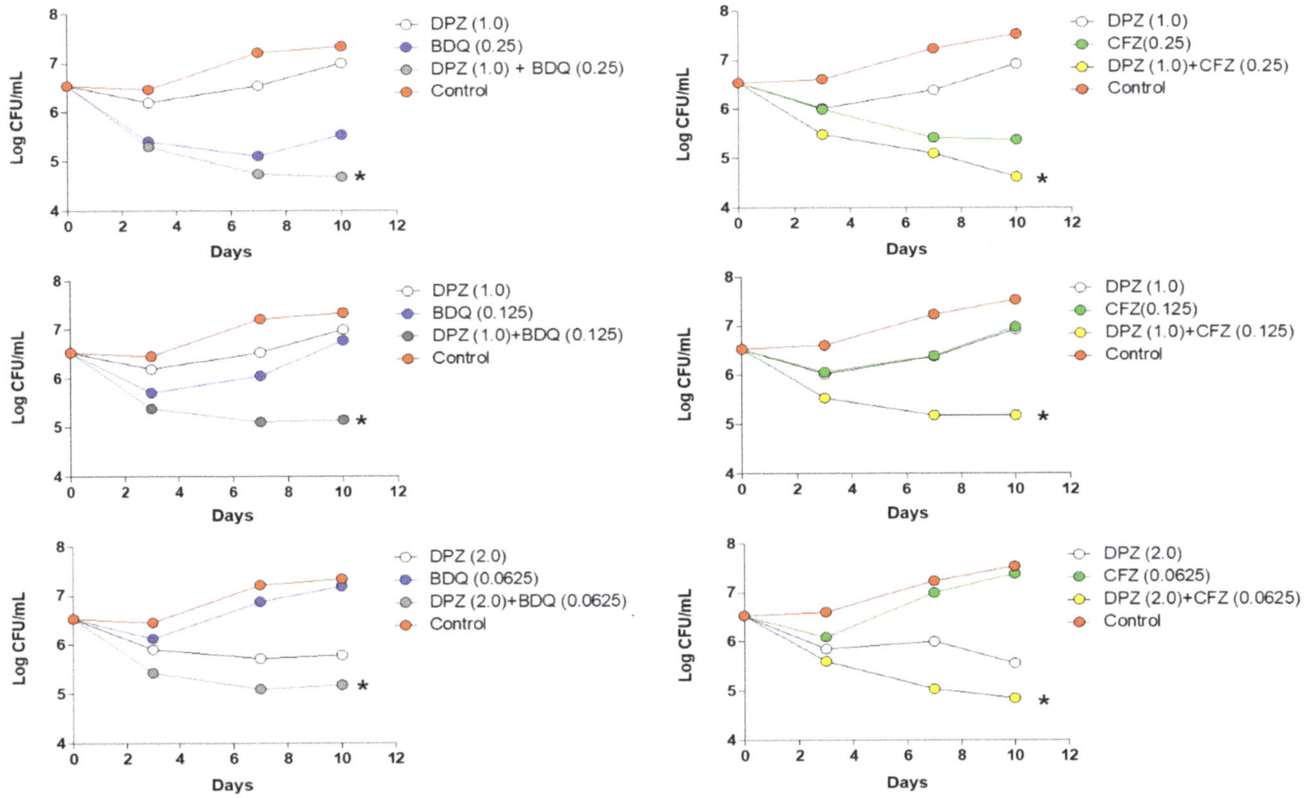

Figure 4. In vitro combination time-kill assay with anti-TB drugs. Viability of *M. tuberculosis* H37Rv was evaluated using combinations of various concentrations of delpazolid and bedaquiline or clofazimine (μg/mL).

Using the MIC against *M. tuberculosis* H37Rv for each drug, changes in colony-forming units (CFU) with monotherapy or combination therapy were evaluated. In addition, based on the MICs, synergistic effects between delpazolid plus bedaquiline and delpazolid plus clofazimine were evaluated at varying doses. Although the CFUs decreased at the MIC of a single drug, regrowth was observed over time. However, when delpazolid was combined with bedaquiline or clofazimine, using the 0.5× MIC of each drug, no regrowth was observed (Figure 4). In addition, the combination of bedaquiline and clofazimine with delpazolid consistently suppressed the growth of *M. tuberculosis* H37Rv, exhibiting high synergistic effects with 1× MIC delpazolid (1 μg/mL) and 0.5 × MIC clofazimine (0.25 μg/mL), resulting in a 2 log CFU reduction in *M. tuberculosis* H37Rv. Synergy between two new antimycobacterial compounds, such as delpazolid and bedaquiline or clofazimine, offers an attractive foundation for a new tuberculosis regimen.

7. Activity of Delpazolid on Nontuberculous Mycobacteria

Nontuberculous mycobacteria (NTM) are naturally occurring organisms found in water and soil. They are associated with biofilm formation, which enhances their disinfectant and antibiotic resistance. Particularly, *Mycobacterium avium* complex and *Mycobacterium abscessus* are the most common causes of pulmonary NTM and deadly pathogens, with high failure rates and relapse rates that may exceed 40% [20]. Although most people are not affected by such pathogens, in some individuals susceptible to conditions such as cystic fibrosis, chronic obstructive lung disease, bronchiectasis, and thoracic skeletal abnormalities, progressive and debilitating disease can occur [21].

A key concern in NTM treatment is the lack of antibiotics appropriate for long-term treatment for diverse NTM pathogens. Here, we evaluated the activity of delpazolid via in vitro susceptibility tests, as shown in the table below (Table 7) [22].

Table 7. MICs of antibiotics against clinical isolates of NTMs.

NTM Species (no. of strain tested)	Antibiotics	Range (μg/mL)	MIC_{50} (μg/mL)	MIC_{90} (μg/mL)
Mycobacterium avium (22)	Delpazolid	8-0.125	2	8
	Linezolid	8-0.125	2	8
	Clarithromycin	>128-≤0.125	>128	>128
Mycobacterium abscessus (20)	Delpazolid	8-0.25	2	8
	Linezolid	16-0.5	4	8
	Clarithromycin	128- ≤0.125	≤0.125	1
Mycobacterium fortuitum (21)	Delpazolid	2-0.25	1	2
	Linezolid	8-0.5	2	8
	Clarithromycin	8-≤0.125	0.25	4
Mycobacterium kansasii (22)	Delpazolid	2-0.25	1	2
	Linezolid	2-0.25	0.5	2
	Clarithromycin	0.125- ≤0.125	≤0.125	≤0.125
Mycobacterium chelonae (20)	Delpazolid	4-0.25	1	2
	Linezolid	8-0.5	2	4
	Clarithromycin	0.2- ≤0.025	0.1	0.2

Delpazolid had MICs similar to those of linezolid against *M. avium*, *M. abscessus*, *M. fortuitum*, *M. kansasii*, and *M. chelonae*, and inhibited NTM proliferation. In particular, delpazolid was effective against several *M. abscessus* strains in vitro and in a macrophage infection model. Acute infections in C57BL/6 mice, delpazolid 100 mg/kg exhibited greater in vivo efficacy than clarithromycin 200 mg/kg, a macrolide that is the main drug currently for *M. abscessus* treatment [12]. Therefore, delpazolid represents a promising novel class of oxazolidinones with improved safety for the treatment of *M. abscessus*.

8. Conclusions

As observed in clinical studies, the greatest advantage of delpazolid over linezolid is the potential for delpazolid to be used in long-term therapies. The development of delpazolid has focused on TB treatment, as this disease requires long-term treatment. In December 2016, LegoChem Biosciences entered into a license agreement with RMX Biopharma for the development, manufacture, and commercialization of delpazolid in China. In addition, delpazolid received an FDA orphan drug designation, a Qualified Infectious Disease Product Designation, and was selected as a Fast Track target drug.

On October 30, 2019, at 'The 50th Union World Conference on Lung Health,' held in Hyderabad, India, LegoChem Biosciences released the interim efficacy and safety results of a phase 2a study on delpazolid. Particularly, the results of a clinical phase 2a early bactericidal activity trial involving 79 Korean patients with drug-susceptible tuberculosis were reported. The findings will be further analyzed to determine the doses appropriate for different patient populations to guide further phase 2a studies. The phase 1 trial revealed that myelosuppression can be reduced, and phase 2a results suggested that delpazolid can replace linezolid as a therapy for TB and reduce the treatment period.

Author Contributions: Conceptualization, Y.L.C. and J.J.; writing, J.J.; review and editing, Y.L.C. and J.J.; visualization, Y.L.C. and J.J.; project administration, Y.L.C. and J.J. All authors have read and agreed to the published version of the manuscript.

Acknowledgments: We thank all those who provided important information that was part of this work. We also thank Tae ho Kim for his assistance in figure preparation.

References

1. Bozdogan, B.; Appelbaum, P.C. Oxazolidinones: Activity, mode of action, and mechanism of resistance. *Int J Antimicrob Agents.* **2004**, *23*, 113–119. [CrossRef] [PubMed]
2. Marchese, A.; Schito, G.C. The oxazolidinones as a new family of antimicrobial agent. *Clin Microbiol Infect.* **2001**, *4*, 66–74. [CrossRef] [PubMed]
3. Moellering, R.C. Linezolid: The first oxazolidinone antimicrobial. *Ann Intern Med.* **2003**, *138*, 135–142. [CrossRef] [PubMed]
4. Millard, J.; Pertinez, H.; Bonnett, L.; Hodel, E.M.; Dartois, V.; Johnson, J.L.; Caws, M.; Tiberi, S.; Bolhuis, M.; Alffenaar, J.C.; et al. Linezolid pharmacokinetics in MDR-TB: A systematic review, meta-analysis and Monte Carlo simulation. *J Antimicrob Chemother.* **2018**, *73*, 1755–1762. [CrossRef]
5. Gerson, S.L.; Kaplan, S.L.; Bruss, J.B.; Le, V.; Arellano, F.M.; Hafkin, B.; Kuter, D.J. Hematologic effects of linezolid: Summary of clinical experience. *Antimicrob Agents Chemother.* **2002**, *46*, 2723–2726. [CrossRef]
6. Choi, Y.; Lee, S.W.; Kim, A.; Jang, K.; Nam, H.; Cho, Y.L.; Yu, K.S.; Jang, I.J. Chung, J.Y. Safety, tolerability and pharmacokinetics of 21 day multiple oral administration of a new oxazolidinone antibiotic, LCB01-0371, in healthy male subjects. *J Antimicrob Chemother.* **2018**, *73*, 183–190. [CrossRef]
7. De Freitas Ferreira, R.; Schapira, M. A systematic analysis of atomic protein-ligand interactions in the PDB. *Medchemcomm.* **2017**, *8*, 1970–1981. [CrossRef]
8. Singh, B.; Cocker, D.; Ryan, H.; Sloan, D.J. Linezolid for drug-resistant pulmonary tuberculosis. *Cochrane Database Syst Rev.* **2019**, *3*, CD012836. [CrossRef]
9. Cho, Y.S.; Lim, H.S.; Cho, Y.L.; Nam, H.S.; Bae, K.S. Multiple-dose Safety, Tolerability, Pharmacokinetics, and Pharmacodynamics of Oral LCB01-0371 in Healthy Male Volunteers. *Clin Ther.* **2018**, *40*, 2050–2064. [CrossRef]
10. Cho, Y.S.; Lim, H.S.; Lee, S.H.; Cho, Y.L.; Nam, H.S.; Bae, K.S. Pharmacokinetics, Pharmacodynamics, and Tolerability of Single-Dose Oral LCB01-0371, a Novel Oxazolidinone with Broad-Spectrum Activity, in Healthy Volunteers. *Antimicrob Agents Chemother.* **2018**, *62*, e00451-18. [CrossRef]
11. Sunwoo, J.; Kim, Y.K.; Choi, Y.; Yu, K.S.; Nam, H.; Cho, Y.L.; Yoon, S.; Chung, J.Y. Effect of food on the pharmacokinetic characteristics of a single oral dose of LCB01-0371, a novel oxazolidinone antibiotic. *Drug Des Devel Ther.* **2018**, *12*, 1707–1714. [CrossRef] [PubMed]
12. Kim, T.S.; Choe, J.H.; Kim, Y.J.; Yang, C.S.; Kwon, H.J.; Jeong, J.; Kim, G.; Park, D.E.; Jo, E.K.; Cho, Y.L.; et al. Activity of LCB01-0371, a Novel Oxazolidinone, against Mycobacterium abscessus. *Antimicrob Agents Chemother.* **2017**, *61*, e02752-16. [CrossRef] [PubMed]
13. Hällberg, B.M.; Larsson, N.G. Making proteins in the powerhouse. *Cell Metab.* **2014**, *20*, 226–240. [CrossRef] [PubMed]
14. McKee, E.E.; Ferguson, M.; Bentley, A.T.; Marks, T.A. Inhibition of mammalian mitochondrial protein synthesis by oxazolidinones. *Antimicrob Agents Chemother.* **2006**, *50*, 2042–2049. [CrossRef] [PubMed]
15. De Vriese, A.S.; Coster, R.V.; Smet, J.; Seneca, S.; Lovering, A.; Van Haute, L.L.; Vanopdenbosch, L.J.; Martin, J.J.; Groote, C.C.; Vandecasteele, S.; et al. Linezolid-induced inhibition of mitochondrial protein synthesis. *Clin Infect Dis.* **2006**, *42*, 1111–1117. [CrossRef]
16. Nagiec, E.E.; Wu, L.; Swaney, S.M.; Chosay, J.G.; Ross, D.E.; Brieland, J.K.; Leach, K.L. Oxazolidinones inhibit cellular proliferation via inhibition of mitochondrial protein synthesis. *Antimicrob Agents Chemother.* **2005**, *49*, 3896–3902. [CrossRef]
17. Jeong, J.W.; Jung, S.J.; Lee, H.H.; Kim, Y.Z.; Park, T.K.; Cho, Y.L.; Chae, S.E.; Baek, S.Y.; Woo, S.H.; Lee, H.S.; et al. In vitro and in vivo activities of LCB01-0371, a new oxazolidinone. *Antimicrob Agents Chemother.* **2010**, *54*, 5359–5362. [CrossRef]
18. Zong, Z.; Jing, W.; Shi, J.; Wen, S.; Zhang, T.; Huo, F.; Shang, Y.; Liang, Q.; Huang, H.; Pang, Y. Comparison of In Vitro Activity and MIC Distributions between the Novel Oxazolidinone Delpazolid and Linezolid against Multidrug-Resistant and Extensively Drug-Resistant Mycobacterium tuberculosis in China. *Antimicrob Agents Chemother.* **2018**, *62*, e00165-18. [CrossRef]
19. Kerantzas, C.A.; Jacobs, W.R., Jr. Origins of Combination Therapy for Tuberculosis: Lessons for Future Antimicrobial Development and Application. *mBio.* **2017**, *8*, e01586-16. [CrossRef]
20. Abate, G.; Hamzabegovic, F.; Eickhoff, C.S.; Hoft, D.F. BCG Vaccination Induces M. avium and M. abscessus Cross-Protective Immunity. *Front Immunol.* **2019**, *10*, 234. [CrossRef]

21. Johnson, M.M.; Odell, J.A. Nontuberculous mycobacterial pulmonary infections. *J Thorac Dis.* **2014**, *6*, 210–220. [PubMed]
22. DeStefano, M.S.; Shoen, C.M.; Sklaney, M.R.; Cynamon, M.H. *The In Vitro Activity of Delpazolid (LCB01-0371) against Several Non-Tuberculous Mycobacteria (NTM)*; (Poster Number AAR-731, Friday, June 21, 2019); ASM Microbe: San Francisco, CA, USA, 2019.

Permissions

All chapters in this book were first published by MDPI; hereby published with permission under the Creative Commons Attribution License or equivalent. Every chapter published in this book has been scrutinized by our experts. Their significance has been extensively debated. The topics covered herein carry significant findings which will fuel the growth of the discipline. They may even be implemented as practical applications or may be referred to as a beginning point for another development.

The contributors of this book come from diverse backgrounds, making this book a truly international effort. This book will bring forth new frontiers with its revolutionizing research information and detailed analysis of the nascent developments around the world.

We would like to thank all the contributing authors for lending their expertise to make the book truly unique. They have played a crucial role in the development of this book. Without their invaluable contributions this book wouldn't have been possible. They have made vital efforts to compile up to date information on the varied aspects of this subject to make this book a valuable addition to the collection of many professionals and students.

This book was conceptualized with the vision of imparting up-to-date information and advanced data in this field. To ensure the same, a matchless editorial board was set up. Every individual on the board went through rigorous rounds of assessment to prove their worth. After which they invested a large part of their time researching and compiling the most relevant data for our readers.

The editorial board has been involved in producing this book since its inception. They have spent rigorous hours researching and exploring the diverse topics which have resulted in the successful publishing of this book. They have passed on their knowledge of decades through this book. To expedite this challenging task, the publisher supported the team at every step. A small team of assistant editors was also appointed to further simplify the editing procedure and attain best results for the readers.

Apart from the editorial board, the designing team has also invested a significant amount of their time in understanding the subject and creating the most relevant covers. They scrutinized every image to scout for the most suitable representation of the subject and create an appropriate cover for the book.

The publishing team has been an ardent support to the editorial, designing and production team. Their endless efforts to recruit the best for this project, has resulted in the accomplishment of this book. They are a veteran in the field of academics and their pool of knowledge is as vast as their experience in printing. Their expertise and guidance has proved useful at every step. Their uncompromising quality standards have made this book an exceptional effort. Their encouragement from time to time has been an inspiration for everyone.

The publisher and the editorial board hope that this book will prove to be a valuable piece of knowledge for researchers, students, practitioners and scholars across the globe.

List of Contributors

Stephani Joy Y. Macalino
Chemistry Department, De La Salle University, 2401 Taft Avenue, Manila 0992, Philippines
OVPAA-EIDR Program, "Computer-Aided Discovery of Compounds for the Treatment of Tuberculosis in the Philippines", Department of Physical Sciences and Mathematics, College of Arts and Sciences, University of the Philippines Manila, Manila 1000, Philippines

Junie B. Billones, Voltaire G. Organo and Maria Constancia O. Carrillo
OVPAA-EIDR Program, "Computer-Aided Discovery of Compounds for the Treatment of Tuberculosis in the Philippines", Department of Physical Sciences and Mathematics, College of Arts and Sciences, University of the Philippines Manila, Manila 1000, Philippines

Hamza Arshad Dar, Tahreem Zaheer, Nimat Ullah and Amjad Ali
Atta-ur-Rahman School of Applied Biosciences, National University of Sciences and Technology, Islamabad 44000, Pakistan

Syeda Marriam Bakhtiar
Department of Bioinformatics and Biosciences, Capital University of Science and Technology Islamabad expressway, Kahuta Road, Zone-V, Islamabad 44000, Pakistan

Tianyu Zhang
State Key Laboratory of Respiratory Disease, Guangzhou Institutes of Biomedicine and Health (GIBH), Chinese Academy of Sciences, Guangzhou 510530, China

Muhammad Yasir and Esam I. Azhar
Special Infectious Agents Unit, King Fahd Medical Research Center, King Abdulaziz University, Jeddah 21589, Saudi Arabia
Medical Laboratory Technology Department, Faculty of Applied Medical Sciences, King Abdulaziz University, Jeddah 21589, Saudi Arabia

Caroline Shi-Yan Foo
Laboratory of Virology and Chemotherapy, Rega Institute, Leuven 3000, Belgium

Kevin Pethe
Lee Kong Chian School of Medicine and School of Biological Sciences, Nanyang Technological University, Singapore 636921, Singapore

Andréanne Lupien
Infectious Diseases and Immunity in Global Health Program, Research Institute of the McGill University Health Centre, Montreal, QC H4A 3J1, Canada
McGill International TB Centre, Montreal, QC H4A 3J1, Canada

Catherine Vilchèze
Einstein College of Medicine, 1301 Morris Park Avenue, the Bronx, New York, NY 10461, USA

Eduardo M. Bruch, Stéphanie Petrella and Marco Bellinzoni
Unité de Microbiologie Structurale, Institut Pasteur, CNRS, Université de Paris, F-75015 Paris, France

Balachandra Bandodkar
Pharmaron Beijing Co., Ltd., 6, Taihe Road, BDA, Beijing 100176, China

Radha Krishan Shandil
Foundation for Neglected Disease Research [FNDR], Plot 20A, KIADB Industrial Area, Doddaballapur, Bengaluru 561203, India

Jagadeesh Bhat and Tanjore S. Balganesh
Gangagen Biotechnologies P Ltd., #12, 5th Cross, Raghavendra Layout, Tumkur Road, Yeshwantpur, Bengaluru 560022, India

Raphael Gries
Department I of Internal Medicine, Division of Infectious Diseases, University of Cologne, 50931 Cologne, Germany
Center for Molecular Medicine Cologne, University of Cologne, 50931 Cologne, Germany

Claudia Sala
Fondazione Toscana Life Sciences, 53100 Siena, Italy

Jan Rybniker
Department I of Internal Medicine, Division of Infectious Diseases, University of Cologne, 50931 Cologne, Germany
Center for Molecular Medicine Cologne, University of Cologne, 50931 Cologne, Germany
German Center for Infection Research (DZIF), Partner Site Bonn-Cologne, 50931 Cologne, Germany

Vadim Makarov
Federal Research Center "Fundamentals of Biotechnology RAS", Leninsky prospect 33, bld. 2, 119071 Moscow, Russia

Katarína Mikušová
Department of Biochemistry, Faculty of Natural Sciences, Comenius University in Bratislava, Mlynská dolina, Ilkovičova 6, 84215 Bratislava, Slovakia

Christian Lienhardt
Unité Mixte Internationale TransVIHMI (UMI 233 IRD–U1175 INSERM, Université de Montpellier)-Institut de Recherche pour le Développement (IRD), 34000 Montpellier, France

Mario C. Raviglione
Centre for Multidisciplinary Research in Health Science (MACH), Università di Milano, Milan, Italy and Global Studies Institute, Université de Genève, 1211 Genève, Switzerland

Rob C. van Wijk, Rami Ayoun Alsoud and Ulrika S. H. Simonsson
Department of Pharmaceutical Biosciences, Uppsala University, Uppsala 75123, Sweden

Hans Lennernäs
Department of Pharmacy, Uppsala University, Uppsala 75123, Sweden

Giulia Degiacomi, Maria Rosalia Pasca, Edda De Rossi, Giovanna Riccardi and Laurent Roberto Chiarelli
Department of Biology and Biotechnology "Lazzaro Spallanzani", University of Pavia, 27100 Pavia, Italy

Juan Manuel Belardinelli
Mycobacteria Research Laboratories, Department of Microbiology, Immunology and Pathology, Colorado State University, Fort Collins, CO 80523-1682, USA

Paolo Mazzarello
Department of Brain and Behavioral Sciences and University Museum System, University of Pavia, 27100 Pavia, Italy

Young Lag Cho
LegoChem Biosciences, Inc., 8-26 Munoyeongseo-ro, Daedeok-gu, Daejeon 34302, Korea

Jichan Jang
Molecular Mechanisms of Antibiotics, Division of Life Science, Research Institute of Life Sciences, Gyeongsang National University, Jinju 52828, Korea

Index

www.ingramcontent.com/pod-product-compliance
Lightning Source LLC
LaVergne TN
LVHW080931210926
848485LV00004B/774